# THERAPEUTIC MEDICAL DEVICES

## Application and Design

# THERAPEUTIC MEDICAL DEVICES

## Application and Design

EDITED BY

ALBERT M. COOK
*California State University, Sacramento*

JOHN G. WEBSTER
*University of Wisconsin, Madison*

PRENTICE-HALL, INC. *Englewood Cliffs, New Jersey 07632*

**Library of Congress Cataloging in Publication Data**
Main entry under title:

Therapeutic medical devices, application and design.

Includes bibliographies and index.
Contents: General concepts / Albert M.
Cook—Cardiac pacing / Paul Citron . . . [et
al.]—Defibrillators / Charles F. Babbs,
Joe D. Bourland—[etc.]
1. Medical instruments and apparatus.
2. Therapeutics—Equipment and supplies.
I. Cook, Albert M. II. Webster, John G.
[DNLM: 1. Equipment and supplies. WB 26 T398]
R856.T44      681'.761      81-5926
ISBN  0-13-914796-9          AACR2

Editorial/production supervision
and interior design by *Daniela Lodes*
Cover design by *Judith A. Matz*
Manufacturing buyer: *Joyce Levatino*

Printed in the United States of America

10  9  8  7  6  5  4  3  2  1

Prentice-Hall International, Inc., *London*
Prentice-Hall of Australia Pty. Limited, *Sydney*
Prentice-Hall of Canada, Ltd., *Toronto*
Prentice-Hall of India Private Limited, *New Delhi*
Prentice-Hall of Japan, Inc., *Tokyo*
Prentice-Hall of Southeast Asia Pte. Ltd., *Singapore*
Whitehall Books Limited, Wellington, *New Zealand*

# CONTRIBUTING AUTHORS

DAVID R. ASCHE

Radiation Oncology Center
Sacramento, CA


DAVID C. AUTH, PH.D., PE

Electrical Engineering Department
Center for Bioengineering
University of Washington, Seattle


CHARLES F. BABBS, M.D., PH.D.

Biomedical Engineering Center
Purdue University
W. Lafayette, IN


JOE D. BOURLAND, PH.D.

Biomedical Engineering Center
Purdue University
W. Lafayette, IN


PAUL CITRON

Medtronic, Inc.
Minneapolis, MN


ALBERT M. COOK, PH.D., PE

Assistive Device Center
Biomedical Engineering Program
California State University, Sacramento

JEFFREY B. COOPER, PH.D.

Bioengineering Unit
Department of Anesthesia
Massachusetts General Hospital
Harvard-MIT Division of Health Sciences
    Technology
Boston, MA


TREVOR B. DAVEY

Biomedical Engineering Program
California State University, Sacramento


EDWIN G. DUFFIN, PH.D.

Medtronic, Inc.
Minneapolis, MN


JOSEPH FETTER

Medtronic, Inc.
Minneapolis, MN


LESTER GOODMAN, PH.D.

Medtronic, Inc.
Minneapolis, MN


RICHARD F. HARVEY, M.D.

Department of Rehabilitation Medicine
University of Wisconsin-Madison

PHILIP H. HEINTZ, PH.D.

*Radiation Oncology Center*
*Sacramento, CA*


TERRY A. HULL, LPT

*Wilford Hall, USAF Medical Center*
*San Antonio, TX*


RONALD W. JODAT, PH.D.

*Department of Electrical Engineering*
*Marquette University*
*Milwaukee, WI*


JOSEPH A. KLEINKORT, LPT

*Wilford Hall, USAF Medical Center*
*San Antonio, TX*


G. GUY KNICKERBOCKER, PH.D.

*Chief Scientist*
*Emergency Care Research Institute*
*Plymouth Meeting, PA*


SANFORD J. LARSON, M.D., PH.D.

*Department of Neurosurgery*
*Medical College of Wisconsin*
*Milwaukee, WI*


EUGENE F. MURPHY, PH.D.

*Office of Technology Transfer*
*Veterans Administration*
*New York, NY*


PETER MORAWETZ, PH.D.

*Medtronic, Inc.*
*Minneapolis, MN*


MICHAEL R. NEUMAN, M.D., PH.D.

*Department of Biomedical Engineering*
*Case Western Reserve University*
*Cleveland, OH*


RONALD S. NEWBOWER, PH.D.

*Bioengineering Unit*
*Department of Anesthesia*
*Massachusetts General Hospital*
*Harvard-MIT Division of Health Sciences*
*    and Technology*
*Boston, MA*


JAMES H. PHILIP, M.D.

*Instructor in Anesthesia Harvard Medical School*
*Junior Associate in Anesthesiology,*
*Affiliated Hospitals Center, Inc.*
*Boston, MA*


ANTHONY SANCES, JR., PH.D.

*Biomedical Engineering*
*The Medical College of Wisconsin*
*Milwaukee, WI*


JOHN S. SKREENOCK

*Project Engineer*
*Emergency Care Research Institute*
*Plymouth Meeting, PA*

# Contents

## Chapter 7 PHYSICAL THERAPY EQUIPMENT    202

## Chapter 8 NEUROMUSCULAR PROSTHETICS AND ORTHOTICS    241

## Chapter 9 INTERNAL PROSTHETICS AND ORTHOTICS    301

# Preface

This book will help you design and use therapeutic medical equipment. It helps you assess those diseases that can benefit from therapeutic devices and predict the patient benefits. For each device it describes the medical problem, details the design of the equipment, and describes the form of energy applied to the patient.

Chapter 1 introduces you to the questions you should ask when using therapeutic equipment. What is the medical problem? What is the equipment output and how do you control it? What effect does this output have on the patient? How should you design this equipment to meet these requirements, including those of safety? Several examples clarify these concepts for you.

Chapter 2 describes one of the most successful collaborations between engineers and physicians—the cardiac pacemaker. You will learn the many abnormal cardiac rhythms and how to design pacemakers for each type of problem. A critical component of pacemaker therapy is following up the patient to determine if it is providing the expected therapy. You will learn this—and also troubleshooting techniques for solving problems that may arise.

We are all familiar with the dramatic way defibrillators can resuscitate hearts that prematurely fail. Chapter 3 teaches you the physiology of cardiac fibrillation and then shows how to optimize the defibrillator design to cure the problem with the least tissue damage.

Pump oxygenators can carry the body through an acute need, such as during open heart surgery. Cardiac assist devices lower the patient work required. Chapter 4 shows you the design of these devices, as well as heart valves, arterial grafts, and the total artificial heart.

Chapter 5 teaches you how electrical stimulation affects nerve and muscle. Then it takes you through the many applications of neural assist devices which are in clinical use.

The biomedical engineer has much to offer for those who cannot see, hear, or speak. Chapter 6 shows you how to design communication systems as well as mobility aids for the sensory impaired.

Chapter 7 shows you how physical therapy can assist in patient rehabilitation. It not only covers the standard techniques of traction, exercise, heat, and nonionizing radiation, but also extends into newer areas such as biofeedback.

Many biomedical engineers are naturally drawn to the design of prosthetic devices, such as replacement for lost limbs. Chapter 8 includes the design of these—and also orthotic devices that assist the body in replacing lost function.

Chapter 9 shows you the problems that arise when you place prosthetic and orthotic devices within the body. It explains the biocompatibility problems which are due to the placement of artificial materials in contact with tissue.

The electrosurgical unit not only cuts tissue during surgery but also provides simultaneous coagulation. Chapter 10 shows you how to choose the proper waveform, design the equipment for safe operation, and perform equipment tests for preventive maintenance.

Chapter 11 provides you with a basic understanding of the use of lasers in medicine. You will learn details of their application in ophthalmology and surgery.

In chapter 12 you will learn not only how anesthesia machines function today, but also how to design an improved man-machine interface to help the anesthesiologist cope with a bewildering array of equipment.

Ventilators are the most important devices for maintaining pulmonary perfusion. Chapter 13 teaches you the design of these devices and their associated gas-delivery systems.

Chapter 14 describes the renal dialysis program, which has present expenditures over $1 billion per year. It teaches you the design of artificial kidneys and the mass transport characteristics of the different membranes and configurations.

The ability to keep premature infants alive has spawned the new discipline of neonatology. In Chapter 15, you learn incubator design, respiratory assist devices, and how to maintain proper nutrition.

A major portion of modern cancer therapy uses ionizing radiation. Chapter 16 teaches you the principles of radiation therapy biology so that you understand radiation therapy.

We assume that you know basic physiology, general chemistry, differential equations, physics, and electronics. Thus the book should be suitable for senior-graduate courses in biomedical engineering.

In addition to students, this book will appeal to practicing clinical engineers, biomedical engineers, nurses, physicians, and other health-care personnel who need to become familiar with medical equipment designed for therapeutic applications.

We would welcome your comments on improvements that would enhance further editions or revisions of this text.

ALBERT M. COOK

*Assistive Device Center*
*Biomedical Engineering Program*
*California State University, Sacramento*
*6000 Jay Street*
*Sacramento, CA 95819*

JOHN G. WEBSTER

*Dept. of Electrical and Computer Engineering*
*University of Wisconsin, Madison*
*1425 Johnson Drive*
*Madison, WI 53706*

# THERAPEUTIC MEDICAL DEVICES

# Application and Design

# 1 General Concepts

*Albert M. Cook*

## 1.1 LEARNING OBJECTIVES

Upon completing this chapter you will be able to:

- Describe the differences in function between diagnostic, monitoring, and therapeutic medical devices.
- Define and discuss the design goals for therapeutic medical devices.
- Relate the use of therapeutic devices to other modes of therapy.
- Describe the effects of therapeutic devices in terms of the energy imparted to the biological system.
- Describe the advantages and limitations of the use of closed-loop control in therapeutic devices.
- Describe the ways that feedback can affect device performance.

This textbook describes therapeutic medical devices. This chapter presents general aspects of these devices and their application. This provides a framework for studying specific devices in more detail in successive chapters. Keep in mind the general goals and design considerations as you evaluate each device presented in following chapters. We also discuss some devices not presented in other chapters.

| Application | Goals |
|---|---|
| Diagnostic devices | Determination of the cause of malfunction due to disease or injury. Minimal change in biological system as a result of measurement (e.g., "non-invasive methods" wherever possible). Precise, quantitative measurements. |
| Therapeutic devices | Implementation of a therapeutic regime involving medical and/or surgical goals which will lead to improved function or alteration in the course of disease. Effect changes in structure and/or function of the biological system with minimal side effects. |
| Monitoring devices | Determination of the progress of therapy and the state of the patient in response to therapeutic regime. Minimal effect on biological system. Determination of trends rather than precise measurements. |

**FIGURE 1.1.** Design goals for diagnostic, therapeutic and monitoring medical devices. There are differences in the interaction of each kind of device with the biological system, and in the type of information obtained from diagnostic and monitoring devices.

## 1.2 DIAGNOSIS, THERAPY, AND MONITORING

Complete medical care involves three distinct but related activities: diagnosis, therapy, and monitoring. The physician determines the cause of physiological abnormality through diagnosis. He uses either medical (e.g., drug) or surgical methods to effect structural and/or functional changes that lead to improved overall function. This process is termed *therapy*. The physician or surgeon also monitors the course of disease or therapy and modifies his actions based on the results. Medical devices exist that are used in each of these phases of medicine. They are generally designed to be adjuncts to other forms of therapy. In some cases, the functions of monitoring and therapy may be combined in one device. Figure 1.1 lists the goals for each of these classes of devices.

### Devices for Diagnosis

Medical devices employed to aid diagnosis are often covered in textbooks and courses dealing with medical instrumentation. These devices are designed to determine physical signs of disease and/or injury without alteration of the structure and function of the biological system. This goal of nonalteration—referred to as a non-invasive measurement—is seldom completely met. Medical instrumentation is, however, designed with this goal in mind. All measurement devices affect the measured system in some way. However, medical instruments are typically designed with great care to reduce the possibility of hazardous effects. There are many textbooks on medical instrumentation (e.g., see Webster, 1978; Geddes and Baker, 1975; and Cobbold, 1974).

### Devices for Therapy

There are significant differences between the requirements for diagnostic and therapeutic devices. While safety is still of prime importance, the criteria used to judge safe operation are dramatically changed. In diagnosis, the criterion is minimal effect on the biological system. Because the goal of therapy is to effect changes, we cannot apply this criterion to therapeutic devices. For these devices we must ensure that the desired therapeutic effect is achieved, but that no unnecessary physical alteration of the biological system occurs.

### Devices for Monitoring

Once the physician starts a therapeutic regime, he must monitor the patient's progress. Devices used in this process are similar to diagnostic devices (some may be identical), but the requirements are slightly different. In diagnosis, very precise measurements are necessary in order to determine the etiology of the disease or injury. In monitoring, we may make less precise measurements because the goal is to determine a trend in patient condition. For example, the bandwidth requirement for diagnosis of heart arrhythmias using the ECG is 0.05 to 100 Hz (Newman, 1978). For monitoring of the heart in the intensive care ward, we reduce the bandwidth to 0.5 to 40 Hz. This reduction in bandwidth accomplishes several purposes. First, the system is less sensitive to noise and artifacts that are more likely to occur in long-term monitoring than in a diagnostic measurement situation. Second, by raising the low-frequency breakpoint, we can minimize the long-term effects of drift caused by the skin–electrode interface. Thus, even though we may use the same equipment for diagnosis and monitoring, we relax some parameters in monitoring situations. But we do not relax safety. For example, electrical safety requirements for monitoring and diagnosis are similar. The requirements may actually be more restrictive if the monitored patient is electrically susceptible (Freeman et al., 1979). Powers and Gisser (1974) describe monitoring principles in detail.

We may indirectly incorporate monitoring instruments into therapeutic devices. This combines the functions of the two classes of devices and may enhance the therapeutic effect. For example, anesthesia equipment may include pressure, volume, and flow indicators (Chapter 12), and defibrillators typically display stored energy (Chapter 3). This type of monitoring plays an important role in the control of therapeutic devices (Section 1.7). Recently developed devices provide some degree of closed-loop control, that is, the output of the device is directly controlled based on monitored parameters. A familiar example of such a system is the demand pacemaker (Chapter 2).

## 1.3 DESIGN GOALS FOR THERAPEUTIC DEVICES

When designing any medical device, we must first consider the medical or surgical goals that the device must help to meet. We must also determine the relationship between the device and other medical and/or surgical treatment procedures. Finally, we must determine how the device will be used and who will use it.

Figure 1.2 shows the major components that comprise a therapeutic medical device. Figure 1.3 shows examples of these components. The output component generates the energy that is actually used for therapy. This energy may take several forms. Section 1.5 presents the major types of energy and the methods for maximizing their therapeutic effect. The output energy enters the biological system via

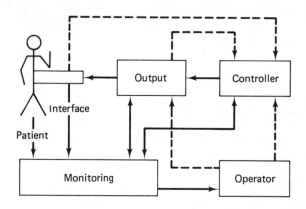

**FIGURE 1.2.** General form for a therapeutic medical device. The interface provides the direct interaction with the patient. This may be through skin contact, implantation or noncontact (e.g. radiation). The output determines the therapeutic effect and implements the functions of the controller. The controller provides operator and/or physiologic control over the output. The dotted lines indicate possible modes of control (*see Section 1.7*).

the interface. The interface may be internal or external, and we must design it to be specific for the type of energy applied. Examples of interfaces include the piezoelectric crystal used in ultrasound therapy (Chapter 7), electrodes used in cardiac pacemakers (Chapter 2), wire loops used for thermal coagulation (Chapter 11), and the breathing circuits used in anesthesia (Chapter 12) and ventilators (Chapter 13). Each of these interfaces is usually a separate system component. The femoral stem on a prosthetic hip (Chapter 9) and the sewing ring on a prosthetic heart valve (Chapter 4) are also interfaces. In some cases the interface does not contact the patient at all. For example, in radiation therapy (Chapter 16) and laser surgery (Chapter 11), the energy is applied through radiation to the biological system.

The controller alters, focuses, and shields the output energy. It adjusts the output level, wavelength, and duration to maximize the therapeutic effect. In sensory aids for reading (Chapter 6), the controller converts printed material to voice output. In ventilators (Chapter 13), the controller provides the desired flow and pressure of air by controlling the output pump. We discuss control of therapeutic devices in Section 1.7.

| Example (Chapter #) | Interface | Output | Controller | Monitoring |
|---|---|---|---|---|
| Ultrasound (7) | Piezoelectric crystal | ac voltage | | Medical exam |
| Ventilators (13) | Patient circuit | Piston or bellows | Electronic or pneumatic circuit | Blood gases, volumes |
| Hip prosthesis (9) | Femur shaft | Mechanical | None | Medical exam via x ray |
| Communication aid (6) | Switch | Visual or auditory | Electronic vocabulary selection | Visual or auditory feedback to user |

**FIGURE 1.3.** Examples of interface, controller, output, and monitoring. In some cases not all components are present (e.g. hip joints). Monitoring may be done by physical exam, user feedback or automatic methods.

Medical devices designed for therapeutic applications may also serve either medical or surgical goals. Examples of devices aiding medical treatment include ventilators (Chapter 13), which control levels of $O_2$ and $CO_2$ in the blood, and hemodialyzers (Chapter 14), which regulate the concentration of toxic substances in the blood. Aids to surgery include anesthesia (Chapter 12), electrosurgical equipment (Chapter 10), and internal orthotics such as bone plates (Chapter 9). Other devices have functions that are only loosely related to other medical and surgical treatment regimes. For example, although radiation therapy (Chapter 16) may be part of an overall oncology program that includes medical (chemotherapy) and surgical components, its effects are direct and separate from these other modes. Likewise, pacemakers (Chapter 2), defibrillators (Chapter 3), and sensory and communication aids (Chapter 6) have direct effects not directly dependent on specific medical or surgical treatment.

## 1.4 DEFINING MEDICAL AND/OR SURGICAL GOALS—THE OUTPUT MODES

Any therapeutic device will aid one or more of the following goals:

1. Maintain or reestablish homeostasis.
2. Alter structure to enhance function.
3. Directly aid function.
4. Replace absent function.

Figure 1.4 shows that each of the devices described in this text falls into one or more of these categories.

### Maintenance of Homeostasis

Homeostasis refers to the ability of the body to act to minimize changes in the internal environment in the presence of changes in the external environment or in the individual (Selkurt, 1976). Homeostatic mechanisms respond to internal changes that are the result of nutritional imbalances, exercise, disease, or trauma. We are most concerned with disease and trauma. Like any other control system, the internal feedback mechanisms of the body have limits over which they are effective. When these limits are exceeded, internal regulation is no longer possible and death may occur rapidly. We often employ medical devices to temporarily compensate for excessive changes in the internal environment of the body.

Examples of homeostatic regulatory mechanisms include: thermoregulation, blood-gas levels, blood-sugar levels, muscle tone, blood pressure, electrolyte balance, and fluid balance. These parameters are kept within normal limits through the interaction of the autonomic nervous system, the circulatory system, the renal system, the respiratory system, and the spleen, liver, and pancreas. If disease or injury affects any of these systems, then this impairs the regulation of the internal environment. Therapeutic medical devices combat this situation in two ways. They may directly substitute for a defective organ system. For example, hemodialyzers (Chapter 14) help overcome abnormalities in electrolyte balance, fluid balance, and

Acute care devices:

| Device | Medical/surgical goal | Chapter |
|---|---|---|
| Cardiac defibrillators | Directly aid function | 3 |
| Balloon pump* | Directly aid function | 4 |
| Blood pump/oxygenators* | Maintain homeostasis | 4 |
| Internal bone plates | Alter structure to aid function | 9 |
| Electrosurgical devices | Alter structure to aid function | 10 |
| Cryogenic, laser, other surgical devices | Alter structure to aid function | 11 |
| Anesthesia equipment | Maintain/alter homeostasis | 12 |
| Ventilators* | Maintain/alter homeostasis | 13 |
| Hemodialyzers* | Maintain/alter homeostasis | 14 |
| Incubators | Maintain homeostasis | 15 |
| Radiation therapy | Alter structure to aid function | 16 |

Chronic care devices:

| Device | Medical/surgical goal | Chapter |
|---|---|---|
| Cardiac pacemakers | Directly aid function | 2 |
| Heart valves | Replace function | 4 |
| Artificial heart | Replace function | 4 |
| Neural assist | Directly aid function | 5 |
| Sensory/communication aids | Replace function | 6 |
| Physical therapy equipment | Directly aid function or alter structure to aid function | 7 |
| Limb prosthetics and orthotics | Directly aid or replace function | 8 |
| Internal joint replacements | Replace function | 9 |

*Also may be used to directly aid function of target organ system.

**FIGURE 1.4.** We must base design goals for therapeutic medical devices on the intended medical and/or surgical effect desired. Each device in this text has a primary mode of operation as shown. Each device also serves primarily acute or chronic care needs.

blood-sugar levels. Ventilators (Chapter 13) help to control blood-gas levels. Balloon pumps (Chapter 4) help overcome deficiencies in central circulatory function. We may also apply therapeutic devices to directly affect overall function. For example, incubators (Chapter 15) compensate for deficiencies in thermoregulation in neonates.

In order to carry out some therapeutic medical procedures, we must depress the regulatory mechanisms of the body. Anesthesia equipment (Chapter 12) depresses the autonomic nervous system and alters the response of the body. For this reason, we may also use other life support systems such as ventilators (Chapter 13) and blood oxygenators (Chapter 4) during the administration of anesthesia.

Because devices in this category are life sustaining, we must design them to be extremely reliable. Monitoring of both device and patient function is critical (Powers and Gisser, 1974). We must design the devices to include key parameters related to the effectiveness of the therapy. Often, monitoring is carried out "off-line." For example, during ventilatory assist (Chapter 13), we typically measure blood gases on a withdrawn sample of atrial, venous, or capillary blood. A second-ary monitoring that is incorporated into the device is measurement of both tidal and minute ventilation. Because changes in the respiratory system may occur over a matter of days and lead to total failure, we must detect subtle changes. When designing monitoring functions for therapeutic devices, we must choose those pa-rameters that are most directly related to the performance of the organ system that the device is aiding. We must choose the parameters that will most quickly indicate a change in patient condition that is life-threatening. Powers and Gisser (1974) present an excellent discussion of these parameters for the circulatory, renal, auton-omic, nervous, and respiratory systems.

## Alteration of Structure to Enhance Function

Many therapeutic procedures require the alteration of structure to enhance function. We commonly use several types of structural alteration. Cutting or severing of tissue is the function of several devices. Cutting usually results in blood loss, so a second structural effect is coagulation. We may also need to destroy tissue that is foreign to the organism. This effect imposes different goals than the first two types of structural change. Therapeutic medical devices often aid these procedures. We must design devices of this type to maximize the structural changes desired and minimize undesirable changes. For example, we can design electrosurgical equip-ment (Chapter 10) to provide clean cutting with minimum blood loss. This requires an understanding of the principles of RF cutting as well as an understanding of the surgical goals.

Alteration of structure is not an end goal in itself but is rather a means to achieve enhanced function. This means that we must emphasize the specificity of the effect and minimize side effects (see Section 1.5).

In all cases the type of structural alteration must be consistent with the medical or surgical goals. We must avoid excessive blood loss, removal of excess tissue, or causing effects that may prolong the healing process. We must also design devices to minimize the total surgical time.

## Direct Aid to Function

Therapeutic medical devices also effect improvement in specific organ system function. We call devices that aid function *orthotic devices* or *orthoses*. Before designing a device for this type of application, we must thoroughly understand the physiology of the organ system being aided. For example, in order to design devices that aid the heart, we must first define the problems in engineering terms. Electrical abnormalities (arrhythmias) require specific design parameters such as stimulus voltage, current, and duration in the pacemaker output (Chapter 2). The type of arrhythmia also dictates the design goals for control. A stable, third-degree heart block requires a different type of device than a second-degree block. Mechanical failure of the heart requires different design goals. The important parameters in designing left ventricular assist devices are stroke volume, cardiac output, and coronary circulation (Chapter 4). Unless we consider these specific requirements early in the design process, the device is unlikely to serve its intended function. Similarly, we must base design specifications for hearing aids on the functional loss experienced by the individual (Chapter 6).

Sometimes devices are lifesaving. For example, we use defibrillators (Chapter 3) when death or severe impairment can occur in a matter of minutes. Other devices improve the quality of a patient's life but are not life-sustaining. For example, we may use neural-assist devices (Chapter 5) to reduce chronic intractable pain. Limb orthotics (Chapter 8) provide for enhanced upper or lower limb function in neuromuscular disease or trauma. We must consider the relationship of the device to the patient's well-being when designing for reliability, safety, ease of use, and overall size and cost. The role of the device in maintaining life versus improving quality of life is the essential criterion in evaluating the design trade-offs between these factors.

### Replacement of Function

In many cases, there is total loss of function due to disease or injury. When a medical device is used as a replacement for lost or absent function, we call it a *prosthetic device* or *prosthesis*. The major design goal is replacement of *function*. The *structure* of the replacement may not resemble that of the biological system at all. For example, prosthetic heart valves (Chapter 4) may utilize floating balls or rotating disks rather than the leaflet structure of the normal valve. It is particularly important to design replacement parts using a functional approach rather than a mimicking of structure. Leaflet prosthetic valves have typically failed because they did not have the structural support of the papillary muscles present in normal valves. Because the prosthesis is totally passive and is controlled strictly by the pressure gradient across the orifice, a leaflet structure has excessive leakage.

Sensory aids (Chapter 6) replace function but rarely replace a structure. We design reading and mobility aids for the blind on the basis of information input required, not on the basis of a photochemical approach similar to the eye. Communication aids (Chapter 6) do not replace speech as it occurs naturally. They replace the essentials of communication by substituting one method for another. The artificial hook (Chapter 8) replaces hand function but does not have the dexterity or structure of the normal hand.

Some devices do copy the structure of the body part to be replaced. For example, the artificial hip (Chapter 9) has a structure that is very similar to the natural hip joint. This is because the function of the hip is structural, and materials exist that can copy the natural structure.

### An Example of Goal-Directed Device Design— Implantable Drug-Delivery Systems

Many therapeutic drugs are most effective when we administer them at a constant rate. The use of oral or injection administration results in a rapid high blood level immediately after the drug is infused, but the drug rapidly decreases in concentration with time. This results in a "peak–valley effect" that has several disadvantages. For example, we must give some drugs (e.g., procainamide) every three hours in order to provide blood levels necessary to avoid irregular heart rhythms. However, immediately following injection, the concentration of this substance reaches blood levels that may be toxic in some patients. If the patient skips one dose (such as during a night's sleep), the levels may reach low values that are hazardous. Continuous infusion would avoid these effects.

Many drugs cannot be given orally because the gastrointestinal system inactivates them. These must be given either by regular injection or by IV therapy. In either case, we must restrict the patient to the hospital during administration of the drug. The medical goal for a therapeutic device for drug infusion is, then, to overcome these two problems by infusing a constant low level of a drug directly into the bloodstream.

Blackshear (1979) and his co-workers have developed an implantable pump to meet this goal. The pump consists of a titanium disk about the size of an ice hockey puck with a weight of 190 g. Figure 1.5 shows that the inside of the disk is

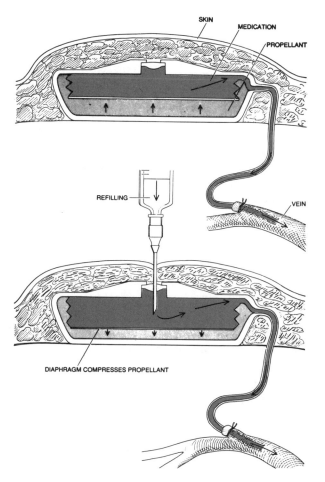

FIGURE 1.5. An implantable pump for drug delivery consists of two chambers. The top chamber holds the drug to be infused, and the lower a propellant. The refilling procedure is also shown. (From Blackshear, Implantable Drug-Delivery Systems, Copyright © 1979, by Scientific American, Inc. All rights reserved.)

divided into two chambers. One of these is filled with a fluorocarbon, which acts as a propellant. A titanium bellows separates this chamber from the second one, which contains the drug solution to be infused. The second chamber has a connection to the patient's vein. The pump provides a constant flow of drug through the basic physical principle that a liquid in equilibrium with its vapor phase exerts a constant vapor pressure at a given temperature, regardless of its volume. The constant temperature of the body ensures that the infusion rate is constant. The pump is installed just beneath the skin in the same manner as a cardiac pacemaker. The nurse can refill it (necessary about every 45 days) with a syringe injected through the skin.

Blackshear has implanted about 20 pumps for the delivery of heparin. They have effectively avoided the formation of clots and the necessity for repeated injections. The levels of heparin are relatively constant over time without the peak-and-valley effect of injections. Another advantage is that we can alter the quantities of drug during the refilling phase. Other uses of this pump are in chemotherapy, administration of antiarrhythmia drugs, and insulin administration in diabetes.

## 1.5 DELIVERED ENERGY—DESIGN OF THE OUTPUT

All effects caused by therapeutic devices are due to the input of energy into the biological system. We deliver this energy through some sort of output transducer, as shown in Fig. 1.2. In some cases the output transducer produces a form of energy that has a direct biological effect. For example, the electrodes in cardiac pacing systems (Chapter 2) produce a current that directly stimulates the myocardium. In other cases there is a second transduction of energy by the biological system, and this secondary form of energy causes the desired biological effect. For example, in therapeutic ultrasound (Chapter 7), the output transducer is a piezoelectric crystal that produces a high-frequency mechanical vibration. The biological effect is due, however, to the secondary thermal energy generated by the vibration. In other cases, the biological system alters the form of the input energy to produce a more effective form. An example of this is the conversion of tactile stimulation in sensory prosthesis to neural signals that are processed by the central nervous system as visual images (Chapter 6). In many cases we do not know the precise mechanism by which a device is able to effect therapy. When this is true, we must design the output based on empirical data rather than on a precise definition of the underlying theory. We must always keep the final biological effect in mind, however, rather than looking just at the primary output of the device.

### Types of Energy Used in Therapeutic Devices

Figure 1.6 lists the major types of energy provided by therapeutic devices together with the primary and possible secondary effects and examples of devices employing each type of energy. Each of these forms of energy has unique effects on living tissue. We discuss them in following chapters. They are all capable of meeting one or more of the medical and surgical goals discussed in Section 1.4. Sometimes a primary form of energy may have accompanying secondary forms that are damag-

| Primary form | Modes of application | Secondary effects | Examples (Chapter #) |
|---|---|---|---|
| Electrical | Electrodes | Thermal, chemical | Pacing (2), defibrillation (3), electrosurgery (10), neural assist (5), sensory aids (6) |
| Mechanical | Direct contact Flow or pressure source External via skin | Thermal, chemical | Heart valves (4), internal orthotics and prosthetics (9), ventilators (13), aortic balloon pump (4), ultrasound (7), sensory aids (6), limb prosthetics (8) |
| Nonionizing radiation | Coherent light Electromagnetic (RF) Noncoherent light | Thermal Chemical | Laser surgery (11), RF diathermy (7), bilirubin light (15), electrosurgery (10) |
| Ionizing radiation | Decaying nuclide X-ray generator | Thermal Chemical | Radiation therapy (16) |
| Thermal | Conduction Convection Radiation | | Incubators (15), physical therapy (7), heart-lung machine (4), ventilators (13) |
| Chemical | Membrane gradient Airflow | | Hemodialysis (14), anesthesia (12), ventilators (13), blood oxygenators (4) |

**FIGURE 1.6.** There are several types of output energy used in therapeutic devices. The modes of application and secondary effects differ with the type of energy supplied.

ing. These secondary forms are usually chemical or thermal. For example, burns may be sustained by patients during electrosurgery (Chapter 10). Another example is the formation of chemical by-products by electrolysis during chronic electrical stimulation (Chapters 2 and 5). We must therefore design the output section of therapeutic devices to control not only the primary form of energy delivered but also to minimize any secondary effects that may occur.

We use the term *electrical energy* to refer to any output that provides current to the biological system via direct physical contact. The output transducer is a pair of electrodes, and we obtain the biological effect by passing current between them. We must design the output transducer to transfer an optimum charge in a given time in order to obtain the desired effect (Chapter 5). Cardiac pacing (Chapter 2) and neural assist (Chapter 5) provide stimulation in a periodic manner over a prolonged period of time. Our design goals for these systems are therefore different from those for electrical output devices that provide a large pulse of energy on a one-shot basis. For example, we use defibrillators (Chapter 3) and electrocautery loops (Chapter 11) to effect an immediate change in the biological system but do not use them chronically. The electrode design and output circuits of these two types of devices are significantly different even though the form of energy is the same. Secondary effects are chemical (due to electrolysis) and thermal. These may lead to burns or the production of toxic substances.

We may impart mechanical energy to the biological system directly to provide structural enhancement. Internal bone plates and prosthetic joints (Chapter 9) have a mechanical energy output that is transferred to the biological system to aid in the loading of the part. Mechanical energy may also be in the form of a generated pressure or flow. Ventilators (Chapter 13) generate an airflow at pressure levels compatible with the respiratory system. Aortic balloon pumps (Chapter 4) generate a pressure that is transferred to the heart to increase blood flow and reduce the work of the heart. Therapeutic ultrasound (Chapter 7) is also a mechanical form of energy. The output crystal vibration transfers energy through the skin to deeper tissues to effect therapy. Principal secondary effects from mechanical energy systems are thermal and chemical. The thermal heating in ultrasound is one example. Ventilators produce secondary blood-gas effects that are partially controllable by the design of the pressure or flow-source output (see Chapter 13). Internal orthotic and prosthetic devices (Chapter 9) may produce chemical breakdown products that are toxic to the body.

Nonionizing radiation includes coherent and noncoherent light and electromagnetic fields. The major difference between this and the previous modes is that the energy is transferred by radiation rather than by direct attachment to the patient. Laser surgery for retinal repair (Chapter 11) is an example of the use of coherent light. Bilirubin lights, used in phototherapy of neonates (Chapter 15), illustrate the use of noncoherent light sources. Electrosurgical devices (Chapter 10) and RF diathermy (Chapter 7) both use electromagnetic radiation and cause a secondary effect of thermal energy generation. In electrosurgery (Chapter 10), the heating effects of the applied energy are crucial for effective coagulation of small blood vessels. Thermal effects can be undesirable as well. For example, electrosurgical devices can cause severe burns near the dispersive or monitoring electrodes if the output is not carefully designed. Chemical effects can also be produced. In the case of bilirubin lights, this is desirable. Electrolysis or evaporation effects are undesirable in electrosurgery, however.

We apply ionizing radiation by controlling the output of decaying nuclides (cobalt for example) or by the generation of high-energy x rays (Chapter 16). We must design the output generator to ensure maximum protection of the operator and patient. Linear accelerators use RF energy to generate the x-ray beam. In ultravoltage x-ray units, direct acceleration methods generate the x rays. In either case, the control is via careful selection of electrical parameters. When we use radionuclides, it is more difficult to control the output of the device. In this case, we must use mechanical design of the carrier to achieve control.

We may obtain thermal effects via convection, conduction, or radiation. Strictly speaking, thermal radiation is an electromagnetic energy form. We list it with thermal because its effect on the biological system is heating. Convection devices provide heating via air flow. An example is the heating of air before it is pumped to the patient in ventilators (13). Incubators employ radiant heating (Chapter 15). Heart–lung machines (Chapter 4) provide conductive heating of the blood prior to pumping it back into the patient.

The existence of a chemical potential due to differing concentrations of a substance produces chemical energy (Chapter 14). This form of energy is employed primarily in dialyzers (Chapter 14). The chemical gradient established across a membrane is responsible for the therapeutic effect. In order to control this type of energy, we must design the output component to vary flow and pressure of dialysate in order to establish the desired gradient. Anesthesia systems (Chapter 12) also use chemical energy as the primary therapeutic form. The mechanical energy of the output pressure or flow source controls the flow of gas to the patient.

## *Energy Levels Employed in Therapeutic Devices*

Energy levels are of prime importance in the use of therapeutic devices. For example, thermal effects may be moderate, as in the case of physical therapy (Chapter 7), or drastic, as in the case of cryosurgery (Chapter 11). In both cases we obtain the desired effect by lowering the temperature, but the final effect is drastically different.

Many of the devices used for therapy employ energy outputs similar to those of their diagnostic or monitoring counterparts. For example, diagnostic ultrasound and therapeutic ultrasound (Chapter 7) both use high-frequency mechanical energy generated by using piezoelectric crystals. The fundamental difference is the power level applied to the tissue. Likewise, diagnostic x-ray systems and some radiation therapy equipment (Chapter 16) both generate x-ray beams. The increased power levels required for therapy place severe restrictions on both the methods of generation and the facilities required for safe operation.

Figure 1.7 illustrates a comparison of energy levels for several modes used in both diagnosis and therapy. The energy required for effective therapy is several orders of magnitude greater than for diagnosis. In the case of ultrasound, the diagnostic power levels are thought to be low enough to cause no biological effect. We express the therapeutic level in terms of cross-sectional area of application because the effect depends on area. For x rays, the therapeutic levels vary over a wide range depending on the generator and the target site within the body (see Chapter 16). The magnitudes are, however, much higher than for diagnosis.

For comparison, Fig. 1.7 shows electrical power levels for electrical impedance plethysmography and cardiac defibrillation and pacing. The mode of application is crucial. The values for pacing are several orders of magnitude lower than those for defibrillation. This is because the defibrillating pulse must pass through the tissues of the chest before reaching the heart. When the energy is applied directly to the heart, the power levels are much less. Another factor is the desired

| Type of energy | Diagnostic or power energy level | Therapeutic energy level |
|---|---|---|
| Ultrasound | $< 1$ mW | 1.5 W/cm$^2$ |
| X-ray | $\sim 50$ keV | (1) 3-25 meV |
| Electrical | (2) 1.6 mW | (3) 20 MW |
| | | (4) 15 mW |

Notes:

1. Depends on mode — see Chapter 16
2. Impedance plethysmography
3. Defibrillation
4. Cardiac pacing — power shown is per pulse delivered

FIGURE 1.7. Diagnostic energy levels are always less than their therapeutic counterparts. The mode of application, bandwidth and method of generation all affect the energy level *(see text)*.

physiological effect. It takes less energy to pace the heart than to depolarize all the ventricular cells simultaneously as required in defibrillation. Electrical impedance plethysmography is also applied externally but requires only small currents for measurement.

## Maximizing the Therapeutic Effect

Therapeutic devices must, in general, restrict the application of energy to a relatively small area in order to maximize the therapeutic effect while leaving normal tissue unaltered. We may accomplish this by shielding, focusing, or by the careful placement of the patient interface. An example of careful placement is the location of the electrosurgical dispersive electrode (Chapter 10) or the placement of defibrillator electrodes to minimize effects on other tissues (Chapter 3). Less obvious is the proper design of a bone plate to ensure adequate distribution of forces while also enhancing mechanical alignment (Chapter 9).

Radiation therapy typically employs shielding (Chapter 16). Using both collimators and lead shields, we can shape the x-ray or gamma-ray beam to maximize the energy level at the tumor and minimize it in normal tissue. We can also use focusing of the energy of the device on a specific region. For example, devices employing lasers for cutting (Chapter 11) maximize the desired effect by taking into account the optical properties of the tissue and focusing the energy at a specific point. Another method of focusing is to deliver energy at a certain frequency. This takes advantage of the frequency response characteristics of the biological tissue and allows us to maximize desired effects and minimize secondary effects. For example, the depth of penetration of x-ray beams is proportional to their wavelength (Chapter 16). Electrosurgery has an output current in the 1-MHz range. This minimizes the biological effect because the thresholds for perception and stimulation are higher at this frequency. We can also choose laser systems (Chapter 11) on the basis of their wavelength to maximize their effect.

We can also control the delivery of energy through mechanical structure of the output. For example, the geometry of the probe drastically affects the energy delivered in thermal electrocautery (Section 11.3). This also applies to mechanical loading in stump sockets for prosthetic limbs (Chapter 8). The design of the socket can provide maximum mechanical stability and control while minimizing the tissue damage due to prolonged contact. We may use the waveshape of flow and pressure patterns in ventilators (Chapter 13) to maximize respiratory effects while minimizing undesirable cardiovascular side effects.

## An Example of Output Design—The Neurourologic Prosthesis

The output component and interface of a therapeutic device often require a careful analysis of the properties of the living system. Most electrical stimulation employed in therapeutic devices takes advantage of the internal conduction of the electrical energy by the biological tissue. Thus, cardiac pacemakers must excite only one part of the myocardium. The rest of the muscle is stimulated by cell-to-cell conduction.

Because skeletal or smooth muscle systems have little cell-to-cell conduction, we must provide multiple stimulators (Timm and Bradley, 1973).

A major result of certain neurological trauma or disease is urinary incontinence. This presents two major design challenges. We must provide a controllable valving system to allow voiding under voluntary control, and a means of completely evacuating the bladder must be available. Electrical stimulation of the bladder can cause contraction and complete voiding. Timm and Bradley (1973) developed a series of small stimulators that were sequentially pulsed. Those near the top of the bladder activated first with a sequential firing of those located closer to the urethra. In this manner, this stimulated the entire bladder. They also carefully designed the electrode pairs to avoid spread of current from one region to an adjacent region. This would result in asynchronous firing and incomplete voiding of the bladder. By a careful design of the stimulators, their timing, and the electrodes, Timm and Bradley were able to effectively stimulate smooth muscle in a predetermined manner.

## 1.6 DEFINING THE RELATIONSHIP TO OTHER MODES OF THERAPY

In order to design a therapeutic device for a specific application, we must understand the other procedures and treatment modalities to be used. We must also consider the interaction of our device with other therapeutic or monitoring equipment.

### Implanted Devices

The successful application of many therapeutic medical devices depends on surgical procedures. For implanted devices, we must understand the surgical capabilities available to "install" the device. Obviously, the size and weight of a cardiac pacemaker package (Chapter 2) must be compatible with the space available for its implantation. More important is the design of the lead system to provide attachment to the myocardium in such a way as to maximize the transfer of electrical energy. Some radiation therapy (Chapter 16) is carried out using implanted (interstitial or intercavitary) devices. When designing the carriers for these implants, we must consider the method of implantation, the anatomic location, and the length of time they will be implanted. The surgical procedures available for implantation determine these parameters.

Other medical devices depend on the preparation of a site within or external to the body. The type of surgical preparation of the stump dictates the design of artificial limbs (Chapter 8). We must design internal hip joints (Chapter 9) to interface as completely as possible with the remaining portion of the femur and acetabulum. Artificial knee designs (Chapter 9) vary widely in the amount of bone that is necessary for attachment. This dramatically affects the long-term effects of device failure. If only a small amount of bone removal is necessary for installation, then failure of the prosthesis may lead only to fusing of the joint. If the surgeon must remove large amounts of bone, then the failure of the device may leave him with few choices for further therapy.

Many implanted devices require a design that allows for tissue attachment and eventual ingrowth of tissue for long-term stability. We must design prosthetic heart valves (Chapter 4) to accommodate this structural attachment. This requires an understanding of the surgical methods of installation. Since most of the defective valve is removed, the surgeon must make attachment around the prosthetic valve structure. Although tissue ingrowth is important, we must also design the valve such that no tissue ingrowth occurs in the flow path. In prosthetic hips (Chapter 9), bone ingrowth into the femoral component is crucial for long-term stability. This requires us to carefully consider the materials used in our design and to understand the surgical preparation of the femoral shaft for installation.

In any surgical procedure, there is the possibility of infection. Implanted devices must be capable of sterilization and there is often concomitant medical treatment with antibiotics following surgery. Impurities in implanted device materials may lead to tissue reactions that compromise both the effectiveness of the device and the patient's condition (Chapter 9). We must also consider the body's natural defense mechanisms. The inflammatory response process (Chapter 9) can severely limit the effectiveness of a device by local edema, formation of fibrous tissue around an implant (including electrodes in pacemaker applications), and walling-off of the implanted device. With circulatory assist devices, there is also the problem of blood coagulation. This often leads to secondary medical treatment when some devices are used. For example, patients who have artificial heart valves implanted must take anticoagulant drugs for the rest of their lives. This affects their activities and may result in complications with other injuries or diseases. The quantity of anticoagulants necessary can be partially controlled by considering this problem during the design process.

### External Devices

Therapeutic medical devices that are applied externally also require consideration of other modes of therapy. For example, a patient suffering from severe pneumonia with empyema (fluid in the thoracic cavity) is subjected to many devices and procedures. If the fluid build-up is large, then we may employ a chest drainage unit (Chapter 13) with a suction device. Because this results in an open wound, the patient is subject to further infection. We also use a drug infusion apparatus (IV unit) for administering antibiotics. Because pneumonia results in significantly reduced lung capacity, we also use oxygen delivery equipment and possibly a ventilator. Because this is a life-threatening situation, we monitor the patient, who is probably in the intensive care unit (ICU). The effectiveness of each device depends on the effectiveness of antibiotic and fluid infusion therapy to reduce further build-up of fluid. The ventilator must be capable of delivering sufficient oxygen and removing sufficient carbon dioxide to prevent blood acidosis. This depends on the effectiveness of both the IV and chest drainage units to reduce the obstructions to breathing and to prevent a worsening of the condition.

Another aspect of interface design is the control required. For communication and control devices (Chapter 6), this requires a knowledge of the remaining function and the role of other devices. For example, if we use hand function to control a device, then we must know the role of body-positioning devices (braces) and hand orthotic devices (Chapter 8). We must design the interface to work with other assistive devices used by the patient. These principles also apply to the design of control systems for upper extremity prosthetic devices (Chapter 8). The method of attaching the device is dependent on the amount of tissue remaining and the sensory and motor capability of the stump.

In addition to meeting one or more of the goals listed above, we can group therapeutic medical devices into either chronic (long-term) or acute (short-term) use categories. These two applications place significantly different constraints on the design of devices. We have shown these categories for each of the devices in Fig. 1.4.

## *Devices Designed for Short-Term Use—Acute Care*

Many therapeutic devices are used in an acute care situation. They are intended to cause an immediate transient effect. Most of these devices are used in conjunction with surgical procedures. For example, we use electrosurgical equipment (Chapter 10), cryogenic surgery devices (Chapter 11), and anesthesia equipment (Chapter 12) as adjuncts to other surgical procedures. In these cases, the device is not the primary mode of therapy, but rather it serves to improve the effectiveness of other procedures.

We use other acute care devices as adjuncts to medical treatment. These devices cause specific effects on the biological system that aid its function during periods of acute illness or injury. Examples of devices of this type are defibrillators (Chapter 3), ventilators (Chapter 13), and radiation therapy equipment (Chapter 16). In each of these cases, the device supplements other medical procedures, but each device has a specific therapeutic effect independent of other procedures.

We always use acute care devices under the control of a trained operator. This relaxes design constraints to some extent because the operator can alter device function as the patient's condition warrants. We usually employ monitoring functions to indicate one of two conditions: failure to operate and abnormalities of operation. Because most devices of this type are life-supporting, monitoring and alarms are very important. An overdriven condition, such as an airway pressure exceeding a preset limit in a ventilator (Chapter 13), may trigger alarms. Indicators that monitor physiological function may also trigger them. Examples of this type are temperature alarms in incubators (Chapter 15) or conductivity meters in hemo-dialyzers (Chapter 14).

We must also design acute care therapeutic devices so that they fail safely if they fail. Freeman et al. (1979) discuss this concept from mechanical design in detail. Basically, it means that any device that fails to function should do so in a manner that does not further injure the patient. For example, if we use an anesthesia machine in a rebreathing mode, it should fail in a manner that allows the patient to either breathe room air or be artificially ventilated (Chapter 12). Likewise, it should fail in a manner that results in too little rather than too much anesthetic agent.

## Devices Intended for Chronic Care

We use a second major class of therapeutic device for long-term or chronic use. These devices, due to their use, have significantly different requirements. We may use some chronic care devices, such as those applied in physical therapy (Chapter 7) or hemodialysis (Chapter 14), in the hospital or clinic with a trained operator present. But most chronic care devices, including some aspects of physical therapy and dialysis, accompany the patient to many different locations. Because a trained operator is not present, considerations of reliability and fail-safe design become much more important.

Monitoring of performance is still a fundamental aspect of chronic care devices, but it is done on a very different basis. The determination of device function is from two sources: the patient and periodic follow-up evaluations. The follow-up evaluations may be measurements of physical performance with an artificial leg (Chapter 8), x rays of an implanted joint (Chapter 9), or ECG recordings that indicate the functioning of a cardiac pacemaker (Chapter 2). We perform each of these types of measures on an infrequent basis and do not monitor device function daily.

We generally intend prosthetic and orthotic devices for long-term use by the patient. They must be capable of operating reliably and safely in a wide variety of environments. For this reason, we must shield cardiac pacemakers (Chapter 2), for example, to reduce the effects of microwave ovens on their performance. Likewise, artificial arms and legs (Chapter 8) must resist moisture, heat, and chemicals.

Because we use orthotic devices with the body part still present, there is generally more structural support available than with a prosthetic device. However, the existence of a nonfunctioning body part (such as a leg, for example) may represent dead weight that the orthosis must support. Orthotic devices also need only supplement the existing function, while prosthetic devices must totally replace the biological system. In some cases, either type of device may be possible and we base the ultimate decision on a careful evaluation of the existing function. An example is the replacement or augmentation of internal joints (Chapter 9).

A major consideration in the design of some chronic care devices is the power consumption of the device. Much of size and weight of many devices is due to the electrical or pneumatic power source required. Devices must be capable of operating over extended periods of time without the need for replacement of a power source. This is particularly important for implanted electrical devices such as cardiac pacemakers and neural assist devices (Chapter 5).

In summary, we must carefully design devices intended for chronic use for safe, effective, and maintenance-free operation. In some cases, the patient's life may depend on such design. In other cases, the patient's livelihood and/or quality of life is at stake.

## 1.7 CONTROL OF THERAPEUTIC DEVICES

The control of therapeutic devices depends on feedback regarding the effectiveness of the therapy. This feedback may be part of an automated system in which sensors directly measure the output and affect the device. More likely with current devices is the use of an *executive control loop* in which a physician, therapist, or nurse monitors the effect of the device and adjusts it accordingly. This is *open-loop control* in engineering terminology. We discuss some general properties of feedback systems in this section and show how they are employed in therapeutic medical devices.

## Open Loop Control of Therapeutic Devices

Most therapeutic medical devices have a control scheme that is *open loop*. By this term we mean that the system output is not internally regulated by the use of feedback. Figure 1.2 shows that there are several types of external feedback that are used. The physician determines the settings of the device necessary to cause the desired therapeutic effect. The therapist or nurse then adjusts the device. A crucial aspect of this process is the continual monitoring of patient and device performance. This monitoring leads to adjustment of machine settings to correct for problems occurring over time.

There are two major disadvantages to this approach. First, the system dynamics are slow. Effects of improper settings may not be apparent for periods of hours, and we may not detect them until we make off-line measurements. For example, in artificial ventilation (Chapter 13), the major monitoring and feedback is based on blood-gas levels. By the time we draw blood and determine the $O_2$ and $CO_2$ concentrations, a period of hours may have passed. When we make a correction, it may be too small or too large. Again, there is no indication of the appropriateness of the change until we analyze a new blood-gas sample. This leads to a total control system that is usually underdamped or overdamped with large amounts of overshoot or undershoot.

The second major problem with open-loop control is a failure to account for changes in the physiological state of the patient over time. We may not see changes in physiological or interface parameters until we carry out off-line sampling. For example, the intra-aortic balloon pump (Chapter 4) depends on a certain pressure "load." If the vascular resistance changes substantially, then the pump may deliver either too high or too low a pressure. With an open-loop system, we would have to note this situation and correct it quickly to prevent either damage to the circulatory system or an inadequate supply of blood.

Closed-loop feedback control systems can compensate for these two deficiencies in open-loop control. There are, however, many problems associated with using closed-loop control.

## Effect of Feedback on Parameter Variation

We define *feedback* as any system that has some form of parameter variation reduction capability. This definition of feedback includes very simple systems in which it may be difficult to define the feedback path. An example of this type of system is the voltage divider shown in Fig. 1.8. For this system, a 10% change in $R_2$ results in a smaller than 10% change in $V_o$. Thus, the system is able to reduce

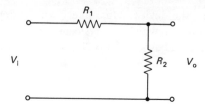

**FIGURE 1.8.** A common voltage divider is an example of the use of feedback to reduce parameter variation.

the internal parameter variation. This effect is not always desirable. For example, if the resistor in Fig. 1.8 were a negative resistance, such as a tunnel diode, then a 10% change in $R_2$ would result in more than a 10% change in $V_o$. By trying to self-calibrate, the system has amplified the parameter variation. Figure 1.9 shows the most general feedback configuration. The controller may actually contain the therapeutic device or the therapeutic device might be the device we wish to control. The signals may be of any form (continuous, sampled, binary, etc.) and in medical applications are normally electrical, mechanical, thermal, fluid, or chemical. The most common reason for applying feedback is to reduce effects due to parameter variation. In a linear continuous closed loop system, overall system change due to internal forward loop parameter variation is reduced by roughly the loop gain (Dorf, 1967). These parameter variations may be due to either the device itself, the physiological system, or the transducers connecting the two. There are several examples of therapeutic devices that demonstrate successful application of this technique. When pacing the heart (Chapter 2), we must ensure that the energy delivered by the pacemaker is constant. Thus, when battery voltage diminishes over time, we increase the duty cycle (pulse width) of the pacemaker to compensate for battery drain. This is a case in which we use feedback to sense the output and correct for changes in device parameters.

Another example of this feedback property is the use of feedback to compensate for compression of the driving bellows in mechanical ventilators that are used for artificial respiration (Bell, 1973). This system is necessary because we must precisely know the amount of air supplied to a patient on each cycle of a ventilator in order to ensure that we achieve adequate minute ventilation (Chapter 13). Ventilators using a bellows as a driving reservoir have the disadvantage that they do not deliver the preset amount of inspired air (tidal volume) at higher pressures due to compression of the bellows itself. We can compensate for this effect by using a feedback system in which we use the system pressure together with machine

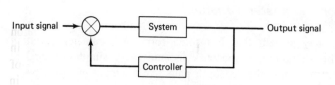

**FIGURE 1.9.** A closed loop feedback system usually consists of a controlled system (plant), a controller (feedback element) and a comparator that provides a difference signal between a desired input and the feedback signal.

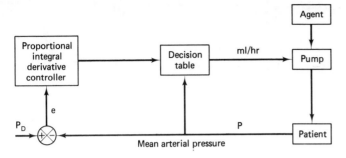

**FIGURE 1.10.** This system provides closed loop control of drug infusion. The desired pressure is 80. The controller and decision table are realized using a digital computer (from Shepard, *IEEE Frontiers in Health Care Conf. 1979*, with permission.)

compliance to calculate a compliance compensation volume. We use this compliance compensation volume and the desired volume setting to generate an error voltage that alters volume delivery. Thus, this system compensates for internal parameter variation.

We may also compensate for changes in the physiological state of the patient by using feedback. An example of this use of feedback is the computer-controlled infusion of drugs to control blood pressure in postsurgical cardiac patients (Shepard et al., 1979). Figure 1.10 shows the system block diagram. The design goal is to reduce mean arterial pressure (MAP) through the infusion of nitroprusside, a fast-acting vasodilator. Control of arterial pressure with this drug requires frequent adjustment of the rate of infusion based on measurement of systematic pressure or MAP. Because the drug is fast-acting, there is a rapid reduction of peripheral vascular resistance when it is administered and the effect subsides quickly when the infusion is stopped. Due to the problems in obtaining adquate control manually, we use automatic feedback control methods.

The control parameter $P_D$ in Fig. 1.10 is the desired pressure. The attending physician or nurse determines this value. The medical goal of the immediate postoperative period is to achieve optimal performance of each physiological subsystem while maintaining adequate reserves with a minimum of pharmacologic intervention. Shepard et al. have established a set of rules to dictate the quantities of drug to be infused under these conditions. These rules bias the infusion of drugs toward minimizing the infusion rate and total amount of agent. They use both feedback, based on a comparison of current MAP and desired $P_D$, and feedforward (used to decrease the MAP when it is 5 mm Hg or more above the set point). Figure 1.11 is a comparison of manually controlled and computer-controlled MAP. The automatic system provides more stable MAP values. In this manner, we use feedback to compensate for variations in unknown biological parameters.

### *Effect of Feedback on System Dynamics*

A second and equally important reason for using feedback is the ability to alter the dynamics of the device, the physiological system, or a combination of the two. The two systems shown in Fig. 1.12 illustrate this property. When we apply voltage to the motor in Fig. 1.12a, the shaft begins to turn and continues to turn ($\theta$ increases)

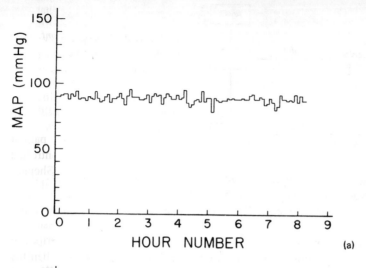

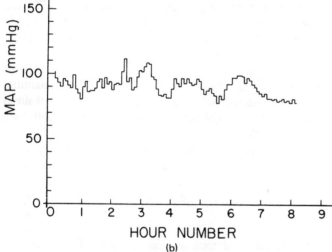

**FIGURE 1.11.** The closed loop system shown in Fig. 1.10 provides more stable control over MAP (a) than manual open loop control provides (b). (From Shepard, *IEEE Frontiers in Health Care,* 1979, with permission).

until we remove the voltage. However, when we apply voltage to the motor with feedback around it (Fig. 1.12b), the motor continues to turn until the position causes the electrical output of the position transducer to be the same as the input voltage. At this time, the motor drive voltage is zero and the motor shaft remains at this position (stationary) until we apply a different voltage.

There are several examples of the application of feedback to therapeutic devices to affect system dynamics. One of the most common applications in this area is the demand pacemaker (Chapter 2). This device monitors the atrial or ventricular electrogram and determines the rate. It compares this rate with a preset rate and energizes the pacemaker if the actual rate falls below the preset level.

We can also use feedback to affect system dynamics in hearing aid design (Chapter 6). Hearing aids include automatic gain control circuits to prevent distor-

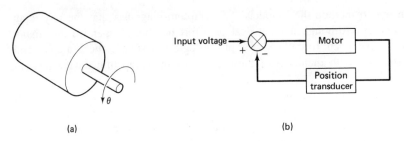

(a)                                    (b)

**FIGURE 1.12.** When we drive a motor in an open loop mode (a) the motor shaft turns until the voltage is removed. When we apply feedback (b) the shaft moves to a desired position determined by the position transducer and input voltage.

tion or overdriving. These circuits use closed-loop feedback to adjust the output to a preset value when the input exceeds a tolerable sound-pressure level. When we design these circuits, the gain must be such that there is adequate response time to avoid missing any auditory information, but the response cannot be too fast or the result is a flutter that causes severe distortion. Proper use of feedback improves system performance by compensating for changes and modifying system dynamics to respond in an optimum way to changes in input signal level.

There are several potential problems associated with the use of these feedback techniques. The first and foremost problem is that feedback intended to reduce error induced by parameter variation also tends to cause undesirable, if not unstable, system dynamics. For example, high loop gains that ensure low error due to internal parameter variations also tend to cause highly undamped system dynamics. The automatic gain control of hearing aids illustrates this point. Therefore, the design of feedback systems must represent a compromise between the two major reasons for using feedback. Fortunately, the design of feedback systems is well defined, at least within the two provisions that a sufficient model of the system to be controlled exists and that a sufficient number of signals may be measured with sufficient accuracy and signal-to-noise ratio to implement the device control. In general, the more insensitivity to parameter variation desired and the more the desired improvement in system dynamics, the more signals that must be measured to provide the control.

These factors, the need for appropriate models and sensors, and the availability of an adequate number of control sites are the major limitations to the successful design of closed-loop control in therapeutic medical devices.

### The Need for Appropriate Models of Physiological Systems

Feedback control systems are generally model-centered systems; that is, they determine the controller output by the available signals and by some mathematical model of the system to be controlled. In medical devices, we may extend the model-centered concept to include the "models" of symptom-diagnosis that the physician employs in therapy. Although a great deal of effort has been expended and many useful models have been formulated for physiological systems, there are several problems associated with inclusion of these concepts in therapeutic device realizations.

In many cases, we base mathematical modeling techniques for physiological systems on very simple, inaccurate physical analogs. We then manipulate the equations derived from these analogs to estimate unknown parameters and optimize some variable relative to a performance index. Many times, we extrapolate these results far beyond the region over which the original analog applied. Examples are the use of simple R-C circuit analogs to evaluate lung performance (Chapter 13) and the calculation of alveolar $CO_2$ based on empirical formulae. Both of these techniques have been used in the design of ventilators (Mitamura et al., 1971; Jain and Guhta, 1972). Neither approach was successful because of the simplicity of the model relative to the dynamics of the respiratory system.

A major problem associated with the use of sophisticated mathematical modeling is the difficulty of implementing the necessary controller in a reasonably-priced design. There are two ways by which we may implement automatic control schemes based on more realistic models. We can use, in hospital environments, on-line computer systems, such as the one used by Shepard et al. (1979). We may also use microcomputer-based controllers when portability and cost are major factors. Klig (1978) and Tompkins and Webster (1981) contain examples of microcomputer control of therapeutic devices.

A second problem associated with the model-centered concept is that we must choose appropriate models. As obvious as this is, its implementation may be difficult. The level of physiological sophistication associated with modeling and that associated with therapy may be vastly different. In addition, the problems of most interest to modelers may not be of prime importance to the clinician. The modeling of the respiratory control system, for example, has received much more attention than the problem of pulmonary mechanics. The latter is of prime concern to chest physicians and respiratory therapists and is the primary consideration in artificial ventilation. Even the existence of models of pulmonary mechanics would not, however, totally solve the problem. Other aspects of ventilation that we cannot infer from models of normal function include such things as the use of positive mouth pressure in artificial ventilation as opposed to the existence of negative internal pressure in normal ventilation. This situation has profound cardiovascular effects that we must also include in the controller model. The case of the kidney also illustrates the difference between therapeutic and physiological models. Areas of prime concern to therapists are pH, electrolyte balance, and removal of toxins and water (Chapter 14). Each of these areas has separate models that we must integrate in order to apply feedback to hemodialysis. Currently, the only feedback used in dialysis is in the executive loop with laboratory blood and urine tests and gross conductivity measurements for determination of electrolyte balance.

An additional problem area is that many mathematical models require signals that may be easily accessible in an experimental animal but that are totally inaccessible in a human patient. Examples include arterial $CO_2$, cardiac output, blood pressure (continuously), resistance and compliance of the alveoli, and so on. The necessity to continuously measure these variables in order to close a feedback loop is a major problem in the design of closed loop therapeutic devices.

Completely automated therapy systems also have medical and legal implications. The control algorithms cannot substitute for good judgment exhibited by a well-trained physician, therapist, or nurse. The physician is ultimately legally responsible for the well-being of the patient. We must design any automated system such that its internal control scheme can be overridden by a human operator.

## The Need for Adequate Sensors

Closed-loop control of therapeutic devices is a combination of monitoring and therapy that requires accurate, stable, noise-free transducers with adequate bandwidth to provide the necessary control signals. Many therapeutic device parameters are set based on the measurement of signals that are not easily monitored continuously. For example, we may measure blood-gas levels accurately off-line, but the design of stable, long-term implantable sensors presents much more difficult problems than the off-line measurements. We can recalibrate off-line systems with every sample and can carefully monitor them to ensure accuracy. A sensor implanted into a vein or artery must provide stable readings over a prolonged period of time. Invasive measurements such as blood gases may also cause infection problems.

The pump system developed by Blackshear (1979) provides an effective method of delivering drugs over prolonged periods of time. This system is ideal for use by diabetics who require a continuous infusion of insulin. Unfortunately, the infusion rate varies with the intake of food and physical activity. We must know the current levels of glucose in the blood in order to set the rate of infusion of insulin. We do not have any adequate glucose detectors that can be used in a control loop. This is the major limitation to a completely implantable artificial pancreas for diabetics. Blackshear has taken an intermediate step of designing a pump with two infusion rates. The patient uses one between meals and the other (a higher rate) when the need for insulin increases. The patient controls these two rates by placing a magnet over a valve located just under the skin.

Closed-loop control of therapeutic devices must wait, in general, for the development of new sensors that can accurately provide feedback signals necessary for control. We can, however, imagine complete systems such as the one in Fig. 1.13. In this system, the patient has a throat swab taken (Fig. 1.13a) and it is injected into the automatic system. The system determines what bacterium is responsible, calculates the desired dose of antibiotic, and administers the drug immediately (Fig. 1.13b). Although this totally automated type of system may be a figment of our imagination now, the availability of better sensors, smarter computer-controlled devices, and appropriate models for therapy delivery will eventually allow us to design such systems. For the present, we must be content to provide the best possible therapeutic device based on our current limited knowledge of both the physiological system and the methods of correcting abnormalities in it.

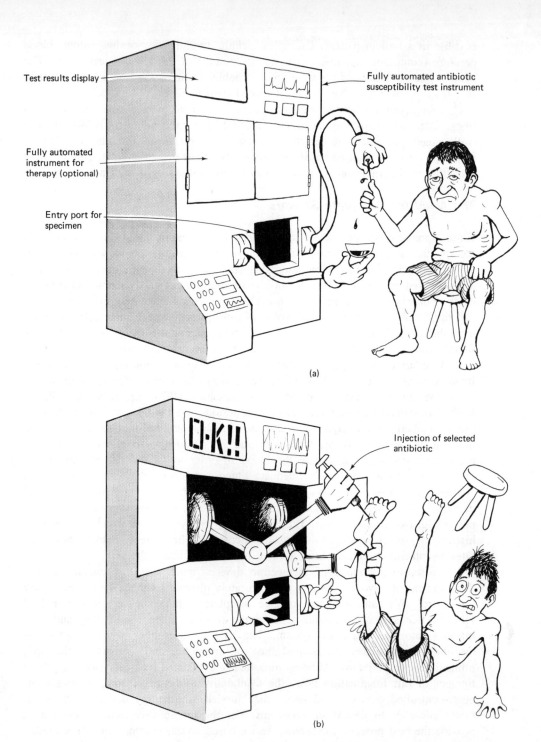

Test results display

Fully automated antibiotic susceptibility test instrument

Fully automated instrument for therapy (optional)

Entry port for specimen

(a)

O·K!!

Injection of selected antibiotic

(b)

**FIGURE 1.13.** An "ideal" fully automated antibiotic test and delivery system. (a) Acquisition of specimen (throat swab) and insertion into entry port of automated antibiotic susceptibility test instrument. (b) After results of fully automated antibiotic susceptibility test are known, the appropriate antibiotic is administered automatically. (From B. Keine, "An evaluation of different methods of measuring antibiotic susceptibilities with a view towards automation", MS Thesis, Biomed. Engr., Calif. State Univ., Sac., 1975).

## REFERENCES

BELL, S. A. (1973). Compliance compensated ventilator system, U.S. Patent #3,729,000.

BLACKSHEAR, P. J. (1979). Implantable drug-delivery systems. *Sci. Am.*, 214(6): 66–73.

COBBOLD, R. S. C. (1974). *Transducers for biomedical measurements.* New York: Wiley.

DORF, R. (1967). *Modern control systems.* Reading, MA: Addison-Wesley.

FREEMAN, J. J., D. L. STONER, J. B. SMATHERS, D. E. CLAPP, and D. D. DUNCAN (1979). Safety Program, in J. G. Webster, and A. M. Cook (eds), *Clinical engineering: Principles and practices.* Englewood Cliffs, NJ: Prentice-Hall.

GEDDES, L. A., and L. E. BAKER (1975). *Principles of applied biomedical instrumentation.* New York: Wiley.

JAIN, V. K., and S. K. GUHTA (1972). A control system for long-term ventilation of the lungs. *IEEE Trans. Bio. Med. Eng.*, BME-19: 47–52.

KLIG, V. (1978). Biomedical applications of microcomputers. *Proc. IEEE,* 66: 151–61.

MITAMURA, Y., T. MIKAMI, H. SUGAWARA, and C. YOSHIMOTO (1971). An optimally controlled respirator. *IEEE Trans. Bio. Med. Eng.*, BME-18: 330–38.

NEWMAN, M. R. (1978). Biopotential amplifiers, in J. G. Webster (ed), *Medical instrumentation: Application and design.* Boston: Houghton Mifflin.

POWERS, S. R., and D. G. GISSER (1974). Monitoring the traumatized patient, *Adv. Biomed. Eng.*, 4: 151–207.

SELKURT, E. E. (ed) (1976). *Physiology.* Boston: Little, Brown.

SHEPARD, L. C., J. F. SHOTTS, N. F. ROBERSON, F. D. WALLACE, and N. T. KOUCHOUKOUS (1979). Computer-controlled infusion of vasoactive drugs in post cardiac surgical patients. *IEEE Frontiers Eng. Health Care:* 280–84.

TIMM, G. W., and W. E. BRADLEY (1973). Technologic and biologic considerations in neuro-urologic prosthesis development. *IEEE Trans. Biomed. Eng.*, BME-20: 208–12.

TOMPKINS, W. J., and J. G. WEBSTER (eds) (1981). *Design of microcomputer-based medical instrumentation.* Englewood Cliffs, NJ: Prentice-Hall.

WEBSTER, J. G. (ed) (1978). *Medical instrumentation: Application and design.* Boston: Houghton Mifflin.

## STUDY QUESTIONS

**1.1** List the differences between diagnostic, therapeutic, and monitoring medical devices.

**1.2** Complete a table similar to Fig. 1.3 for cardiac pacemakers, intra-aortic balloon pumps, upper extremity prosthetic devices, and hemodialyzers.

**1.3**   List the major types of energy that have a therapeutic effect and give an example of a device employing each.

**1.4**   Compare the energy levels required for microwave diathermy and microwave diagnosis.

**1.5**   List two or three examples of designs that maximize the therapeutic effect of a particular energy source (other than those listed in Section 1.5).

**1.6**   Read the paper by Burton et al. [*Med. Instru.*, 11(4), 217–20, 1977] describing the development of urethral occlusive techniques. What were the design goals employed? How were they derived? Describe the three artificial sphincter designs and list the differences between them. Why are all three models available clinically?

**1.7**   List three ways in which surgical procedures affect the design of therapeutic devices. Given an example of each.

**1.8**   What are the major differences between devices intended for chronic care and those for acute care? Compare defibrillators and cardiac pacemakers.

**1.9**   What does *fail-safe design* mean? How is this employed in the design of ventilators?

**1.10**  Both anesthesia delivery systems and ventilators supply air to the patient. However, these two systems have different medical goals. Discuss these goals in terms of the status of the patient, the requirements for delivery of air (and gases such as oxygen and anesthetics), and monitoring systems used.

**1.11**  What types of monitoring of device and patient performance are utilized with external prosthetic devices?

**1.12**  Compare orthotic and prosthetic devices in terms of general design goals. Include the presence or absence of supporting anatomic parts, the control signals available, and degree of functional replacement.

**1.13**  Clark et al. (*IEEE Trans. Biomed. Eng.*, BME-20, 404–12, 1973) propose a closed-loop control system for intra-aortic balloon pumping. What control scheme did they use? Why was it chosen over other possible schemes? What were these results as compared to open-loop balloon pumping? What was the system performance index used, and how was it chosen? Draw a block diagram of the hardware required for this system. What are the limitations to using a microcomputer to implement the control algorithm?

**1.14**  Drack et al. [*Med. Instru.*, 13(2), 78–81, 1979] describe an automated cardiac resuscitator. What are the medical design goals on which this system is based? How is closed-loop control employed? What are the medical–legal problems involved in this use of closed-loop control? How successful is this system? Would you want it used on you? Why or why not?

**1.15**  A number of solid-state sensors have been described. Conduct a review of the literature and determine if any sensors are suitable for the long-term monitoring of arterial $pCO_2$. Design a hypothetical closed-loop ventilator based on the best available sensor.

# 2 Cardiac Pacing

*Paul Citron*
*Edwin G. Duffin*
*J. Fetter*
*Lester Goodman*
*Lawrence W. Shearon*

## 2.1 LEARNING OBJECTIVES

Upon completing this chapter you will be able to:

- Describe normal and abnormal cardiac electrical activity.
- Draw a block diagram of a pacemaker and describe the function of each block.
- Describe how sensing and stimulation thresholds vary with time and trade characteristics.
- Identify pacemakers by their generic letter code.
- Select the proper pacemaker for each patient pathology.
- Perform test measurements during implant and during follow-up.
- Troubleshoot pacemaker failures and recommend corrective action.

## 2.2 INTRODUCTION

The implantable artificial cardiac pacemaker replaces or supplements the physiological electrical system that normally initiates and controls cardiac contraction.

If the natural pacemaker of the heart fails to act, or if the natural conduction system of the heart does not operate properly, an external stimulus applied in the proper location of the heart and at appropriate times can restore proper function.

The design and construction of pacemaker systems is thus governed by the objective of reliably and safely applying electrical impulses to a suitable location of the heart at appropriate intervals, when—and only when—they are required.

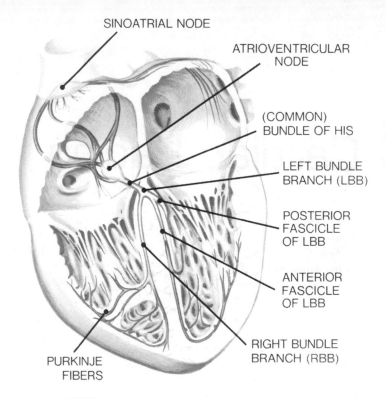

SINOATRIAL NODE

ATRIOVENTRICULAR NODE

(COMMON) BUNDLE OF HIS

LEFT BUNDLE BRANCH (LBB)

POSTERIOR FASCICLE OF LBB

ANTERIOR FASCICLE OF LBB

RIGHT BUNDLE BRANCH (RBB)

PURKINJE FIBERS

**FIGURE 2.1.** The human heart.

## 2.3 NORMAL AND ABNORMAL CARDIAC ELECTRICAL ACTIVITY

### *The Normal Heart*

Figure 2.1 shows the normal heart. The cardiac electrical system includes the following major components: sinoatrial (SA) node, internodal conduction pathways (atrial), atrioventricular (AV) node, HIS bundle, left and right bundle branches, and Purkinje fibers. Spontaneous depolarization of the cells in the sinoatrial (SA) node, the natural cardiac pacemaker, initiates electrical activity (Wellens et al., 1976). This depolarization repeats at rates between 60 and 100 beats per minute in the normal resting heart. Activity then spreads over the left and right atrial conducting pathways. This causes atrial muscle contraction and pumping of blood into the ventricular chambers. This atrial electrical activity produces a small deflection, the *P wave,* in the body-surface electrocardiogram (ECG). The atrioventricular (AV) node then conducts the electrical signal. This group of fibers provides a conduction delay, which allows completion of atrial depolarization and realization of the atrial contribution to ventricular filling before initiation of ventricular activity. After exiting the AV node, electrical activity passes via the HIS bundle and left and right bundle branches to the finely dispersed Purkinje fibers, ultimately reaching the ventricular myocardium. This produces ventricular muscle contraction and ejection of blood into the aorta and pulmonary artery. The body surface ECG displays a large deflection, the *QRS complex,* during ventricular depolarization.

In summary, the SA node sets cardiac rate while the conducting fibers and AV node interlink the cardiac chambers in a fashion that provides proper temporal sequencing for effective hemodynamic performance. Disturbances in either impulse formation or conduction can compromise cardiac performance. Utilization of an electronic cardiac pacemaker can yield an approximation to normal function.

### The Dysrhythmic Heart

Cardiac rhythm disturbances can result either from defective impulse formation or from improper conduction. Some of these abnormal rhythms, such as atrial or ventricular fibrillation, cannot be improved with available pacemakers (see Chapter 3). Those that can clearly benefit from pacemaker therapy include: sinus arrest, sinus block, symptomatic sinus bradycardia, third-degree AV block, symptomatic Mobitz Type II block, and bradytachy syndrome. In addition, some atrial and ventricular ectopic rhythms (rhythms that originate elsewhere than in the SA or AV node) and tachycardias can be managed with appropriate pacing modalities. Figure 2.2 summarizes the salient features of arrhythmias for which pacemaker implantation is clearly indicated. Bilitch (1971) summarizes cardiac arrhythmias.

## 2.4 PACEMAKER DESIGN

Cardiac pacing has evolved at an exceptional rate over the past 20 years by virtue of the collaboration of teams of engineers and physicians. This section discusses several aspects of modern pacing technology of importance to the engineer.

The cardiac pacing system consists of three basic components: (1) the pulse generator, (2) the lead/electrode, and (3) the heart itself. To understand and use cardiac pacing, we must comprehend the structure, function, and interrelationships among these components.

The pulse generator (PG) may be external or implantable. In either case, it comprises a power source and a set of electronic components that can be divided into distinct functional parts (Fig. 2.3). The oscillator produces timed electrical impulses to stimulate the atrium, the ventricle, or both. The output circuit delivers energy via the lead/electrode assembly to the heart. The amplifier accepts signals resulting from depolarization events from the heart via the lead/electrode assembly and distinguishes spontaneous atrial and ventricular depolarization from other signals such as environmental electromagnetic signals emanating from machinery and appliances.

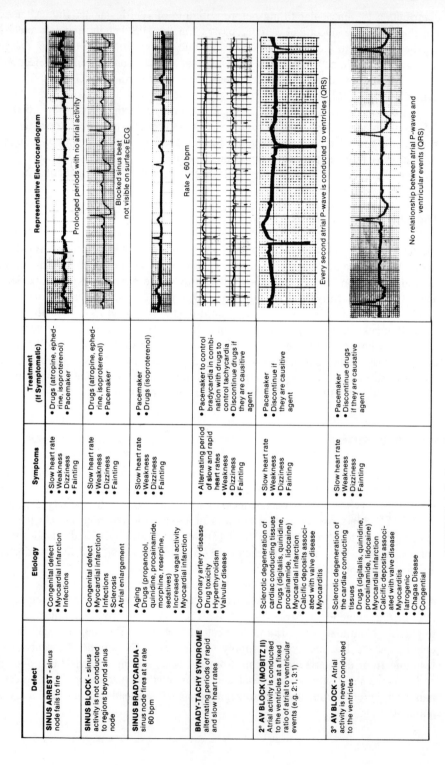

| Defect | Etiology | Symptoms | Treatment (If Symptomatic) | Representative Electrocardiogram |
|---|---|---|---|---|
| **SINUS ARREST** - sinus node fails to fire | • Congenital defect<br>• Myocardial infarction<br>• Infections | • Slow heart rate<br>• Weakness<br>• Dizziness<br>• Fainting | • Drugs (atropine, ephedrine, isoproterenol)<br>• Pacemaker | Prolonged periods with no atrial activity |
| **SINUS BLOCK** - sinus activity is not conducted to regions beyond sinus node | • Congenital defect<br>• Myocardial infarction<br>• Infections<br>• Sclerosis<br>• Atrial enlargement | • Slow heart rate<br>• Weakness<br>• Dizziness<br>• Fainting | • Drugs (atropine, ephedrine, isoproterenol)<br>• Pacemaker | Blocked sinus beat not visible on surface ECG |
| **SINUS BRADYCARDIA** - sinus node fires at a rate 60 bpm | • Aging<br>• Drugs (propanolol, quinidine, procainamide, morphine, reserpine, sedatives)<br>• Increased vagal activity<br>• Myocardial infarction | • Slow heart rate<br>• Weakness<br>• Dizziness<br>• Fainting | • Pacemaker<br>• Drugs (isoproterenol) | Rate < 60 bpm |
| **BRADY-TACHY SYNDROME** alternating periods of rapid and slow heart rates | • Coronary artery disease<br>• Drug toxicity<br>• Hyperthyroidism<br>• Valvular disease | • Alternating period of slow and rapid heart rates<br>• Weakness<br>• Dizziness<br>• Fainting | • Pacemaker to control bradycardia in combination with drugs to control tachycardia<br>• Discontinue drugs if they are causative agent | |
| **2° AV BLOCK (MOBITZ II)** Atrial activity is conducted to the ventricles at a fixed ratio of atrial to ventricular events (e.g. 2:1, 3:1) | • Sclerotic degeneration of cardiac conducting tissues<br>• Drugs (digitalis, quinidine, procainamide, lidocaine)<br>• Myocardial infarction<br>• Calcific deposits associated with valve disease<br>• Myocarditis | • Slow heart rate<br>• Weakness<br>• Dizziness<br>• Fainting | • Pacemaker<br>• Discontinue if they are causative agent | Every second atrial P-wave is conducted to ventricles (QRS) |
| **3° AV BLOCK** - Atrial activity is never conducted to the ventricles | • Sclerotic degeneration of the cardiac conducting tissues<br>• Drugs (digitalis, quinidine, procainamide, lidocaine)<br>• Myocardial infarction<br>• Calcific deposits associated with valve disease<br>• Myocarditis<br>• Iatrogenic<br>• Chagas Disease<br>• Congenital | • Slow heart rate<br>• Weakness<br>• Dizziness<br>• Fainting | • Pacemaker<br>• Discontinue drugs if they are causative agent | No relationship between atrial P-waves and ventricular events (QRS) |

**FIGURE 2.2.** Heart arrhythmias requiring the use of a pacemaker.

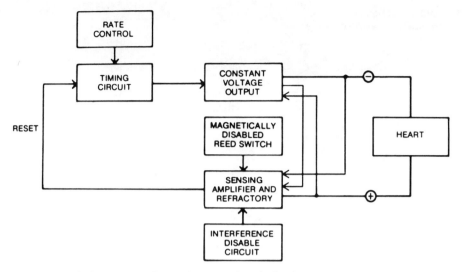

**FIGURE 2.3.** Block diagram of typical pulse generator.

The implantable pulse generator (IPG) consists of the electronic circuit and the power source, or battery, packaged together in a single container constructed of metal or polymer with a connector block to interface with the lead.

## *Oscillator*

The oscillator performs the basic timing operations and controls the rate of cardiac stimulation. Two significant time intervals are the pulse interval (PI) and pulse duration (PD) (see Fig. 2.4). The pulse interval, typically set between 750 and 1000 ms, establishes the basic pacing rate (80 to 60 pulses/min). Pulse duration is the time during which energy is delivered to the heart, typically a very small part of the pulse interval.

Typical pulse durations are 0.5 to 2.0 ms. Pulse duration and pulse amplitude, PD and A, determine the amount of energy delivered to the heart and thus primarily establish power source drain.

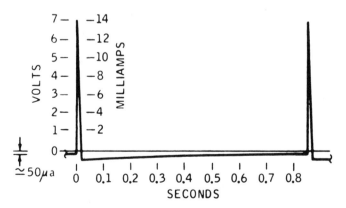

**FIGURE 2.4.** Pulse interval and pulse duration in the output of a typical pulse generator.

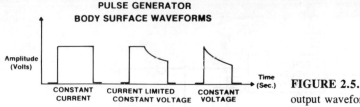

PULSE GENERATOR
BODY SURFACE WAVEFORMS

Amplitude
(Volts)

Time
(Sec.)

CONSTANT     CURRENT LIMITED     CONSTANT
CURRENT      CONSTANT VOLTAGE    VOLTAGE

**FIGURE 2.5.** Characteristic output waveforms.

## Pulse Output Circuit

The output circuit performs a dual function. It delivers energy to the electrode/heart system and isolates the timing circuits from external interference, thereby protecting the patient from untoward electrical events.

Two basic output circuits are used, capacitor charge and capacitor discharge. The capacitor charge circuit provides stimulation energy by charging a capacitor in series with the heart/electrode circuit. Because charging is done through a high resistance, this arrangement is often termed *constant current*. A capacitor discharge mode provides energy by discharging a capacitor across the heart/electrode circuit via a low resistance. Hence, we can use the term *constant voltage* here.

*Current-limited constant voltage* combines constant current and constant voltage; it operates as a constant current source with a short initial plateau followed by an exponential voltage decay. Although each of these circuits possesses particular technical features, as yet no specific electrophysiological differences, acute or chronic, have been observed. The output circuit in conjunction with the power source determines the amplitude of the output pulse. Each output circuit has a characteristic output waveform (see Fig. 2.5).

## Sensing Amplifier

The amplifier is the IPG control element. It receives electrical signals from the heart (electrogram) and discriminates between ventricular depolarization (R wave) and other components (P waves, T waves, noise, etc.). The discrimination process involves a complex interrelationship between amplitude and frequency content of the detected electrogram (see Fig. 2.6). Upon sensing cardiac depolarization ((P wave or R wave), the amplifier generates appropriate timing signals to control the sequencing of the oscillator and output circuitry.

This "sensing" characteristic conveys the test signal amplitude required to inhibit (or trigger) a pulse generator for a given pulse width. Tacitly assuming that this test signal resembles the actual R wave in terms of amplitude and spectral content, we can use it to determine which combinations of amplitude and frequency cause the amplifier to "sense."

## Power Supply

Historically, a rechargeable nickel-cadmium cell powered the first IPG. The rechargeable system, with its potential for extended longevity and reliability, had obvious appeal, but inherent disadvantages, particularly those arising from the pa-

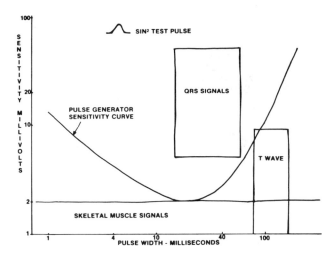

**FIGURE 2.6.** Relationship between sensitivity and pulse width.

tient's need to frequently recharge the batteries, precluded widespread adoption.

**Mercury-Zinc.** Before 1976, mercury-zinc systems were used in approximately 98% of all IPGs.

The most common mercury-zinc battery was the Mallory RM-1. The RM-1 cell is a right circular cylinder, 1.6 cm in diameter (see Fig. 2.7a). The electrodes are concentric cylinders (see Fig. 2.7b). The core is the anode, which is a pressed, powdered zinc composition amalgamated with mercury. The cathode is mercuric oxide.

The RM-1 maintains an open circuit cell voltage of 1.35 V with a capacity of 1000 mAh. At typical pacemaker current drains, the voltage of the mercury-zinc system is essentially constant (see Fig. 2.8) over its total theoretical capacity. Theoretical capacity, however, is rarely achieved. Clinical pacemaker applications use four to six batteries.

**Lithium.** Limitations of the mercury-zinc systems spurred development of alternate electrochemical power sources for pacemaker applications. Most notable are lithium anode systems with a variety of cathode materials. Lithium cells are now the most commonly used energy source in IPGs.

The lithium iodide cell, currently the most commonly used of a variety of lithium batteries, contains a lithium anode and an organic polymer cathode (polyvinyl pyridine iodide), which serves as a bonding agent for excess iodine (see Fig. 2.9).

The low self-discharge rate of lithium systems implies long shelf and operating life. Self-discharge processes depend on cell geometries and current drain.

**Nuclear.** Nuclear conversions are betavoltaic or thermoelectric. The betavoltaic process converts the energy of beta particles emitted by a radioisotope, usually promethium-147, directly into electrical energy using a silicon p-n junction. (This system is no longer in use because the half-life of promethium-147 is so short that lithium systems will last much longer.)

In the thermoelectric nuclear system, plutonium decays to produce heat, which is absorbed by the canister enclosing the cell. The source and sink are used

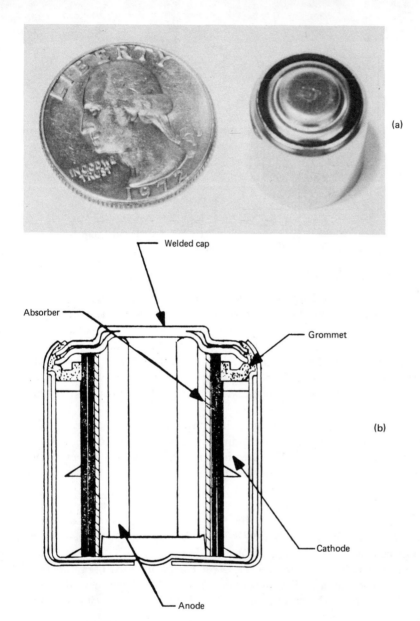

Welded cap

Absorber

Grommet

(a)

(b)

Cathode

Anode

**FIGURE 2.7.** (a) Mallory RM-1 cell; (b) Cross section of cell.

to maintain dissimilar conducting or semiconducting materials at different temperatures, thereby producing a potential gradient via the Seebeck effect. When the ends of material B are connected through a load, as shown in Fig. 2.10, current flows.

This nuclear system is theoretically capable of providing adequate electrical energy to power an IPG for 10 to 20 years. Present experience with implanted radioisotopic IPGs now extends through nine years.

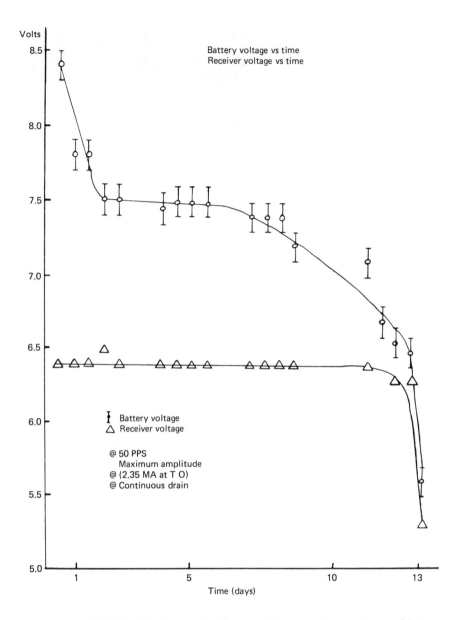

**FIGURE 2.8.** Illustrative diagram of the typical dependence of battery voltage on time compared with that of a device (receiver) powered by the same battery.

Plutonium nuclear power sources have the longest proven reliability to date. Cost, the perceived risk of radiation, and regulatory considerations, however, have precluded widescale application.

**Alternate Power Sources.** Biologic, thermoelectric, piezoelectric, and photoelectric sources have been considered, but none have merited clinical application

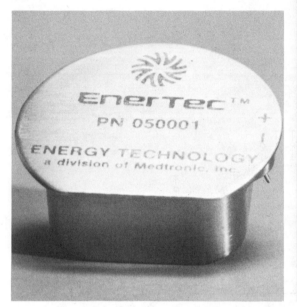

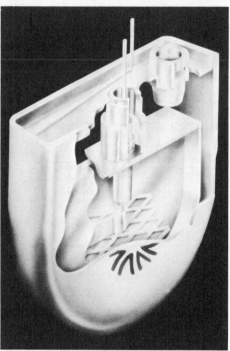

**FIGURE 2.9.** (a) Lithium iodide cell. Note contouring of outside envelope to fit interior of pulse generator; (b) cutaway view of a lithium iodide cell.

because of limited energy capacity. New systems may, however, be developed in the course of time and be adopted.

**Battery Capacity Ratings.** The difficulty of relating the operating time of a pacemaker to the capacity of its battery is due in part to the different methods utilized to establish capacity ratings for the power source. An understanding of the differences between the estimated capacity of a battery and that which will actually be realized requires consideration of polarization (a rate-dependent process) and self-discharge (a time-dependent process). These phenomena in turn are specific to the chemistries involved as well as the battery design. Capacities may be categorized as one of the following three types: (1) *theoretical capacity* (based upon a physical model, i.e., stoichiometric), (2) *experimental capacity* (based upon accelerated discharge tests, i.e., rated capacity), and (3) *formal capacity* (based upon a combination of experimental data and a mathematical model). Some of these will be described in an effort to demonstrate the difficulty of accurately projecting longevities.

Figure 2.11 shows these capacity ratings for a typical lithium battery. Of particular importance is the dependence of capacity on the application's current drain. It is clear that optimal capacity requires matching the electrical design of the pacemaker with the characteristics of the battery.

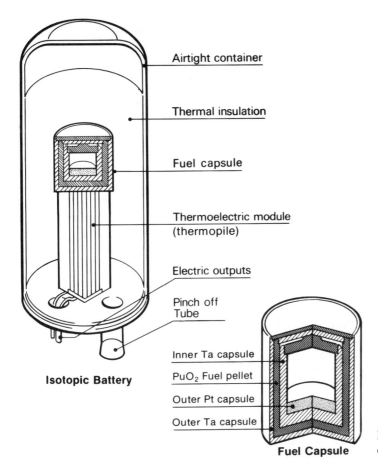

Airtight container

Thermal insulation

Fuel capsule

Thermoelectric module
(thermopile)

Electric outputs

Pinch off
Tube

**Isotopic Battery**

Inner Ta capsule

$PuO_2$ Fuel pellet

Outer Pt capsule

Outer Ta capsule

**Fuel Capsule**

**FIGURE 2.10.** Typical nuclear cell. See text.

## *Lead System*

The pacemaker lead system comprises two distinct components: the body (conductor and insulator) and the electrode. Also, some type of mechanism for affixing the electrode to the heart may be part of the lead body or part of the electrode. Lead system performance is measured by two parameters: pacing threshold and sensing threshold. The pacing (stimulation) threshold indicates efficiency of energy transfer from the pacing system to the heart. The sensing threshold measures the sensitivity of the pacing system to signals transferred via the lead system to the IPG.

**Construction.** Lead systems may be transvenous or myocardial. Modern transvenous leads incorporate a multifilar conductor wound as a coil molded within a silicone or polyurethane sheath (see Fig. 2.12). The coil lumen permits the introduction of stylets or guide wires, which facilitate the insertion of the lead into the proper heart chambers via selected venous routes, for example, cephalics, internal or external jugular, femoral, and so on (Smyth et al. 1976; Kleinert et al., 1977).

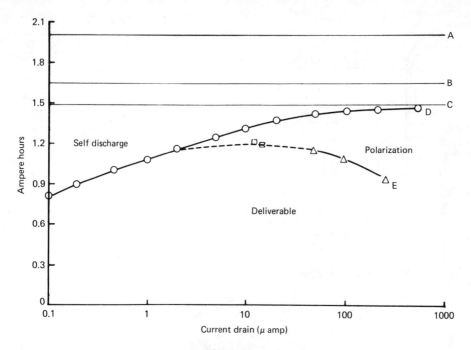

**FIGURE 2.11.** Battery capacity vs. discharge rate.

      A = Stoichiometric capacity.

      B = Capacity corrected for charge transfer complex loss.

      C = Maximum available capacity.

      D = Capacity corrected for self-discharge loss.

      E = Capacity corrected for polarization losses. The deliverable capacity is the curve defined by D at the low rates and E at the higher rates.

         Myocardial leads attached to the outside heart muscle are similar except that the conductor may be comprised of multiple ribbons of wire wound into a configuration known as *tinsel wire* (see Fig. 2.13). Recent improvements in coil construction have virtually eliminated the flexural superiority of tinsel wire; therefore, several manufacturers utilize multifilar coils for both transvenous and myocardial leads.

         Most conductor coil materials used today are forms of platinum, platinum-iridium, or nickel alloys, for example, Eligiloy and MP35N. Tinsel wire is usually made from platinum-iridium ribbons. These represent a compromise between electrical conduction, mechanical flexural, and corrosion properties. Materials presently under development should improve both electrical and mechanical performance.

         Insulator materials used in permanently implanted leads have, until recently, been restricted to biocompatible forms of silicone rubber. These have performed well over time, although recently introduced polyurethane insulators have offered significant improvements in terms of size reduction and mechanical performance.

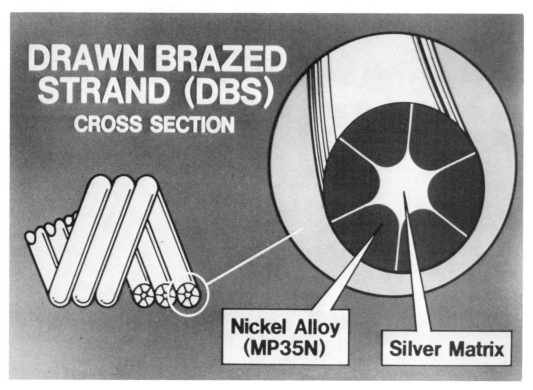

FIGURE 2.12. Construction of a multifilar conductor lead.

**Attachment.** All leads require that the electrode portions be attached or in close proximity to the myocardium. In early days, leads were sutured directly to the myocardium (see Fig. 2.14). Modern leads do not require suturing (see Fig. 2.15) because other methods such as screws or helices have been devised.

Transvenous leads, considered to be less traumatic to implant than myocardial

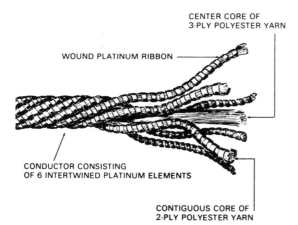

CENTER CORE OF
3-PLY POLYESTER YARN

WOUND PLATINUM RIBBON

CONDUCTOR CONSISTING
OF 6 INTERTWINED PLATINUM ELEMENTS

CONTIGUOUS CORE OF
2-PLY POLYESTER YARN

FIGURE 2.13. Construction of a "tinsel" conductor lead.

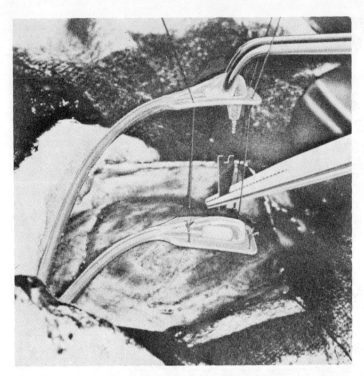

**FIGURE 2.14.** Method of affixing electrodes on the heart's surface.

leads, have historically exhibited instability, particularly soon after insertion. The most disturbing problem with transvenous leads has been dislodgement. Flanges located near the distal end of the lead have been developed, which enhance fibrosis and myocardial tissue engagement, thereby yielding improved stability (see Fig. 2.16). Recent lead configurations using tines (Fig. 2.17) have substantially reduced the incidence of lead-related regenerations from over 20% to less than 5%.

### Electrodes

The electrode is the interface between the pacemaker and the heart. Electrode design has been largely empirical. However, objective criteria do exist. First, because current drain is directly related to surface area of the electrode, small-tip (less than 15 mm² area) electrodes are preferred. Second, because current density in proximity to viable tissue is a primary determinant of myocardial stimulation, electrodes should exhibit concentrated, uniformly-distributed current density. This requirement also favors small-tip electrodes.

Both requirements are offset, however, by the high source impedance of small surface area electrodes. High source impedances result in reduced R-wave or P-

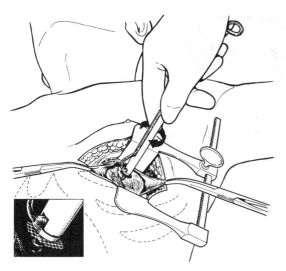

**FIGURE 2.15.** Method of affixing a screw-in electrode on the heart's surface.

wave amplitude transmission to the sense amplifier(s). Numerous electrode designs that strike a balance between these constraints (see Fig. 2.18) are available.

Figure 2.19 shows that generator and leads may be unipolar or bipolar. *Unipolar* implies one electrode in the heart, which is usually the cathode, and a second electrode away from the heart, the indifferent electrode, which is usually the anode and usually formed by the metal housing of the pacemaker. *Bipolar* implies that both electrodes are in the heart, or on the surface of the heart with a typical interelectrode spacing of 15–30 mm.

**Stimulation and Sensing Thresholds.** The performance of a lead system is given by two measures: the pacing (stimulation) threshold and the sensing threshold.

*Pacing threshold* is defined as the minimum amount of energy required to stimulate the heart under prescribed conditions. Thresholds depend upon several factors, as summarized in Fig. 2.20.

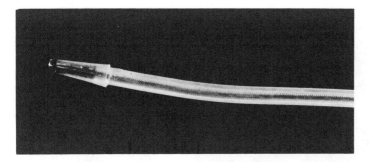

**FIGURE 2.16.** Typical flanged transvenous lead. Note flange.

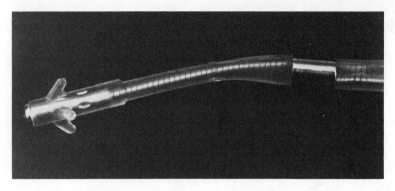

**FIGURE 2.17.** Typical tined transvenous lead. Note tines.

Figure 2.21 shows voltage thresholds as a function of pulse width, which demonstrates the characteristic strength-duration relationship typical of cardiac muscle. Thresholds can be measured in terms of current, charge, and energy. Typical IPG output pulses fall near the "knee" portion of this characteristic. This is deliberate in order to maintain stimulation when battery voltage drops by providing automatic pulse-width widening.

Alternatively, we might determine stimulation thresholds as functions of time and electrode surface area. The characteristic threshold rises and peaks in approximately a two- to four-week period and then stabilizes at a steady value. This chronic level is about two to three times the acute value for large-tip electrodes (but four to five times the acute value for small-tip electrodes). These factors can, however, be misleading because small-tip electrodes may exhibit substantially lower acute thresholds than large-tip electrodes. They thereby maintain a lower level chronically.

The second performance measure, the *sensing threshold,* is defined as the minimum amount of cardiac electrical energy required to inhibit a demand pacemaker or trigger a synchronous pacemaker. It, too, is a complex function of several variables. Figure 2.22 lists various factors that affect sensing threshold.

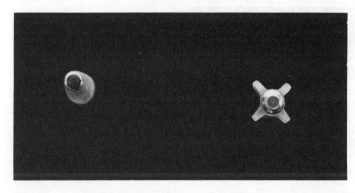

**FIGURE 2.18.** Electrode design for optimal stimulating and sensing.

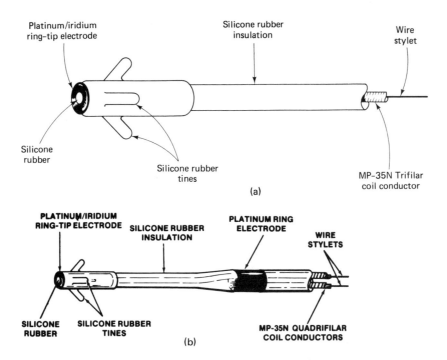

**FIGURE 2.19.** (a) Unipolar lead; (b) Bipolar lead.

Because the environment is electrically noisy, and IPGs are intended to detect cardiac signals as low as 750 $\mu$V, shielding and selective filtering are utilized in most modern pacemakers to assure immunity from common sources of electromagnetic interference. Continuous wave interference above 40 Hz, resulting from current leakage from 50- to 60-Hz line-powered instruments, can cause the pulse generator to revert to fixed-rate pacing. If such interference is modulated or pulsed, mimicking the R wave, it can suppress the output of a demand pulse generator.

## FACTORS AFFECTING STIMULATION THRESHOLDS

- Electrode
  - Material
  - Surface Area
  - Geometry
  - Position—Relative to Stimulatable Tissue
- Lead Insulator Material
  - Thrombogenic Properties
  - Mechanical Characteristics
- Lead Conductor
  - Material—Mechanical Characteristics
  - Geometrical Configuration
- Lead Maturity
- Anodal vs. Cathodal Stimulation
- Pulse Amplitude/Duration
- Drug/Electrolyte Balance

**FIGURE 2.20.**

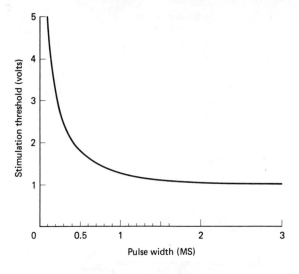

**FIGURE 2.21.** Stimulation threshold voltage vs. pulse width.

Turning off the source or moving away from it should return the pulse generator to normal operation.

Electrosurgical units used on patients with implanted pulse generators may cause ventricular fibrillation if current from the electrosurgical unit is carried by the lead system into the heart (see Chapter 10). Some pacemakers might stop pacing at low to medium levels of electrosurgical current. At higher settings of pulsed electrosurgical current, some pacemakers may produce output stimuli at the electrosurgical current pulse rate. Unipolar pacemakers are more susceptible than bipolar to the electrosurgical current due to the wider effective gap between electrodes; however, some bipolar devices may also be affected under certain conditions. Categorical statements about effects of electrosurgery cannot be made because various models of pacemakers react differently due to variations in electrical design.

When using electrosurgical equipment, it is suggested that:

## FACTORS AFFECTING
## SENSING THRESHOLDS

- Electrode/Tissue Interface Impedance
  - Electrode
    - Material
    - Surface Area
    - Geometry
    - Position—Relative to Stimulatable Tissue

  - Lead Insulator Material
    - Thrombogenic Properties
    - Mechanical Characteristics

- Acute to Chronic Shift in R-Wave Morphology

- Disease

- Pharmacologic Factors

- Electromagnetic Interference—EMI

**FIGURE 2.22.**

1. Electrosurgical units always be used intermittently with bursts no longer than two or three seconds.

2. The return electrode of the electrosurgical unit must be placed near the active electrode. Electrosurgical current return via a path that closely parallels the pacing system leads must be avoided.

Exposure to diagnostic x-ray and fluoroscopic radiation generally does not affect most pacemakers.

Defibrillator discharges of 400 J may damage the pacemaker; paddles should be placed as far from the pulse generator as possible. Further, it is recommended that pacemaker function be verified following each defibrillation episode and that patients be closely observed for at least 24 hours following defibrillation. Defibrillator currents may conduct preferentially along the implanted leads, resulting in high-current densities at the tissue-electrode interface with consequent searing or scarring of tissue, resulting in increased thresholds and possible loss of capture.

Many modern pacemakers are not affected by microwave ovens or diathermy. However, therapeutic diathermy should not be used directly over a pacemaker because internal components may be damaged by heating.

Questions regarding electrical interference should be addressed first by reference to the manufacturer's technical manual.

### Semiconductor Technologies

Early IPGs were constructed with discrete resistors, capacitors, and transistors. The emergence of thick- and thin-film technologies, as well as microprocessor methods, has revolutionized pacemaker design.

Continuing efforts to reduce size, weight, and power consumption have been facilitated by monolithic integrated circuit technologies. These include TTL (transistor-transistor-logic), I²L (integrated injection logic), CMOS (complementary metal oxide semiconductor), MOS (metal oxide semiconductor), and MOSFET (metal oxide semiconductor field effect transistor) technologies.

Application of these new technologies has permitted a reduction in both mass and size, while increasing functionality from the large (200-g) asynchronous pacemakers available in the early 1960s to small (40-g) multimodal units now available (Fig. 2.23).

**Programmability.** Rate and output-adjustable pacemakers have been available since the late 1960s. Primitive "programmable" systems required the passage of a needle (Keith Needle) through the skin and into a potentiometer for adjustments.

Subsequent developments enabled noninvasive adjustment of rate, pulse width, and pulse amplitude. Rotating or pulsed magnetic fields can effect such noninvasive adjustments.

Modern programmable systems employ combinations of constant or pulsed magnetic fields and/or pulsed RF (radio frequency) coded signals to implement noninvasive programming. Parameters such as sensitivity, mode (unipolar or bipolar), polarity, refractory period, as well as rate, amplitude, and duration, can be

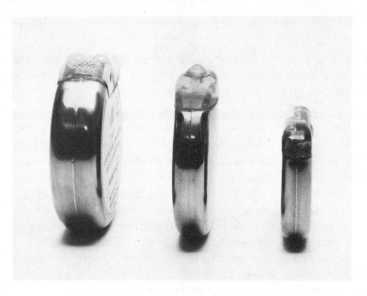

**FIGURE 2.23.** Size decrease of typical pulse generators in the course of approximately ten years. Note that, as the size decreases, the versatility increases.

adjusted. Programming of escape intervals in combination with specific rates is available for the most sophisticated dual chamber systems.

**Physiological Pacing.** Several innovative pacing systems, requiring both atrial and ventricular lead systems, have been developed and others proposed. Common to these is an effort to provide atrioventricular synchrony and physiological control of rate. We can obtain a flavor for these forms through a brief explanation of the available pacemaker types and those currently in clinical evaluation.

## 2.5 TYPES OF PACEMAKERS AND THEIR APPLICATION

### Pacemaker Identification Codes

The identification of pacing systems can be simplified by using the generic code suggested by Parsonnet et al. (1974). The code is a sequence of three characters that conveys the features of the pacemaker. The first character identifies the *chamber paced*—A for atrium, V for ventricle, D for dual-chamber pacing. The second character identifies the *chamber sensed*—A for atrium, V for ventricle, D for dual-chamber sensing. The third character denotes the *mode of response*, if applicable—I for inhibited or blocked output in response to a sensed signal, T for triggered or synchronized output. O is used where the identification character is not pertinent. VOO, for example, designates a ventricular stimulating device that does not sense intrinsic activity and thus does not modify its output in response to spontaneous events. VAT describes a ventricular stimulating pacemaker whose output is triggered by sensed atrial signals. It should be noted, however, that this code is undergoing revision to accommodate newer pacemaker types.

## Asynchronous Pacemakers

**Function.** The basic pacemaker system is asynchronous with respect to the ECG. It consists of a pulse-forming network (oscillator) and a lead system for connection to the heart. The purpose is to provide a fixed-rate train of stimuli to the atria (AOO) or ventricles (VOO) irrespective of and unresponsive to intrinsic cardiac activity. Because the output from VOO and AOO devices is so regular, these are often incorrectly referred to as fixed-rate pacemakers.

Radio-frequency-coupled asynchronous pacing systems deserve mention. These consist of a small, implanted, passive receiver/decoder to which heart leads are connected and an external battery-powered transmitter used to power and program the receiver. Systems of this type received much early attention because the implanted portion was much smaller than the self-powered devices of that period (Stephenson et al., 1959; Camilli et al., 1962). RF-coupled pacers offered increased reliability and the patient had less exposure to surgery. Although RF pacemakers are no longer used for maintenance of heart rate, interest in these devices continues for the management, with rapid pacing, of certain episodic refractory tachycardias (Kahn et al., 1970).

**Clinical Application.** Clinical use of AOO devices is rare. They can be useful for patients concurrently demonstrating (1) stable sinus bradycardia or absolute pacemaker dependence, (2) a normal HIS-Purkinje system, and (3) improved hemodynamics with temporary atrial pacing. Atrial pacing is contraindicated in cases of atrial paralysis.

VOO pacemakers may be indicated in cases of complete AV block, given no intrinsic competitive rhythms and total pacemaker dependence. Those patients with complete antegrade *and* retrograde AV block and sinoatrial node dysfunction that is manifest as sinus bradycardia, sinoatrial block, or atrial fibrillation may also be candidates for VOO pacing. Retrograde AV atrial activation, upon ventricular stimulation, may cause inappropriate contraction sequences and pronounced hypotension. Patients considered for VOO pacing include those who would benefit little from cardiac output enhancement because of general infirmity. Less than 5% of patients are estimated to be candidates for VOO pacemakers.

## Demand Pacemakers

**Function.** Many patients demonstrate periods of spontaneous cardiac activity during which artificial pacing may be inappropriate. Lacking the means to sense intrinsic cardiac activity, asynchronous pacemakers may compete with spontaneous rhythms. Competitive pacing may produce symptomatic hypotension (low blood pressure), ventricular tachycardia, or ventricular fibrillation (Furman, 1973). With a properly designed electrogram-sensing element (amplifier) as described in Section

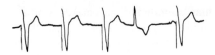

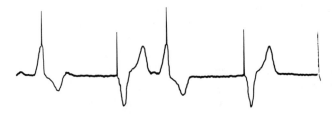

**FIGURE 2.24.** Typical electrograms with: (a) inhibited demand pacemaker, and, (b) triggered demand pacemaker.

2.4, the pacemaker can be made responsive to intrinsic activity. The demand pacemaker produces stimuli at a preset fixed rate (nominally 1,000–800 ms interstimulus or escape interval). Electrograms detected by the amplifier modify the basic escape interval of the oscillator in one of two ways. In the case of *inhibited* demand devices, electrograms occurring within the interstimulus interval reset the oscillator so that the next pacemaker stimulus occurs at the preset escape interval following intrinsic activity (Fig. 2.24a). No stimuli are produced when the intrinsic rate is greater than the preset rate of the pacemaker. When spontaneous activity is faster than the pacemaker escape interval in *triggered* demand pacemakers, an output stimulus occurs during the absolute refractory period of the tissue (i.e., that period when tissue is unresponsive to electrical stimulation) (Fig. 2.24b). Demand pacemakers of the triggered or inhibited types may be applied to either the atria (AAT, AAI) or to the ventricles (VVT, VVI).

    **Clinical Application.** AAI and AAT Pacemakers are often indicated in sick sinus syndrome with no attendant HIS-Purkinje disease where cardiac output is improved by atrial contribution (Benchimol et al., 1965; Samet et al., 1966; Befeler et al., 1971).

    Ventricular demand pacemakers may be indicated in complete AV block when periods of normal conduction or spontaneous ventricular rhythms may exist and when the hemodynamic benefit of atrial systole is judged unnecessary (Paeprer et al., 1977). Demand systems, in particular the VVI, are indicated for patients with atrial fibrillation who manifest faster rhythm than that of the pacemaker in response to stress or exercise.

## *Atrial Synchronous Pacemakers*

    **Function.** Atrioventricular dissociation can occur during periods of stimulation using asynchronous or demand ventricular devices (VOO, VVT, VVI). In the majority of patients demonstrating normal sinus node function treated with ven-

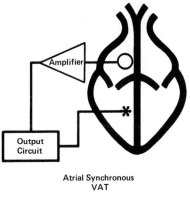

Atrial Synchronous
VAT

* = Stimulation
o = Sensing        **FIGURE 2.25.**

tricularly programmed pacemakers, the cardiac output decrement due to AV dissociation may not be obvious. However, the ability to augment ventricular stroke volume in response to physical activity may be markedly improved by synchronizing ventricular stimulation to atrial systole, thereby taking advantage of the atrial contribution to cardiac output (Nathan et al., 1963; Samet et al., 1966; Karlof, 1975). The atrial (P-wave) synchronous pacemaker (VAT) consists of an atrial-sensing amplifier and a ventricular-stimulating oscillator connected to the heart as shown in Fig. 2.25. Every time the pacemaker detects an atrial electrogram, it triggers the ventricular oscillator. This produces a stimulus after an interval that mimics the normal atrioventricular delay interval (Fig. 2.26). Sensed atrial electrograms may be absent because of atrial lead displacement during atrial fibrillation or sinus arrest. The atrial synchronous pacemaker then operates as an asynchronous ventricular pacemaker (VOO) at a preset basic rate.

Figure 2.27 shows another version of the atrial synchronous device, the atrial synchronous ventricular inhibited pacemaker. In addition to the functional elements of the VAT pacemaker, this device has a second sensing amplifier intended to sense intrinsic ventricular activity and inhibit the ventricular oscillator when necessary. In the absence of sensed atrial electrograms, this device functions as an inhibited ventricular demand pacemaker (VVI). During periods of normal sinus rhythm, without normal ventricular response, this device behaves as a VAT pacemaker.

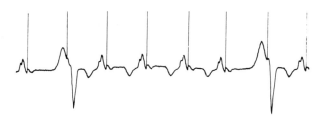

**FIGURE 2.26.** Typical electrogram with a VAT pacemaker.

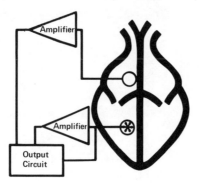

Atrial Synchronous Ventricular Inhibited

$$VD\frac{T}{I}$$

\* = Stimulation
○ = Sensing

**FIGURE 2.27.**

When normally conducted ventricular complexes or ventricular ectopic activity occurs, the device's oscillator is inhibited for that cycle in a manner similar to a VVI device, as shown in Fig. 2.28.

The application of atrial pacemakers has been expanding as their therapeutic benefits have emerged. The contribution of the atrial contraction to cardiac output is reported in the range of 10–30%. P-wave-synchronous pacing helps achieve a physiologically governed rate variability.

VAT P-wave-synchronous pacemakers (Fig. 2.25) do, however, present certain problems. They do not monitor ventricular activity and might be triggered by an ectopic focus in the ventricle. They also function as asynchronous pacemakers if atrial sensing is lost and present the small but real danger of pacing into the T wave, which in certain circumstances may produce ventricular tachycardia or fibrillation. The system shown in Fig. 2.27 obviates these problems.

**Clinical Application.**   Atrial synchronous pacemakers are indicated in complete or intermittent heart block with normal sinus node function where the hemo-dynamic benefit of the properly timed atrial systole is helpful (Karlof, 1975). These patients may exhibit AV block, which frequently develops upon exercise. Atrial synchronous devices are contraindicated in sick sinus syndrome or atrial fibrillation.

### *AV Sequential Pacemaker.*

The AV sequential pacemaker utilizes two bipolar pacing leads, one atrial and one ventricular. Sensing occurs only through the ventricular lead; intrinsic atrial activity without AV conduction has no effect on IPG function.

An AV sequential pacemaker consists of two separate oscillator/output circuits sharing a common power source. Both oscillators, atrial and ventricular, are simul-taneously reset by an R wave sensed via the ventricular pacing lead or are reset by

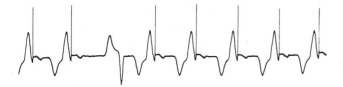

**FIGURE 2.28.** Typical electrogram with a VDT/I pacemaker.

output pulses from the ventricular oscillator. Thus, escape intervals for both oscillators are measured from the same sensed R wave or ventricular output pulse.

Figure 2.29 shows operations of a currently available programmable AV sequential pulse generator.

1. When the patient's spontaneous R-to-R interval is shorter than the pulse generator atrial escape interval, both atrial and ventricular oscillators are reset by the sensed ventricular depolarization, and the unit produces no output pulses (inhibited mode).

2. When the R-to-R interval exceeds the pulse generator atrial escape interval, an atrial output is emitted. If the patient's P-R interval is shorter than the pulse generator AV sequential (delay) interval, the conducted R wave resets the ventricular oscillator before its escape interval elapses (atrial pacing only mode).

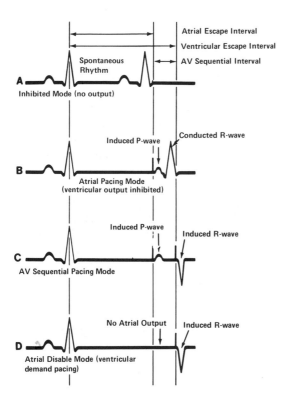

**FIGURE 2.29.** See text. Programmable AV sequential pacemaker.

3. After an atrial output pulse, if the patient's P-R interval exceeds the pulse generator AV sequential interval (i.e., the ventricular oscillator escape interval elapses), a ventricular output pulse is emitted (AV sequential pacing mode).

4. The AV sequential pulse generator can be programmed to a mode of operation in which the ventricular oscillator escape interval is set for 70 ppm pacing and the atrial output is disabled. In this mode, the pulse generator functions as a ventricular pacing, ventricular-inhibited pulse generator (atrial disable mode).

The AV sequential pacemaker allows noninvasive programming of the atrial/ventricular escape interval to any of several preestablished combinations, including the atrial disable mode.

In this device, the combination of both transmitted radio-frequency code pulses and the presence of a magnetic field are required for programming to occur.

**Clinical Application.**  DVI pacemakers are indicated in sick sinus syndrome with accompanying His-Purkinje disease or in AV block with accompanying evidence of abnormal sinus node function when hemodynamic benefit from correctly placed atrial systole is demonstrated (Fields et al., 1973).

## Fully Automatic Pacemaker Systems

**Function.**  Advances in technology have permitted the development of highly sophisticated pacemaker systems that combine features and operational modalities previously only available in separate devices. This becomes relevant because, over the course of a patient's disease process, the conduction disorder for which a particular type of pacemaker was originally implanted may change significantly.

The so-called fully automatic pacemaker combines the operational features of the atrial demand (AAI), AV sequential (DVI), and atrial synchronous ventricular inhibited devices. This advanced device automatically adjusts its output stimulus pattern to maintain a 1:1 atrioventricular contraction sequence (Rogel and Mahler, 1971).

In the event of: (1) a slow atrial rhythm with normal ventricular conduction, this device stimulates the atrium only; (2) a slow atrial rhythm with prolonged ventricular conduction, this device stimulates the atria and ventricles sequentially separated by a time delay mimicking the AV delay; (3) an atrial contraction falling within the normal rate range (e.g., 60–140 bpm), the pacemaker stimulates the ventricles in response to each atrial contraction; and (4) normal atrial rate and normal ventricular conduction, the pacemaker is fully inhibited. Figure 2.30 summarizes these features.

Extensions of cardiac pacing into the control of ventricular and supraventricular tachyarrhythmias are now being investigated. Such applications will, without doubt, soon become an integral part of cardiac pacing technology and valuable additions to the armamentarium with which physician and engineer, together, attack refractory problems of cardiac dysfunction.

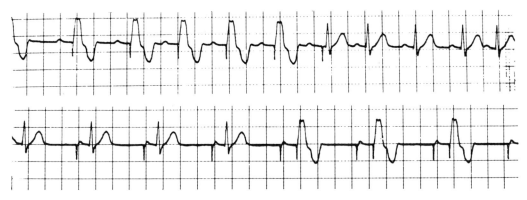

**(Continuous ECG Strip)**

FIGURE 2.30. See text. "Fully automatic" pacemaker.

## 2.6 PACEMAKER ASSESSMENT: IMPLANT, FOLLOW-UP PROCEDURES, TROUBLESHOOTING

### *Implant*

The engineer may participate in a pacemaker implant procedure in the catheterization laboratory or operating room. He is an active member of the clinical team.

To achieve a successful pacemaker implant, specific evaluating procedures must be performed. These include confirmation of proper pacemaker performance before implantation, electrical evaluation of electrode placement during the implantation procedure, and confirmation of total system performance prior to discharging the patient from the operating room.

**Testing the Pacemaker.** The pacemaker should be tested prior to implantation to assure proper device operation and performance. The following instruments are used to evaluate pacemaker performance.

> *Pacing System Analyzer.* This multipurpose device is an instrument for measuring stimulation thresholds, intracardiac signals, and evaluation of pacemaker system operation. The typical analyzer is used to evaluate the pulse generator parameters listed in Fig. 2.31.
>
> *Pacemaker Programmer.* The programmer is used to confirm proper operation of the programmable pacemaker through its range of parameters.

**Testing Lead (Catheter) Placement.** After the pacemaker lead (the catheter) has been placed, tests should be performed to assure proper electrode contact with viable heart tissue.

The measurements outlined in Fig. 2.31 include the stimulation threshold and the amplitude of the intracardiac electrogram obtained from a pacing systems analyzer or similar device. (An external pacemaker may be used to obtain these

| Pacemaker parameter* | Measurement units | Typical values |
|---|---|---|
| Pulse amplitude | Peak voltage (V) or current (mA) delivered across a known load. | 5 V or 10 mA across 500 Ω. |
| Pulse interval | Interval between pacing stimuli or equivalent rate (ms or pulses per minute). | 857 ms (70 ppm) |
| Pulse width | Duration of the stimulus artifact (ms). | 0.5 ms |
| Sensing amplifier | Signal value required to inhibit or trigger the pulse generator circuit of a demand pacemaker. | 2 mV |

*Other parameters such as hysteresis, refractory period, and pacing mode can also be tested to determine device integrity.

**FIGURE 2.31.** Pacemaker parameters.

measurements, although the results may not be directly related to implantable pacemaker performance due to limitations of parameter adjustment.) Typical values are shown in Fig. 2.32.

The following conventional electronic test equipment can also be used for these measurements but is much less convenient, particularly because of the need for electrical isolation:

- *Oscilloscope (battery-operated with storage preferred).* Used to display the intracardiac atrial or ventricular electrogram.

- *Oscilloscope Camera.* Attached directly to the oscilloscope front panel to obtain permanent records.

- *Isolation Amplifier.* To provide patient isolation where required.

- *Electrocardiogram (ECG) Recorder.* Used to obtain permanent recordings of the intracardiac electrograms. Most ECG recorders will inscribe a signal reduced in amplitude by 20–50% from that seen on an oscilloscope because of the recorder's limited high-frequency response.

| Parameter | Measurement (units) | Typical values |
|---|---|---|
| Threshold | Minimum voltage (V) and current (mA) required to consistently produce cardiac depolarizations. (Lead resistance can be calculated using voltage and current threshold values.) | 0.6 V, 1.2 mA |
| Intracardiac electrogram* | Atrial or ventricular electrogram amplitude (mV), and slew rate (V/s). | 12 mV (ventricular) 4 mV (atrial) 0.5 to 2.0 V/s. |

*Intracardiac electrogram ST elevation has sometimes been used as an indicator of adequate lead/tissue contact. This ST elevation is produced by cardiac injury currents, caused by the lead tip impacting viable heart tissue. However, newer more flexible leads cause less irritation yielding smaller or nonexistent elevation thereby eliminating the value of monitoring ST signal change to evaluate lead placement.

**FIGURE 2.32.** Typical values of threshold and electrogram.

| Test | Verifies | Equipment |
|---|---|---|
| Electrocardiogram | — System sensing and capture.<br>— Power source status (via rate of stimulation)<br>— Pacing mode relative to patient's current ECG status. | ECG machine and (1) magnet (converts most IPGs to asynchronous mode), (2) carotid sinus massage (slows patient's heart rate). |
| Rate/Pulse width monitoring | — Power source status<br>— Programmed settings | Pacemaker monitor or frequency counter and (1) magnet, (2) carotid sinus massage. |
| Chest wall stimulation | — Status of sense amplifier in pulse generator (normal demand generator will be inhibited, triggered generators will track external signals).<br>— Underlying patient rhythm (by inhibiting pacemaker output). | ECG machine and external pacemaker. |
| Waveform analysis | — Stimulus artifact amplitude and duration to detect power source depletion.<br>— Output waveform to detect lead or IPG defect. | Oscilloscope and magnet. |
| Telephone transmission of pacemaker signals and ECG | Remote evaluation of items listed in Figure 2.2 | Telephone pacemaker monitor and transmitter. |

**FIGURE 2.33.** Test equipment used for evaluating pacemakers.

**System Validation.** When the lead has been connected to the pacemaker, system tests should be conducted to assure proper pacemaker operation. These tests should be performed before the pacemaker pocket is surgically closed.

The test instruments used to evaluate the integrity of the pacemaker and lead follow:

- *Pacemaker Programmer.* Used to program the pacemaker to those parameters that are physiologically most beneficial to the patient and to confirm that the system responds to programming.

- *Electrocardiogram Recorder.* Used to confirm appropriate periods of pacing, sensing, and capture.

- *Test Magnet.* It may be necessary to apply a permanent magnet over the pulse generator if the patient's intrinsic rhythm is inhibiting the pacemaker. (Typical implanted pacemakers operate in an asynchronous or other defined test mode when a magnet of sufficient field strength is placed over the device.)

## Follow-Up

Verification of proper pacemaker system operation should be performed periodically. This routine follow-up can be accomplished in the physician's office, a pacemaker clinic, or by telephone transmission of appropriate pacemaker data. These checkups are designed to detect improper sensing or pacing, early power source depletion, and effectiveness of the pacing modality and parameters. The test equipment and its application in evaluating the integrity of the pacemaker system is given in Fig. 2.33.

| Pulse generator: | Model, manufacturer, characteristics, and specifications, implant data |
| Lead: | (Same) |
| Patient: | ECGs, X rays of pacing system, pacing system measurements at implant, records of prior evaluations, electrolyte levels, and drug regimens. |

**FIGURE 2.34.** Component parts of the pacemaker/patient system.

Most modern pacemakers are designed to signal power source depletion by changes in rate and pulse duration. Typically, rate will remain relatively constant throughout the effective pacemaker service life and then decrease approximately 10% when the power source voltage has dropped approximately 25%. (The rate may continuously decrease proportionally to the decrease in voltage supply to a

A. Noninvasive

| Troubleshooting tool | Function |
| --- | --- |
| Electrocardiogram recorder | Provides rate, stimulus efficacy, and sensing data. |
| X Ray | Show pacemaker position, lead connection, displacement, or broken wires. |
| Oscilloscope | Display pacemaker output artifacts via ECG chest electrodes (bipolar 5–30 mV), (unipolar 30–120 mV). |
| Magnet | Conversion of demand pulse generator to asynchronous operation. |
| Chest-wall stimulation | Provides an external signal via ECG chest electrodes to test pacemaker sensing. |
| Carotid sinus massage | Slows the patient's heart below the rate which inhibits the demand pacemaker. |
| Pacemaker monitor or Universal counter/timer | Provides an accurate digital readout of the rate and pulse duration. |
| Manipulation of the pulse generator in the pocket | To check for loose lead connections or lead problems |
| Programmer | Program the pacemaker parameters, to provide an indication of the source of a potential problem (e.g., alter sensitivity to evaluate oversensing of T waves). |

B. Invasive

| | |
| --- | --- |
| Pacing system analyzer | Check stimulation thresholds, intracardiac electrogram amplitude, pacemaker parameters. |
| External pacemaker | To take threshold or sensing data and provide temporary pacing while implantable system is being tested. |
| Oscilloscope (battery powered with storage preferred) | Display electrogram, and any electrical artifacts which may be present on lead (e.g., myopotential, intermittent electrical discontinuities). |
| Electrocardiogram recorder | Provides a permanent recording of the electrogram. |

**FIGURE 2.35.** Instrumentation used to evaluate pacemakers.

| Cause | Techniques of recognition | Corrective action |
|---|---|---|
| Lead displacement | • X-ray comparison (AP and lateral)<br>• Test threshold by programming pulse width or amplitude of IPG output.<br>• Test threshold with pacing systems analyzer or external pacemaker.*<br>• 12-lead (ECG). | • Reposition or replace lead if possible; otherwise, abandon lead and place new one. |
| Exit block | • Same as above. | • Reposition or replace lead if possible; otherwise, abandon lead and place new one.<br>• Use high output pulse generator or program IPG output to high energy level. |
| Perforation | • X-ray comparison.<br>• Test threshold by programming IPG output.<br>• ECG comparison.<br>• Test threshold with pacing system analyzer or external pacemaker.*<br>• Patient symptoms (hiccoughs, diaphragmatic twitching, pericardial rub). | • Gently retract the electrode. |
| Battery depletion | • Rate decrease of 5 to 10 bpm (with or without magnet depending on pacemaker).<br>• Pulse width increase (in some pacemakers).<br>• Pacemaker monitor. | • Check IPG with analyzer and if depleted, replace. |
| Lead insulation failure | • ECG analysis (change in amplitude of stimulation spikes).<br>• Test threshold with pacing systems analyzer (failure indicated by high current and low impedance).* | • If the fracture is accessible, repair with tip end replacement or medical grade adhesive; otherwise, abandon or remove old lead and place new one. |
| Lead fracture with insulation failure | • ECG analysis (change in amplitude and direction of stimulus spikes).<br>• Test threshold with pacing systems analyzer (failure indicated by intermittent high and low readings).* | • Repair if possible<br>• Abandon or remove lead and place new one. |
| Defibrillation effects | • ECG analysis.<br>• Threshold programmer test.<br>• Analyzer threshold test (temporary or permanent rise in threshold).* | • Rise in threshold may be temporary or permanent. Monitor patient for 24 h and if no change, abandon and/or remove the old lead and replace it with a new one. |
| Inappropriate pacemaker output | • ECG analysis (loss of capture). | • Reprogram the pulse width or amplitude to value which achieves continuous capture. |

*Invasive

**FIGURE 2.36.** Failure to capture in pacemaker systems.

specified end-of-life rate in some pacemakers). Additionally, in many pacemakers a progressive increase in pulse duration serves as a secondary power-source-depletion indicator. In some pacemakers that maintain constant stimulation energy, as battery voltage declines the pulse duration steadily widens to as much as twice that of its initial setting.

Some recent pacemakers include a telemetry system that can be interrogated while the patient is in the clinic or via transmission over the telephone. The pacemaker parameters can be compared to the initial implant parameters and to current actual performance, facilitating detection of inappropriate function or undocumented changes in parameters as a result of reprogramming.

It is essential during the evaluation process to have immediate access to

| Cause | Techniques of recognition | Corrective action |
|---|---|---|
| **For All Pacemakers:** | | |
| Loose pacemaker Lead connection | • ECG analysis (no stimulus artifacts or erratic/intermittent appearance or artifacts).<br>• X ray (of pacemaker).<br>• Manipulate the pacemaker in the pocket. | • Tighten connection. |
| Fractured lead | • ECG analysis (no stimulus artifacts or erratic/intermittent appearance of artifacts).<br>• X ray.<br>• Manipulate the pacemaker in the pocket. | • Repair if possible.<br>• Change to unipolar configuration if bipolar and good threshold on one electrode.<br>• Abandon or remove old lead and place new one. |
| Pacemaker failure | • ECG analysis (no stimulus artifacts).<br>• Pacemaker monitor. | • Test pacemaker and replace if defective. |
| Electromagnetic interference (EMI) | • Patient experiences slow heart rate. | • Implant different pacemaker system (bipolar, asynchronous).<br>• Advise patient to avoid EMI source. |
| **For Demand Pacemakers:** | | |
| Muscle inhibition | • ECG analysis (myopotentials present during periods of nonpacing). | • Program to a less sensitive setting.<br>• A change to bipolar pacemaker. |
| Sensing electrogram from wrong chamber | • ECG analysis (pacemaker timing reset by atrial events or T waves if ventricular pacemaker, or reset by R wave if atrial pacemaker. | • Program to aless sensitive setting.<br>• Reposition the lead. |
| Concealed ventrivular activity | • ECG analysis. | • Increase the pacemaker rate to over drive the spontaneous rate. |
| Cross talk (A–V sequential systems) | • ECG analysis. | • Program to a lower sensitivity setting.<br>• Reposition the lead which is detecting the crosstalk. |

**FIGURE 2.37.** Incomplete pacing failures in pacemaker systems.

pacemaker specifications and data recorded during the implant procedure. This will prevent delays and misinterpretation of data.

When performance does not conform to pacemaker system specifications, appropriate troubleshooting and correction procedures must be followed.

### Troubleshooting

The patient and the pacemaking hardware must be regarded as a set of interactive components comprising a single system. If a problem is suspected, a troubleshooting procedure is indicated.

**Troubleshooting Data.** The patient and pacemaker comprise a single system. Obtaining and reviewing the data shown in Fig. 2.34 will prove useful.

**Troubleshooting Tools.** The tools necessary to evaluate pacemaker system problems fall into two basic categories: noninvasive and invasive. The preferred approach is to use noninvasive methods, reserving invasive approaches for intractable cases. The tools and their function are shown in Fig. 2.35.

| Cause | Techniques of recognition | Corrective action |
|---|---|---|
| Lead displacement | • ECG analysis.<br>• Measure electrogram with PSA*.<br>• Evaluate electrogram with oscilloscope.* | • Reposition the lead. |
| Poor lead placement | • ECG analysis.<br>• Measure electrogram with PSA.*<br>• Evaluate electrogram with oscilloscope.* | • Reposition the lead. |
| Pacemaker failure | • ECG analysis.<br>• No response to chest wall stimulation (CWS).<br>• Test IPG with PSA.* | • Replace the pacemaker. |
| Electromagnetic interference (EMI) | • Patient experienced slow heart rate or dizziness. | • Replace IPG with bipolar or asynchronous device, or reprogram sensitivity or mode.<br>• Advise patient to avoid EMI source. |
| Apparent failure due to refractory periods | • ECG analysis—(intermittent rate slow down by sensing T waves (or R waves with an atrial demand pacemaker) or failure to sense PVCs. | • Reprogram the refractory period.<br>• Replace the pacemaker with a unit having the correct refractory period. |
| Inadequate pacemaker sensitivity | • ECG analysis.<br>• Measure pacemaker sensitivity with PSA.*<br>• Measure electrogram with PSA or oscilloscope.* | • Program the pacemaker to a higher sensitivity.<br>• Reposition the lead.<br>• Replace the pacemaker (with a higher sensitivity unit if needed). |

*Invasive

**FIGURE 2.38.** Sensing failures in pacemaker systems.

| Cause | Techniques of recognition | Corrective action |
|---|---|---|
| **All Pacemakers:** | | |
| Circuit failure | • ECG analysis (no stimulus artifact). <br> • Oscilloscope (connected to ECG electrodes). <br> • Pacing system analyzer test of pacemaker.* <br> • Pacemaker monitor. | • Replace the pacemaker. |
| Rate change (slowdown or runaway) | • ECG analysis. <br> • Pacemaker monitor. <br> • Pacing system analyzer.* | • Replace the pacemaker if runaway; if minor drift in circuit parameters, probably no correction required. |
| Electromagnetic interference (EMI) | • Patient experiences change in heart rate. | • Implant different pacemaker system (bipolar, asynchronous). <br> • Advise the patient to avoid EMI source. |
| Battery depletion | • Pacemaker monitor: <br>    – Rate decrease of 5 to 10 bpm (with or without magnet depending on pacemaker). <br>    – Pulse width increase (with some pacemakers). <br> • Pacing system analyzer test of IPG.* | • Replace the pacemaker. |
| **Demand Pacemakers:** | | |
| Hysteresis | • ECG analysis shows two distinct pacing intervals: a shorter one between repetitive stimuli and a longer escape interval following sensed activity. Rate regular with magnet. | • None needed if pacemaker has hysteresis. |
| Hairline lead fracture | • ECG analysis (change from a normal to a small or nonexistent spike or irregular pacing intervals). <br> • X ray. <br> • Manipulate the pacemaker in the pocket. | • Repair if possible. <br> • Change to unipolar configuration if bipolar and good threshold on an intact site. <br> • Abandon or remove old lead and place new one. |
| Loose pacemaker lead connection | • ECG analysis (change in direction and amplitude of spikes or irregular pacing rate). <br> • X ray (of pacemaker). <br> • Manipulate the pacemaker in the pocket. | • Tighten connections. |
| Muscle inhibition | • ECG analysis (myopotentials present during periods of irregular pacing). | • Program to a less sensitive setting. <br> • Change from a unipolar to a bipolar pacemaker. |
| T-wave sensing | • ECG analysis. (Rate on the ECG is slow. Magnet application restores normal rate.) | • Reprogram to longer refractory time. <br> • Reprogram to a less sensitive setting. <br> • Replace the pacemaker with a low-sensitivity one. |
| P-wave sensing | • ECG analysis (Rate on the ECG is slow. Magnet application restores heart rate.) | • Reprogram to less sensitivity. <br> • Replace the pacemaker with a low-sensitivity one. |
| Concealed ventricular activity | • ECG analysis. | • Increase the pacemaker rate to over drive the spontaneous rate. |

*Invasive

**FIGURE 2.39.** Inappropriate alterations in pacing rate in pacemaker systems.

**Types of System Malfunction.** There are four categories of pacemaker system malfunction: intermittent or complete noncapture, intermittent or complete nonpacing, malsensing, or pacing at an altered rate.

1. *Intermittent or Complete Noncapture.* There are times when a pacemaker emits a stimulus that fails to reliably depolarize cardiac tissue. Figure 2.36 lists the causes, recognition techniques, and methods of resolution for intermittent or complete *noncapture*.

2. *Intermittent or Complete Nonpacing.* The category of *nonpacing* covers those situations where there is no paced artifact visible in the records.

   Figure 2.37 defines the causes, recognition techniques, and methods of resolution for the problem of intermittent or complete *nonpacing*.

3. *Sensing Failure.* Most pacemakers include sensing circuitry that can either fail to sense desired signals or can sense signals that should not be detected. In either case, the pacemaker will generate inappropriate pacing stimulus sequences. Figure 2.38 lists the causes of inappropriate sensing, recognition techniques, and methods of resolution.

4. *Alterations in Pacing Rates.* Figure 2.39 lists the causes, recognition techniques, and methods for resolution of inappropriate alterations in pacing rate.

## REFERENCES

BEFELER, B., L. S. COHEN, F. J. HILDNER, R. P. JAVIER, O. S. NARULA, and P. SAMET (1971). Atrial contribution to ventricular function in the sitting position. *Chest,* 60: 240.

BENCHIMOL, A., L. G. ELLIS, and E. G. DIMOND (1965). Hemodynamic consequences of atrial and ventricular pacing in patients with normal and abnormal hearts. *Amer. J. Med.,* 39: 911.

BILITCH, M. (1971). *A Manual of cardiac arrhythmias;* Boston: Little, Brown & Co.

CAMILLI, L., R. POZZI, and G. DRAGO (1962). Remote heart stimulation by radio frequency for permanent rhythm control in the Morgagni-Adams-Stokes syndrome. *Surgery* 52: 765.

CASTILLO, C. A., B. V. BERKOVITS, A. CASTELLANOS, L. LEMBERG, G. CALLARD, and J. R. JUDE (1971). Bifocal demand pacing. *Chest,* 59: 360.

CITRON, P., and E. DUFFIN (1979). Implantable pacemakers for management of tachyarrhythmias. *Herz,* 4: 269.

FIELDS, J., B. V. BERKOVITS, and J. M. MATLOFF (1973). Surgical experience with temporary and permanent A-V sequential demand pacing. *J. Thoracic Cardiovasc. Surg.,* 66: 865.

FISHER, J. D., R. MEHRA, and S. FURMAN (1978). Termination of ventricular tachycardia with bursts of rapid ventricular pacing. *Amer. J. Cardiol,* 41: 94.

FURMAN, S. (1973). Therapeutic uses of atrial pacing. *Amer. Heart J.,* 86: 835.

GREENBERG, P., M. CASTELLANET, J. MESSENGER, and M. H. ELLESTAD (1978). Coronary sinus pacing. *Circulation,* 57: 98.

KAHN, M., E. SENDEROFF, J. SHAPIRO, S. B. BLEIFER, and A. GRISHMAN (1970). Bridging of interrupted A-V conduction in experimental chronic complete heart block by electronic means. *Amer. Heart J.,* 59: 548.

KARLOF, I. (1975). Haemodynamic effect of atrial triggered versus fixed rate pacing at rest and during exercise in complete heart block. *Acta Med. Scand.,* 197: 195.

KLEINERT, M., M. BOCK, and F. WILHEMI (1977). Clinical use of a new transvenous atrial lead. *Amer. J. Cardiol.* 40: 237.

NATHAN, D. A., S. CENTER, C. Y. WU, and W. KELLER (1963). An implantable synchronous pacemaker for the long term correction of complete heart block. *Amer. J. Cardiol.,* 11: 362.

NATHAN, D. A., S. CENTER, R. E. PINA, A. MEDOW, and J. W. KELLER (1966). The synchronous pacer in the therapy of Adams-Stokes disease, in L. DREIFUS and W. LIKOFF (eds.): *Mechanisms and therapy of cardiac arrhythmias,* 510–522. New York: Grune and Stratton.

OGAWA, S., L. S. DREIFUS, P. N. SHENOY, S. K. BROCKMAN, and B. V. BERKOVITS (1978). Hemodynamic consequences of atrioventricular and ventriculoatrial pacing. *PACE,* 1: 8.

PAEPRER, J., I. THORMANN, and M. NASSERI (1977). Cardiac pacing in the sick sinus syndrome, in Y. WATANABE (ed): *Cardiac pacing,* 200–203. Amsterdam: *Excerpta Medica.*

PARSONNET, V., S. FURMAN, and N. P. D. SMYTH (1974). Implantable cardiac pacemakers status report and resource guideline. *Circulation,* 50: A-21.

ROGEL, S., and Y. MAHLER (1971). The universal pacer. A synchronized-demand pacemaker. *J. Thoracic Cardiovasc. Surg.,* 61: 466.

SAMET, P., C. CASTILLO, and W. H. BERNSTEIN (1966). Hemodynamic sequelae of atrial, ventricular and sequential atrioventricular pacing in cardiac patients. *Amer. Heart J.,* 72: 725.

SCHECHTER, D. C. (1972). Background of clinical cardiac electrostimulation. *N. Y. State J. Med.,* 72: 605.

SMYTH, N. P. D., P. CITRON, J. M. KESHISHIAN, J. M. GARCIA, and L. C. KELLY (1976). Permanent pervenous atrial sensing and pacing with a new J-shaped lead. *J. Thoracic Cardiovasc. Surg.* 72: 565.

STEPHENSON, S. E., P. C. JOLLY, H. W. BAILEY, W. H. EDWARDS, and L. H. MONTGOMERY (1959). Evaluation of the P-wave external cardiac stimulation. *Surg. Forum,* 10: 612.

WELLENS, H. J. J., K. I. LIE, and M. J. JANSE (eds) (1976). *The conduction system of the heart,* Philadelphia: Lea & Febiger.

# STUDY QUESTIONS

**2.1**  What are the basic components of a pacing system? Describe the role of each in forming a total system.

**2.2**  What is the basic difference in electronic design between a *"constant-current"* and *"constant-voltage"* pulse output circuit? Why are the quotation marks used to describe these circuits?

**2.3** What significant characteristics of the electrogram affect detection of the cardiac signal by the sensing amplifier? Propose some design specifications for an atrial and a ventricular sensing circuit and contrast the requirements imposed on the amplifier.

**2.4** Make a table comparing mercury-zinc, lithium, and nuclear power sources in terms of mode of storage, voltage, capacity, size, and life. Also include factors such as weight, safety, and cost. You will need to conduct a literature search.

**2.5** Describe the major lead system designs currently used. Contrast different approaches from the electrical and mechanical design requirements and the surgical implantation methods perspective. Include materials, bipolar versus monopolar systems, and mechanical stress parameters in your analysis.

**2.6** Define stimulation threshold. What factors affect this parameter? How are thresholds determined? What is the role of the strength-duration curve and electrode surface area in determining thresholds?

**2.7** What is sensing threshold and what parameters affect it? What design constraints do the signal levels and environment place on sensing circuits?

**2.8** Describe the major effects that electrosurgical equipment has on pacemaker function. How can these effects be reduced?

**2.9** Refer to Chapters 3 and 10 and relate pacemaker operation and design to use considerations for defibrillators and electrosurgical equipment. How does the design of one of these three systems affect the other two?

**2.10** How are programmable pacemakers designed? What parameters are varied and why were those chosen?

**2.11** Explain the pacemaker identification code. Why was it adopted? What are its limitations?

**2.12** List each of the types of pacemakers. Include the circuit components required (e.g., pulse generator, timing, sensing amplifier, etc.), clinical indications for its use, and the identification codes that apply.

**2.13** Contrast the timing and control circuit specifications required for demand versus atrial synchronous pacemakers. When is each clinically indicated?

**2.14** What are the advantages of the AV sequential pacemaker over other types of synchronized circuits? When is this type used?

**2.15** What are the major failures noted in pacemaker systems? How are they determined in the pacemaker clinic?

**2.16** Describe the methods for testing a newly implanted pacemaker. How do these differ from the methods used during follow-up evaluations?

**2.17** Describe how you would distinguish among the four types of pacemaker system failures described in Section 2.6.

# 3 Defibrillators

*Charles F. Babbs*
*Joe D. Bourland*

## 3.1 LEARNING OBJECTIVES

Upon completing this chapter you will be able to:

- Explain the generation of ventricular fibrillation according to the circus motion theory.
- Predict the consequences of atrial versus ventricular fibrillation for the patient.
- Describe three clinical settings in which a defibrillator may be used.
- Discuss three measures of defibrillator shock intensity.
- Draw the output circuits for a capacitor-discharge defibrillator, a trapezoidal waveform defibrillator, and a damped sine wave defibrillator.

## 3.2 PHYSIOLOGY OF CARDIAC FIBRILLATION

### Introduction and History

Ventricular fibrillation, the most dangerous cardiac arrhythmia, is a common immediate cause of death in patients with heart, lung, or kidney disease. During this arrhythmia, there is random, uncoordinated contraction of multiple areas of muscle in the cardiac ventricles. When viewed directly, the heart appears as a shimmering mass of tissue. Upon close inspection multiple, unsynchronized waves of contraction and relaxation can be seen transversing the ventricular surface in random directions. Coordinated beating does not occur and, because the ventricles are the main pumping chambers of the heart, the circulation of blood to the brain, the heart itself, and other vital organs comes to a standstill. Ventricular fibrillation causes certain death if resuscitative measures and definite therapy are not begun within 3–5 min (Stephenson, 1974). Spontaneous defibrillation of the ventricles virtually never occurs in humans.

## Mechanism of Fibrillation: The Circus Motion Theory

The simplest theory describing a mechanism for ventricular fibrillation is the *circus motion* theory. Figure 3.1 shows the development of a "circus motion" in rings of myocardium. Purkinje fibers first stimulate subendocardial muscle fibers of the ventricles, so that the impulse normally spreads from subendocardial muscle to the epicardial surface (Fig. 3.1a). The tissue is completely excited, and further spread of the impulse is impossible because ventricular muscle is refractory for about 300 ms after excitation. Hence, such a normally conducted impulse cannot become self-propagating.

A typical premature ventricular contraction (PVC) is also not self-propagating in a normal heart. An impulse arising from a single focus in the ventricular wall and spreading in all directions will coalesce on the side of the heart opposite its origin and annihilate itself due to the refractoriness of the converging masses of recently excited tissue (Fig. 3.1b).

However, in injured hearts containing patchy areas of refractoriness, PVCs are more dangerous. Figure 3.1c shows that an impulse arising from an irritable focus at the edge of an injured area is blocked in one direction due to prolonged refractory period in the injured tissue. The impulse therefore travels only clockwise around the ventricular wall. Traveling at 50 cm/s, such an impulse would close the loop around a 5-cm-diameter ventricle (16 cm in circumference) in 320 ms. This is adequate time for the muscle first stimulated by the PVC to recover sufficiently to be excited by the "re-entrant" impulse. Under these conditions, a self-propagated "circus motion" of excitation develops, and the impulse conducts around and around the myocardium.

Failing hearts may be both injured and dilated. This prolongs the time available for recovery of the initially excited myocardium and so enhances the probability of development of circus motions. Figure 3.1d shows that the path length for potential circus motions is longer in an enlarged heart. For example, in a dilated 8-cm-diameter ventricle (25 cm in circumference), a blocked unidirectional impulse requires 500 ms to travel completely around the wall. This allows ample time for recovery of initially refractory fibers.

**The Impulse Wavelength.** Figure 3.1 shows that the impulse conduction velocity multiplied by the refractory period gives the length of the strip of refractory myocardium. We define the product of conduction velocity and effective refractory period as the "wavelength" of the impulse of depolarization. A normal value for the impulse wavelength in mammals is about 10–30 cm (Hoffman and Cranefield, 1960). Figure 3.1d shows that if the impulse wavelength is less than the ventricular circumference, then the development of circus movements becomes possible, especially in the presence of patchy areas of refractoriness caused by ische-

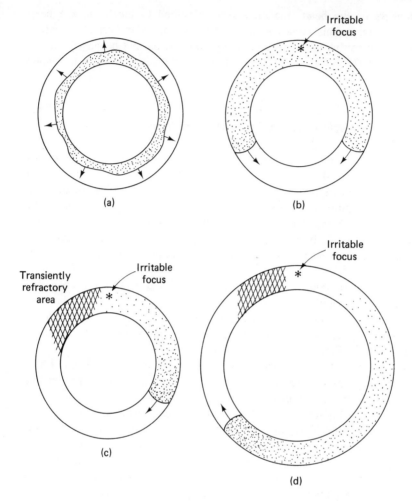

**FIGURE 3.1.** Development of circus motion pattern of ventricular excitation. (a) Normal excitation via subendocardial Purkinje fibers. (b) Excitation during a typical PVC, originating at an irritable focus. (c) Excitation by a PVC originating at the edge of a transiently refractory area, leading to a self-perpetuating circus motion. (d) Development of a circus motion in a dilated heart.

mia, cooling, or rapid, repetitive stimulation. On the other hand, small hearts of circumference less than 10–30 cm (diameter less than 3–10 cm) may be unable to sustain fibrillation according to the circus motion theory. Rabbits possess hearts with dimensions equal to or below the theoretical limit for circus motion, and indeed smaller rabbit hearts will not sustain fibrillation at normal body temperatures whereas larger rabbit hearts may continue to fibrillate (Geddes, 1970).

**The Relation of Circus Motions to Fibrillation.** If a circus motion of the type diagrammed in Fig. 3.1 occurred circumferentially about the long axis of a left

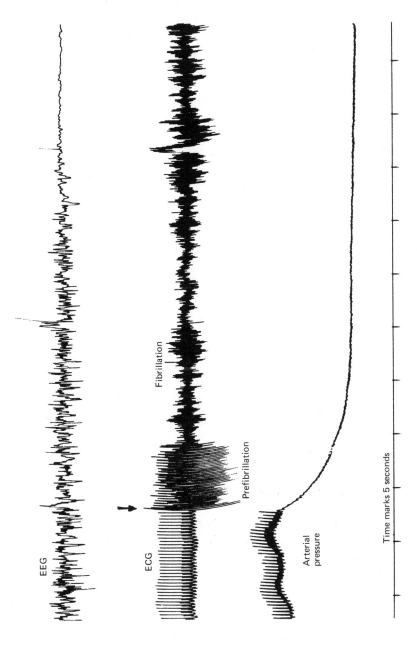

EEG

ECG

Fibrillation

Prefibrillation

Arterial pressure

Time marks 5 seconds

**FIGURE 3.2.** Physiologic events of ventricular fibrillation. Electroencephalogram (EEG) showing brain activity, electrocardiogram (ECG), and arterial blood pressure records. Electrical stimulation at arrow produces fibrillation. The ECG becomes chaotic, brain activity ceases in 30 s, and blood pressure falls toward zero.

ventricle composed of uniformly excitable tissue, the rhythm known as ventricular flutter would be present. Ventricular flutter usually exists only for a short time and usually degenerates into fibrillation. Because of the asymmetrical geometry of the heart, the depolarization wavefront of a circus motion soon breaks up into multiple wavefronts upon encountering the junction between right ventricular free wall and interventricular septum, the mitral and tricuspid valve rings, or islands of refractory tissue. Soon the closed-loop pathways permitting ventricular re-excitation become multiple, convoluted, and everchanging as true ventricular fibrillation develops.

In summary, sustained fibrillation in cardiac muscle requires a large enough mass, an adequately slow propagation velocity, and a short enough refractory period so that recovered tissue is always encountered by advancing excitation.

### Atrial Fibrillation and Its Consequences

The atria are the supercharging antechambers of the heart. Atrial fibrillation decreases cardiac output because the added ventricular filling provided by the atria is abolished. During atrial fibrillation, arterial blood pressure is high enough to perfuse vital organs. Patients may live almost normally for many years with uncorrected atrial fibrillation. In contrast, ventricular fibrillation is a cause of sudden death.

### Ventricular Fibrillation and Its Consequences

The ventricles are the main pumping chambers of the heart. During ventricular fibrillation, the heart no longer pumps blood and vital organs lose perfusion. As soon as the ventricles begin to fibrillate, blood pressure falls to zero (Fig. 3.2). Organs and tissues that require an uninterrupted supply of blood deteriorate rapidly. The first organ to sustain permanent damage is the brain. Within about 3–5 min, permanent brain damage occurs if nothing is done to restore the circulation. Death occurs in a matter of only a few more minutes (Stephenson, 1974). Defibrillation of the ventricles is a lifesaving procedure.

## 3.3 PHYSIOLOGY OF CARDIAC DEFIBRILLATION

Defibrillation, which is the abolition of fibrillation, requires resynchronization of the ventricular muscle cells. In the early 1930s, Kouwenhoven and associates at Johns Hopkins University, while studying the mechanism of death by accidental electrocution, discovered a remarkable fact. While low-intensity ac shocks to the heart could cause fibrillation, higher intensity shocks to the same heart could abolish fibrillation. Upon review of the literature, they found the neglected reports of the French investigators Prevost and Batelli, who had encountered the same phenomenon in 1899. After Kouwenhoven's discovery, Beck et al. (1947) successfully used ac shocks applied directly to the heart to defibrillate human patients. Zoll et al. (1956a, 1956b) successfully used ac shocks for transchest defibrillation in man.

Several investigators (Gurvich and Yuniev, 1947; Lown, 1962; Edmark, 1963) later confirmed that very brief dc shocks of high intensity also were able to defibrillate the heart. Moreover, dc current defibrillation had the advantage that it could be used for atrial cardioversion. Thereafter, dc defibrillators quickly became standard equipment in hospitals.

## Mechanism of Defibrillation

Electrical defibrillation works by producing a uniform state of ventricular excitability. The defibrillating shock stimulates all excitable tissue, including tissue just ahead of the multiple wavefronts of circus motion in the fibrillating heart. This blocks propagation of any circus motion. The shock brings a critical mass of ventricular muscle to the refractory state, and fibrillation cannot proceed. Usually the heart is able to beat synchronously immediately after electrical defibrillation.

For an individual cardiac cell, the defibrillating shock need be no stronger at the cellular level than that delivered by a pacemaker. In this sense, a defibrillator is a stimulator much like a large-scale cardiac pacemaker. In theory, therefore, the defibrillating shock need not be damaging to the heart. Small currents (a few milliamperes) are required for cardiac pacing because the surface area of pacing electrodes is relatively small (a few square millimeters). To pace the heart, we need to stimulate only a small area of tissue adjacent to the electrode because the excitation subsequently spreads throughout an entire cardiac chamber (see Figure 3.1b). To stimulate the entire heart for the purpose of defibrillation, we require electrodes roughly a thousand times larger in area. Accordingly, to produce the same current density as required for pacing, defibrillation requires roughly a thousand times as much current. Animal studies (Geddes, 1970) and human data (Guinn et al., 1974) have shown that in order to defibrillate the ventricles during surgery with electrodes directly on the heart, we need a few amperes of current.

With electrodes applied across the chest in man-sized animals, we require several tens of amperes to defibrillate (Bourland et al., 1978a) because much of the current passes around the heart rather than through the heart. Transchest defibrillation may require several thousand volts to achieve adequate current through the chest. These transchest shocks may seem very strong, and possibly dangerous. However, for the cardiac muscle cell, defibrillator shocks are not necessarily any more harmful than pulses from a cardiac pacemaker, provided the current density is roughly uniform.

## Electrical Dose

With present technology, it is impractical to apply measured doses of current because the resistance of the chest to current flow varies greatly from one subject to another. We cannot predict in advance the current that will flow for a given energy setting. We can, however, precisely measure the voltage to which the defibrillator is charged. Thus we can calculate the energy stored in the defibrillator before the shock is delivered. This latter measure, known as *stored energy,* has been the traditional measure of defibrillator shock intensity.

The stored energy in a defibrillator is independent of the subject's chest resistance. If the internal resistance of the defibrillator is small—a situation that is not necessarily true (Babbs and Whistler, 1978)—most of the stored energy will be delivered to the patient. Although the fraction of stored energy that is actually delivered is somewhat dependent upon subject resistance, it is much less dependent upon subject resistance than is the current. The actual relationship is:

$$U_{\text{delivered}} = U_{\text{stored}} \times \frac{R_s}{R_d + R_s}$$ (3.1)

where  $U$ = energy,
  $R^s$ = subject resistance,

and  $R_d$ = defibrillator internal resistance.

The energy dose delivered to the patient (the "delivered energy") is a fraction (typically about ¾) of the stored energy (Babbs and Whistler, 1978).

Because it is fairly easy to estimate the energy that will be delivered without accurate knowledge of chest resistance, dosing by energy would appear to be a relatively straightforward matter. For example, we might imagine that a simple dosage scheme of so many joules per kilogram would suffice. What is more, mathematical modeling by Schuder et al. (1975) predicts that if transchest electrodes of diameter proportional to the chest circumference are used, the delivered energy per kilogram should be a constant for geometrically similar subjects, regardless of their size.

### Other Factors Influencing the Electrical Dose

There are many factors in addition to body weight that influence the strength of shock necessary to defibrillate the ventricles. We previously mentioned the most important of these factors—the transchest resistance to current flow. Transchest resistance (also called *apparent impedance*) may vary considerably from individual to individual. Chest impedance values measured by Machin (1978) in adult men during in-hospital defibrillation ranged from 25–105 $\Omega$. Nine percent of 175 measured impedance values were less than 40 $\Omega$, and 20% of measured impedance values were greater than 70 $\Omega$. The mean value was 58 $\Omega$, not far from the usually assumed value of 50 $\Omega$. But, because chest impedance in man varies over a fourfold range, the voltage and energy settings required to produce an adequate current for defibrillation vary proportionally.

There are other subject-dependent factors that influence dose and that we cannot control in advance of defibrillation. These may include heart size, chest conformation, disease states such as myocardial infarction, blood gas, and electrolyte disturbances, and the presence of some drugs. The quantitative effects of these variables are under investigation.

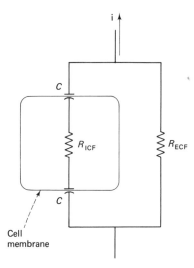

**FIGURE 3.3.** Simple electrical analog for heart muscle cell and surrounding extracellular fluid (ECF). The cell membrane is modeled as a capacitance and the intracellular fluid (ICF) as a resistance.

## The Strength-Duration Curve for Defibrillation

Studies with all current waveforms used to date have shown that two factors, shock intensity and duration, are of importance in effecting defibrillation. The function that describes the trade-offs required between strength and duration sufficient to produce a just adequate defibrillating current is known as a *strength-duration curve*.

A cardiac cell membrane is bathed on one side by extracellular fluid and on the other by intracellular fluid. Both contain electrolytes and are relatively good conductors. The membrane contains a large percentage of lipids, which are relatively poor conductors. Hence, the cell membrane and its environment comprise two conductors separated by an insulator, that is to say, a capacitor. Figure 3.3 shows a simplified model of a cardiac cell and surrounding extracellular fluid as a capacitor in parallel with a resistor.

We can consider the source of the defibrillating shock as a current source. This is a reasonable representation for a stimulating source of a single cell when we recognize that a great number of cells are in series with the cell being modeled. Therefore, changes in the voltage across the cell have little effect on the current flow. The equation representing this simple model of a cardiac cell is:

$$i = C\frac{dv}{dt} + \frac{v}{R}$$

*(3.2)*

where $i$ is the amplitude of the current source, $R$ and $C$ are the resistance and capacitance of the cell membrane, and $v$ is the voltage across the membrane. In order to stimulate a cell, the voltage across the cell membrane must change by $v_t$ volts, where $v_t$ is the difference between the resting membrane potential and the "firing" threshold of the cell. Solution of equation 3.2 for a rectangular current pulse of duration $d$ and of threshold intensity yields

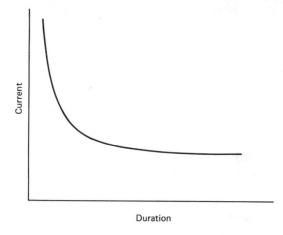

Current

Duration

FIGURE 3.4. Strength-duration curves. Solid line from theoretical equation (3.4).

$$v_t = iR \ (1 \ - \ e^{-d/RC})$$

*(3.3)*

Rearranging equation 3.3 gives the relationship between intensity of the stimulating source $i$ and its duration $d$ as shown in equation 3.4.

$$i = \frac{v_t/R}{1 - e^{(-d/RC)}}$$

*(3.4)*

If we extend the concepts developed above for a single cell to a mass of tissue, we can represent the relationship between the intensity of a stimulus and its duration as

$$i = \frac{b}{1 - e^{(-d/a)}}$$

*(3.5)*

where $a$ and $b$ are constants characterizing the tissue and electrode configuration employed. Equation 3.4 describes a strength-duration curve, as shown in Fig. 3.4.

Because successful cardiac defibrillation requires simultaneous stimulation of a sufficient number of cells, it seems reasonable that a similar strength-duration curve for cardiac defibrillation may exist. Indeed, using an equation of the form of equation 3.5, Geddes et al. (1970) have demonstrated strength-duration curves for transchest ventricular defibrillation. Bourland et al. (1978a) have demonstrated a similar strength-duration curve for ventricular defibrillation with a catheter-based electrode system.

We may measure shock intensity in terms of either delivered current, energy, or charge. Figure 3.5 shows typical current, energy, and charge versus duration relationships. There are three different electrical quantities that we can use to describe an "optimum" pulse of defibrillating current; these are *minimum current*, *minimum energy*, and *minimum charge*. For example, if we adopt defibrillation with minimum energy as a criterion, then there is a duration for minimum energy. If we select minimum charge, then we require the shortest possible duration pulse of current.

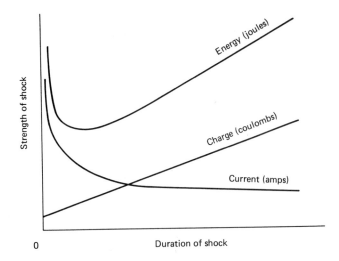

**FIGURE 3.5.** Strength-duration curves in terms of energy, charge, and current compared. Duration for minimum strength shock depends upon the measure of shock intensity.

## Current Waveforms

The first generation of defibrillators used several cycles of 60-Hz ac to defibrillate. These defibrillators strongly stimulated skeletal muscle and delivered an excessive amount of energy. It was not long before the advantages of the damped sine wave defibrillator were recognized. Prior to the 1970s, the damped sine wave defibrillator had no rival. In the 1970s, new defibrillators generated a truncated-exponential waveform, sometimes called a trapezoidal waveform, by shorting a discharging capacitor. The design of the defibrillators was based on the pioneering work of Schuder et al. (1966). Following the introduction of the truncated-exponential defibrillator into clinical practice by Anderson and Suelzer (1976), a controversy existed over the merits of the two types of defibrillators. A fundamental question that had to be answered before the controversy could be resolved was: What is an appropriate basis for comparison of different waveforms?

Our group (Bourland et al., 1978a) obtained strength-duration curves for ventricular defibrillation in the dog via a catheter-based electrode system. We tested truncated-exponential waveforms with four values of tilt (*tilt* is defined as the percent decrease in current during the pulse) and measured intensity of the defibrillating shock in terms of the initial current, which is equal to the peak current of a truncated-exponential waveform. Curves for waveforms that had tilts of less than 5%, 50%, 65%, and 80% are shown in Fig. 3.6a.

For a given duration, we must increase initial current as we increase tilt for the two waveforms to be equally effective in defibrillating the ventricles. However, if we select average current as the measure of shock intensity, the curves for the four values of tilt are very close to one another, as shown in Fig. 3.6b. This implies that the average current required to defibrillate is independent of tilt. Interestingly, the average current for a truncated-exponential and a damped sine wave required to defibrillate animal ventricles via transchest electrodes is approximately the same (Bourland et al., 1978b). Note that waveforms can be compared on the basis of their average current only if their duration is the same.

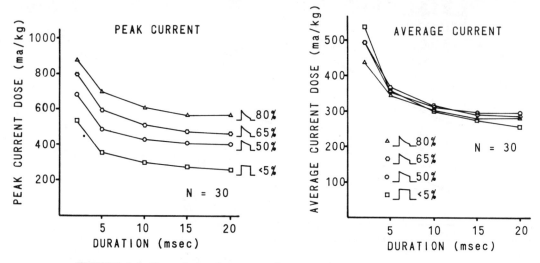

**FIGURE 3.6.** Strength-duration curves for catheter defibrillation with waveforms of varying tilt. (a) Peak current is the measure of intensity. (b) Average current is the measure of intensity.

The *average current law* for defibrillation is: If a damped sine and a truncated-exponential wave, or two truncated-exponential waves with different tilt, have the same average current, then they will be equally effective in defibrillating the ventricles, provided they are of the same duration.

In addition to choosing the waveform and duration for a pulse of defibrillating current, we must establish the amplitude of the defibrillating stimulus for a given defibrillation attempt. We can consider that a given defibrillator selection of the shock amplitude is analogous to selection of the dose of a drug. This "dose concept" implies that a stronger defibrillating shock is required to defibrillate larger hearts. In one form or another, clinicians use the dose concept. Those who are most aware of it are pediatric cardiologists who have learned that children require less output from a defibrillator than adult subjects (Gutgesell et al., 1976). In practice, physicians are aware of the dose concept and use less energy for children than for adults.

## 3.4 USES OF DEFIBRILLATORS

We use defibrillators for three purposes: (1) ventricular defibrillation at the time of thoracic surgery—that is, direct heart defibrillation; (2) cardioversion, that is, the termination of arrhythmias with a synchronized countershock; and (3) emergency ventricular defibrillation.

### *Direct Heart Defibrillation*

Surgeons use a defibrillator for terminating ventricular fibrillation in the hearts of patients who have undergone elective ventricular fibrillation during thoracic surgery. In many types of cardiac surgery supported by a heart-lung machine, it is desirable to fibrillate the ventricles. Fibrillation achieves a stationary operative field that facilitates rapid completion of the surgical procedure and also decreases the probability of air or blood emboli entering the circulation. The surgeon can intentionally fibrillate the ventricles by the application of low-intensity alternating current shocks through electrodes that are applied to the ventricular epicardium. He or she can then perform surgery in the absence of cardiac beating and then can electrically defibrillate the ventricles with sterile paddle electrodes.

Failure of the defibrillator to function properly is potentially catastrophic. We may waste valuable time in locating and transporting a second defibrillator to the operating site. A spare set of sterilized electrodes should be on hand to prevent delay in defibrillation. The spare electrodes must be properly mated to the defibrillator—often a nontrivial practical problem.

The surgeon usually places the electrodes laterally (one on each side of the ventricles) or one on the anterior surface and one on the posterior surface of the ventricles. Gentle compression of the heart between the electrodes squeezes blood from the ventricular chambers allowing defibrillation with lower energy.

Ventricular defibrillation is successful in nearly 100% of patients in the prepared and controlled operating room environment. Low energy usually defibrillates (Guinn et al., 1974) and it is not necessary to greatly increase energy if the first shock fails to defibrillate. On the contrary, higher energy is almost certainly detrimental in such cases.

## Elective Defibrillation

Elective defibrillation, or cardioversion, is the use of synchronized electrical shock for treatment of arrhythmias other than ventricular fibrillation. Such arrhythmias include atrial fibrillation, atrial flutter, paroxysmal atrial tachycardia, junctional (A-V node) tachycardia, and ventricular tachycardia. Some of the enthusiasm for this technique has decreased with the finding that many of the patients who are cardioverted to normal sinus rhythm will subsequently revert to their abnormal rhythm. However, cardioversion is a significant and important therapeutic procedure for treating many patients with cardiovascular disease. It is very effective for the treatment of acute tachyarrhythmias, particularly those that may be life-threatening; and it is really the only alternative for treating patients with chronic supraventricular arrhythmias that do not respond to drug therapy.

We should attempt cardioversion when the causative mechanism for the arrhythmia has been removed. For example, if atrial fibrillation is caused by a valve lesion and we surgically replace the valve, then we should perform electrical cardioversion. Because atrial function may be improved and atrial size may decrease after surgery, sinus rhythm may be long-lasting.

For elective treatment of arrhythmias, we usually combine the use of dc shock with drug therapy. It is common practice to utilize drug therapy as a first course of action for most non-life-threatening tachyarrhythmias, because this may help to maintain the sinus rhythm. If the cardioversion is unsuccessful, the patient may discontinue the selected drug. Just prior to applying the shock, we usually give patients intravenous diazepam, or some other tranquilizing agent.

**Cardioversion Procedure.** Set the defibrillator in the synchronized mode and apply conducting paste to the metal defibrillating electrodes. Use a low-resistivity paste and avoid smearing paste on the chest wall except directly under the electrode. Do not inadvertently apply a bridge of paste between the two electrodes, or current will flow through this short-circuiting paste and little will pass through the subject.

**Overall Success.** The most disappointing aspect of atrial cardioversion is the number of patients who revert to their arrhythmia within a short time. Although we can convert over 90% of patients to sinus rhythm after cardioversion, multiple studies have documented that success rates are only 30% for persistence of sinus rhythm for periods of 36 months or more (Resnekov, 1973). This has resulted in some decrease of enthusiasm for the use of electric shock for treating atrial tachyarrhythmias.

### Emergency Defibrillation

Emergency defibrillation is one component of medical care necessary for the sudden death syndrome. *Sudden death syndrome* is the sudden and unexpected cessation of cardiac function and respiration. The American Heart Association has developed a widely accepted program for the treatment of sudden death. The immediate care of the patient who has sudden death syndrome is called cardiopulmonary resuscitation (CPR). CPR is a technique used to maintain respiration and circulation until we can apply definitive care. The goal of CPR is to prevent irreversible brain damage. Definitive care includes drug administration and defibrillation, which comes under the category of advanced life support, for which CPR is the first step. Defibrillation (and therefore the defibrillator) is part of the advanced life support technique.

**Overall Success.** Survival following closed-chest resuscitation ranges from 0 to 82% with a mean value of 16% (Stephenson, 1974).

## 3.5 DEFIBRILLATOR DESIGN

A variety of defibrillator designs have been used to generate shocks adequate to defibrillate the cardiac ventricles. As we have observed, in the case of transchest defibrillation, a peak current of tens of amperes may be required to defibrillate the adult human heart. Furthermore, because the resistance to defibrillating current is typically 50 $\Omega$, the voltage across defibrillating electrodes may exceed 3,500 V. Therefore, defibrillators are generators that must produce high peak power but that are required to do so only for a short time.

**AC Defibrillators.** Zoll et al. (1956a) were the first to successfully defibrillate a human patient with transchest electrodes, and the defibrillator they used was an ac defibrillator. Early ac defibrillators were, in essence, nothing more than step-up power transformers with timing circuits to limit the duration of output current. A simplified circuit of an ac defibrillator is shown in Fig. 3.7. Line voltage [120 V (rms), 50 or 50 Hz] was stepped up by the transformer to, typically, 720 V. Current was permitted to flow for 250 ms in early models, but it was found that a

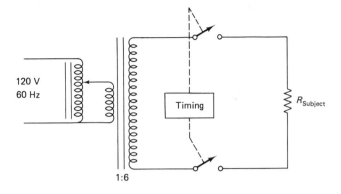

AC Defibrillator

**FIGURE 3.7.** AC defibrillator.

100-ms pulse of current is equally effective. Hence, the output of later ac defibrilla-tors consisted of 5 or 6 cycles of sinusoidal voltage and typically had an amplitude of 720 V. Assuming a transchest resistance of 50 $\Omega$, a typical output current was almost 15 A. Because the 6:1 transformer required to increase the 120-V line voltage to the required 720-V output voltage also increases the line current by approximately the same factor, the danger of melting fuses or tripping circuit breakers was a problem. Transformers capable of handling such high power at line frequencies are necessarily large and heavy. Consequently, ac defibrillators were large, heavy devices and were not well suited for portable applications.

**Capacitor Discharge Defibrillators.** Prevost and Battelli (1899c) were first to successfully defibrillate the cardiac ventricles of the dog by discharging a capacitor through electrodes placed directly on the heart. The capacitor discharge defibrillator is elegant in its simplicity, as shown in Fig. 3.8. The defibrillator consists of a power supply, an energy-storage capacitor, and a relay. The output voltage (and current) from a capacitor discharge defibrillator decays exponentially with time and is given by equation 3.6.

$$v = V\,e^{-t/RC} \qquad\qquad (3.6)$$

where   $v$ is the output voltage

  $V$ is the voltage to which the capacitor is charged

  $t$ is time

  $R$ is the resistance of the subject

  $C$ is the capacitance of the energy-storage capacitor

In the above expression, it has been assumed that the internal resistance of the defibrillator is much smaller than the subject resistance, and may be ignored.

  Although, theoretically, the current in an R-C circuit decays to zero only after

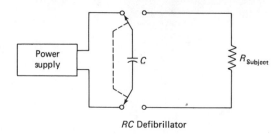

RC Defibrillator

**FIGURE 3.8.** Capacitor-discharge defibrillator.

an infinite time, a convenient measure of the duration of an exponentially decaying waveform is the time constant of the circuit, which is the product, $RC$, of the resistance and capacitance of the circuit. (Current decays to 37% of its initial peak value in one time constant.) Geddes (1970) demonstrated that minimum current is required to defibrillate the canine ventricles when the time constant of the defibrillating circuit is 3.5–5 ms.

Although the capacitor discharge defibrillator is highly desirable because of its simplicity, adverse side effects of the capacitor discharge waveform have caused this defibrillator design to be abandoned for human applications. Tacker et al. (1978) demonstrated a high incidence of atrioventricular block following direct-heart defibrillation with a capacitor discharge defibrillator. Peleska (1963) demonstrated that the high peak current produced by the capacitor discharge defibrillator depresses myocardial muscle fibers. Schuder et al. (1966) suggested that refibrillation may be precipitated by the exponential "tail" of the capacitor discharge waveform if the time constant is too long.

**RLC Defibrillators.** The defibrillator design that has gained widest clinical acceptance is the RLC defibrillator. The RLC defibrillator is identical to the RC defibrillator except that an inductor is connected in series with the energy-storage capacitor and the subject. Gurvich and Yuniev (1947) found that placing an inductor in the output circuit reduced the peak current required to defibrillate the cardiac ventricles of animal subjects. Lown (1962) reported similar reduction in peak current requirements when an inductor was inserted in the output circuit of a defibrillator designed for transchest human defibrillation.

A simplified circuit for an RLC defibrillator is shown in Fig. 3.9. Adding an inductor to the RC defibrillator changes the output waveform from a simple exponential to a damped sine wave. The current in the RLC defibrillator circuit is given by equation 3.7.

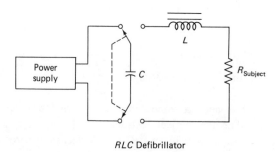

RLC Defibrillator

**FIGURE 3.9.** RLC defibrillator.

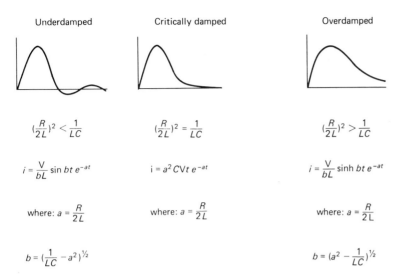

| Underdamped | Critically damped | Overdamped |
|---|---|---|

$(\frac{R}{2L})^2 < \frac{1}{LC}$ $\qquad$ $(\frac{R}{2L})^2 = \frac{1}{LC}$ $\qquad$ $(\frac{R}{2L})^2 > \frac{1}{LC}$

$i = \frac{V}{bL} \sin bt\, e^{-at}$ $\qquad$ $i = a^2 CVt\, e^{-at}$ $\qquad$ $i = \frac{V}{bL} \sinh bt\, e^{-at}$

where: $a = \frac{R}{2L}$ $\qquad$ where: $a = \frac{R}{2L}$ $\qquad$ where: $a = \frac{R}{2L}$

$b = (\frac{1}{LC} - a^2)^{1/2}$ $\qquad\qquad\qquad\qquad$ $b = (a^2 - \frac{1}{LC})^{1/2}$

**FIGURE 3.10.** Solutions for the RLC defibrillator circuit.

$$\frac{d^2i}{dt^2} + \frac{R}{L}\frac{di}{dt} + \frac{1}{LC}i = 0 \qquad\qquad (3.7)$$

The initial conditions are: (1) the current flowing in the inductor is zero; and (2) the voltage across the capacitor is the voltage, $V$, to which it has been charged. The output current can be either underdamped, critically damped, or overdamped, depending on the selection of the component values in the defibrillator and on the resistance of the output circuit (which includes the resistance of the subject). Figure 3.10 summarizes the solutions for equation 3.7. Typical component values for the RLC defibrillators are $C = 16\ \mu F$ and $L = 100$ mH.

**Trapezoidal Defibrillators.** Schuder et al. (1967) showed that less peak current is required to defibrillate with a rectangular pulse than with a damped sine wave. In a waveform comparison study, Schuder et al. (1971) also demonstrated that, if the top of the rectangular pulse is permitted to tilt, the efficacy of the shock is not greatly reduced.

A simplified circuit for a trapezoidal defibrillator is shown in Fig. 3.11. The trapezoidal waveform can be generated by truncating an exponentially decaying current. An advantage of the trapezoidal defibrillator design is that no inductor is required. The trapezoidal defibrillator is, in essence, an RC defibrillator in which the output current is interrupted within a time constant or two of its initiation. Theoretically, the output current could be interrupted by opening the output switch, $S_1$. Because output current and voltage may be high at the time of truncation, design of reliable, small devices to implement $S_1$ has proven difficult. However, by adding a second switch, $S_2$, the output current can be truncated. Because $S_2$ is in parallel with the subject, closing $S_2$ shorts the voltage applied to the subject. Silicon-controlled rectifiers (SCRs) that can withstand the voltage and current requirements of trapezoidal defibrillator designs are available.

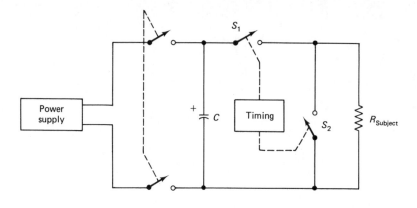

Trapezoidal defibrillator

**FIGURE 3.11.** Truncated exponential waveform defibrillator.

## 3.6 FUTURE DEVELOPMENTS

**Automatic Sensing of Chest Resistance.** The peak output current from damped sine and truncated-exponential waveform defibrillators varies inversely with the resistance in the defibrillating circuit, because these defibrillators generate the output waveform by connecting a charged capacitor to the subject. (An inductor is between the energy-discharge capacitor and the subject in a damped sine wave defibrillator). The observations of Machin (1978) suggest that the peak current delivered to a human subject may vary by a factor of 6 or more for the same energy setting on a defibrillator control. If we must achieve a threshold current in order to defibrillate, then perhaps a defibrillator that can automatically sense chest resistance and act as a current source would be a more effective therapeutic device.

**Automatic and Implantable Defibrillators.** One of the most exciting (and certainly the most controversial) ideas in ventricular defibrillation is the creation of a completely automatic defibrillator. It contains circuitry that detects the onset of ventricular fibrillation and, without the assistance of a human operator, applies a pulse of defibrillating current. Two practical forms for such a device have been proposed. In one, the automatic defibrillator is outside of the body and communication with the heart is via a transvenous catheter that incorporates the fibrillation-sensing system and the defibrillating electrodes. In the other concept, the defibrillator is totally implanted within the subject. A group of investigators at the Sinai Hospital and the Johns Hopkins University in Baltimore, led by M. Mirowski, is developing an automatic defibrillator. It is $87 \times 65 \times 32$ mm and weights 299 g. It has an output of 10 joules and employs electrodes located either on a transvenous catheter or placed directly on the apex and base of the heart. This device identifies fibrillation by monitoring the cardiac electrical activity recorded from the defibrillating electrodes. It differentiates the ECG and then analyzes the voltage waveform to identify the absence of isopotential segments. Additional processing consists of identifying the percentage of time spent by the signal between two amplitude limits. Once the presence of ventricular fibrillation is detected, the device delivers the defibrillating pulse via the ECG sensing electrodes.

It will not be long before surgeons will select suitable high-risk patients in the coronary-care unit for automatic defibrillation. Automatic defibrillation will probably enter clinical practice first with the transvenous catheter electrode in the right ventricle. Much valuable experience with this approach will lead to better identification of the candidates who can benefit from the surgical implantation of an automatic defibrillator.


# REFERENCES

ANDERSON, G. J., and J. SUELZER (1976). The efficacy of trapezoidal waveforms for ventricular defibrillation. *Chest,* 70: 293.

BABBS, C. F., and S. J. WHISTLER (1978). Evaluation of the operating internal resistance, inductance, and capacitance of intact damped sine wave defibrillators. *Med. Instrum.* 12: 34–37.

BECK, C. S., W. H. PRITCHARD, and H. S. FEIL, (1947). Ventricular fibrillation of long duration abolished by electric shock. *JAMA,* 135: 985–86.

BOURLAND, J. D., W. A. TACKER, and L. A. GEDDES (1978a). Strength-duration curves for trapezoidal waveforms of various tilts for transchest defibrillation in animals. *Med. Instrum.,* 12: 38–41.

BOURLAND, J. D., W. A. TACKER, L. A. GEDDES, and V. CHAFFEE (1978b). Comparative efficacy of damped sine wave and square wave current for transchest ventricular defibrillation in animals. *Med. Instrum.,* 12: 42–45.

EDMARK, K. (1963). Simultaneous voltage and current waveforms generated during internal and external direct current pulse defibrillation. *Surg. Forum,* 14: 262–64.

GEDDES, L. A. (1970). Electrical ventricular defibrillation. *Cardiovasc. Res. Ctr. Bull.,* 10: 3–42.

GEDDES, L. A., and W. A. TACKER (1971). Engineering and physiological considerations of direct capacitor-discharge ventricular defibrillation. *Med. Biol. Eng.,* 9: 185–99.

GEDDES, L. A., W. A. TACKER, J. MCFARLAND, and J. BOURLAND (1970). Strength-duration curves for ventricular defibrillation in dogs. *Circ. Res.,* 27: 551–60.

GOLD, J. H., J. C. SCHUDER, H. STOECKLE, T. A. GRANBERG, S. Z. HAMDANI, and J. M. RYCHLEWSKI (1978). Comparison of transthoracic square-wave defibrillation experience in the dog and calf. *Med. Instrum.,* Proc. 2nd Purdue Cardiac Defib. Conf.

GUINN, G. A., W. A. TACKER, L. A. REYES, F. L. KOROMPAI, and L. A. GEDDES (1974). Quantitation of required energy for direct human cardiac defibrillation. *Circulation,* 50(3): 229.

GURVICH, N. L., and G. S. YUNIEV (1947). Restoration of heart rhythm during fibrillation by a condenser discharge. *Am. Rev. Soviet Med.,* 4: 252–56.

GUTGESELL, H. P., W. A. TACKER, L. A. GEDDES, J. S. DAVIS, J. T. LIE, and D. G. MCNAMARA (1976). Energy dose for ventricular defibrillation of children. *Pediatrics,* 58(6): 898–901.

HOFFMANN, B. F., and P. F. CRANEFIELD (1960). *Electrophysiology of the heart.* New York: McGraw-Hill.

KERBER, R., and W. SARNAT (1977). Influence of body weight and heart weight on the success of defibrillation. *Circulation,* 55(Suppl III): 97.

LOWN, B. (1962). A new method for terminating cardiac arrhythmias: The use of synchronized capacitor discharge. *JAMA* 182: 566.

MACHIN, J. W. (1978). Thoracic impedance of human subjects. *Med. Biol. Eng. Comput.,* 16: 169–78.

PELESKA, B. (1963). Cardiac arrhythmias following condenser discharges and their dependence upon strength of current and phase of cardiac cycle. *Circ. Res.,* 13: 21–32.

PREVOST, J. L., and F. BATTELLI (1899a). Death by electric currents (alternating current). *CR Acad. de Sci.,* 128: 668–70.

PREVOST, J. L., and F. BATTELLI (1899b). Death by electric discharge. *CR Acad. de Sci.,* 129: 651–54.

PREVOST, J. L., and F. BATTELLI (1899c). Some effects of electric discharge on the hearts of mammals. *Comptes Rendus,* CXXIX, 129: 1267–68.

RESNEKOV, L. (1973). Present status of electroversion in the managment of cardiac dysrhythmias. *Circulation,* 17: 1356–63.

SCHUDER, J. C., J. H. GOLD, H. STOECKLE, T. A., GRANBERG, and K. A. LIES (1978). Defibrillation in the calf with 70 ampere truncated and untruncated exponential stimuli. *Proc. AAMI Annu. Meeting:* 238.

SCHUDER, J. C., G. A. RAHMOELLER, S. H. NELLIS, H. STOECKLE, and J. W. MACKENZIE (1967). Transthoracic ventricular defibrillation with very high amplitude rectangular pulses. *J. Appl. Physiol.,* 22: 1110–14.

SCHUDER, J. C., G. A. RAHMOELLER, and H. STOECKLE (1966). Transthoracic ventricular defibrillation with triangular and trapezoidal waveforms. *Circ. Res.,* 19: 689–94.

SCHUDER, J. C., H. STOECKLE, and J. H. GOLD (1975). Effectiveness of transthoracic ventricular defibrillation with square wave and trapezoidal waveforms. *Proc. Cardiac Defibrillation Conf.,* Purdue Univ.

SCHUDER, J. C., H. STOECKLE, J. A. WEST, and P. Y. KESKAR (1971). Transthoracic ventricular defibrillation in the dog with truncated and untruncated exponential stimuli. *IEEE Trans. Biomed. Eng.,* 18: 410–15.

STEPHENSON, H. E. (1974). *Cardiac arrest and resuscitation.* St. Louis: C. V. Mosby.

TACKER, W. A., and L. A. GEDDES (1980). *Electrical defibrillation.* Boca Raton, FL: CRC Press.

TACKER, W. A., G. A. GUINN, L. A. GEDDES, J. D. BOURLAND, and F. L. KOROMPAI (1978). The electrical dose for direct ventricular defibrillation in man. *J. Thoracic Cardiovasc. Surg.,* 75: 224–26.

ZOLL, P. M., A. J. LINENTHAL, W. GIBSON, M. H. PAUL, and L. R. NORMAN (1956a). Termination of ventricular fibrillation in man by externally applied electric countershock. *New Eng. J. Med.,* 254: 727–32.

ZOLL, P. M., A. J. LINENTHAL, L. R. NORMAN, M. H. PAUL, and W. GIBSON (1956b). Treatment of unexpected cardiac arrest by external electric stimulation of the heart. New Eng. J. Med., 254: 541–46.

# STUDY QUESTIONS

**3.1** An RLC defibrillator contains the following components:

$$C = 32 \ \mu F$$

$$L = 50 \ mH$$

The internal resistance (most of which is the resistance of the inductor coil) of the defibrillator is 15 $\Omega$.

(a) At what subject resistance is the output waveform critically damped?

(b) Plot a graph of energy delivered to the subject versus subject resistance, for subject resistance from 0 to 200 $\Omega$.

**3.2** The energy stored on the capacitor of a trapezoidal defibrillator before initiation of the output pulse is:

$$U_i = 0.5 \times C \times V_i^2$$

where   $C$ is the capacitance of the energy storage capacitor

and   $V_i$ is the voltage to which the capacitor is charged

At the end of the pulse, the energy remaining on the energy storage capacitor is:

$$U_f = 0.5 \times C \times V_f^2$$

where $V_f$ is the voltage on the energy storage capacitor at the time the current is truncated.

(a) Design a defibrillator that delivers the same energy to subjects with different resistances.

(b) Derive an expression for the duration of the output pulse.

# Cardiovascular Prostheses and Assist Devices

**4**

*Trevor B. Davey*
*Edward A. Smeloff*

## 4.1 LEARNING OBJECTIVES

Upon completing this chapter you will be able to:

- Describe the basic anatomy and physiology of the cardiovascular system.
- Discuss procedures used in cardiovascular medicine with cardiologists and cardiovasular surgeons.
- Describe those cardiovascular abnormalities that require prostheses or assist devices.
- Define and discuss the design parameters associated with various cardiac protheses and assist devices.

## 4.2 INTRODUCTION

Diseases of the heart and circulatory system account for more deaths in the United States than any other cause. Most major hospitals have extensive facilities devoted to the care of patients having cardiovascular problems. Industry and government spend hundreds of millions of dollars annually on research, development, and manufacture of devices used to treat cardiovascular diseases. There is a high probability that any graduate of a biomedical engineering program will at some time in his professional career become involved in technical problems associated with cardiovascular disease. In this chapter we introduce the biomedical engineer to the material necessary for an understanding of cardiovascular medicine and develop design parameters associated with various cardiac prostheses and assist devices.

## 4.3 ANATOMY AND PHYSIOLOGY

### Heart

Homeostasis, the constant and optimal environment of the body, requires the body to control concentrations of nutritive, hormonal and waste materials, tensions of respiratory gases, and temperature. Cellular activity is continuous and, in order to maintain this optimum environment, there must be an uninterrupted flow of blood. The function of the cardiovascular system is to supply this continuous flow and it is the heart that pumps the blood (Selkurt, 1976). Cardiac output, the flow of blood from the heart, and systemic arterial blood pressure are determined by the input pressure to the heart (central venous pressure), cardiac rate and contractility, and the total resistance of the peripheral vessels.

The human heart (Fig. 4.1) is suspended in the thoracic cage, at its base, by the great vessels. It has an asymmetrical position with its apex directed anteriorly, inferiorly, and about 60° towards the left (Netter, 1969). The heart has four chambers, two thin-walled atria on top and two thick-walled ventricles below. The atrial and ventricular septa divide it into right and left halves. The fibrous skeleton of the heart separates the atria from the ventricles and is also the mounting base of the four heart valves. The bundle of His passes through this skeleton, providing a conduction path between the atria and ventricles to the Purkinje fibers, which are the excitation conductors to the ventricular tissues. On a radiograph of the chest, the right ventricle lies anteriorly, with the left cardiac border formed by the left ventricle and the right border formed by the right atrium.

Venous blood returning to the right side of the heart first enters the easily expanded right atrium. It then passes through the tricuspid valve into the right ventricle. Contraction of the right ventricle moves the blood through the pulmonary valve into the lungs via the pulmonary arteries. The pulmonary capillaries approximate the alveoli to oxygenate the blood. The oxygenated blood then returns in the pulmonary veins to the left atrium. The mitral valve lies between the left atrium and left ventricle. The blood leaves the left ventricle through the aortic valve and flows into the aorta, which is the principal high-pressure arterial distribution system.

The heart valves function as check valves, permitting primary flow in one direction with a minimal amount of backflow or regurgitation. They are essentially passive, responding to the flow of blood. The aortic and pulmonary valves (also called semilunar valves) are similar in shape, each having three half-moon cusps or flaps attached symmetrically around the valve rings. The cusps are thin, flexible, tough membranes consisting primarily of collagen-reinforced endothelium. The tricuspid and mitral valves (sometimes called the atrioventricular valves) consist of cusps, chordae tendinae, and papillary muscles (Fig. 4.2). The atrioventricular

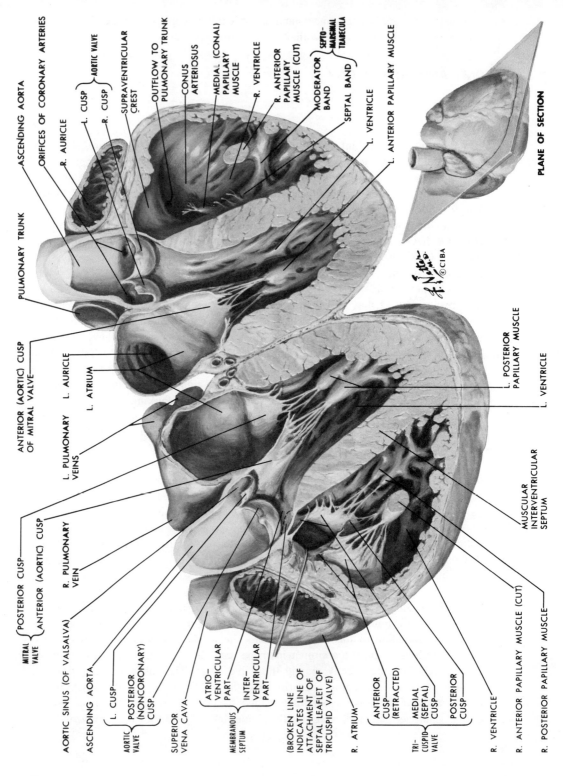

MITRAL {POSTERIOR CUSP
VALVE {ANTERIOR (AORTIC) CUSP

ANTERIOR (AORTIC) CUSP
OF MITRAL VALVE

AORTIC SINUS (OF VALSALVA)

ASCENDING AORTA

AORTIC {L. CUSP
VALVE {POSTERIOR (NONCORONARY) CUSP

SUPERIOR VENA CAVA

MEMBRANOUS SEPTUM {ATRIO-VENTRICULAR PART
{INTER-VENTRICULAR PART

(BROKEN LINE INDICATES LINE OF ATTACHMENT OF SEPTAL LEAFLET OF TRICUSPID VALVE)

R. ATRIUM

TRI-CUSPID VALVE {ANTERIOR CUSP (RETRACTED)
{MEDIAL (SEPTAL) CUSP
{POSTERIOR CUSP

R. VENTRICLE

R. ANTERIOR PAPILLARY MUSCLE

R. POSTERIOR PAPILLARY MUSCLE

MUSCULAR INTERVENTRICULAR SEPTUM

L. VENTRICLE

L. POSTERIOR PAPILLARY MUSCLE

L. PULMONARY VEINS

L. AURICLE

L. ATRIUM

R. PULMONARY VEIN

PULMONARY TRUNK

ASCENDING AORTA

ORIFICES OF CORONARY ARTERIES

R. AURICLE

AORTIC VALVE {L. CUSP
{R. CUSP

SUPRAVENTRICULAR CREST

OUTFLOW TO PULMONARY TRUNK

CONUS ARTERIOSUS

MEDIAL (CONAL) PAPILLARY MUSCLE

R. VENTRICLE

R. ANTERIOR PAPILLARY MUSCLE (CUT)

MODERATOR BAND {SEPTO-MARGINAL TRABECULA
SEPTAL BAND

L. VENTRICLE

L. ANTERIOR PAPILLARY MUSCLE

PLANE OF SECTION

ANTERIOR PAPILLARY MUSCLE

ANTERIOR CUSP (RETRACTED)

MEDIAL (SEPTAL) CUSP

POSTERIOR CUSP

F. Netter M.D. ©CIBA

valves are larger in area than the semilunar valves, resulting in lower pressure gradients during ventricular filling (diastole). During ventricular ejection (systole), there are greater forces on these larger orifices. The added support from the cordae tendinae and papillary muscles prevent eversion into the atria.

The smoothly rounded base of the cusps of the aortic valve reduces sharp angles and excessive eddying of blood that can lead to thrombus formation. There is a bulge in the wall of the aorta above and behind each of the cusps of the aortic valve called the sinus of Valsalva. During systole, the valve leaflets do not become flattened against the sinus walls. This prevents excessive flexing stresses and also eliminates possible interference with flow to the two coronary arteries located near the top of the sinuses. Fluid-dynamic force studies show that the sinuses of Valsalva have an important role in valve closure. The space behind each cusp permits an inflow–outflow vortical motion to be established when the valve opens. The pressure distribution associated with the vortical flow during the deceleration phase of the forward flow causes the cusps to move toward apposition, which results in a more rapid closure (Talbot and Berger, 1974). A similar effect occurs with the mitral valve, where a vortical flow develops within the ventricle through the combination of a starting vortex shed by the valve cusps on opening and the recirculation produced when the flow from the valve impinges on the apex of the ventricle. During systole, there is also an inward movement of the left ventricular wall, which decreases the cross-sectional area of the closed mitral valve. This reduces the stresses on this valve. There is also a small movement of the aortic (anterior) cusp of the mitral valve towards the left ventricular wall, which provides a smooth outflow path for blood flow through the aortic valve.

The pumping action of the heart is complex and involves a reduction in both diameter and length with the apex and base moving towards each other. There are additional factors affecting the emptying of the right ventricle, including a bellows-like action and a "left-ventricular aid" caused by a change in the curvature of the ventricular septum (Selkurt, 1976).

Figure 4.3 shows events of the cardiac cycle in the left heart. The cycle has seven phases (Selkurt, 1976), which are determined by relaxation and contraction states during systole and diastole.

Cardiac output, about 5.5 l/min in the average-size man, varies with heart rate, end-diastolic volume (preload), and end-systolic volume. The difference between end-diastolic volume and end-systolic volume is stroke volume. Stroke volume multiplied by heart rate equals cardiac output.

Heart rates in a normal adult at rest may vary from 40–100 beats/min. Because filling time decreases with increased heart rate, cardiac output decreases when heart rates exceed 60 beats/min unless compensatory mechanisms cause an increase in contractility. The heart reaches maximum cardiac output at about 180 beats/min.

FIGURE 4.1. (Facing page) Cross-section of the heart. © Copyright 1969 CIBA Pharmaceutical Company, Division of CIBA-GEIGY Corporation. Reproduced, with permission, from *The CIBA Collection of Medical Illustrations* by Frank H. Netter, M.D. All rights reserved.

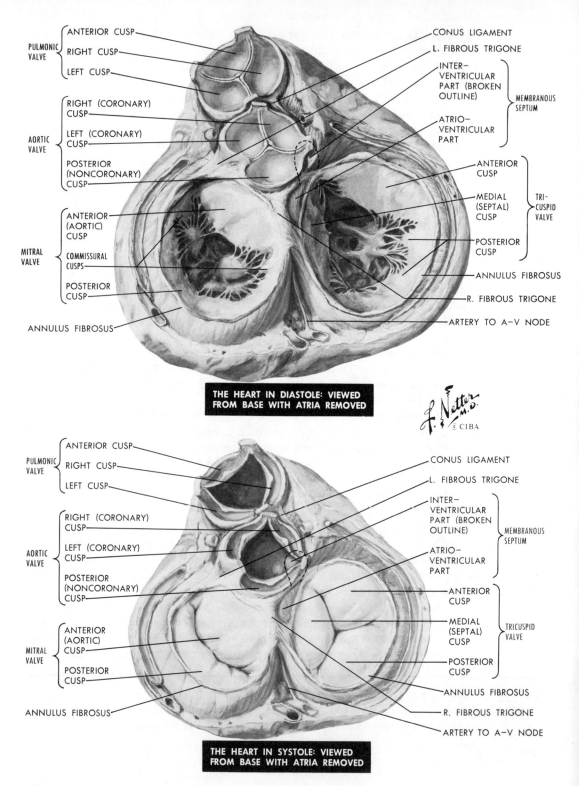

PULMONIC VALVE
- ANTERIOR CUSP
- RIGHT CUSP
- LEFT CUSP

AORTIC VALVE
- RIGHT (CORONARY) CUSP
- LEFT (CORONARY) CUSP
- POSTERIOR (NONCORONARY) CUSP

MITRAL VALVE
- ANTERIOR (AORTIC) CUSP
- COMMISSURAL CUSPS
- POSTERIOR CUSP

ANNULUS FIBROSUS

CONUS LIGAMENT

L. FIBROUS TRIGONE

MEMBRANOUS SEPTUM
- INTER-VENTRICULAR PART (BROKEN OUTLINE)
- ATRIO-VENTRICULAR PART

TRI-CUSPID VALVE
- ANTERIOR CUSP
- MEDIAL (SEPTAL) CUSP
- POSTERIOR CUSP

ANNULUS FIBROSUS

R. FIBROUS TRIGONE

ARTERY TO A–V NODE

**THE HEART IN DIASTOLE: VIEWED FROM BASE WITH ATRIA REMOVED**

PULMONIC VALVE
- ANTERIOR CUSP
- RIGHT CUSP
- LEFT CUSP

AORTIC VALVE
- RIGHT (CORONARY) CUSP
- LEFT (CORONARY) CUSP
- POSTERIOR (NONCORONARY) CUSP

MITRAL VALVE
- ANTERIOR (AORTIC) CUSP
- POSTERIOR CUSP

ANNULUS FIBROSUS

CONUS LIGAMENT

L. FIBROUS TRIGONE

MEMBRANOUS SEPTUM
- INTER-VENTRICULAR PART (BROKEN OUTLINE)
- ATRIO-VENTRICULAR PART

TRICUSPID VALVE
- ANTERIOR CUSP
- MEDIAL (SEPTAL) CUSP
- POSTERIOR CUSP

ANNULUS FIBROSUS

R. FIBROUS TRIGONE

ARTERY TO A–V NODE

**THE HEART IN SYSTOLE: VIEWED FROM BASE WITH ATRIA REMOVED**

*Cardiovascular Prostheses and Assist Devices*

End-diastolic volume, the volume of the ventricle before systole, varies with filling time, the effective filling pressure, distensibility of the ventricles, and atrial contraction.

Filling time is dependent on heart rate. The transmural pressure gradient, which is the pressure difference between the inside of the ventricles and the pressure outside, determines the effective filling pressure. This pressure gradient varies with the rate of venous return and the amount of negative thoracic pressure. The pericardium, which is not distensible, limits the magnitude of the end-diastolic volume.

End-systolic volume, the amount of blood remaining in the ventricle following systole, is determined by the arterial pressure load (afterload) and the strength of the intrinsic capability of the myocardial muscle to shorten and generate force (cardiac contractility).

Many factors influence contractility. Heart muscle tissue has the ability to increase work output independently of changes in fiber length or hormonal factors (homeometric autoregulation). This requires an increased supply of oxygen. Cardiac muscle contracts with greater tension if it is stretched. This is the Frank-Starling relationship (heterometric autoregulation). This is an important factor in maintaining a balanced output from the right and left ventricles. However, because end-diastolic volume is normally near maximum at rest, this does not have a significant effect on cardiac output over short periods of time. If the heart becomes dilated due to chronic disease as in ventricular hypertrophy, there are opposing effects. Myocardial viscosity and elastic forces are reduced tending to permit improved ventricular function. This is counterbalanced by the fact that a large heart requires a greater tension to eject a unit volume of blood against a given pressure (Laplace relation). Thus, a large hypertrophied heart often leads to cardiac failure.

An index of cardiac performance, $V_{max}$, measures the force–velocity relationship of contracting heart muscle. It is an application of the Hill model (Urschel and Sonnenblick, 1972) to the intact heart and is based on several assumptions that cannot directly be checked. Two major assumptions are: (1) during the isovolumetric contraction phase of the heart cycle, there is no significant muscle fiber shortening or ventricular shape change, that is, contraction is also isometric; (2) for isometric contraction, the differential of wall stress with time equals the differential of ventricular pressure with time. Calculations with these assumptions give the velocity of a contractile element, $V_{CE} = (dP/dt)/KP$, where $P$ is the left ventricular pressure and $K$ is a constant. Some investigators recommend use of developed pressure $P_D$ equal to $P$ minus EDP (end-diastolic pressure) to ensure independence of the index from preload. Plotting $V_{CE}$ versus $P_D$ during the isovolumetric phase and extrapolating the curve to zero pressure gives a value for $V_{max}$. There has not been a general clinical acceptance of $V_{max}$ as a determinant of cardiac performance, but it is widely used in biomedical research investigations.

---

FIGURE 4.2. (Facing page) Valves in open and closed positions, detailed valvular relationships. © Copyright 1969 CIBA Pharmaceutical Company, Division of CIBA-GEIGY Corporation. Reproduced, with permission, from *The CIBA Collection of Medical Illustrations* by Frank H. Netter, M.D. All rights reserved.

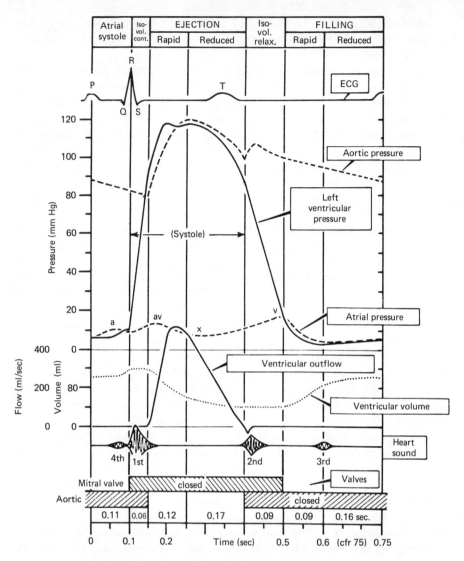

**FIGURE 4.3.** Events of the cardiac cycle. From *Physiology,* Selkurt; Little, Brown and Company.

Adequate coronary blood flow is essential for supplying sufficient oxygen to the myocardial cells. Although the heart can extract more oxygen from the blood and increase its efficiency, the principal mechanism for increasing oxygen availability is dilation of the coronary arterioles. Flow is also increased by a higher systemic arterial pressure. However, when the heart contracts during systole, the intramural (intramuscular) pressure may exceed arterial pressure, which causes coronary occlusion and stops blood flow. Therefore, 60–90% of blood flow in the coronary arteries occurs during the relaxation (diastolic) portion of the heart cycle, an important design consideration in heart assists where one objective is to increase coronary perfusion.

We can approximate the time rate of cardiac work (power) by multiplying the mean arterial pressure by the cardiac output. At rest, a cardiac output of 5.5 l/min and a mean arterial pressure of 95 mm Hg gives 69.6 J/min (1.2 W) of power in the left ventricle. The output of the right ventricle is about $\frac{1}{7}$ of this. Assuming an average cardiac efficiency of 20%, the input power to the heart is about 400 J/min (7 W). This requires approximately 20.6 ml/min of oxygen or 8% of the total body requirement.

## Vessels

The aorta and large arteries are heavy-walled vessels containing relatively large amounts of elastin and collagen in addition to smooth muscle. If we compare the large veins to their arterial counterparts, we note that they have larger diameters and thinner walls, which is consistent with their function as low-pressure conduits. The arteries contain about 10% of the total blood volume, the heart 10% and the large veins about 21%. The remaining volume is distributed in the capillaries, venules, and small veins.

The systemic arteries act as pressure reservoirs. The contracting left ventricle rapidly ejects blood into the aorta and other arteries, which become distended because their walls are elastic. During diastole when inflow to the system stops, the wall tension in the arteries continues to drive the blood through the peripheral arteries with a mean pressure of about 90 mmHg. When an artery bifurcates, the cross-sectional area of its branches exceeds that of the parent vessel. Thus, the aorta of a 80-kg man with a diameter of 2 cm and a cross-sectional area of 3 cm$^2$ has a total flow area of about 800 cm$^2$ in the arterioles.

The arterial pressure and velocity pulses are complex (Talbot and Berger, 1974). They are influenced by the geometry of the vessels, which taper and often curve and branch, the vessel distensibility, which is visco elastic in nature, and the physical properties of blood. The viscosity of blood has been found to be non-Newtonian both at very low and very high shear rates. The latter effect is small so that if shear rates exceed 100 s$^{-1}$, a constant Newtonian viscosity can be assigned to whole blood. Quantitative estimates of flow and pressure gradients can be made assuming the flow is steady and nonpulsatile. Peak Reynolds numbers in the circulatory system are approximately 3000–5000. These occur in the aortic root. Thus, for most analyses, the assumption of laminar flow is valid and pressure gradients can be calculated by Poiseuilles' equation.

Many investigators have attempted to analyze the pulsatile flow characteristics of blood in arteries and veins, although no complete satisfactory analysis exists at this time. Womersley, in 1957, included the effects of wall elasticity, fluid viscosity, and the coupling between fluid and wall motion and restraint of longitudinal motion of the wall, called tethering. However, his analysis, using Fourier techniques, does not correctly predict the evolution of the pulse contour observed in humans as the pulse travels from the heart to the extremities of the body. This is because it does not take fully into account vessel geometry. Anliker obtained good correlation with physiological data by using a one-dimensional flow that includes the effects of elastic and geometric taper, friction, and branching (Kenner, 1972).

## Blood

**Clotting.** Blood is a heterogeneous, non-Newtonian suspension of cellular elements in a complex aqueous continuous phase called plasma. Red cells (erythrocytes), which contain hemoglobin, are 97% of the total cell volume. White cells (leukocytes) of various categories make up less than 0.2% of the total cellular fraction and are involved in the immune reaction to foreign substances. The other formed elements are platelets, which are part of the blood-clotting mechanism. The plasma contains proteins, lipids, and carbohydrates.

Clot formation (thrombosis) involves the coagulation factors, which are numbered according to the order of their discovery I through XIII. (VI is not used). All of the factors, which are triggered in specific sequences, involve proteins except IV, which is a calcium ion (Sherry et al., 1969).

We can divide the coagulation mechanism into intrinsic and extrinsic pathways. A variety of stimuli trigger the intrinsic pathway. These include the contact of blood with glass and many other foreign materials, disturbances in blood flow such as stagnation or excessive turbulence, and hereditary disorders. When blood contacts an injured blood vessel, this triggers the extrinsic pathway. Both pathways represent the same basic interaction of platelet, plasma, and tissue factors (Ocumpaugh and Lee, 1971).

Sawyer et al. (1969) have shown that red cells and platelets have a negative surface potential in blood and also the intact intima of a blood vessel is negative to the adventitia. Injury alters this potential difference. There are inherent inhibitors in the blood that control clotting at each stage. Heparin, a natural anticoagulant, exhibits a high negative charge, which removes or depresses the $Ca^{++}$ ions necessary for the activation of prothrombin, one of the clotting factors.

**Hemolysis.** Hemolysis causes the liberation of free hemoglobin into the bloodstream through damage to the red blood cells. Evidence for the presence of intravascular hemolysis includes elevated serum hemoglobin, virtual absence of haptoglobin reduction in red blood cell life span, and the presence of fragmented cells in the circulating blood (Blackshear, 1972). Normally, red blood cells, which are produced in the bone marrow, live for 120 days and then are scavenged by the reticulo-endothelial system. Two factors usually cause mechanical hemolysis. One is the hammer and anvil effect, where the cells are physically crushed. The other factor is the abrasion or friction effect. Cells that come in physical contact with surfaces of foreign materials in the bloodstream adhere and become anchored. Exposure to shear stresses in excess of 4 $N/cm^2$ (40,000 dynes/$cm^2$) for short durations (1–100 ms) exceed the yield strength of the red cell membranes. Moderate shear stresses of 0.1–0.2 $N/cm^2$ (1,000–2,000 dynes/$cm^2$) caused by fluid turbulence can result in bulk hemolysis unrelated to interaction with walls if maintained for durations in excess of several seconds. Hemolysis can trigger the extrinsic clotting reaction and may also saturate the kidney, which leads to uremia.

**Cardiovascular Diseases.** Cardiovascular diseases may be congenital or acquired. About 70% of valve defects are due to rheumatic fever or bacterial endocarditis. The defect may be stenosis, where the valve becomes thickened and heavily calcified. This severely restricts blood flow. If the valve does not close properly and allows excessive regurgitation, the defect is called insufficiency. These problems may occur in any of the four heart valves but are much more common in the left side of the heart and involve either the aortic or mitral valve or both.

Atherosclerosis of the blood vessels reflects the accumulated effect of many factors acting over a lifetime and often is clinically mainifested only when complications such as thrombosis or aneurysms occur. Factors related to this disease include hypertension, smoking, obesity, diet, age, exercise, and genetic makeup. On arterial walls it causes deposition of sclerotic plaques, which, depending on their location, may lead to serious heart damage and death.

Heart failure where there is inadequate cardiac output occurs for a number of reasons. The principal ones include: (1) primary diseases of the myocardium, as in coronary artery disease, which may lead to myocardial infarction; (2) interference with the pumping or filling of the ventricles due to valvular disease or arterial hypertension; and (3) interference with systemic venous return, as in the case of hemorrhage or shock, pericardial tamponade, or tricuspid stenosis. When heart failure is accompanied by an abnormal increase in blood volume and interstitial fluid, this is called congestive heart failure (Selkurt, 1976).

## 4.4 CLINICAL ASPECTS

### Cardiovascular Diagnostic Procedures

Radiological techniques constitute the primary examination modality for evaluation of cardiac disease. Cineangiography provides us with chamber size, degree of pericardial, cardiac and coronary calcification, and data concerning the function and hemodynamics of the heart. Cardiac angiography is a procedure whereby we inject a radiopaque substance into the bloodstream at different locations and take x-ray motion pictures. Injection of contrast medium into the coronary arteries (cinecoronary arteriograms) reveals the location and severity of plaque build-up. Injection just downstream to a heart valve gives an indication of the amount of regurgitation through the valve. Release in a chamber upstream to the valve shows the degree of stenosis and also permits calculation of chamber volume at any time in the cardiac cycle and determination of ejection fraction (Jacobson and Webster, 1977). Calculation of ventricular volume requires the assumption that the ventricle is an ellipsoid of revolution whose measurements are taken from the x-ray projections. We can compute ventricular dynamics by using minute tantalum markers surgically attached to the ventricular walls to mark left-ventricular wall motion. Daughters et al. (1977) show good correlation for the two methods. Isotopic scanning techniques recently have expanded the ability to evaluate cardiac function.

Evaluation of valvular disease is also based on measuring pressure gradients and effective valve area. We can measure pressures in all four chambers of the heart and in the great vessels by positioning either a liquid-filled catheter or a miniaturized transducer during fluoroscopy. Resulting data permit calculation of valve gradients (Webster, 1978). To position the catheter in the left atrium, we must pass it retrograde through both the aortic and mitral valve. Therefore, cardiologists, in some patients, prefer to measure left atrial pressure by measuring pulmonary wedge pressure. This technique uses an inflated balloon-tipped, flow-directed catheter (Swan-Ganz). The cardiologist positions it without fluoroscopy into a small pulmonary artery where it wedges, blocking local flow. Because of the small pressure gradient across the capillary bed, the measured pulmonary wedge pressure is a replica of delayed mean atrial pressure. Calculation of pressure gradients requires shifting the pressure curves to the same time base.

For stenotic valves, we calculate effective valve orifice area using the Gorlin equation. This equation is based on hydraulic equations for steady flow through a sharp-edged orifice and requires measurement of cardiac output (using Fick, dye, or thermodilution methods) and valve gradients as previously described.

The equation is

$$VA = \frac{CO}{(C)\,(HR)\,(DFP)\,\sqrt{\Delta P}}$$

where  $VA$ is effective valve area

$CO$ is cardiac output

$HR$ is heart rate

$DFP$ is diastolic filling period (mitral valve)
        systolic ejection period (aortic valve)

$\Delta P$ is valve pressure gradient

$C$ is a constant that converts units and includes a discharge coefficient, which is different for each valve site. For a stenotic mitral valve, $C$ is 37.9–40 if pressures are in mm Hg, heart rate in beats/min, cardiac output in l/min, and diastolic filling period in s/beat (Hammermeister et al., 1973). $C$ is 44.5 for stenotic aortic valves.

We may also use echocardiography to study cardiac function. This technique utilizes ultrasound frequencies of 1–10 MHz at low power levels to visualize tissue and fluid interfaces. This method has the advantage of being noninvasive, providing a safe and simple procedure for studying the motion of valves and heart-wall movement. We can also use ultrasound to measure blood velocity in arteries and detect air embolism in the heart (Borik et al., 1973).

## Cardiovascular Surgery

Prior to 1954 and the introduction of cardiopulmonary bypass, surgical correction for heart disease was not widely practiced. The heart–lung machine allowed direct surgical approach to all areas of the heart. It led to the development of many new techniques, including procedures to replace defective heart valves, bypass coronary occlusions, and close atrial and ventricular septal defects.

In cardiopulmonary bypass (Fig. 4.4), cannulas inserted in both vena cavae or directly into the right atrium shunt venous blood returning to the heart to an extracorporeal circuit. The blood then flows into the oxygenator, where it picks up oxygen and eliminates carbon dioxide. The oxygenator may contain a heat exchanger for controlling blood temperature or the heat exchanger may be a separate device in the circuit. A pump then returns blood through a filter and bubble trap into a cannula connected to the aortic arch. The blood instead may be returned to a femoral artery, but this requires retrograde flow in the aorta, which results in an increased risk of dislodging arteriosclerotic plaques and causing embolism. The surgeon cross-clamps the aorta just above the sinuses of Valsalva, which isolates the heart and lungs. Cross-clamping of the aorta causes anoxic arrest of the heart. A drip of chilled Ringers solution containing Xylocaine is perfused into the base of the aorta near the coronary arteries. This prevents damage to the myocardial tissue during the period of interrupted coronary blood flow. Because a small quantity of blood from the bronchial arteries returns to the arrested heart in the pulmonary veins, the surgeon must vent the left ventricle with a small cannula in the apex to prevent dilatation. The cannula may also be positioned through the pulmonary vein across the mitral valve into the left ventricle. The heat exchanger in the heart–lung machine reduces body temperature to approximately 28°C. For most surgeries, the pump-oxygenator supports the patient for about an hour. Toward the end of the procedure, the surgeon rewarms the heart. Often it begins a normal rhythm as soon as the surgeon removes the cross-clamp from the aorta. It may be necessary to employ electrical defibrillation. The vent tube is used to remove entrapped air left in the heart following cardiotomy. Once normal beat and pressure have been established, the surgeon removes the cannulas from the vena cavae and aortic arch and closes the chest.

In open-heart surgery, a midline sternotomy usually exposes the heart. If a mitral valve is to be replaced, the approach is through the left atrium. An aortic valve replacement involves a transverse aortotomy just above the valve. For occlusive disease of a coronary artery, a section of removed saphenous vein bypasses the diseased area. Often, an electromagnetic flowmeter checks the flow in the vein graft.

## 4.5 ENGINEERING ASPECTS

### Material Selection

Proper selection of materials for devices to be used in the human body depends upon many factors (see Chapter 9). These must include an evaluation of the mechanical and physical properties necessary to achieve the desired function and an assessment of the compatibility of the material to the body environment. Design considerations should also ensure methods are available for production, quality control, sterilization, packaging, and delivery of these devices. The geometry of the devices inserted in the cardiovascular system may be critical in determining biocompatibility.

**Compatibility.** A major concern whenever we place a device constructed of

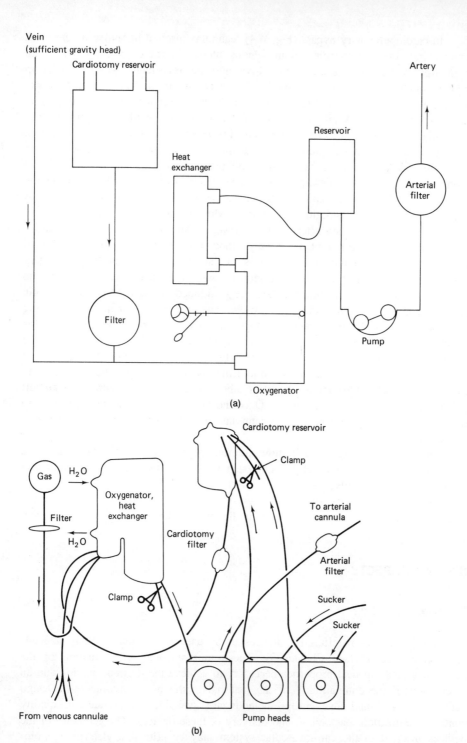

**FIGURE 4.4.** Cardiopulmonary bypass equipment set-up for a) membrane oxygenator b) bubble oxygenator.

foreign materials in the cardiovascular system is thromboembolism. Thrombus formation is the result of complex chemical reactions that occur at the blood–foreign-surface interface. The reaction rate is controlled by the interaction of patient, surface, and hemodynamic transport properties. Investigators have examined the physical and chemical properties of foreign surfaces that might relate to thrombus formation. They have examined surface roughness, wetability, surface charge, and streaming potential (Williams, 1971). It is impossible to predict with certainty the effect of materials on blood, although some guidelines are known. Consequently, we must base the use of any material on its clinical history. In the case of metals where tissue ingrowth is not a factor, they must be nonthrombogenic, corrosion resistant, highly polished, and scrupulously clean (Sawyer et al., 1969). Experience has shown that few metals meet all these criteria. Commercially pure titanium and a cobalt-chromium molybdenum alloy called stellite 21 have been used successfully in heart valves. Pyrolytic carbon, a ceramic, is very strong, wear resistant, and nonthrombogenic. The thromboresistant quality of pyrolytic carbon is due to its ability to maintain an intermediate absorbed layer of protein at the carbon-blood interface. This simulates the natural vascular lining without causing the appreciable alteration in protein molecules that trigger the intrinsic clotting mechanism (Bokros et al., 1975).

Polymers have been used more extensively than metals in devices that are immersed in the blood stream. Dacron, Teflon, silicone rubber, polypropylene, and polyurethane are materials that are suitable for long-term use in cardiovascular prostheses because of their nonthrombogenic, nontoxic, stable properties. If we desire endothelial tissue in-growth, as in the case of arterial grafts or the sewing cuffs of heart valves, the physical nature of the fabric is as important as the chemistry of the material in determining suitability. Textiles are quickly covered with a clot when placed in the bloodstream. The clot is organized into intima so that after a period of time, which varies with different species, the blood is no longer in contact with any foreign material. This reduces the possibility of thromboembolism. The amount of hemolysis caused by a material is also related to its surface roughness. For example, Dacron velours in arterial grafts cause excessive blood-cell damage. The ideal physical characteristics for the fabrics of a sewing cuff are a pore size from 90–125 $\mu$m and an open area range from 38–48% (Clark, 1974).

Medical-grade silicone rubber is used for indwelling catheters and the occluders of heart valves. As in the case of pyrolytic carbon, the nonthrombogenic properties of silicone rubber are related to its ability to absorb proteins from the blood so that its surface is altered. This results in reduced platelet adhesion.

Other important mechanical properties are tensile and shear strength, Young's modulus of elasticity, ductility and brittleness, fatigue and wear resistance, and corrosion potential.


## Hemodynamics

Both stagnation and excessive turbulence can lead to clot formation. Blood, because of its rheological properties, increases its viscosity by a factor of 5 to 10 times when arterial velocity decreases to zero. This increase is caused by the formation of protein bridges linking one red cell to another (Wells, 1969) and is related to thrombosis. In arteries where there is a lesion in the normally smooth intimal layer, particularly at branches of the aorta, thrombi originate with significant frequency. Thus, any device in the bloodstream should not have surfaces that are normal to flow, as this produces stasis. Changes in flow geometries such as bends, sudden contractions or expansions that result in separation can also result in stasis.

Excessive turbulence causes hemolysis. Red blood cells contain ADP and erythrocytin, a clot-promotion factor. These are released into the plasma when the red cell is damaged. The ADP and erythrocytin initiate platelet-adhesion aggregation and coagulation, which results in clot formation.

Talbot and Berger (1974) showed that endothelial cells on the aortic wall will be damaged if wall-shear stresses exceed 0.04 $N/cm^2$ (400 dynes/cm$^2$). Platelets do not adhere to intact endothelial cells, but they do become attached to subendothelial connective tissue that is composed of collagen, elastin, and smooth muscle. Thus, the lesion may lead to thrombus formation. This is particularly important in the design of prosthetic valves. Using a laser-Doppler anemometer for in vitro measurements, Yoganathan et al. (1978) reported shear stresses at the aortic wall in excess of 0.1 $N/cm^2$ (1000 dynes/cm$^2$) for flow rates of 167 ml/s (10 l/m) with some valve designs. This is one explanation for reports of aneurysms forming in the aortic roots of some patients with tilting disc-type valves. There are also reports of intimal thickening involving not only the ascending aorta and proximal coronary arteries but also the entire coronary bed in patients with many different types of prosthetic valves, particularly those that have central occluders.

## Testing

Because geometries and the biological environment are extremely complex, we must base design solutions for cardiovascular prostheses and assist devices primarily on testing rather than analysis. The testing of these devices includes three phases: (1) in vitro, (2) animal, and (3) human (Swanson and Clark, 1977). In vitro testing involves flow studies, durability tests, including fatigue and wear, and acoustical studies (Koorajian et al., 1969). Although testing in machines and animals prior to clinical trial often indicates potential design problems and contributes to their solution, it is also very important to understand the limitations of such tests.

**In Vitro Tests.** Mechanical testing devices that duplicate the heart or other components of the cardiovascular system must follow the laws of similarity. We must scale parameters such as shape, dimensions, flow rates, pulse rates, viscosity, density, and pressure curves close to normal physiological values. Heart simulators are an example of in vitro testing devices that are used to study prosthetic heart valves. These systems can determine pressure gradients, regurgitation, power consumption, areas of stasis and excessive turbulence, shear rates and show occluder motion in valves (Wieting et al., 1969).

Heart simulators or pulse duplicators as they are often called are designed to test valves in the aortic and/or mitral position (Smeloff et al., 1969). The two valve sites are quite different and we must base valve chambers on models of human hearts. Dimensions of the aortic root and left ventricle are obtained by injecting RTV silicone rubber into cadaver hearts and measuring the casting. We then machine these dimensions into a Plexiglas block to obtain a three-dimensional model of the aortic root. We keep the outside surface of the Plexiglas flat to eliminate distortion when photographing. A sac-type variable speed pump simulates the left ventricle. The pump drive operates through a cam or is programmed electrically to give physiological pressure curves and flow rates. We simulate systemic load by using flexible tubing for the aorta and discharging through a sponge that is compressible. A water–glycerol mixture (37% glycerol by volume) provides viscosity, density, and Reynolds number consistent with the values for blood.

We use this type of set up to visualize flow patterns in different types of valves. Collimated light passing through a slit illuminates suspended particles in the fluid. A high-speed camera provides photographs of areas of stasis and high turbulence. For pulsatile flow, transducers measure pressure gradients. Pressure-tap location is very important because we should measure pressure in regions where flow transition disturbances are negligible (Swanson and Clark, 1976). An electromagnetic flowmeter determines flow rates and regurgitation.

Rainer et al. (1977) used this type of test set up to analyze valve dynamics. They mounted three microminiature strain gages on the struts of an aortic ball valve cage to measure strain deformation. They compared values obtained from a valve inserted in an animal. In vivo forces were on the average 54% less than those obtained on the pulse duplicator. This is because the dampening effect of resilient tissue in the animal partially absorbs the forward impact of the poppet striking the cage leg as compared to the rigid mounting of the valve in the in vitro case.

Note that although most pulse duplicators are similar, there are small design differences in valve-chamber shape and pressure-tap location. Therefore, absolute values of pressure gradients obtained with different systems vary and comparisons may not be valid.

Fatigue and wear testers that determine durability are another class of in vitro testing devices. Because cardiovascular prostheses must often last for 10 years or more in the body, we conduct most testing of this type at highly accelerated frequencies. This generally eliminates heart simulators as suitable devices and requires some compromise on pressure and flow conditions with respect to physiological valves. If we simulate the cycle pressure amplitude and there is a full valve excursion when testing heart valves for durability, then we can obtain useful data on fatigue and wear characteristics. If durability tests are being conducted on polymers, they should be continuous and at 37°C. However, these kinds of tests cannot take into account changes with time in surface characteristics of materials reacting with blood or those due to tissue deposition. Thus, wear studies involving sliding and rotational friction may indicate the location of problem areas but not give realistic time data (Tabor, 1977). For example, in vitro tests on cloth-covered valves did not predict major clinical cloth wear problems encountered later with this type of prosthesis (Korrajian et al., 1969; Ranier et al., 1977).

**In Vivo Tests.** Animal tests of prostheses and assist devices have been done in many species, although those on dogs and calves are the most common. Sheep and pigs have also been suggested, but there is little experience with their use in procedures involving open-heart surgery. No animal, of course, has a cardiovascular system identical to man. Dogs have a more severe clotting mechanism than humans; their aortic root is very small and the tissue is very fragile, so that valves are usually tested only in the mitral position. Calves have been used for valve testing in both the mitral and tricuspid positions and occasionally in the aortic area (Braunwald and Bull, 1969). They are the usual test animal for heart assists and artificial mechanical hearts (Kolff and Lawson, 1975). Calves have a similar mechanism for the development of tissue layers on cloth, but the time rate is much faster. Two weeks in the calf is equivalent to 3 months in the human (Braunwald and Bull, 1969). Calves also have a rapid growth rate, which presents a problem for long-term studies of mechanical hearts. It is very difficult or impossible to simulate human cardiac disease in animals; thus, testing of devices under actual disease conditions is not possible. For example, the dog rarely develops arteriosclerosis and has a highly developed collateral coronary artery system, so that infarctions are very difficult to induce, even if the coronaries are artificially plugged or ligated. Although animal tests will give useful data on design, the ultimate test must be in man. It has been suggested that "a medical device is safe when its use is safer than the disease process for which it is used and it is the best device available for the purpose" (Beall, 1977). The testing of prostheses in humans is now governed by Public Law 94-295, the Medical Device Amendments Act of 1976 (Shaffer and Gordon, 1979). Specific procedures for heart valve testing have been proposed by the Association for the Advancement of Medical Instrumentation.

## 4.6 PUMP-OXYGENATORS

For technical reasons, intracardiac surgery normally requires the heart to be fibrillating or arrested during the operative procedures. In order to sustain life, we must pump the blood externally. The anatomical and physiological interactions of the heart–lung complex require the lungs to be bypassed also and their function included in the extracorporeal circulation. A heart–lung machine includes pumps, an oxygenator, a heat exchanger to control blood temperature, filters, and a bubble trap (Fig. 4.5). The machine may have four or five separate pump heads. Venous blood is shunted to the pump-oxygenator usually by gravity. However, some procedures may require a pump. A separate pump also sucks blood from a vent tube in the left ventricle and another pump head may operate a suction cannula. Arterial blood return requires a fourth pump head and a fifth head may be used as a spare.

### Roller Pumps

Roller pumps are used almost exclusively for nonpulsatile circulation of blood in pump-oxygenators. This pump uses a variable-speed, rotating armature. It compresses the walls of circular tubing and moves the blood in one direction (Wesolowski, 1966). Because the blood is contained entirely in sterile, disposable

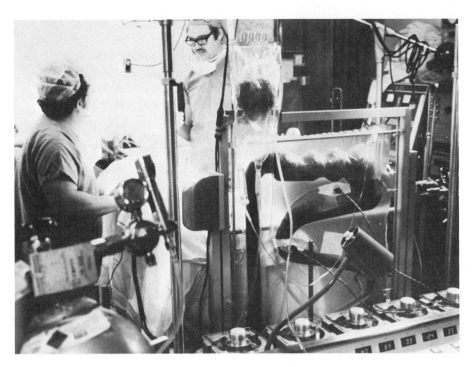

**FIGURE 4.5.** Cardiopulmonary bypass with a bubble oxygenator—operational set-up.

tubing, it does not directly contact the rollers. The outflow of the pump is proportional to the rotational speed of the rollers and therefore we can easily control it during surgery. Roller pumps do cause shear stresses in the blood that result in hemolysis, and so we must restrict their use to periods of a few hours.

We can minimize hemolysis if we take the following precautions (Myers and Parsonnet, 1969):

1. Use stiff vinyl plastic tubing instead of pliable rubber tubing. This reduces relative movement between the tube walls and the roller.
2. Use the largest diameter of tubing possible.
3. Use a nonocclusive setting for the roller. This also reduces tube wear.
4. Use lubricants such as silicone jelly or spray both inside and outside the tube to reduce blood damage and prolong tube life.

## Oxygenators

There are two groups of oxygenators, direct blood–gas contact and membrane. In both designs, we should have systems with the following features: (1) minimal blood trauma, (2) safety and reliability, (3) low cost, and (4) small blood-priming volumes. These design criteria are ultimately related to gas-exchange efficiency, which in turn is dependent on the relative rates of oxygen uptake and carbon dioxide removal. These rates should be physiologically balanced so that oxygen uptake exceeds carbon dioxide removal by approximately 30%.

**Direct Contact.** Direct blood–gas contact oxygenators are either film or bubble construction. They provide large surface areas for exposure of the blood to an atmosphere in which oxygen and carbon dioxide exchange is governed by the relative partial pressures. The film oxygenator has venous blood flowing over either a stationary surface such as wire mesh or on a moving surface such as a partially submerged spinning disc or cylinder. In bubble oxygenators, oxygen gas is dispersed directly into the entering venous blood at the bottom of a column. The resulting foam is then coalesced in a reservoir. The blood must then pass through a filter and bubble trap before it is returned, to ensure any remaining bubbles are removed. Figure 4.6 shows a hybrid oxygenator design where a combination of gas-bubble action and stable laminar blood-film flow permits rapid, effective gas exchange at oxygen to blood flow rates of about 1:1. This disposable system incorporates a venous side heat exchanger constructed of epoxy-coated aluminum. This surrounds the oxygenating column to regulate blood temperature during gas exchange and reduces the possibility of gas embolic formation.

**Membranes.** Direct contact of gaseous oxygen and blood causes blood trauma, mainly by denaturing plasma proteins and damaging the blood cells. This limits perfusion times to a few hours. When a thin semipermeable membrane separates the blood and gas phases, interfacial forces are reduced and damage to the proteins and formed elements is minimal. This allows the possibility of longer-term (i.e., several days) perfusion (Dorson and Vorhees, 1974). This may be vital in the treatment of some circulatory and respiratory diseases. It also has application in specialized areas such as organ preservation and transplantation.

Membrane oxygenators simulate the natural lung by dividing the blood flow into many membrane-lined thin films to provide the high surface-to-volume ratios necessary for rapid gas exchange. The membranes may be flat plates or closely spaced tubes. However, the membrane materials available to date cannot be fabricated to the scale of the natural lung and efficiencies are relatively low. Efficiency can be improved if there is convective mixing turbulence in the blood film. Therefore, many designs use geometries that induce secondary flow patterns or incorporate mechanical agitation.

**Design Criteria.** Analytic techniques for design of both direct contact and membrane type oxygenators have been developed (Spaeth, 1973, and Lightfoot, 1974). Analysis requires quantitative description of blood flow and gas diffusion. The chemical reactions between oxygen, carbon dioxide, and blood must also be specified in order to fully describe the convective gas transfer. Local chemical equilibrium is assumed to simplify calculation, a valid assumption for oxygenators designed with oxygen as the rate-limiting species. This includes all direct contact and some membrane systems.

Three general models representing increasing levels of mathematical complexity can be used to describe convective gas transfer in blood: macroscopic, coupled macroscopic-microscopic, and statistical. Although not suitable for actual design because of their complexity, these general models form the basis for simplified models that describe three limiting cases of general behavior. These are:

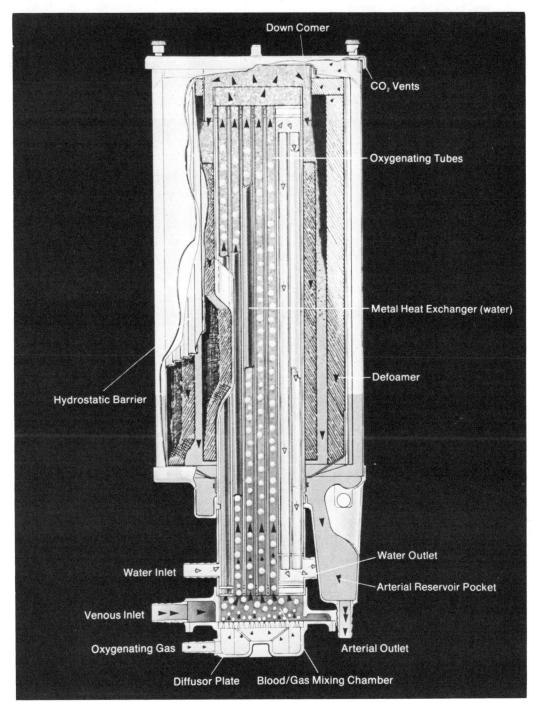

Down Comer

CO₂ Vents

Oxygenating Tubes

Metal Heat Exchanger (water)

Defoamer

Hydrostatic Barrier

Water Outlet

Arterial Reservoir Pocket

Water Inlet

Venous Inlet

Oxygenating Gas

Arterial Outlet

Diffusor Plate    Blood/Gas Mixing Chamber

**FIGURE 4.6.** Combined film-bubble oxygenator. Courtesy, William Harvey Corporation.

1. Gas exchange is limited by high resistance to convective diffusion in the blood—*blood-limited*. This condition is present in direct contact oxygenators and in some membrane oxygenators that have highly permeable membranes.

2. Gas exchange is limited by high resistance to diffusion in the membrane—*membrane-limited*. This occurs when either a low-permeability membrane is used or when the blood is well mixed, creating a very low blood-side resistance.

3. Gas exchange may become reaction-limited if transport through the membrane and fluid phase is very efficient—*reaction-limited*. This condition has not been achieved in present designs.

Calculations of oxygen transfer rates across blood–gas interfaces in direct contact oxygenators involve conditions of high Schmidt numbers, low interfacial stress, short contact times, and constantly deforming mass transfer surfaces. The Schmidt and Nusselt numbers are dimensionless mass transfer coefficients significant in similarity calculations. The Nusselt number ($h_D L/D$) and the Schmidt number ($\nu/D$) are functions of the Reynolds number ($VL/\nu$) where

$h_D$ = mass transfer coefficient

$D$ = diffusivity

$\nu$ = kinematic viscosity

$L$ = characteristic length

$V$ = velocity

Assuming a blood-limiting case with local equilibrium conditions, the mass of oxygen transferred across an element of reference area $dS_0$ in the time $\lambda$ for the above conditions is given by the following equation:

$$\frac{dm_{O_2}}{dS_0} = \frac{\lambda a (P_I - P_V)\, D_{O_2,B}\, (N_{u_{\text{local}}})}{L}$$

where $a$ = solubility of oxygen in blood $\cong 0.3 \times 10^{-4}$ ml[STP]/ml-mm Hg

$P_I$ = partial pressure of oxygen at the interface (mm Hg)

$P_V$ = partial pressure of oxygen in venous blood (mm Hg)

$D_{O_2,B}$ = diffusivity of oxygen in blood $\cong 0.8 \times 10^{-5}$ cm$^2$/s

$L$ = characteristic length (cm)

$N_{u_{\text{local}}}$ = local Nusselt number

$$= -\pi(O)' \sqrt{\frac{L^2}{D_{O_2,B}\, \lambda}} \; \sqrt{\frac{1}{\lambda} \int_0^{\lambda} \left(\frac{S}{S_0}\right)^2 d\lambda}$$

where $\pi(O)' = [44.6 + \sqrt{3.81 \times 10^3 - (83.5\ P_V)}]\ [P_I]^b$

$\qquad b \qquad = -0.5\ [\sin\ (1.02 + \dfrac{P_V}{67.1})]$

$\qquad \dfrac{S}{S_0} \quad = $ degree of blood film surface stretch $\cong 1$ for rigid rotation

These equations can be used over the range:

$$20 < P_V < 40 \text{ mm Hg}$$
$$70 < P_I < 760 \text{ mm Hg}$$

Typical physiological conditions are $P_I = 100$ mm Hg and $P_V = 40$ mm Hg. During bypass, the values are approximately 700 and 40 mm Hg respectively.

This technique has been used successfully to estimate the performance of a Kay-Cross disc oxygenator (Lightfoot, 1974).

Mass transfer in membrane oxygenators involves conditions of high Schmidt numbers, high interfacial stresses, retarded flow near the interface, and fixed interfacial geometry. The coupled phenomena of diffusion through both the solid (membrane) and fluid (blood) phases must be considered simultaneously. The gas-phase mass-transfer resistance can be neglected. Although current designs use highly permeable silicone rubber membranes, induced secondary flow patterns mix the blood sufficiently to cause gas transfer conditions to be membrane-limited. Analysis and experience have shown that in blood-limited oxygenators, too much carbon dioxide is removed whereas in membrane-limited oxygenators, too little carbon dioxide is removed. Therefore, in the latter case, the rate-limiting species is carbon dioxide and this must be the design-controlling factor. For a membrane-limited system with two parallel plate silicone rubber membranes, the oxygenator length required to reduce the partial pressure of the carbon dioxide in blood from $P_O$ to $P_L$ is given by

$$L = \frac{K\ Q_B\ t}{2W\ Da_{CO_2,M}}\ \ln\left(\frac{P_0}{P_L}\right)$$

where $K$ is a proportionality constant $\approx 2.5 \times 10^{-4}$ mol $\cdot$ liter$^{-1}$ $\cdot$ mm Hg$^{-1}$

$\qquad Q_B \qquad$ = blood flow rate (ml/s).

$\qquad t \qquad\quad$ = thickness of the membrane (cm)

$\qquad W \qquad$ = width of plates (cm)

$\qquad Da_{CO_2,M}$ = permeability of the membrane to carbon dioxide

$\qquad\qquad\qquad$ = $8.33 \times 10^{-11}$ mol $\cdot$ cm$^{-2}$ $\cdot$ min$^{-1}$ $\cdot$ mm Hg$^{-1}$ $\cdot$ cm

A similar analysis for a silicone rubber tube gives the following equation:

$$L = \frac{K \ Q_B \ \ln\left(\frac{R_o}{R_i}\right)}{2 \ \pi \ Da_{CO_2,M}} \ln\left(\frac{P_0}{P_L}\right)$$

where $R_o$ = outside radius of the tube (cm)

$R_i$ = inside radius of the tube (cm)

The priming volume $V_p$ for a parallel plate system with $N$ identical plates is given by the equation:

$$V_p = N \ (WhL)$$

Substituting for the product $(WL)$ from the above equation:

$$V_p = \frac{h \ (K \ Q_T \ t)}{2 \ Da_{CO_2,M}} \ln \left(\frac{P_0}{P_L}\right)$$

where $h$ = plate spacing (cm)

$Q_T$ = total blood flow (ml/s)

= $NQ_B$

This equation shows that priming volume is independent of the number of plates used in the design. Thus, the oxygenator can be designed for minimum pressure gradient by using many short channels in parallel, limited only by the practical consideration of manifolding a large number of channels. Priming volume can be further minimized by using thinner membranes and small gap spacing.

The corresponding equation for a silicone rubber membrane-limited oxygenator with multiple tube construction and a reduction in partial pressure from 50 mm Hg to 40 mm Hg is

$$V_p = 2.8 \times 10^{-8} \left[\frac{Q_T \ R_i^2}{Da_{CO_2,M}}\right] \ln \left(\frac{R_o}{R_i}\right)$$

One measure of overall oxygenator efficiency is the ratio of total flow rate of priming volume = $Q_T/V_p$ = 336 $(h)(t)$ for a membrane-limited parallel plate system using silicone rubber.

The efficiency for a normal resting man with pulmonary blood flow of 3,000 ml/min and a lung capillary volume of about 100 ml is 30 min$^{-1}$. During exercise, the efficiency may increase to 150 min$^{-1}$. A 25-$\mu$m silicone rubber parallel plate membrane oxygenator with membrane-limiting gas exchange has an efficiency of about 12 min$^{-1}$. Multiple silicone rubber tubes with $R_i$ = 0.012 in., $R_o$ = 0.025 in. have an efficiency of 17.5 min$^{-1}$.

Careful biomedical engineering design can increase the mass transfer efficiency per unit area in artificial lungs (oxygenators) to almost compensate for the inherent advantage of the enormous interfacial area resulting from the microstructure of the natural lung.

## 4.7 HEART VALVES

Many concepts have been proposed and tried as replacements for defective human heart valves. Ball and disc valve designs have proven to be reliable long-term mechanical substitutes and the advantages of porcine xenograft prostheses have led to their extensive use. However, no one has developed the perfect heart valve prosthesis. Such a design would have to contain all the features of normal human valves plus be completely resistant to disease. No known substitute material can meet these requirements. Thus, heart valve design requires a trade-off of various factors to achieve an optimal solution.

### *Mechanical*

**Configurations.** Ball and disc valves have an occluder that sits in an orifice to prevent backflow in the closed position. It moves out of the orifice to a retaining structure in the open position. The occluder may be a spherical ball, a free floating flat or streamlined lens that moves essentially perpendicular to blood flow, a flat hingeless tilting disc that rotates 60–70° to the open position, or flat leaflets that move parallel to blood flow when the valve opens (Fig. 4.7).

The different configurations each have advantages. The ball valve is durable, has good hemodynamics to minimize gradients and hemolysis, and has the longest history of clinical use (Davey and Smeloff, 1977). Disc valves have the advantage of lower profiles, which may be particularly important in mitral valve replacement with a small left ventricle. This prevents cage strut impingement on the ventricular septum and helps to retain a good left ventricular outflow path. Caged disc valves exhibit the poorest hemodynamics, which results in relatively high gradients and hemolysis, although these problems can be reduced by using a streamlined double-cone lens (Cooley, 1977). Hingeless pivoting disc valves have good hemodynamics with lower hemolysis and pressure gradients than other disc configurations (Lillehei, 1977; Bjork, 1977). However, they require specific orientation in the valve annulus and may cause excessive shear rates in small aortic roots (Sauvage, 1977; Yoganathan et al., 1978). All mechanical prostheses require permanent use of anticoagulant agents to keep thromboembolism at acceptable levels.

**Design Criteria.** Each valve configuration has specific design requirements. General criteria applicable to all mechanical valves are:

1. Hemodynamic properties must ensure adequate forward flow with minimal pressure gradients and regurgitation. The characteristics of blood flow through a prosthetic valve depend on the shape and size of flow areas in the valve and related anatomical structures, and the type of occluder used. We must consider several flow

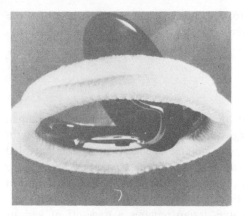

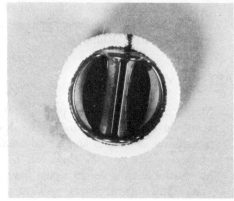

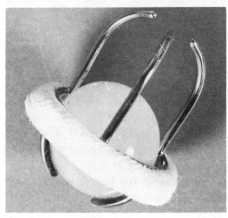

**FIGURE 4.7.** Mechanical-
heart valve prostheses: Bottom
left; Smeloff mitral ball valve.
Top left: Bjork-Shiley tilting disc
valve. Top right: St. Jude medical
leaflet valve.

areas. The primary area is the orifice in the valve ring, which must be as large as
possible. Closely related to the orifice area is the tissue annulus area. The ratio
($A_{\text{tissue}}$) : ($A_{\text{orifice}}$) should be minimized to ensure minimal obstruction of flow. The
shape of the orifice is also important. We must avoid a sharp-edged orifice because
of the vena contracta effect. Instead, all edges should be curved for streamlined
flow, which minimizes turbulence. A secondary area is the flow area created
between the occluder and the valve ring when the valve is open. In a ball valve,
this is the lateral area of the frustum of a right circular cone and it should not be
less than the primary orifice area. In ball valves, another important flow area is
present in the aortic root between the occluder and the sinus wall when the ball is
in the open position. If this area is small, as in the case of a large diameter ball and
a small aortic root, the valve causes stenosis. There may be excessive shear rates at
the wall, which cause damage to the endothelium.

We can study hemodynamic properties using pulse duplicator techniques
described earlier. Unusual behavior in valves such as ball bounce and lateral
wobble, disc cocking, and excessive occluder closing times can be observed if inlet
flow is closely modeled to physiological conditions.

2. The valve must not be thrombogenic or cause damage to blood elements.

Thrombus formation and hemolysis are dependent on hemodynamics, material characteristics, and valve geometry. Stasis, which causes thrombus formation, can occur if there is flow separation from a surface or if a surface projects normal to the flow. Valve cages must have curved orifice throats and no crossing struts to avoid these conditions. Because cloth–metal interfaces often lead to thromboembolism, these areas must be constantly washed during all phases of the cardiac cycle. We can accomplish this by allowing a small regurgitation when the valve is closed.

Excessive turbulence and high shear stresses cause damage to red cells, denaturation of lipoprotein, and contribute to thrombogenicity. They also lead to higher pressure gradients. The shape and location of the occluder influence this. A flat lens perpendicular to flow will cause greater turbulence than a ball. A tilted disc has areas of turbulence and stasis that vary with the opening angle of the disc. This requires a design trade-off because closing time is also related to opening angle. If the opening angle is too large, there is a delay in closing that allows excessive regurgitation.

3. Ideally, a valve prosthesis should last for 20 to 30 years, although 10 years without degeneration has been considered satisfactory. The heart beats approximately 42 million times a year and materials may fail due to fatigue and wear stresses or because they are not inert in blood.

We can avoid fatigue failure of metals by proper design and quality control. Inadequate stress relief, impurities, and poor grain microstructure are potential causes of problems. Accelerated fatigue tests of cage struts give realistic data on durability of these components.

Wear is more difficult to predict and depends on many factors, including lubrication, adhesion, material transfer, and relative hardness (Kar and Bahadur, 1977). Although in vitro tests may give some indication of wear strength, it is impossible to simulate the blood environment and its effect on materials. Silicone rubber balls in valves rotate randomly and their surface is lubricated by blood so that sliding wear on metal struts is insignificant. Silicone rubber lens in disc valves failed, however, because the disc could not rotate and this concentrated wear at one point. Pyrolytic carbon discs that have sufficient wear strength solved this wear problem. Complete covering of valve cages with Dacron or polypropylene cloth was utilized clinically with the expectation that endothelization of the cloth would decrease thromboembolism. Because tissue ingrowth was not fully developed for several months, excessive cloth wear occurred in aortic valves with silicone rubber balls. Fabric destruction was more severe in valves with metal balls and there was also evidence of mitral valve wear (Ranier et al., 1977). Similarly, experience has shown that wear of a silicone rubber ball rubbing against a suture or cloth on the strut or calcified tissue can reduce its diameter sufficiently to allow escape from the cage.

Early ball valves with silicone poppets had severe problems because of ball variance. Ball variance is defined as faceting, shrinking, and even splitting of the ball and has been associated with absorption of complex lipids into the silicone rubber (Carmen and Mutha, 1972). Studies have correlated this problem with the amount of turbulence in the valve orifice and the cure time and temperature of the silicone rubber. Proper design of the orifice and a low-temperature cure has made incidence of this problem negligible. Hollow metal balls, both titanium and stellite, introduced as alternatives for dimensional stability, caused high hemolysis rates.

4. The valve should not interfere with cardiac function. This is primarily related to the overall dimensions of the valve. With a small left ventricular cavity sometimes associated with mitral valve stenosis, a large cage impinges on surrounding structures of the heart. If the valve is too large, there are excessive shear rates and high gradients in small aortic roots. In these situations, low-profile valves having disc or leaflet configurations have an advantage. In a ball valve, we can reduce overall size by using the full-orifice concept, in which ball diameter and orifice diameter are essentially equal. For a given orifice size, the ball diameter is smaller than that necessary for an orifice-seating valve. This allows use of a shorter cage and results in a faster closing response because of the reduced inertia.

5. Valve attachment must be simple and secure. All present valves use Dacron or Teflon cloth rims, which allow tissue ingrowth for anchoring. Interrupted suture techniques are safer, although continuous sutures reduce the number of knots required. Paravalvular leaks are usually caused by tissue failure rather than suture breaks. However, suture placement may affect valve performance (Ranier et al., 1977). We may reduce tissue failure by using Teflon felt pledgets for suture butresses, but this can cause early hemolysis and late fibrosis.

6. We must design valves to allow manufacturing and quality control standards consistent with their medical use. We must consider sterilization procedures and their effect on materials. Because the size of valve required cannot be determined prior to surgery, several different sizes must be available and, consequently, they may undergo repeated sterilization. We require suitable designs for valve holders, obdurators for sizing, and packaging, as well as complete instructions for their use.

7. Patients with prosthetic valves should experience significant improvement in cardiac function and be able to lead relatively normal lives. The prosthesis should not restrict activities or lead to patient discomfort. The valve must operate independent of body position. In ball valves, the specific gravity of poppets should be close to that of blood (1.04). Noise associated with occluder movement must not be audible, as this can lead to psychological problems. Cost should be kept reasonable to ensure acceptability.

## *Bioprosthesis*

A major problem associated with prosthetic heart valves is the need for anticoagulant therapy to prevent thromboembolism. Tissue valves were originally designed to act as a framework for host fibroblast infiltration that would lead, in time, to complete regeneration of the valve and potentially eliminate the requirement of anticoagulants. This concept, although theoretically possible, was not successful, as cellular ingrowth was often inflammatory in the untreated tissue (Carpentier, 1977). Research was then directed toward developing chemical treatments to prevent graft-tissue collagen degeneration and using fabric covering over the outer sheath to prevent host cell penetration. Although general design requirements for bioprotheses are similar to those outlined previously for mechanical valves, there are special considerations.

**Tissue Preparation.** Studies have shown that aortic porcine valves are similar in size and most suitable as replacements for human valves even though there are anatomical differences. In the animal, the intraventricular wall extends to the base of the right coronary cusp and acts as a support. Mounting structures for the valves must take this into account.

Several substances were tried as preservatives to reduce antigenicity and improve long-term stability. These included different solutions of mercury salts, formaldehyde, and glutaraldehyde. The chemical treatments, which are temperature dependent, caused new cross-linkages to form in collagen molecules or reinforced existing ones. Animal testing and clinical experience showed the glutaraldehyde-preserved xenograft had the best durability.

**Stent Design.** The mounting structure or stent must preserve normal function and absorb stresses. Therefore, the valve requires a flexible stent that is carefully shaped to the configuration of the donor valve (Fig. 4.8). The resilient stent can be made from a noncorrosive metal wire or plastic that is completely covered by a Dacron or Teflon cloth sleeve, to which the tissue graft is sutured. We may use felt packing to protect the cloth and suture from wearing on the stent. The cloth sleeve also supports the rim used to suture the valve to the annulus. Cloth placed over the tissue graft along the stent minimizes reaction from bioprosthesis antigens. The struts preserve natural cusp size and have a slight asymmetry to incorporate the muscular part of the right coronary cusp into the stent.


## Clinical Experience

Well over 200,000 mechanical and tissue valves have been implanted in humans. The mechanical prostheses, primarily ball and disc configurations, have the longest clinical history. Valve-related complications are generally due to thromboembolism, valvular leakage due to suture separation at the annulus, or bleeding secondary to anticoagulant therapy. Experience gained with the Smeloff-Cutter ball valve over a 10-year period is an example of the results obtained (McHenry et al., 1978). The study included 83 aortic valve and 130 mitral valve replacements. There were 25 aortic and 16 mitral valve late deaths, with half occurring in the first year following surgery. Seventy-five percent survived 5 years or more. Fourteen late deaths, 6 aortic and 8 mitral, had valve-related complications. In patients with aortic valve replacement, 79% improved by one or more categories according to American Heart Association criteria, and similarly 81% of the mitral valve replacement showed improvement. Thromboembolism occurred in 3% of the aortic valve and 9.5% of the mitral valve replacements for an overall 5.2%. Lefrak and Starr (1979) and Sarma et al. (1977) reported average pressure gradients of 14 mm Hg in aortic and 5.2 mm Hg in mitral valve replacements.

Over 30,000 glutaraldehyde-fixed porcine valves have been implanted with a maximum clinical history of about 7 years. Clinical data indicate a good early survival rate and low rates of thromboembolism, although anticoagulant therapy

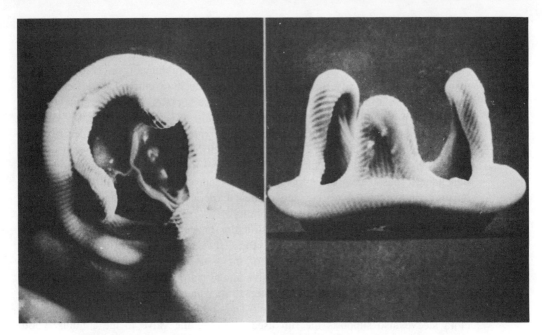

**FIGURE 4.8.** Porcine Bioprosthesis. Left: Top View. Right: Side View.

recommendations are still being evaluated. Bioprostheses have relatively small orifice areas. This causes significant stenosis, especially in the smaller sizes, and results in excessive pressure gradients. Design modifications, in which the leaflet containing the septal shelf has been replaced by a leaflet from another valve, have resulted in significantly lower gradients (Wright, 1977). No one has determined the life expectancy of these valves. Clinical studies have shown that porcine xenografts are not biologically inert in man (Spray and Roberts, 1977) and their durability may be limited to about 10 years due to structural stresses in the leaflets (Clark and Swanson, 1979).

## 4.8 ARTERIAL GRAFT PROSTHESES

Replacement of arteries with tubes made from synthetic materials was first reported in 1954 (Edwards, 1978). Despite design improvements utilizing new fabricating techniques and materials, a prosthetic graft that maintains flexibility and luminal integrity in all instances is not yet available. In small (less then 8 mm) vessel grafts, such as those used in coronary artery bypass, saphenous vein autograft is still considered the standard and prosthetic vascular grafts are used only if there are no alternatives.

Vascular grafts should be fabricated from materials in accordance with these design criteria:

1. They should be seamless and available in various sizes.

2. The material must have low porosity to control blood loss.

3. The material should not fray or ravel, be easy to handle, and permit suturing without cuffs wherever it is cut by the surgeon.

4. The tube must be flexible and not kink when bent.

5. The design must provide for bifurcations and branches.

6. Permanent synthetic suture material must be used to ensure long-term integrity of the anastomosis.

Dacron and Teflon are used for graft materials. The cloth can be woven or knitted. An important property of the cloth is porosity. Weaving permits a lower porosity. This is necessary to prevent excessive bleeding in thoracic aortic replacement when heparin anticoagulation is used. However, in vessels smaller than the aorta, embolization of the neointima with subsequent occlusion has occurred at higher rates in tightly woven grafts. Consequently, grafts for vessels in the abdomen and extremities are made from knitted cloth that must be preclotted. To reduce the possibility of kinks in the cloth, the tubes are permanently crimped during manufacture. However, fibrous tissue ingrowth will cause the implant to become rigid and lose its ability to resist kinking. The use of prosthetic grafts to replace arteries that are frequently flexed, such as those that cross the knee joint, is not recommended.

Antithrombogenicity of a graft is determined by the degree of neo-intimal healing in the graft. If there are even small unhealed granulation areas, clotting of the stagnant blood is rapid. Graft designs were developed that tried to promote tissue ingrowth by using single- and double-velour construction. Clinical results were not satisfactory, particularly in the smaller sizes.

Low porosity, extruded polytetrafluorethylene (PTFE) is a recently developed material that purportedly allows tissue ingrowth about the microfilaments. Our experience with this graft as a single layer has shown almost uniform dilatation and aneurysm formation with thrombosis or rupture. A two-layer laminated graft of this material has given better clinical results but continues to have disappointing evidence of late occlusion. Preserved umbilical cord veins have recently been introduced as a homologous graft and warrant evaluation. They require careful preparation and washing out of the preservative to avoid thrombotic occlusion.

## 4.9 HEART ASSISTS

Design and development of cardiac assist devices that relieve acute or chronic heart failure is a current, top-priority research goal. Objectives range from temporary left-ventricular support systems for patients that cannot be weaned from cardiopulmonary bypass to permanently implanted devices for assisting hearts in chronic failure.

Most concepts use counterpulsation or auxiliary left ventricles (Kaufman et al., 1968). In counterpulsation, an additional pulse is applied in the aorta during diastole to increase coronary blood flow and decrease heart work by lowering afterload. This is effective in some acute situations. Auxiliary ventricles that take over the pumping work of the left heart are used in chronic applications where long-term or permanent assistance is necessary.

Development of cardiac assist devices is complicated by the fact that design criteria must sometimes be based on clinical requirements that are not fully specified because of unknown physiological factors. Consequently, a system that meets specifications may not provide effective support in all recommended clinical applications.

### Counterpulsation

The most widely used and simplest clinical assist device for cases of shock and low cardiac output is the intra-aortic balloon (Kolff and Lawson, 1975). The surgeon introduces a nonthrombogenic smooth polyurethane balloon attached to an external pumping system by a catheter through the femoral artery. It passes into the descending thoracic aorta with the balloon tip reaching the aortic arch. The balloon is rapidly inflated by a gas during early diastole and deflated during early systole. An ECG input synchronizes inflate and deflate times with the cardiac cycle (Fig. 4.9). Inflation in diastole augments arterial diastolic or coronary perfusion pressure; deflation in systole reduces the aortic impedance to ventricular ejection. These actions improve metabolic supply–demand ratios in the ischemic heart and reduce the possibility of an infarct, or minimize its size if one occurs.

Although simple in concept, intra-aortic balloon counterpulsation effectiveness depends on many factors. These include the relationships between aortic instantaneous impedance and blood flow, balloon volume and left-ventricular ejection, and timing. Thus, optimal use of this equipment requires reliable and easily read monitoring systems for recording ECG and arterial blood pressure so the system can be tuned to individual patient requirements. Electrical safety considerations, possible balloon leaks, complications related to arterial cannulation, and operator training are problems that must be considered during system design. A subcommittee of the American Society for Artificial Internal Organs recommends standards to cover balloon and catheter design, timing and safety requirements, console design, and packaging, training, maintenance, and service specifications (Kennedy, 1974).

If we use a single cylindrical balloon, the ends of the balloon inflate first, which traps blood and subjects the proximal aorta to pressures far exceeding normal physiological levels (Jones, 1972). We can limit this phenomenon, called *bubble trapping,* by dividing the balloon along its length into a number of segments, usually three, and inflating the compartments selectively by using orifices of different diameters. The balloon diameter should be slightly smaller than the diameter of the aorta. Balloon volumes for clinical use usually range from 20 to 40 ml. Gas pressures from the compressor-vacuum pump usually do not exceed 250 mm Hg with a normal range of 0–100 mm Hg. The gas used for balloon inflation can be helium or carbon dioxide. Helium is safer because it diffuses quickly through the arterial wall due to its small molecular size. It will also give the highest response time. Carbon dioxide released into the blood increases pH levels and could cause acidosis.

Precise timing is critical in all counter-pulsation augmentation systems. Variations of a few milliseconds can be important. Because triggering is based on ECG timing and has to be coordinated with arterial pressure, we must compensate for time delays associated with different transducer locations when adjusting the inflate

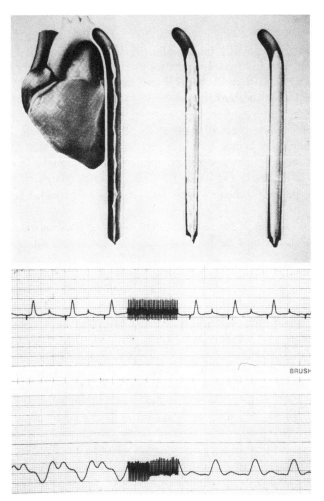

BRUSH

**FIGURE 4.9.** Intra-aortic balloon inserted in the descending aorta. Courtesy, Roche Medical Electronics Inc. and Avco Medical Products. Top: Expansion cycle of balloon. Middle: ECG showing inflate and deflate markers. Bottom: Arterial pressure curve with the balloon operating (left) and turned off (right).

cycle. A simple rule of thumb helps to avoid serious timing errors. Divide the arterial pressure tracing from the systolic peak to the dicrotic notch into three equal zones. The balloon pressure pulse for the inflate cycle must not coincide with the first zone adjacent to the peak pressure as this will initiate inflation too soon. If the pressure transducer is in a femoral artery, the mark should fall in the middle zone. The third zone is for placement of the transducer in the aorta (McCusker and Davey, 1979).

We may operate the intra-aortic balloon continuously for several months or use it intermittently with the deflated balloon remaining in the aorta. The deflated balloon should not remain in the aorta for more than 20 minutes or clots may be formed. If there is loss of signal or system failure, the equipment must deflate the balloon and give an alarm. Manual operation is necessary when arrhythmias, which prevent automatic triggering, occur. The design should include provision for battery operation in the event of a power failure.

## Left Heart Bypass

Left-ventricular assist devices have potential for long-term assistance of hearts in chronic failure for periods ranging from a few months to two years or longer. Chronic implantation requires systems that are portable and suitable for placement in or near the thoracic cavity. Current designs bypass the left ventricle by cannulating blood from the apex of the left ventricle and returning it to the descending aorta. Major components under development include the blood pump, energy converter, internal and external power sources, and support equipment (Fig. 4.10). The specific design objectives are a system that will pump blood at a rate of 10 l/m with an average pressure of 120 mm Hg (150 mm Hg peak) for a period of two years. This equals 2.66 W of power. Ultimately, the duration may be extended to ten years.

**Blood Pumps.** Most blood pumps for left-ventricular assist applications are based on pusher plate principles and may be pneumatic, hydraulic, or cam driven (Poirier et al., 1977; Washizu et al., 1977; Moise et al., 1978). The pump outer housing can be constructed from titanium with external dimensions of 10.8 × 4.2 cm. Inner diaphrams are smooth or textured polyurethane or polyolefin rubber. Pusher plate mechanisms can achieve an efficiency of 78%. Internal pump flow patterns must be studied to ensure elimination of stasis and excessive turbulence (Igo et al., 1978). Pumps require two valves—one each at the inflow and outflow tracts. There are both mechanical and biological valve designs. The inlet cannula design and insertion technique is also important. The surgical procedure must be quick, simple, and not result in any significant myocardial injury. For this purpose, there is a coring knife designed with a special double-edge guillotine cutting mechanism (Alexander et al., 1978). Pump capacity should be sufficient to allow total bypass, although minimal flow through the aortic valve is desirable to reduce the possibility of thromboembolism. Pump ejection occurs during the diastolic phase of the cardiac cycle and controls to synchronize pump action with the heart should be provided because asynchronous operation at a fixed rate is less efficient. Control can be triggered by the QRS complex in the ECG, monitoring of pusher plate positions or its time derivative, or by using a position switch and measuring pressure differentials in the actuator circuit. In the latter design, we require no electronic monitoring because a reduced pressure in the actuator output line indicates the end of cardiac systole and established pump rate. Stroke volume during pump filling is sufficient to handle all blood coming from the left ventricle so that the pump can adjust itself to different flow requirements.

**Energy Converters.** Both electrical and thermal designs have been studied. Two electrical concepts are based on the use of brushless, dc motors operating at 28 V. One design uses a direct-connected cam to drive the pusher plate in the blood pump and achieves an overall efficiency of about 30% (Poirier et al., 1977). The cam profile is exponential to optimize $dP/dt$ characteristics. Another design has an electrohydraulic system with a gear pump using silicone oil flowing through a spool valve to operate the blood pump. This system also uses a linear magnetic coupling between the converter and pump to allow hermetic sealing of the two components

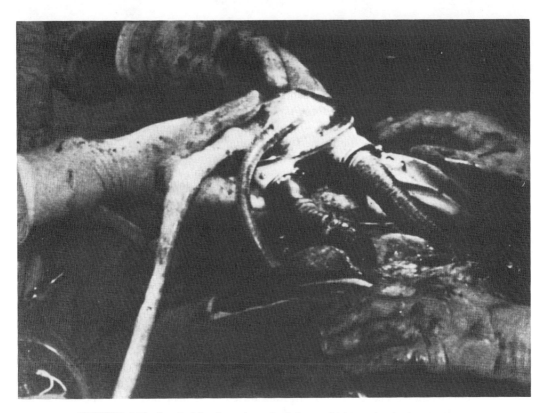

**FIGURE 4-10.** Surgical implantation of a left-ventricular assist device in a calf. Courtesy, Aerojet Energy Conversion Company.

without using a metal bellows. Because all exposed metal surfaces are titanium, the design has good biocompatability. Efficiencies approaching 40% may be possible with this concept (Moise et al., 1978). The volume of the converter is approximately 0.13 l and it weighs 350 g.

Electrical systems require rechargeable external batteries and should include an emergency internal battery. Power is supplied with percutaneous leads or a transcutaneous transformer. Conduits, which transfer energy percutaneously through several layers of tissue, must be designed to prevent infection and allow for biological reactions around the device. Intact skin transformers with implanted secondary coils require tightly coupled magnetic structures that are compatible with anatomical and physiological constraints.

A thermal system uses a modified Stirling cycle with helium as the fluid. This concept could use a radioisotope heat source, which would eliminate the need for an external power pack. It can also be adapted to utilize a melting salt heat source with periodic electrical heater recharge. The converter uses a double-acting pneumatic actuator to drive the pusher plate type blood pump and also uses a linear magnetic coupling between the two components. Efficiency is approximately 15%.

## Clinical Experience

Physicians have accumulated considerable clinical experience using intra-aortic balloon pumps for both surgical and medical indications. In surgical cases, the most common application involves patients unable to be weaned from pump-oxygenators. They have also been used for postoperative shock and poor ventricular function (ejection fraction less than 0.40). Medical indications include cardiogenic shock and preinfarction angina. In a case study involving 65 surgical and 29 medical applications over a 4-year period, survival of patients with cardiogenic shock and post-pump oxygenator failure was enhanced (Lefemine et al., 1977). Also, results and operability of poor-risk patients with reduced ejection fraction, intractable angina, and recent myocardial infarction are improved. Effectiveness is limited by a significant number of cases in which the balloon could not be placed by the femoral or iliac route. Complications involving circulation to the legs are common and can lead to gangrene. In a few cases, amputation was required, especially when there were diseased arteries and low cardiac output. A modified balloon that includes a central lumen to allow pressure monitoring, injection of contrast medium, and passage of a guide wire may improve the efficacy and safety of these devices (Wolfson et al., 1978). The use of anticoagulants, although still being evaluated, is not generally recommended during balloon operation.

There have been less than 100 reported cases of left-ventricular assist devices being used clinically (Norman and Bregman, 1978). Designs are still being evaluated with tests conducted in animals, primarily calves. In addition to system effectiveness, studies are investigating different implantation sites, internal fixation methods, and heat dissipation and vibration problems.

Configurations adaptable to human use have been studied in calves and cadavers. Cadaver studies alone can be misleading because of shrinkage and easy displacement of nonfunctioning organs. Feasible anatomical sites include areas in the intrathoracic, intraperitoneal, and parathoracic regions. Assist system components coated with silicone rubber and covered with a Dacron velour have been placed in a pouch between muscles in a calf without migration occurring (Moise et al., 1978).

The blood circulation can be used to dissipate the heat. Studies have shown that the calf can tolerate at least 50 W being released into the circulation without problems (Sandberg et al., 1970). Additional cooling effects through the skin and muscle can be obtained if the parathoracic location is used (Washizu et al., 1977).

## 4.10 TOTALLY ARTIFICIAL HEARTS

Although we have emphasized the development of a heart assist, research has also continued on the design of a totally artificial heart. Substantial progress has been made. Survival times exceeding 5½ months have been achieved with calves. This suggests that these devices may ultimately be suitable for human use.

## Design Criteria

Most concepts replace only the ventricles and leave the atrial walls intact. Pneumatically driven ellipsoidal sac-type pumps driven by an external air supply are used. Intrinsic control of the pump maintains adequate blood flow if a soft shell is used for the outer wall of the pump (Smith et al., 1975). The wall collapses during diastole to ensure a full chamber but does not extend beyond a certain limit in systole. Thus, the pump output matches input and this eliminates the need for complex electronic instrumentation. A pump of this design with a 120-ml stroke volume and 120 beats per min frequency had an output of 14 l/min.

It is important that the materials used in the diaphragm and pump housing minimize thrombus formation. One design has the entire blood interface surface, including the housing inner lining and blood diaphragm, cast from smooth, air-dried polyurethane (Jarvik et al., 1977). A pump diaphragm fabricated from gelatin-coated polyolefin yields good results. Blood contact surfaces of the pump housing are made with glutaralydehyde-treated bovine pericardium (Tsushima et al., 1977).

Valve selection for these pumps is also important in reducing thromboembolism. Outflow valves have been made from bovine aortic and pulmonary valves, while inflow valves have been either Bjork-Shiley mechanical prostheses or trileaflet biological valves made from human dura matter.

Extensive monitoring systems, which include telemetry, have permitted continuous evaluation of test animals, even during exercise. Airlines of 1.3 to 1.4 cm o.d. polyurethane tubing, coated on the outside with Dacron velour and tunneled subcutaneously for 30 cm before crossing the skin, have remained almost free of infection problems.

Low cardiac output was the most common cause for terminating animal experiments. Contributing factors included: (1) Pannus formation in the inflow tracts; (2) fibroplasia of the left ventricular outflow tract; (3) large body weight; and (4) inflow valve limited filling.

Three phases have been observed in animals involved in long-term survival tests: (1) surgical postoperative; (2) maintenance; and (3) terminal deterioration. A researcher suggests that clinical use of an artificial heart in humans not be attempted unless the patient can expect to benefit from a prolonged period of good health combined with rapid postoperative recovery and minimal terminal suffering (Jarvik et al., 1977).

## REFERENCES

ALEXANDER, J. E., J. ROBINETTE, R. GRIFFITH, and K. CAMPBELL (1978). A modified knife for apical coring in LVAD implantation studies. Trans. Am. Soc. Artif. Internal Organs, XXIV: 324–27.

BEALL, A. C., Jr. (1977). Who protects our patients, and from what? *Med. Instrum.*, 11 72–73.

BJORK, V. O., (1977). The history of the Bjork-Shiley tilting disc valve. *Med. Instrum.*, 11. 80–81.

BLACKSHEAR, P. L. (1972). Mechanical hemolysis in flowing blood, in V. C. Fung, N. Perrone, and M. Anliker (eds), *Biomechanics: Its foundations and objectives.* Englewood Cliffs, NJ: Prentice-Hall.

BOKROS, J. E., et al. (1975). Carbon in prosthetic devices. Deviney, M. L., and T. M. O'Grady (eds.), Petroleum derived carbons. *ACS Symp. Series:* 21.

BORIK, S., T. B. DAVEY, B. KAUFMAN, E. A. SMELOFF, and G. E. MILLER (1973). A new method for intraoperative detection of intracardiac air prior to discontinuance of bypass. *Ann. Thoracic Surg.*, 16: 344–48.

BRAUNWALD, N. W., and B. S. BULL (1969). Factors controlling the development of tissue layers on fabrics, in L. A. Brewer (ed), *Prosthetic heart valves.* Springfield, IL: Charles C Thomas.

CARMEN, R., and S. C. MUTHA (1972). Lipid absorption by silicone rubber heart valve poppets in-vivo and in-vitro results. *J. Biomed. Mat. Res.*, 6: 327–46.

CARPENTIER, A. (1977). From valvular xenograft to valvular bioprosthesis (1965–1977). *Med. Instrum.*, 11: 98–101.

CLARK, R. E. (1974). New principles governing the tissue reactivity of prosthetic materials. *J. Surg. Res.*, 16: 510–22.

CLARK, R. E. and W. M. SWANSON (1979). Durability of prosthetic heart valves *in vitro* and *in vivo*, in A. P. Yoganathan, E. C. Harrison, and W. H. Corcoran (eds), *Proc., Symp. on prosthetic heart valves. AAMI,* 443–52.

COOLEY, D. A. (1977). The quest for the perfect prosthetic heart valve. *Med. Instrum.*, 11: 82–84.

DAUGHTERS, G. T., N. B. INGELS, E. B. STINSON, E. L. ALDERMAN, and C. W. MEAD (1977). Computation of left ventricular dynamics from surgically implanted markers. *Proc. San Diego Biom. Symp.*, 16: 97–101.

DAVEY, T. B., and E. A. SMELOFF (1977). Development of a cardiac valve substitute: The Smeloff-Cutter prosthesis. *Med. Instrum.*, 11: 94–97.

DAVEY, T. B., and E. A. SMELOFF (1979). Design and testing of prosthetic heart valves, in D. N. Ghista and E. van Vollehoven (eds), *Cardiovascular engineering.* Verlag Gerhard Witzstrock Gmbh: 476–89.

DORSON, W. J., and M. VORHEES (1974). Limiting models for the transfer of $CO_2$ and $O_2$ in membrane oxygenators. *Trans. Am. Soc. Artif. Internal Organs,* XX: 219–25.

EDWARDS, W. S. (1978). Arterial grafts, past, present, and future. *Arch. Surg.*, 11: 1225–35.

HAMMERMEISTER, K. E., J. A. MURRAY, and J. R. BLACKMON (1973). Revision of Gorlin constant for calculation of mitral valve area of left heart pressures. *Br. Heart J.*, 35: 392–96.

IGO, S. R., C. W. HIBBS, R. TRONO, C. H. EDMONDS, and J.C. NORMAN (1978). Theoretical design considerations and physiologic performance criteria for an improved intracorporeal (abdominal) electrically-actuated long-term left ventricular assist device (E-type ALVAD) or partial artificial heart. *Cardiovascular disease,* Bull. Texas Heart Inst., 5(2): 172.

JACOBSON, B., and J. G. WEBSTER (1977). *Medicine and clinical engineering.* Englewood Cliffs, NJ: Prentice-Hall.

JARVIK, R. K., D. B. OLSEN, T. R. KESSLER, J. LAWSON, J. ENGLISH, and W. J. KOLFF, (1977). Criteria for human total artificial heart implantation based on steady state animal data. *Trans. Am. Soc. Artif. Internal Organs,* XXIII: 535–42.

JONES, R. T. (1972). Fluid dynamics of heart assist devices, in Y. C. Fung, M. Perrone, and M. Anliker (eds), *Biomechanics: Its foundations and objectives.* Englewood Cliffs, NJ: Prentice-Hall.

KAR, M.K., and S. BAHADUR (1977). Micromechanism of wear at polymer-metal sliding interface. *Wear of materials.* A.S.M.E.: 501–9.

KAUFMAN, B., T. B. DAVEY, A. C. HUTLEY, G. E. MILLER, and E. A. SMELOFF (1968). Development of mechanical heart assists. *A.S.M.E.:* 68–WA/BHF-4.

KENNEDY, J. H. (1974). Report of the ASA 10 subcommittee on intra-aortic balloon augmentation. *Trans. Am. Soc. Artif. Internal Organs,* XX: 775–79.

KENNER, T. (1972). Flow and pressure in the arteries, in Y. C. Fung, M. Perrone, and M. Anliker (eds), *Biomechanics: Its foundations and objectives.* Englewood Cliffs, NJ: Prentice-Hall, 381–434.

KOLFF, W. J., and J. LAWSON (1975). Status of the artificial heart and cardiac assist devices in the United States. *Trans. Am. Soc. Artif. Internal Organs,* XXI: 620–38.

KOORAJIAN, S., D. D. KELLER, W. R. PIERIE, A. STARR, and R. HERR (1969). Criteria and systems for testing artificial heart valves in vitro, in L. A. Brewer (ed), *Prosthetic heart valves.* Springfield, IL: Charles C. Thomas.

LEFEMINE, A. A. (1977). Left ventricular bypass — An experimental and clinical experience. *Trans. Am. Soc. Artif. Internal Organs.,* XXIII: 326–30.

LEFRAK, E. A., and A. STARR (1979). *Cardiac valve prostheses,* New York: Appleton-Century-Crofts.

LIGHTFOOT, E. N., JR. (1974). *Transport phenomena and living systems.* New York: Wiley-Interscience.

LILLEHI, C. W. (1977). Heart valve replacement with the pivoting disc prosthesis: Appraisal of results and description of a new all-carbon model. *Med. Instrum.,* 11: 85–94.

MCCUSKER, D. R., and T. B. DAVEY (1979). Intra-aortic balloon pumping, a teaching system. *Proc. AAMI Annu. Meeting.,* 170.

MCHENRY, M. M., E. A. SMELOFF, and T. B. DAVEY (1978). Ten-year experience with the Smeloff-Cutter heart valve prosthesis. *Today's Clinician,* Jan: 44–47.

MOISE, J. C., J. M. FOERSTER, R. J. FAESER, and J. W. HELLWIG (1978). Development of compact thermal and electrical energy converters for left heart assist systems. *Trans. Am. Soc. Artif. Internal Organs,* XXIV: 77–83.

MYERS, G. H., and V. PARSONNET (1969). *Engineering in the heart and blood vessels.* New York: Wiley.

NETTER, F. H. (1969). *The CIBA Collection of Medical Illustrations, The Heart, Vol. V.* Summit, N.J.: CIBA Pharmaceutical Co., Div. of CIBA Corp.

NORMAN, J. C., and D. BREGMAN (1978). Mechanical circulatory support: Evolving perspectives. *Trans. Am. Soc. Artif. Internal Organs,* XXIV: 782–87.

OCUMPAUGH, D. E., and H. L. LEE (1971). Foreign body reaction to plastic implants, in *Biomedical polymers.* New York: Marcel Dekker.

POIRIER, V., D. GERNES, and M. SZYCHER (1977). Advances in electrical assist devices. *Trans. Am. Soc. Artif. Internal Organs,* XXIII: 72–79.

RANIER, W. G., R. A. CHRISTOPHER, and T. R. SADLER (1977). Some comments on heart valve testing and other observations. *Med. Instrum.*, 11: 104–6.

SANDBERG, G. W., F. N. HUFFMAN, and J. C. NORMAN (1970). Implantable nuclear power sources for artificial organs. 1. Physiologic monitoring and pathologic effects. *Trans. Am. Soc. Artif. Internal Organs*, XVI: 172–79.

SARMA, R., E. J. ROSCHKE, E. C. HARRISON, W. A. EDMISTON, and F. Y. K. LAU (1977). Clinical experience with the Smeloff-Cutler aortic valve prosthesis: An 8-year follow-up study. *Am. J. Cardiol.*, 40(3): 338–43.

SAUVAGE, L. R. (1977). Prosthetic valves 1977: A retrospective analysis and a look to the future. *Med. Instrum.* 11: 107–9.

SAWYER, P. N., S. SHRINIVASON, M. E. LEE, J. G. MARTIN, T. MURAKAMI, and B. STANCZEWSKI (1969). The influence of the metal interface charge on long-term function of prosthetic heart valves, in L. A. Brewer (ed), *Prosthetic heart valves*. Springfield, IL: Charles C Thomas.

SELKURT, E. E. (ed) (1976). *Physiology*. 4th ed. Boston: Little, Brown.

SHAFFER, M. J., and M. R. GORDON (1979). Clinical engineering standards, obligations and accountability. *Med. Instrum.*, 13: 209–15.

SHERRY, S., K. M. BRINKHOUS, E. GENTON, and J. M. STENGLE (1969). *Thombosis*. Washington, DC: National Academy of Sciences.

SMELOFF, E. A., T. B. DAVEY, and B. KAUFMAN (1969). Patterns of blood flow through artificial valves, in L. A. Brewer (ed), *Prosthetic heart valves*. Springfield, IL: Charles C Thomas.

SMITH, L., G. SANDQUIST, D. B. OLSEN, G. ARNETT, S. GENTRY, and W. J. KOLFF (1975). Power requirements for the A.E.C. artificial heart. *Trans. Am. Soc. Artif. Internal Organs.*, XXI: 540–44.

SPAETH, E. E. (1973). Blood oxygenation in extracorporeal devices: Theoretical considerations. *CRC Crit. Rev. Bioeng.*, 1(4): 383–417.

SPRAY, T. L., and W. C. ROBERTS (1977). Structural changes in porcine xenografts used as substitute cardiac valves. *Am. J. Cardiol.*, 40: 319–30.

SWANSON, W. M., and R. E. CLARK (1976). Testing of prosthetic heart valves. *A.S.M.E.*, 76-WA/Bio,:3.

TABOR, D. (1977). Wear, a critical synoptic view. Wear of Materials. *A.S.M.E.*, 1977: 1–11.

TALBOT, L., and S. A. BERGER (1974). Fluid-mechanical aspects of the human circulation. *Am. Scientist*, 62: 671–82.

TSUSHIMA, N., S. KASAI, I. KOSHIMO, G. JACOBS, N. MORINAGA, T. WASHIZU, R. KIRALY, and Y. NOSÉ (1977). 145 days survival of calf with total artificial heart (TAH). *Trans. Am. Soc. Artif. Internal Organs*, XXIII: 526–33.

URSCHEL, C. W., and E. H. SONNENBLICK (1972). Determinants of cardiac performance, in Y. C. Fung, M. Peronne, and M. Anliker (eds), *Biomechanics: Its foundations and objectives*. Englewood Cliffs, NJ: Prentice-Hall.

WASHIZU, T., R. WHALEN, W. MORINAGA, H. HARASAKI, N. TSUSHIMA, K. OUCHI, K. HAYASHI, J. SNOW, R. SUKALAC, G. JACOBS, R. KIRALY, and J. NOSÉ (1977). Parathoracic left ventricular assist device (PVAD). *Trans. Am. Soc. Artif. Internal Organs*, XXIII: 301–8.

WEBSTER, J. G. (ed) (1978). *Medical instrumentation: Application and design.* Boston: Houghton Mifflin.

WELLS, R. E. (1969). Rheologic aspects of stasis in thrombus formation, in *Thrombosis.* Washington, DC: National Academy of Sciences.

WESOLOWSKI, S. A. (1966). Roller pumps. *Mechanical devices to assist the failing heart.* Washington, DC: National Academy of Sciences.

WIETING, D. W., C. W. HALL, D. LIOTTA, and M. E. DEBAKEY (1969). Dynamic flow behavior of artificial heart valves, in L. A. Brewer (ed), *Prosthetic heart valves.* Springfield, IL: Charles C Thomas.

WILLIAMS, D. F. (1971). The effect of materials on blood. *Bio-Med. Eng.* 6: 205.

WOLFSON, S., D. L. KARSH, R. A. LANGOU, A. S. GEHA, G. L. HAMMOND, and L. S. COHEN (1978). Modification of intra-aortic balloon catheter to permit introduction by cardiac catheterization techniques. *Am. J. Cardiol.,* 41: 733–38.

WOMERSLEY, J. R. (1957). Oscillatory flow in the arteries: The constrained elastic tube as a model of arterial flow and pulse transmission. *Phys. Med. Biol.,* 2: 178–87.

WRIGHT, J. T. M. (1977). A pulsatile flow study comparing the Hancock porcine xenograft aortic valve prosthesis, models 242 and 250. *Med. Instrum.,* II: 114–17.

YOGANATHAN, A. P., W. H. CORCORAN, and E. C. HARRISON (1978). Wall shear stress measurements in the near vicinity of prosthetic heart valves. *J. Bioeng.,* 2: 369–79.

## STUDY QUESTIONS

**4.1**  Mr. C. E. Gar was diagnosed as having mitral valve stenosis. Left-heart catheterization showed a diastolic filling period of 34 s/m and a pressure gradient of 34 mmHg based on the pulmonary wedge pressure. Cardiac output, measured by the dye-dilution method, was 5.3 l/m for a heart rate of 75 beats/m. Calculate the valve area using the Gorlin equation.

**4.2**  Mr. Gar's mitral valve was replaced with a prosthetic ball valve. His cardiologist wished to check the Gorlin equation for mitral valves by comparing the known orifice area of the mechanical valve against the area calculated from the equation, with data obtained from left-heart catheterization after valve replacement. Would you expect good correlation from these calculations?

**4.3**  Following coronary artery bypass surgery, blood flow in the vein graft can be checked by an electromagnetic flowmeter. How would you calibrate a flow probe used for this purpose?

**4.4**  Search the medical literature for a new prosthetic heart valve concept. Develop a testing protocol for this design, including both in vitro and in vivo tests.

**4.5**  List material properties (physical, chemical, and electrical) that are significant in determining the antithrombogenic qualities of substances immersed in the blood-stream.

**4.6**  During cardiopulmonary bypass, why is the ascending aorta normally cross-clamped when the heart is fibrillated or arrested?

**4.7**  How are large diameter (greater than 8 mm) woven Dacron grafts reinforced to prevent kinking?

**4.8** What physical properties of helium make it the preferred gas for inflating intra-aortic balloons?

**4.9** Why is a small amount of carbon dioxide included in the oxygen being supplied to a bubble oxygenator?

**4.10** A parallel plate silicone rubber membrane oxygenator with two membranes 40 $\mu$m thick and 20 cm wide has a blood flow of 750 ml/s. Calculate the length of membrane required if the partial pressure of the carbon dioxide in the blood is to be reduced from 45 to 30 mm Hg.

**4.11** Based on maximum efficiencies for LVAD components, estimate the power requirements for an external battery pack to be supplied for a normal man.

**4.12** Calculate $V_{max}$ for a normal left ventricular pressure curve.

# 5 Neural Assist Devices

*Ronald W. Jodat*
*Sanford J. Larson*
*Anthony Sances, Jr.*

## 5.1 LEARNING OBJECTIVES

Upon completing this chapter you will be able to:

- Describe the methods in which electrical stimulation affects the functioning of the nervous system.
- Relate design characteristics of neural assist devices to desired physiological effects.
- Define the characteristics of an effective neural stimulator.
- Describe the use of neural stimulators for pain relief, motor control, and electrotherapeutic sleep devices.

## 5.2 INTRODUCTION

Excitable tissue that comprises our nerve and muscle masses responds to a variety of stimuli, such as heat, light, sound, pressure, and chemicals. It also responds to electrical stimuli. During the functioning of excitable tissue, ionic species—principally sodium and potassium—move rapidly across membranous boundaries, which undergo transient alterations in permeability. This movement constitutes a flow of electrical current. These currents flow through resistive media and produce potential fields on the surface of the body. We can also reverse the process and apply an external electrical stimulus. This establishes an ionic current field in regions with excitable tissue.

## 5.3 NEURAL ASSIST DEVICE APPLICATIONS

### History of Neural Assist Devices

The earliest use of electricity in a medical therapeutic application involved the torpedo fish or electric ray fish. These fish have special organs for separating and storing electric charge. Early Roman physicians recommended the electrical discharge of the torpedo fish as a treatment for pain.

During the eighteenth and nineteenth centuries, voltaic piles or faraday generators provided more convenient forms of electrical power sources. Then, electrotherapy emerged as a separate discipline. During the last half of the nineteenth century, many different electric therapeutic machines became available. Some were based on electrostatic principles, some employed the voltaic pile source to deliver galvanic current, while others used induction machines to deliver current referred to as *faradic*.

As a result of the widespread experimentation with electricity in medical applications, there emerged by the mid-1900s two very useful electrical stimulation devices that are widely used today. These are the defibrillator and the cardiac pacemaker (see Chapters 2 and 3). The continual evolution of the pacemaker over the past two decades has led to improved and more reliable units capable of being implanted in the body. Electrical stimulation for cardiac pacing is the most highly developed and widespread application area at the present time.

The success of cardiac pacing along with the technology developed for the production of this unit has extended to other applications. Cardiac pacemakers have evolved from external units to implantable types powered by radio-frequency coupling of an external power source and eventually to implantable units with completely self-contained long-term power sources. New areas of application can immediately benefit from these advances.

### Modern Applications

The more recent clinical applications of electrical stimulation include:

1. Treatment for chronic and intractable pain, where the use of drug therapy is undesirable or no longer effective.
2. Peripheral nerve stimulation to control respiratory and urinary functions.
3. Cerebellar stimulation for control of disorders in motor function, including epilepsy.
4. Auditory and visual prostheses.
5. Therapeutic sleep treatments.

### Types of Stimulation Devices

Regardless of the application, all systems for electrical stimulation consist of the basic elements shown in Fig. 5.1. The source of power may be self-contained within a totally implantable unit or located externally. The waveform generator

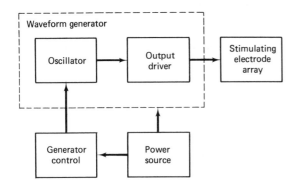

**FIGURE 5.1.** Major functional components of an electrical stimulation system.

transforms the raw power from this source into an effective stimulating waveform. Its output feeds the stimulating electrode array. The control generator may be as simple as an on/off switch, involve the programming of stimulus rate and/or intensity, or depend on the feedback of information from the stimulated or related structures.

In some applications, all of the four major components are actually external to the body, with the applied stimulus using surface electrodes. Development efforts are directed toward totally implantable units. This progression parallels that of the development of cardiac pacemakers but is proceeding at a more rapid rate. As our understanding of the factors that affect a particular stimulation application grow, we can design for the complete implantation of all of the functional elements of a stimulating system.

## 5.4 ELECTRICAL STIMULATION OF NERVES AND MUSCLES

### *Excitation by Electrical Currents*

Nerves and muscles are stimulated by the direct application of current to the target tissue. A sufficient amount of charge per unit area must be displaced across the cell membrane in order to raise the transmembrane potential to its firing threshold. Hodgkin and Huxley (1952) found that the required shock strength is 10–100 nC/cm². Charge transfers of these magnitudes, when delivered by current pulses of 1 ms duration, require current densities of 10–100 $\mu$A/cm². These current densities are established by pulse generators that supply current through electrode configurations specifically designed for each application. The proximity of the electrodes to the target tissue determines how much the current will spread to surrounding tissue and, therefore, be reduced in density. Consequently, the amount of current that must be supplied by the generator is typically in the range of 1–50 mA.

Excitable tissue will respond to current pulses of different amplitude and time durations as described by the strength-duration curve of that tissue. For a given effect, this curve relates the stimulus strength to its required time of application. The proper measure of stimulus strength is current density. Because current density measurements are difficult to perform, users often report peak or average current

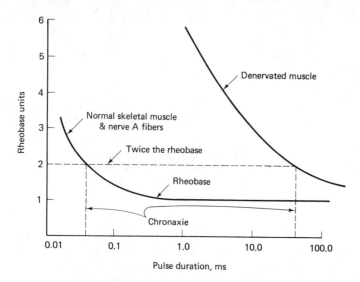

**FIGURE 5.2.** Strength-duration characteristics of nerve and muscle.

levels. A probe design for current density measurements is described by Jarzembski et al. (1970).

Figure 5.2 shows the typical hyperbolic shape of the strength-duration curve that results from the transmembrane resistance and capacitance properties of the excitable tissue. The rheobase is the minimum stimulus strength that is capable of eliciting a response. If we apply a stimulus whose amplitude is twice the rheobase, then its duration must equal the chronaxie to achieve the same response. If through disease or injury the nerve connections to a muscle are impaired, the muscle can still be stimulated directly. Direct excitation of muscle requires greater stimulating currents, as indicated by the denervated muscle curve in Fig. 5.2.

To be effective, the stimulating pulse width must be on the order of the chronaxie time of the target tissue. Nerves that propagate action potentials fast have short chronaxie values. In man, the large motor nerve fibers have a chronaxie of 200 $\mu$s and conduct an impulse of 50 m/s while small sensory nerves have a chronaxie of 20 ms.

Pulse generators used to deliver the stimulating pulses are preferably of the constant current type with adjustable current output levels. The impedance seen by the generator consists of the electrode impedance in series with the tissue impedance. The series combination of these two impedances can range from 300–3,000 $\Omega$ and is primarily determined by electrode area. Large surface area electrodes present low impedances with the residual 300 $\Omega$ attributed to the bulk tissue. Small surface area electrodes for implant applications tend toward the higher figure of 3,000 $\Omega$. In order to deliver 10 mA to this range of load impedances, the voltage compliance of the source must range from 3–30 V, respectively. Implantable power sources of 3 V are possible, but a 30-V source would require voltage conversion circuits. It is important, therefore, to maintain a low value of load impedance when using constant-current generators.

The impedance presented by the tissue mass to be stimulated is fixed by the resistive and dielectric properties of tissue. The impedance presented by the stimulating electrodes can be minimized by increasing their surface area. However, by increasing the area, the current density is decreased and spread over a large, less specific volume of tissue.

## Tissue Response to Electrical Stimulation

We now discuss how excitable tissue responds to electrical stimulation from two viewpoints. The first is the desired or therapeutic response and the second covers the undesirable responses or reactions.

Electrical stimulation of neuromuscular tissue produces the following desired responses:

1. Initiate or block conduction of action potentials along nerve pathways.
2. Stimulate contraction of specific muscle groups.
3. Induce a state of anesthesia.

To accomplish these effects, a sufficient current density must be established at a specific site for a given length of time. This will cause a translocation of a specific amount of charge across the tissue boundary. Charge transfer in regions far from the stimulating electrodes is determined by four factors: current magnitude, time of application, electrode geometry, and tissue impedance. The first three factors are controllable by design, only the last factor relates to tissue characteristics.

The volume of tissue "seen" by the stimulating electrode array is not all of the same type. Because it is not homogeneous, the total current divides, with regions of lower impedance conducting a larger portion of the current. This fact dictates whether surface or implanted electrodes are required. If the target tissue is at a great depth or surrounded by low-impedance structures, then implanted electrodes will be more effective.

The electrical characteristics of excitable membranes can be modeled by a parallel resistor–capacitor combination. The impedance of this combination decreases at the higher frequencies. For effective stimulation, current pulses should have a pulse width approximately equal to the membrane's electrical time constant.

The undesirable responses include reactions at the electrode–tissue interface, abnormal functioning of the stimulated tissue, or unpleasant side effects. We will first consider reactions at the electrode.

After implantation, an electrode becomes encapsulated by a thin layer of fibrous tissue. This nonreactive tissue increases the effective surface area of the electrode and thereby reduces current density and raises the stimulation threshold. This process takes place over a 2–4 week period and stabilizes, providing that the electrode material is nontoxic. The passage of current through these encapsulated electrodes can cause changes in the electrodes and surrounding tissues.

Destruction of tissue surrounding the electrodes must be avoided for successful long-term stimulation. Tissue damage can be caused by the evolution of gas or heat generation under high-current-density stimulation. Toxic materials can be produced by otherwise nontoxic electrodes through chemical reactions. Four distinct types of reaction are:

1. Electrolysis of water.
2. Oxidation of electrode metal.
3. Oxidation of saline.
4. Oxidation of organic compounds.

Damage from these reactions can be minimized by operating the electrodes in a reversible manner with respect to these reaction mechanisms.

Because the reaction mechanisms are electronic charge transfer processes, constant-current stimulus generators exert better control than constant-voltage types. The constant-current generators will deliver their design current to varying load impedances within its voltage compliance range. In contrast, constant-voltage generators will deliver currents that are determined by the biological impedance values.

Studies of the blood–brain barrier (BBB) performed by Mortimer et al. (1970) provided guidelines for waveform parameters under constant-current stimulation. There were three important findings. The first is that platinum electrodes could deliver eight times more energy than stainless steel types before BBB breakdown was observed. Second, an optimal pulse width of 400 $\mu$s was determined. This optimum value was determined with a preparation in which the motor nerve of a cat's gastrocnemius muscle is stimulated with a 60 pps (pulse per second) constant voltage source. The pulses were made biphasic by capacitive coupling. The third finding was a maximum allowable energy density of 50 mW/cm$^2$. This limit applies to platinum electrodes, 400 $\mu$s pulse widths and a pulse repetition rate from 10–100 pps.

## 5.5 TECHNIQUES OF ELECTRICAL STIMULATION

### Mechanism of Action

The beneficial effects of electrical excitation depend on establishing sufficient density with an effective temporal pattern in a specific target region. In most applications, we know neither these parameters nor the mechanisms by which the electrical currents produce their therapeutic effects. Not all patients with apparently similar presenting symptoms are equally benefited by electrical stimulation.

Electrical stimulation can inhibit transmission of neural pulses, as in a nerve blockage. It can also excite neurons or nerve fibers. We can characterize the successful techniques on the basis of the stimulation waveform parameters and the stimulation objective.

**Relief of Pain.** Techniques used to produce an analgesic effect depend on the type and origin of the pain. Pain can arise from sources related to the peripheral portion of the nervous system or have its origin at higher levels in the central nervous system (CNS). In addition to its source, we can divide pain into acute or chronic types. We do not understand just how pain is perceived by the central nervous system. Early concepts of pain-specific pathways have given way to the Gate theory of Melzack and Wall (1965), which postulates a mechanism that modulates pain information as it flows to the CNS. For peripheral nerves, we more clearly understand the technique of transmission blockage.

We can group the electrical stimulation for the relief of pain into three distinct approaches. The first involves a direct effect on the painful area. By establishing a tingling sensation in an area of pain, we can achieve relief of chronic type pain in many but not all cases. We use a method known as transcutaneous electrical neural stimulation (TENS). An external unit with surface electrodes provides the stimulation. A second method uses direct stimulation of the spinal cord with implanted electrodes. Effective pain relief without side effects is highly dependent on electrode design and placement. The third approach uses stimulation at higher levels in the brain. Electrode placement is critical. The advantage of stimulating at these higher centers of pain transmission is that it has yielded successful treatment of all pain types.

**Correction of Motor Function.** Coordinated and directed application of electrical stimulation can restore motor function in certain pathological conditions. Functional neuromuscular stimulation can be put into four broad categories:

1. Lower motor neuron lesions.
2. Upper motor neuron lesions without increased muscle tone.
3. Upper motor neuron lesions with spasticity and rigidity.
4. Movement disorders as in tremor.

We can electrically stimulate at two different levels. One level is restoration of coordinated sequential movements in denervated muscle or intact neuromuscular systems with impaired upper motor drive. A second level corrects for the spasticity or rigidity conditions that result from overactive motor neurons. We describe this area later.

**Restoration of Sensory Function.** Development of electrical stimulation techniques to restore sensory inputs primarily address vision and hearing functions. The major problems that confront these efforts involve the mapping and application of the sensory information to the appropriate areas of cortex (Section 6.9).

### Characteristics of Stimulating Waveforms

How do we select a stimulation waveform for a specific application? The waveform is pulsed and has a pulse repetition rate or frequency, a stimulating pulse width or duration, and an amplitude or intensity. The important measure of stimulus strength is the charge density (current $\times$ time/area) established at the point of excitation.

Typical charge densities effective in stimulation of sensimotor and cerebellar cortex are in the range of 10–300 $\mu C/cm^2$ (Larson et al., 1976). In addition, the pulsed waveform may be monophasic or biphasic. In the case of radio-frequency-coupled devices, the pulse may consist of a burst of the carrier signal. Each parameter influences the overall effectiveness of the waveform.

**Waveform Pulse Duration.** Nerve cell stimulation requires the establishment of sufficient current density in the target area for a length of time dictated by the tissue chronaxie. Tissue excitability as described by strength-duration curves, when superimposed with a curve describing pulse energy, clearly dictates the choice of pulse width. Generally, pulse widths less than 100 $\mu$s or more than 600 $\mu$s require more energy than those within this band.

**Waveform Pulse Amplitude.** The pulse amplitude required to deliver the necessary charge density depends on the size of the stimulating electrodes and the degree of spread of the current in the tissue between electrodes and target. Although the stimulus generator may be of constant voltage or constant current design, it is convenient to speak in terms of total current as a measure of stimulus intensity. In these terms, typical generator output capabilities are from 0–60 mA. Commercially available voltage outputs range from 0–180 V. Higher outputs are required when the stimulus is applied with surface electrodes.

**Waveform Repetition Rate.** Repetition rates reported in the literature range from 1–350 pps. Characteristics of stimulation rates effective in various applications are:

1. Low stimulation rates such as 1 pps find application in cardiac pacing.
2. Stimulation of muscles is limited to a maximum of 50 pps as rates above this produce tetany with rapid fatigue.
3. Low-duty-cycle waveforms help to maintain charge balance at electrode-tissue interfaces and thereby minimize tissue damage. A 10% duty factor is common. This permits 100 pps for pulses of 1 ms duration.
4. Stimulation of the brain at the higher rates (above 200 pps) sometimes produces noxious side effects.

## 5.6 DESIGN CONSIDERATIONS FOR NEURAL ASSIST DEVICES

All systems designed for electrical stimulation consist of the functional components shown in Fig. 5.1. Systems vary as to which functional components are grouped together. However, all of the following five elements are required for a complete stimulation system:

1. Stimulating electrode configuration.
2. Output driver circuit.
3. Oscillator circuit.
4. Generator control circuit.
5. Power source.

## Electrodes for Stimulation

The function of the electrode is to convert the electronic current flow that exists in the connecting metallic conductors into an ionic current for passage through biological tissues. For chronic stimulation, the metal–tissue interface must function over long periods of time without causing damage to the surrounding tissue. Effective application of electrodes depends on an understanding of the electrochemical activity taking place at the metal–tissue interface.

When we place a metal in contact with an electrolyte (interstitial fluids), thermodynamic forces act to bring the metal phase into electrochemical equilibrium with the liquid phase. The equilibrium condition results from a balancing of the electrostatic and diffusional forces acting on each chemical species. This is a dynamic equilibrium in that the net transfer of charge is zero even though individual counterbalancing charge transfers are taking place. We can measure the electrical potential difference across the interface. Because this potential changes in response to attempts to pass currents across the junction, its impedance properties fluctuate also. The pulse generator output must be compatible with the interface impedance.

System design for long-term stimulation of excitable tissue in clinical applications using implanted metal electrodes depends, among other factors, on the tissue–metal interface. Stimulation activity requires that electrical currents flow across this interface. A charge transfer mechanism operates at the metal–tissue interface to sustain current flow.

Electrodes are also used to record bioelectric signals from tissue masses. Although most electrodes can function both in stimulating and recording modes, specific and unique designs for these two applications exist. Recording electrode designs are directed toward minimizing and stabilizing the offset potential at the electrode–tissue interface. Current levels are extremely low (nanoamperes) because of the use of high-input-impedance sensing amplifiers (Newman, 1978). We choose chlorided silver electrodes for recording applications. In contrast, stimulating electrodes operate in the relatively high milliampere range and are usually driven by constant current generators. At these large currents, there is great electrochemical activity at the electrode surface and, therefore, we use an inert metal such as stainless steel or platinum (Dymond, 1976).

With high stimulation currents, electrode behavior is very nonlinear. Figure 5.3 shows an equivalent linear circuit for low-current-density conditions based on the physical mechanisms involved.

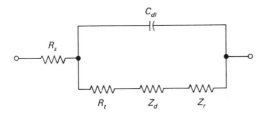

**FIGURE 5.3.** Equivalent circuit of metal-electrolyte interface.

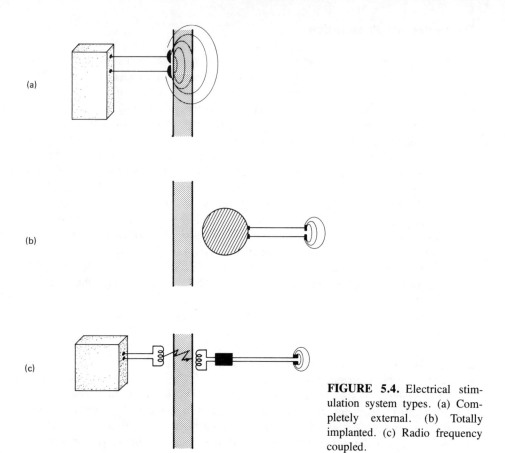

(a)

(b)

(c)

**FIGURE 5.4.** Electrical stimulation system types. (a) Completely external. (b) Totally implanted. (c) Radio frequency coupled.

$R_s$ represents the resistance of the bulk electrolyte away from the interface region. When we place an electrode in an electrolyte solution, ions are attracted to the metal surface and a double layer of charge forms. Capacitance $C_{dl}$ accounts for that charge accumulation. The three remaining impedances are series connected and represent mechanisms controlling the movement of charge across the interface.

## *Power Sources*

We can distinguish electrical stimulation systems by their power source. Figure 5.4a shows the completely external system. The unit may be line-operated but battery operation is more common. We usually use this type with body surface electrodes in a procedure known as transcutaneous electrical stimulation. We may also use these units subcutaneously with needle electrodes.

Figure 5.4b shows the totally implanted unit. It is powered by batteries that may be rechargeable. The unit could also be made programmable. Figure 5.4c shows the partially implanted units. They use radio-frequency coupling of energy to an implanted receiver, which rectifies the pulsed RF signal and applies it to the stimulating electrodes. We prefer this last type for chronic implanted electrodes because the external waveform generator provides easy control of repetition rate, amplitude, and width of the stimulating pulse.

Contemporary practitioners initially chose radio-frequency coupling of the stimulating waveform. It has the advantages of direct application of the stimulating electrodes to the target area and small size of implanted electronics and has the feature of external programming of rate, pulse width, and amplitude. The next most important design is the transcutaneous unit. Its initial use was as a screening tool to noninvasively identify patients who could benefit from an implanted unit. During exploratory use of the transcutaneous unit, some patients obtain pain relief. Physicians now prescribe these units for self-stimulation. Designs that are totally implanted are relatively new. They require rechargeable power sources because the energy consumption is greater than the familiar cardiac pacemaker application by two orders of magnitude. Programmability is necessary because the effective stimulation waveform varies from patient to patient and varies during the course of treatment in a given patient.

## Waveform Generators—The Output Circuit

The oscillator generates pulse waveforms, while the output driver circuit boosts them to sufficient stimulus strength. The characteristics of waveforms that have provided helpful therapeutic stimulation are:

Pulse repetition rate:   10–350 Hz

Pulse width        :   100 $\mu$s to 1 ms

Pulse amplitude     :   10–50 mA

Combinations of pulse width and repetition rate yield a 10% duty factor. We review various output circuit designs used for delivering stimulus pulses to excitable tissue. Because the impedance presented to the output driver by the electrodes and intervening tissue is typically 500–1,000 $\Omega$, special techniques are required to operate from low-voltage battery-type power sources (3–9 V) and still deliver high output currents (10–50 mA).

A basic technique commonly used in heart pacemakers is the capacitor discharge circuit (Figure 5.5). With the transistor cut off, the output capacitor charges through a circuit that includes the tissue. With the transistor driven into saturation by the trigger pulse applied to its base, the capacitor discharges and stimulates the tissue. The tissue impedance in series with the electrode impedance determines the current that flows. For a total load impedance of 500 $\Omega$ and a power supply of 9 V, a peak current is limited to 18 mA. Because the output capacitor is large (5 $\mu$F), only 4% of the charge is lost at a pulse duration of 200 $\mu$s. Thus, this circuit functions as a constant-voltage source. At a charging time constant of 55 ms, this design can only achieve a pulse repetition rate of about 4 Hz.

Some designs use a Darlington pair at the output for current amplification, but

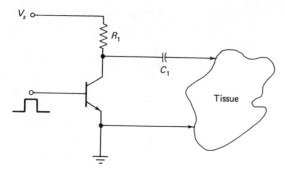

**FIGURE 5.5.** Capacitor discharge output circuit.

the supply voltage limits these, too. In order to achieve output voltages greater than the supply voltage, we must use some type of dc-to-dc converter or transformer coupling.

Units that transmit their stimulus pulse on a radio-frequency carrier to an implanted receiver have vastly different output circuits. The receiver detects and rectifies the transmitted stimulus signal. The amplitude of the stimulus pulse delivered to the tissue depends on the degree of coupling between the transmitting and receiving antennas. Figure 5.6 shows a typical receiver circuit. $L_1$ and $C_1$ form a tank circuit tuned to the carrier frequency, while $D_1$, $R$, and $C_3$ form the detector and low-pass filter. Capacitor $C_2$ maintains capacitive coupling while the diode conducts. The inductor is usually 15–20 turns of #34 AWG wire coiled 2.54 cm in diameter. An inductor this size, in parallel with a 10-nF capacitor, operates at 450 kHz.

Another important form of output circuit is one that is amplitude programmable. A low-power CMOS control section first generates a pulse waveform. This drives an output amplifier, whose gain can be programmed by switching resistor values. A typical circuit uses a Darlington connection, which provides the high gain necessary to transform the CMOS signal into a high-current-level pulse waveform. High gain at low collector current bias is provided by 2N930 transistors. A split supply voltage permits biphasic pulses for charge balancing. Varying base-current drive permits amplitude control. Output current amplitude with a 5-V supply working into a load of 500 $\Omega$ is 10 mA maximum. In order to achieve higher output currents, we require higher voltage power supplies or some form of dc-to-dc conversion.

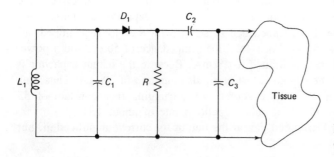

**FIGURE 5.6.** Radio-frequency-receiver-type stimulator.

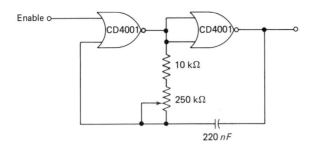

Enable o—

10 kΩ

250 kΩ

220 nF

**FIGURE 5.7.** CMOS oscillator circuit.

## Generator Control Circuits

The span of controls that are found in stimulator designs range from a basic on/off switch on a fixed stimulus unit to a fully programmable unit. Because all patients do not respond to electrical stimulation in the same manner, it is important to be able to vary the characteristics of the stimulation waveform. Parameters that are under user control in some designs are:

1. Output pulse amplitude.
2. Pulse duration.
3. Pulse repetition frequency.

A resistor–capacitor oscillator using complementary metal-oxide–semiconductor NOR gates forms the basic variable pulse-rate generator. Figure 5.7 shows a design that yields pulse rates of 5–200 Hz. The CD4001 chip functions with power-supply voltages as low as 3 V, which is desirable for small low-power designs. This circuit yields a pulse waveform with equal on/off times.

Figure 5.8 shows the section which adds pulse duration control. Pulse widths of 150–350 $\mu$s are possible.

## 5.7 SYSTEMS IN CLINICAL USE

### Transcutaneous Stimulation

Electrical stimulation of peripheral nerves for the relief of pain with electrodes applied to the surface of the body is called transcutaneous electrical neural stimulation (TENS). This approach is based on the previously mentioned gate theory of pain perception. This gate control mechanism modulates sensory inputs before they evoke pain perception. The postulate is that stimulation of the fast conducting A-B fibers inhibits smaller, slower conducting C fiber sensory inputs.

The value of TENS for the relief of pain was discovered during early usage of this form of stimulation as a screening technique for the selection of patients for implantable pain relief devices. About one third of patients suffering from chronic intractable pain can benefit from TENS (Linzer and Long, 1976). In these patients, effective placement of the stimulating electrodes produces a tingling sensation in the painful area. We position the electrodes so that the area of pain is located between

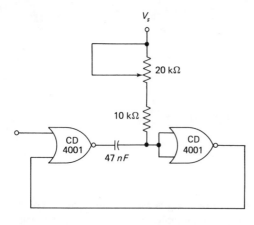

**FIGURE 5.8.** CMOS pulse duration control.

them or stimulate a perhipheral nerve that projects to that area. We must often perform considerable experimentation to find effective electrode locations and optimal stimulation waveform parameters.

Stimulus generators for use in TENS usually have controls for varying pulse width (50–1000 $\mu$s), pulse frequency (20–200 Hz) and output voltage (0–150 V). The output is usually a capacitively coupled bidirectional pulse waveshape.

In those patients reporting excellent pain relief (Linzer and Long, 1976), the stimulation current was 25–60 mA, pulse width was 50–100 $\mu$s, repetition frequency was 15–60 Hz, and charge injected per pulse was 1.5–2.5 $\mu$C.

The pattern of stimulation treatment times depends on the location of patient electrodes and type of pain. A 3-h period of stimulation three or four times daily is typical. Although the total daily stimulation time varies from 15 min to 24 h with an average time of 10.2 h (Linzer and Long, 1976), the average duration of relief following cessation of stimulation is 3.5 h.

The technique of transcutaneous electrical neural stimulation has proven useful in the relief of a variety of types of chronic pain, especially those involving the lumbar section of the spine. The pain etiology commonly involves herniated disks, peripheral neuropathy, injury, arthritis, and strain. TENS is also effective in the relief of acute pain arising postoperatively. Hymes et al. (1974) reported that postoperative pain following various abdominal and thoracic procedures was reduced 60–80%. In addition, electrical stimulation was found to significantly reduce the incidence of postoperative complications such as atelectasis and ileus. Reported stimulation patterns were: rate, 100–150 Hz; pulse widths, 250–400 $\mu$s; and output level, 20–35 mA.

Electrodes used in TENS should be relatively large (4 cm$^2$) to reduce current densities at the skin surface. Because the application times are relatively long, the development of a skin rash at the stimulation site is the most frequent complication.

### *Spinal Cord Implants*

In the late 1960s, neurosurgeons found that electrical stimulation of the spinal cord could relieve certain types of chronic intractable pain. Early applications placed the stimulating electrodes on the dorsal surface of the spinal cord as the gate theory suggests. Stimulation of the ventral surface also provides good pain relief. However, currents passed through multiple electrodes from posterior to anterior columns suppress pain with lower current levels, reduce undesirable paresthesias, and maintain stable thresholds over long time periods.

We do not completely understand the mechanism of pain suppression that results from passage of electrical current. Application of currents to the spinal cord may create a neuronal block in the cord beneath the stimulating electrodes. Clinical studies in which somatosensory evoked potentials were recorded before, during, and after spinal cord stimulation suggest that electrical stimulation produces a depolarizing block beneath the electrodes. Persistence of the block after the current is turned off suggests chemical effects in addition to the immediate electrical effects. Pain relief appears to be related to interference with transmission over fibers of the spinothalamic tract.

The stimulus generator used in these studies supplied capacitor-coupled pulses of 0.1–1.0 ms duration at repetition rates between 10 and 200 Hz with pulse amplitudes up to 4 mA. A common operating point was 250-$\mu$s pulse width at 100-Hz repetition rate and 1-mA output. Linzer and Long (1976) also give an example treatment protocol with the patient self-administering the stimulation for 30-min periods, 3 times each day.

Undesirable side effects of cord stimulation include paresthesias, new areas of pain, muscle contractions, and decreased sensory and joint rotation perception. These side effects result from the spread of the stimulating current to other tracts in the cord. We should avoid stimulation of the corticospinal tract. Good electrode design and surgical positioning can control the current spread.

Electrodes for spinal cord stimulation are multielectrode arrays of three or five platinum disks, 2 mm in diameter. A silicone rubber backing holds these in line and separates them by 4 mm center to center. For single surface applications, the disks are of alternate polarity (Fig. 5.9a), while for currents driven across the cord they are all of the same polarity (Figure 5.9b). Multiple electrodes yield lower and more uniform current densities and less shunting of current.


## Brain Stimulation for Pain Reduction

Although many types of pain can be effectively treated at peripheral sites by surgical techniques or the application of electrical currents, there exist many other types of pain that originate in the central nervous system. Also, we cannot easily treat pain involving cranial and upper-cervical nerves by peripheral methods. Early surgical approaches were aimed at central nerve pathways by making thalamic lesions in the area of the central median nucleus and pulvinar. This technique provided only temporary pain relief (6–12 months) and carried the risk of complications from the destruction of neural tissue.

There are two types of electrical stimulation of the central nervous system based on the site of stimulation. These two stimulation types produce different physiological effects. In the first type, we stimulate the primary sensory nuclei of the thalamus, the ventral posterior medialis (VPM) or lateralis (VPL), or the

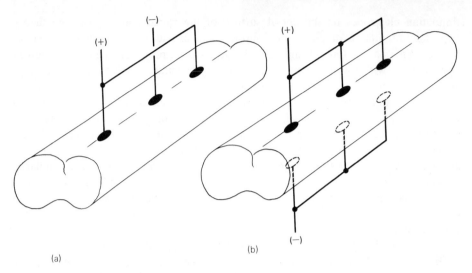

**FIGURE 5.9.** Electrode arrays for spinal cord stimulation. (a) Single surface application. (b) Across-the-cord application.

internal capsule. In the second type, we stimulate the periventricular and peri-aqueductal gray matter, where pain inhibitory systems are located (Fig. 5.10).

**Thalamic Nuclei and Internal Capsule Stimulation.** This type of stimulation effectively controls neurogenic pain from the nervous system or denervated areas of the head and neck. But, it is less effective on externally driven pain arising from pathological processes in the body periphery. Pain relief by this method is short-lived after switching the stimulation off; therefore, we require almost continuous stimulation. It produces paresthesia in the area of pain control. An interrupted ramp stimulation is more efficient than a train of pulses.

**Stimulation of Gray Matter.** Stimulation of periaqueductal gray matter in the brain stem produces strong analgesia but is accompanied by highly noxious side effects. Periventricular stimulation produces weaker analgesia but is better tolerated. Stimulation for a 30-min period provides relief for 6–24 h and is effective for both neurogenic and externally driven pain. Patients that require a high level of stimulating current experience side effects caused by the spread of current to nearby structures. These include nystagmus, a smothered feeling, and temperature paresthesia.

Waveform parameters found to be effective are pulse widths of 150 $\mu$s and repetition rates of 25–50 Hz. At these low frequencies, an increase in stimulation voltage produces the same effect as an increase in frequency.

### Cerebellar Implants

The cerebellum lies at the back of the skull behind the brain stem and below the cerebrum. Its name means "lesser brain" and it is involved in coordination and equilibrium activities. These functions are confined to a thin layer of gray matter known as cerebellar cortex. This layer has many folds and wrinkles to increase its

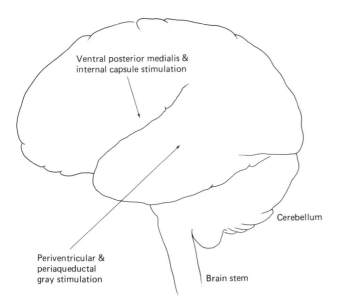

Ventral posterior medialis & internal capsule stimulation

Periventricular & periaqueductal gray stimulation

Brain stem

Cerebellum

**FIGURE 5.10.** Brain stimulation sites.

surface area. Within this layer, the neuronal pattern and interconnections are common to all vertebrates.

The cerebellum coordinates muscle movements initiated by motor centers of the cerebrum and the body's proprioceptive organs. The fundamental circuit of the cortex involves seven different nerve elements. Action potentials or impulses are conducted to the cortical layer by two afferent or input systems: climbing fibers and mossy fibers. The only output or efferent system is the collection of axons from Purkinje cells. The remaining four cell elements, the Golgi, granule, basket, and stellate cells, conduct over short distances between cells. Figure 5.11 shows the spatial distribution of the nerve elements in cerebellar cortex.

Excitation patterns are determined mostly by inhibitory-type neurons. For example, assume that a stimulus is applied to the cortical surface as it would be with implanted electrodes. This activates a small bundle of parallel fibers, which excite the dendrites of all the cells (Purkinje, stellate, basket, and Golgi types) below. Excitation of both basket and stellate cells serves to project the original stimulation of the parallel fibers to additional Purkinje cells, but in an inhibitory manner. Golgi cell excitation also has an inhibitory effect. It inhibits granule cells whose axons are the parallel fibers originally stimulated. Therefore, golgi cells are the negative feedback path that terminates the excitation sequence. This leaves the excitation of Purkinje cells that are directly beneath the parallel fibers as the sole output of the cerebellar cortex.

Note that Purkinje cells can be excited by stimulation of their associated climbing fiber. The Purkinje cell responds with a burst of high-frequency action potentials over a 20-ms time span. This response is strong enough to override all ongoing activity.

Electrical cerebellar stimulation is effective in the treatment of epilepsy,

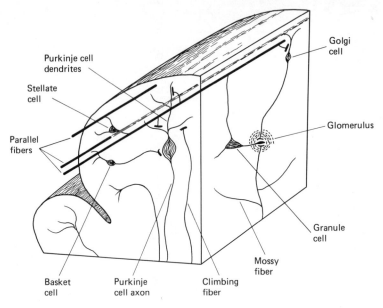

**FIGURE 5.11.** Nerve elements of cerebellum.

cerebral palsy, and motor dysfunction such as spasticity and hypertonus. Cooper (1973a) reported the first clinical use. Although the majority of cases are successfully treated with drugs or brain lesioning, cerebellar stimulation has been used in place of or in conjunction with those forms of treatment.

Results from two areas of neurophysiological research that involved the application of currents to the surface of the cerebellum have suggested the clinical use of this form of therapy. Electrical stimulation of the cerebellum was found to have an effect when decerebrate preparations were used. Transection of the midbrain between the superior and inferior colliculi produces decerebrate rigidity characterized by exaggerated postural tone in antigravity muscles. Muscle control by motor and premotor areas of the cerebral cortex is lost. Stimulation pulses at repetition rates of 30–300 Hz inhibited ipsilateral extensor muscle tone when applied to the anterior lobe of the cerebellum. Pulse rates of 2–10 Hz increased rigidity. Moruzzi (1950) summarizes the results from several authors.

The second area of research that suggested the therapeutic value of cerebellar stimulation involved epileptic discharges. These were also found to be inhibited by pulsed currents of 100–300 Hz applied to the anterior lobe and pyramis of the cerebellum.

At the present time we do not know the specific mechanism by which the stimulating current exerts its effect. Experiments to date suggest three mechanisms. Reimer et al. (1967) suggest that the surface-applied currents spread to cerebellar nuclei or their efferent fibers. Julein and Halpern (1972) believe that the stimulating current increases Purkinje cell activity, which inhibits excitatory outputs of the cerebellar nuclei. Bantli et al. (1976) suggest that the stimulation excites neurons in the ascending reticular formation by antidromic activation of cerebellar afferents.

## Functional Electrical Stimulation

Devices that supplement or replace lost function in neurologically impaired individuals are called neural prostheses. A neural prosthetic technique that utilizes electrical excitation of neural tissue for the inward transmission of control information is termed functional electrical stimulation (FES). FES devices are currently used in the following applications (Hambrecht and Reswick, 1977).

**Foot Drop Correction.** Many patients with cerebrovascular disease, multiple sclerosis, or spinal cord injury experience problems with their gait patterns. The gait problem of foot drop during the swing phase can often be corrected by an external electrical stimulator and surface electrodes. These units are known as peroneal braces. A switch in the heel area of a shoe's inner sole senses the lifting of the heel at the beginning of the leg's swing phase. This information is used to electrically stimulate and cause contraction of dorsiflexor muscles of the foot until the heel again contacts the ground. Some stimulator units can automatically cycle the stimulation sequence to provide therapy for bedridden patients. The success of these external units has made the development of implantable units unnecessary.

**Bilateral Stimulation for Gait Improvement in Cerebral Palsy Children.** The gait pattern of some cerebral palsy children with motor dysfunction of the lower extremities can only be corrected by FES techniques. In this application, the peroneal nerves of each leg are alternately stimulated under contralateral control.

**Correction for Idiopathic Scoliosis.** Curvature of the spine with unknown cause and no evidence of mechanical deficiencies in the joints, ligaments, or tendons of the spinal column is termed idiopathic scoliosis. Stimulation with surface electrodes of the paravertebral muscles on the convex side of the spine has a strong effect on the deformity. This represents an application of FES in postural mechanisms.

**Diaphragm Pacing by Phrenic Nerve Stimulation.** Long-term stimulation (3 years) of the phrenic nerve is useful in the management of chronic hypoventilation. This condition results from brain lesions of the respiratory center, injury to the cervical cord, or cervical cord lesions such as produced by poliomyelitis. Quadriplegic patients are also candidates for this form of ventilatory support. For long-term stimulation, the pulse-generating unit is implanted. Patients require stimulation from 10–24 h per day. The energy required for constant stimulation dictates the use of an external power source. The stimulating electrode is of bipolar, insulated design that encircles the phrenic nerve in the thoracic region. This electrode type minimizes the spread of stimulating current and, therefore, reduces side effects. The stimulation waveform is more complex than previously discussed applications. It consists of a series, for the duration of inspiration, of 150-$\mu$s pulses of increasing amplitude with the rate of increase and inspiration duration under control by the external transmitter.

**Restoration of Micturation Reflex.** The evolution of electronic means for simulating the micturation reflex has proceeded from direct excitation of the bladder's detrusor muscle layer to include volume sensing and regulation of urethral outflow resistance. More recent investigations involve direct stimulation of the spinal cord at the $S_1$–$S_3$ level. Because neurologic dysfunction of the urinary bladder is a common occurrence in multiple sclerosis, spinal cord injury, and Parkinson's disease, continued development of FES systems for this application is important. The reader is referred to Chapter 1 for a discussion of a micturation reflex system.

**Multichannel Stimulation of Leg Muscles.** Multichannel stimulation units required in applications involving dynamic assistance during the stance phase in addition to the swing phase of walking are under development. Clinical results of a six-channel unit were reported by Strojnik et al. (1979). Three groups of flexion and extension muscles were stimulated in a timed sequence. The sequence is initiated with the closure of the heel switch in the one affected leg. With FES, patients can transfer three times more body weight to their disabled leg and double their gait velocity. Major design challenges in multichannel applications involve:

1. Elimination of cross-channel stimulation.

2. Rejection of false triggering from accidental mid-sequence floor contact.

3. Adaptation of stimulus sequence to altered gait velocity requirements

Future developments and improvements in the use of multichannel stimulators in walking applications require increased knowledge and measurements of normal patterns.

## 5.8 FUTURE DEVICES FROM CURRENT RESEARCH

### Electrotherapeutic Sleep Devices

Robinovitch et al. (1914) made the earliest report of the therapeutic benefits of electrical sleep as a treatment for insomnia. Electrotherapeutic sleep or electrosleep (ES) is a special area of application under the more general term *electronarcosis*. Electronarcosis is the term used to describe any phenomenon induced during the passage of electrical currents through the head. Reynolds (1971) describes an electronarcosis family tree. Electronarcosis is divided into three major subdivisions: electroanesthesia, electrosleep, and electrotherapy. The last division is further separated into convulsive and nonconvulsive types.

Electrical currents are commonly applied to the head to correct for severe mental disturbances. Electroconvulsive therapy uses 70–130 V of 60-Hz ac applied for a short time (100–500 ms). The resulting current flow of 1 A or more produces convulsions and loss of consciousness. Tietz et al. (1946) reported a treatment for schizophrenia using 60-Hz ac maintained at 100 mA for up to 30 min. With the development of pulsed waveform generators in the 1950s, nonconvulsive electrotherapy was possible. These generators had controls for pulse-repetition rate, current amplitude, direct current bias, and pulse polarity. With this generation of equipment, a time-averaged current of 10 mA produced an effect. That effect was most often unconsciousness, and it was termed *electrosleep* (Banay, 1952).

The present form of electrosleep that developed in the 1960s resulted from continual experimental reduction of average currents along with increased application times. Now electrosleep treatments typically employ an average current of 500 $\mu$A applied for 1 h or more.

Electroanesthesia is the attempt to electrically produce the equivalent of chemically induced surgical anesthesia. This can be accomplished with pulsed current peaks of 5–50 mA depending on technique. Basic research and developments in electroanesthesia help to guide electrosleep investigations.

**Electrosleep Generators.**   Workers have proposed many different waveforms and electrode placements. This has resulted from a lack of specific knowledge on the basic mechanism of action by which the current produces the sleep state. The waveform most frequently employed is the unbiased rectangular wave known as the Leduc type. The original waveform had a 10% duty cycle, a 100-Hz repetition rate, and a 1-ms pulse duration. Repetition rates between 3–300 Hz have also been employed. A dc bias is sometimes added, which increases the average current.

In addition to the Leduc-type rectangular wave, the following waveforms or techniques are used:

- Sinusoidal waves of 20–10,000 Hz.
- White noise band-limited to 1–50 kHz superimposed on a dc bias.
- Interference currents consisting of two sinusoidal waves of slightly different frequencies each applied to its own pair of electrodes. This waveform produces a resultant wave harmonically varying at one half the difference frequency.
- Bursts of high-frequency waves consisting of 3-ms pulses of 100-kHz sine waves.
- Rotating polarization current, which is made up of two sine waves of the same frequency but with a 90° phase difference. When applied to electrode pairs whose axes are orthogonal, this waveform produces a rotating field at the same frequency.

**Applications.**   Brown (1975) summarizes commercially produced devices. These instruments are mostly high-output-impedance devices. They function as constant current generators with the current level selected by the operator and applied to the subject through large-surface-area electrodes between frontal and occipital locations. The operator increases the current level until the subject perceives a tingling sensation. He adjusts current level and pulse frequency to minimize unpleasant sensations. The electrodes must maintain good contact as intermittent contact produces shocks. Saline-soaked gauze sponges are usually used under the electrodes. Treatment times vary from several minutes to several hours.

Electrosleep is most often applied in the treatment of insomnia and to alleviate the psychiatric symptoms of anxiety, depression, and irritability. Soviet investigators active in this field for the past 30 years report electrosleep therapy to be effective in the treatment of chronic alcoholism, hypertension, hypothalamic disorders, and peptic ulcers, to mention a few.

**Mechanism.** We do not understand just how the electrical currents produce the sleep state. The Soviet viewpoint is based on the theories of Pavlov. He postulated that each nerve cell can exist for a time in a special phase of inhibition, influencing nearby cells and thereby leading to sleep by the radiation of inhibition. He thought it possible to obtain sleep with a weak external physical stimulus that is rhythmic, monotonous, and of long duration. An electric current is one such stimulus. Alternative explanations involve the direct effects of the applied current on some intracranial structure or on sensory tracts of the brain stem.

**Effects.** Basic studies have shown that about 35% of the externally applied current reaches the brain tissue with the rest being shunted by the scalp, skull, and cerebral spinal fluid layer. For a current waveform of 10 mA peak, the resulting current density in brain tissue is 30–50 $\mu A/cm^2$, with electric field intensities approximately 200 mV/cm. Although the current density is an order of magnitude below what is necessary to produce unresponsiveness in electroanesthesia procedures, the electric field strength is an order of magnitude greater than those reportedly able to modify spontaneous neuronal firing patterns. Thus, electrosleep currents are capable of producing neurophysiological modifications.

More recent discoveries involve physiological effects. Electrosleep currents inhibit gastric acid secretion in man. Kotter et al. (1975) report a 30% average reduction in gastric acid output 30 min after application of 900 $\mu A$ average current (1 ms pulses, 100 Hz repetition rate). Rosenthal (1973) reports increased serum thyroxine and catecholamines along with minor alterations in 17 ketosteroids following the transcranial application of current. Because these effects are other than sleep-inducing, the term *transcranial electrotherapy* (TCET) has come into common usage.

**Current Status.** Electrosleep is in widespread use throughout the Soviet Union. It has been applied in the treatment of a variety of psychiatric and psychosomatic disorders for over 30 years. Articles began to appear in the United States in the early 1960s. However, electrosleep has not been equally well accepted here. There exists a need for more basic research into measurable biological changes produced by the transcranial passage of currents at the electrosleep level. Reported hormonal changes caused by ES currents have opened a new area of investigation.

## Spinal Cord Injury

Functional electrical stimulation can potentially help high-level spinal cord injury patients exert voluntary control over paralyzed muscles. Initial experimental efforts are directed toward finger control in quadriplegics (Peckham et al., 1976). Paralyzed muscles lack functional afferent and efferent nervous system connections. Restoration of function, therefore, requires the existence of muscles that will respond to electrical stimulation and a feedback mechanism to monitor and guide performance.

Following paralysis, muscles atrophy and weaken. These muscles can be made functional with low-frequency (15-Hz) stimulation exercise programs. Although feedback control systems are readily designed with current technology, their resulting complexity limits application to basic single-degree-of-freedom hand movements. Three-dimensional locomotion is for future development.

# REFERENCES

BANAY, R. S. (1952). Electrically induced sleep. *Confinia. Neurol.,* 12: 356–60.

BANTLI, H., J. R. BLOEDEL, and D. TOLBERT (1976). Activation of neurons in the cerebellar nuclei and ascending reticular formation by stimulation of the cerebellar surface. *J. Neurosurg.,* 45: 539–54.

BROWN, C. C. (1975). Electroanesthesia and electrosleep. *Am. Psychologist,* 30: 402–10.

BRUMMER, S. B. and M. J. TURNER (1977). Electrochemical considerations for safe electrical stimulation of the nervous system with platinum electrodes. *IEEE Trans. Biomed. Eng.,* BME-24: 59–60.

COOPER, I. S. (1973a). Effects of chronic stimulation of anterior cerebellum on neurological disease. *Lancet,* 1: 206–13.

COOPER, I. S. (1973b). Effect of stimulation of posterior cerebellum on neurological disease. *Lancet,* 1: 1321–29.

COOPER, I. S., E. CRIGHEL, and J. AMIN (1973). Clinical and physiological effects of stimulation of the paleocerebellum in humans. *J. Am. Geriat. Soc.,* 21: 40–43.

DYMOND, A. M. (1976). Characteristics of the metal–tissue interface of stimulation electrodes. *IEEE Trans. Biomed. Eng.,* BME-23: 274–80.

GEDDES, L. A., and L. E. BAKER (1968). *Principles of applied biomedical instrumentation.* New York: Wiley.

HAMBRECHT, F. T., and J. B. RESWICK (eds) (1977). *Functional electrical stimulation— Applications in neural prostheses.* New York: Marcel Dekker.

HODGKIN, A. L., and A. F. HUXLEY (1952). Quantitative description of membrane current and its application to conduction and excitation in nerve. *J. Physiol.,* 117: 500–44.

HYMES, A. C., D. E. RAAB, E. G. YONEHIRO, G. D. NELSON, and A. L. PRINTY (1974). Acute pain control by electrostimulation. *Adv. Neurol.* 4: 761–67.

JARZEMBSKI, W. B., S. J. LARSON, and A. SANCES, JR. (1970). Evaluation of specific cerebral impedance and cerebral current density. *Ann. N.Y. Acad. Sci.,* 120: 476–90.

JULEIN, R. M., and L. M. HALPERN (1972). Augmentation of cerebellar Purkinje cell discharge rate after diphenylhydantoin. *Epilepsia,* 13: 377–85.

KOFFLER, S. W., and J. G. NICHOLLS (1977). *From neuron to brain.* Sunderland, MA: Sinauer.

KOTTER, G. S., E. O. HENSCHEL, and W. J. HOGAN (1975). Inhibition of gastric acid secretion in man by the transcranial application of low density pulsed current. *Gastroenterology,* 69: 359–63.

LARSON, S. J. (1975). A comparison between anterior and posterior spinal implant systems. *Surg. Neurol.,* 4: 180–86.

LARSON, S. J., A. SANCES, JR., J. F. CUSICK, J. MYKLEBUST, E. A. MILLAR, R. BOEHMER, D. C. HEMMY, J. J. ACKMANN, and T. J. SWIONTEK (1976). Cerebellar implant studies. *IEEE Trans. Biomed. Eng.,* BME-23: 319–28.

LINZER, M., and D. M. LONG (1976). Transcutaneous neural stimulation for relief of pain. *IEEE Trans. Biomed. Eng.,* BME-23: 341–45.

MELZACK, R., and P. WALL (1965). Pain mechanisms: A new theory. *Science,* 150: 971–78.

MORTIMER, J. T., C. N. SHEALY, and C. WHEELER (1970). Experimental non-destructive electrical stimulation of the brain and spinal cord. *J. Neurosurg.,* 32: 553–59.

MORUZZI, G. (1950). Effects at different frequencies of cerebellar stimulation upon postural tonus and myotatic reflexes. *Electroencephal. Clin. Neurophysiol.* 2: 463–69.

MORUZZI, G., and R. S. Dow (1958). *The physiology and pathology of the cerebellum.* Minneapolis: U. Minn. Press.

NASHOLD, B. S. (1975). Dorsal column stimulation for the control of pain: A three year follow-up. *Surg. Neurol.,* 4: 146–47.

NEWMAN, M. R. (1978). Biopotential amplifiers, in J. G. Webster (ed), *Medical instrumentation: Application and design.* Boston: Houghton Mifflin.

PECKHAM, P. H., J. T. MORTIMER, and E. B. MARSOLAIS, (1976). Upper and lower motor neuron lesions in the upper extremity muscles of tetraplegics. *Paraplegia,* 14: 115–21.

REIMER, G. R., R. J. GRIMM, and L. S. Dow (1967). Effects of cerebellar stimulation on cobalt induced epilepsy in the cat. *Electroenceph. Clin. Neurophysiol.,* 23: 456–62.

REYNOLDS, D. V. (1971). A brief history of electrotherapeutics, in D. V. Reynolds and A. E. Sjoberg (eds.) *Neuroelectric research.* Springfield, IL: Charles C Thomas.

RICHARDSON, D. E., and H. AKIL (1977). Pain reduction by electrical brain stimulation in man. *J. Neurosurg.,* 47: 184–94.

ROBINOVITCH, L. G., J. T. GWATHMEY, and C. BAKERSVILLE (1914). *Anesthesia.* New York: Appleton.

ROSENTHAL, S. H. (1973). Alterations in serum thyroxine with cerebral electrotherapy. *Arch. Gen. Psychiatr.,* 28: 28–29.

RUCH, T. C., H. D. PATTON, J. W. WOODBURY, and A. L. TOWE (1966). *Neurophysiology.* Philadelphia: W. B. Saunders.

STROJNIK, P., A. KRALJ, and I. URSIC (1979). Programmed six-channel electrical stimulator for complex stimulation of leg muscles during walking. *IEEE Trans. Biomed. Eng.,* BME-26: 112–16.

TIETZ, E. B., G. N. THOMPSON, and A. VAN HARREVELD (1946). Electronarcosis, its application and therapeutic effect in schizophrenia. *J. Nerv. Ment. Dis.,* 103: 144–65.

VAN OVEREEM HANSEN, G. (1979). EMG—Controlled functional electrical stimulation of the paretic hand. *Scand. J. Rehab. Med.,* 11: 189–93.

VODOVINIK, L., U. STANIC, A. KRALJ, R. ACIMOVIC, F. GRACANIN, S. GROBELNIK, P. SUHEL, C. GODEC, and S. PLEVNIK (1977). Functional electrical stimulation in Ljubljana, in T. F. Hamerecht and J. B. Reswick (eds), *Functional electrical stimulation—Applications in neural prostheses.* New York: Marcel Dekker.

## STUDY QUESTIONS

**5.1**  List the major functional components of an electrical stimulation system.

**5.2**  Name three clinical applications of electrical stimulation.

**5.3**  Define the terms *chronaxie* and *rheobase*.

**5.4**  What is the range of pulse repetition rates used in transcutaneous, total implant, and radio-frequency-coupled electrical stimulation of the nervous system?

**5.5**  What determines the minimum effective pulse width of a stimulus waveform?

**5.6**  List the types of reactions that can occur at a tissue–electrode interface when transferring current.

**5.7** In what units is electrical stimulus strength measured?

**5.8** Develop the impedance function from the metal–electrolyte equivalent circuit.

**5.9** Name three stimulation sites that are effective for pain suppression.

**5.10** What are the advantages and disadvantages of transcutaneous versus implanted stimulating electrodes?

**5.11** What magnitude of impedances do implanted stimulating electrodes present to the output of the pulse generator?

**5.12** List the present applications of the neural prosthetic technique known as functional electrical stimulation.

**5.13** How is nerve-impulse propagation velocity related to its chronaxie value?

**5.14** What effects are produced when the cerebellum is electrically stimulated?

**5.15** Discuss the merits of constant-voltage versus constant-current type stimulators.

# 6 Sensory and Communication Aids

*Albert M. Cook*

## 6.1 LEARNING OBJECTIVES

Upon completing this chapter you should be able to:

- Describe the function of the major parts of the speech mechanism.
- Define language and list the major components.
- Describe the major approaches to sensory substitution with advantages and disadvantages of each.
- Describe devices used by the blind for reading and mobility.
- Describe the design and use of hearing aids and aids for the deaf.
- Describe the major approaches to communication aids.

## 6.2 INTRODUCTION

The sensory systems of vision and audition provide the majority of information that we receive about our environment. These two systems account for the major input of information necessary for learning, asthetic pleasure, and recreation. Much of this sensory information is directly related to written or spoken language. Individuals with severe motor system dysfunction may also have a loss of communicative ability. Thus, we include language and speech in this chapter. We primarily deal with current technology that is *available* to individuals with sensory and/or communication handicaps. We also address research directions being actively pursued.

## 6.3 SENSORY AND COMMUNICATIVE SYSTEM FUNCTION AND DYSFUNCTION

We assume that the reader is familiar with the basic physiology of sensory input via the visual and auditory systems. If not, you should consult a basic physiology text such as Selkurt (1976). Kline (1976) presents a biomedical engineering view of sensory function. In this section we concentrate on sensory dysfunction and the basics of speech and language that are fundamental to sensory and communicative aids.

### Speech and Language

We distinguish between the terms *speech* and *language*. Language refers to a system of arbitrary symbols that are organized according to a set of rules. This set of symbols may be the familiar alphabetic written language or spoken language or it may be a set of pictographic symbols conveying meaning (such as hieroglyphics) or a set of hand movements such as sign language. Speech is the oral expression of language. Individuals may have disabilities affecting speech and/or language. A deaf individual generally also has difficulty with expressive language via speech and a blind individual may be unable to use the standard form of manual language (writing). Likewise, the deaf individual may not have access to spoken language and the blind person to written language. Recently, aids have also been developed for individuals with adequate sensory function but with impaired speech and/or language abilities.

**The Speech Production System.**  There are four fundamental components of the speech production system: an air supply (the respiratory system), voicing (the vocal folds), articulation and resonance (the soft and hard palate, tongue, lips, teeth, jaw, alveolar ridges, pharynx, and nasal passage), and central nervous system control (motor control of all components and formation of expressive language components). A fifth part of the system that is vital to successful operation is feedback via the auditory system. We must simulate each of these components in synthetic speech such as that used in reading aids (Section 6.5) or communication devices (Section 6.9).

The well-controlled supply of air is important in order to cause the vocal folds to vibrate. These folds have an average fundamental frequency of 110 Hz and 220 Hz in males and females respectively. They are located behind the thyroid cartilage (Adam's apple). The vibration is actually a complex mechanical pattern. The resonant cavities of the mouth, throat, and nose further modify its quality. We refer to this process of causing the vocal folds to vibrate in a prescribed pattern as *phonation*.

Several disabilities commonly affect the speech mechanism. In addition to deafness, which interrupts the feedback mechanism, dysfunction may occur at any point in the production system. Central nervous system disorders such as cerebral palsy, stroke, or other neurological disease may limit the control of respiratory muscles or prevent the control of the articulators (termed apraxia). When the articulating structures are directly involved, we call the dysfunction *dysarthia*. Respiratory diseases such as emphysema or asthma may also inhibit speech production. Growths on the vocal folds, for example, due to cancer, may inhibit their ability to resonate properly or may lead to the removal of the larynx (vocal folds) (Section 6.9).

**The Structure of Language.** The processing of information received via reading or hearing (receptive language) and the output of language via speech or writing (expressive language) are very complex processes that are not well understood. The form of language is quite variable from speech to writing to sign language, but the fundamental information content is relatively constant. The major variables in the different forms of language are speed and efficiency of presentation. These are controlled by an interaction of central nervous system elements (Gershwind, 1972), peripheral sensors, and output elements. We do not know the exact manner in which the brain processes language, and many fundamental questions regarding this process play a significant role in the design of sensory and communicative aids.

There are five basic components of language: phonology, morphology, syntax, semantics, and pragmatics. Phonology refers to the sounds used in any particular language and the rules for organizing them. The phoneme is the smallest distinctive group or class of sounds in a language that is considered equivalent. A set of approximately 60 phonemes can produce all words in English text. Phonemes are not the same as letters. Phonemes are spoken and letters are written. A word with five letters may have three phonemes. For example, we break the word "night" into its three sounds (phonemes): (1) *n*, (2) *igh*, and (3) *t*. Characteristics that affect more than one phoneme are the prosidic features (also called suprasegmental features). Combinations of these features produce what most people refer to as intonation and stress in speech.

Morphology refers to the meaningful units of a language (morphemes or morphs) and the rules of organizing them. Free morphemes may stand alone (e.g., dog). Bound morphemes connect with a free morpheme (e.g., __er). A *word* is an articulate sound or series of sounds that symbolize, communicate, have meaning, and are used alone as a unit of language.

Syntax provides the rules for organizing words and other longer related units into meaningful utterances. Grammar refers to morphology and syntax and is the set of rules for speaking and/or writing a given language. The parsing (breaking a sentence down into parts and explaining the grammatical form, function, and interrelation of each part) is an example of a grammatical rule.

Semantics refers to the relation between words and their meanings. Pragmatics is the relation between language and language users. These terms are particularly important in considering the substitution of one receptive language mode for another (Section 6.4) or in the development of alternative communication systems (Section 6.9).

We refer to dysfunctions in language by the general term of *aphasias*. Aphasia is not a specific disability but, rather, a general term. We use specific divisions for difficulty in writing (agraphia), difficulty in reading (alexia), reduced ability to remember names (anomia), and inability to associate meaning with one or more classes of symbols (asymbolica).

Clearly, it is the information content that makes language useful. This concept lies at the heart of the development of sensory aids. Studies of the ways in which information is processed by the brain from various sense organs have yielded only sketchy data. These studies do indicate, however, that the form or structure of the language elements is crucial to efficient processing by the brain (e.g., see Nye, 1970 and 1968). The various sense organs and their associated central nervous system processing are adapted to dealing with information in a particular form and at a particular rate. The substitution of one sense for another (see Section 6.4) places constraints on the structure of information presented as well as on the rate of processing. One factor is clear. The brain does not process language by using the simplest elements (e.g., letter-by-letter or phoneme-by-phoneme) but, rather, deals with larger units such as syllables or whole words (Allen, 1971; Kirman, 1973). In order to achieve rapid rates of information input for reading (see Section 6.5), sensory aids must present language in units larger than single letters. Likewise, for efficient and rapid output of language for nonvocal individuals, language units must be correspondingly large (words or phrases).

## Visual Impairment

Visual impairment is typically related to either visual acuity as measured by the Snellen test chart or to the range of the visual field. *Economic blindness* is defined as a corrected visual acuity of 20/200 or visual acuity of more than 20/200 if the visual field subtends an angle no greater than 20° (Allen, 1971). Allen (1971) has described the difficulties that this definition presents in designing sensory aids and in identifying specific segments of the visually impaired population who might benefit from a particular sensory aid.

Although there are no exact figures on the prevalence of blindness as defined above, several studies have provided data ranging from 290,000 to 1,090,000 (Allen, 1971). The wide variance in these data is the result of the way in which they were collected and the definitions employed to include or exclude individuals from the population. Allen states that there are probably a core of 100,000 blind individuals who could benefit from sensory aids.

The majority of blind individuals (about 65%) are over 65 years of age. This is indicative of the leading cause of blindness: senile degeneration. Other causes include diabetes and multiple disabilities of children and the aged. Visual impairment may be the result of direct ocular defect (such as disease affecting the retina) or neural (such as diseases or injuries affecting the brain). Allen (1971), Mann (1974), and Nye and Bliss (1970) contain detailed discussion of the blind population and the "blindness system" that attempts to serve their needs.

## Auditory Impairment

Hearing deficits are less obvious than visual impairments. For this reason, less effort has been expended in this area in terms of developing sensory aids. Estimates of the incidence of hearing impairment vary widely, but there are approximately

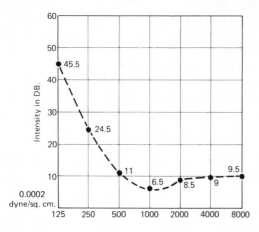

**FIGURE 6.1** This curve relates sound intensity (ordinate) to frequency for equivalent perceived loudness. Each value is referenced to $20\mu$ Pa. Adopted by the International Standards Organization. Reprinted with permission of Reston Publishing Co., Inc., a Prentice-Hall Company, 11480 Sunset Hills Road, Reston, VA.

13.5 million individuals with some degree of hearing loss (Elliott, 1978). Of these, perhaps 300,000–600,000 are functionally deaf. Contrary to popular belief, the deaf obtain relatively little information from lip reading, and only about 10% of the deaf population can effectively use this technique. The vast majority of the deaf population use sign language and the most common type of auxiliary aid used by the deaf is interpreters who have normal hearing and facility with sign language.

**Measurement of Hearing Loss—Audiometry.** The primary method used by audiologists to determine the degree and type of hearing loss is the audiogram. Pure tone threshold audiometry is the most common of the several types of audiometry (Thomas, 1974). This test presents to the ear pure tones representing the major frequencies associated with human speech (124, 250, 500, 1,000, 2,000, 4,000, and 8,000 Hz) and the subject indicates when he hears the tone. To establish the threshold, we raise the amplitude of the tone in 5-dB increments until it is perceived, then lower it in increments until it is not heard. The threshold is the amplitude at which the subject hears the tone 50% of the time. Because the frequency response of the ear is not flat across the range of test tones, we normalize each tone to a standard reflecting the response of the ear. Figure 6.1 shows this standard, which has been established by the International Standards Organization (ISO). The vertical axis of this plot is the intensity in decibels necessary to achieve the same perceived loudness at all frequencies. Thus, it takes 39 dB greater intensity at 125 Hz than at 1,000 Hz for the same perceived loudness. We refer all decibel levels to a standard pressure of 20 $\mu$Pa.

Figure 6.2 shows a typical audiogram. We plot each ear separately, and in plotting the result take into account the ISO curve. Thus, the plot indicates a loss of 50 dB in the left ear at 125 Hz and a 45-dB loss in the right ear at this frequency. This means that we applied an amplitude of 45 + 49.5 dB to this ear and the subject detected it 50% of the time. These curves form the basis for determination of hearing loss and also define goals for hearing aid design (see Section 6.8). Thomas (1974) discusses other types of audiometry.

**Hearing Loss.** Individuals with hearing deficit are typically placed into one of four categories (Mann, 1974). These are: (1) conductive loss associated with

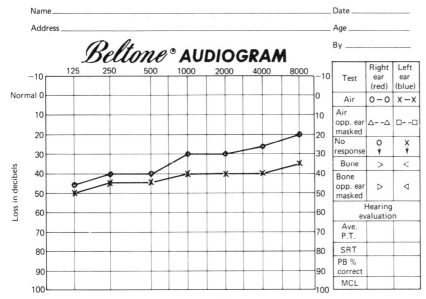

Name _____  Date _____

Address _____  Age _____

By _____

## *Beltone*® AUDIOGRAM

This audiogram plotted to ASA 1951 values

| Test | Right ear (red) | Left ear (blue) |
|---|---|---|
| Air | O – O | X – X |
| Air opp. ear masked | △– -△ | □– -□ |
| No response | O ↓ | X ↓ |
| Bone | > | < |
| Bone opp. ear masked | ▷ | ◁ |
| Hearing evaluation | | |
| Ave. P.T. | | |
| SRT | | |
| PB % correct | | |
| MCL | | |

**FIGURE 6.2** This is a typical pure tone audiogram for a hearing test. The left and right ears are plotted separately. Reprinted with permission of Reston Publishing Co., Inc., a Prentice-Hall Company, 11480 Sunset Hills Road, Reston, VA.

pathological defects of the middle ear, tympanic membrane, or ear canal; (2) sensioneural loss associated with defects in the cochlea or auditory nerve; (3) central induced damage to the auditory cortex of the brain; and (4) functional deafness where the problem is not physical but psychological.

Individuals with less than 60 dB hearing loss of the sensioneural type are the major candidates for hearing aids. Often, a hearing loss is restricted to specific frequency ranges. Greater than 60-dB loss usually precludes the use of a hearing aid and is a functional cutoff for defining deafness.

## 6.4 FUNDAMENTAL APPROACHES TO SENSORY AIDS

All sensory aids must have at least three components: an environmental sensor, an information processor, and a user display interface (Nye and Bliss, 1970). This applies to orthotic devices (e.g., hearing aids) as well as to prosthetic devices (e.g., canes). In some cases, the information processor is very simple, and other cases employ a computer system. The environmental sensor responds to the information normally detected by the defective sensor. The display interface presents information in the same form as the defective sensor when used as an orthotic device. When the sensor is totally nonfunctional, the display interface must present information via an alternative sensory pathway.

## Enhancement or Replacement of Sensory Function

Sensory orthotic devices represent a "gain" problem that depends on the degree of residual function present in the damaged sensory system. Examples of devices in this category are hearing aids (Section 6.8) and closed-circuit television systems for enlarging print and improving contrast (Section 6.5).

The age of the bionic man has created a great deal of public interest in providing replacements for body parts, including sensory systems. Unfortunately, technology has not been able to keep up with television writers and only a few prosthetic sensors have been developed. The most promising is the cochlear implant for aural rehabilitation. Section 6.10 describes this system.

## Use of an Alternative Sensory Pathway

Sensory substitution is necessary when the sensor has total dysfunction. Familiar uses of this method are braille for the blind and sign language for the deaf. Unfortunately, there are fundamental differences between the various sensory systems in both the method of transducing information and the subsequent processing by the central nervous system. These differences are major limitations in the design and successful application of sensory prosthetics. Tactile and auditory systems are used for replacement of the visual system, and visual and tactile systems are used for auditory substitution.

Both the visual and auditory systems process language. The substitution of auditory information for visual or vice versa presents some problems, but they are generally not as severe as those provided by tactile substitution.

**Tactile Substitution.**   There have been many attempts to use tactile substitution as an alternative for either visual or auditory function. The visual system processes information in a spatial mode (Nye and Bliss, 1970). By this we mean that visual information transmitted to the central nervous system retains its orientation relative to other information in space. The auditory system is temporally organized (Kirman, 1973). Auditory information has a unique time relationship that gives it meaning. Tactile information is both spatially and temporally organized (Kirman, 1973). Neither spatial nor temporal cues are adequate, by themselves, to provide effective tactile information processing. For example, the fingers are capable of very fine resolution of features in objects such as coins. However, in order to distinguish a nickel from a dime using only the fingers, we must manipulate the coins. In this way we can determine the important features and identify the coin. If we place two coins on a table and put a hand on top of each coin without moving it, identification is extremely difficult.

We can illustrate the differences between tactile and visual input of information for such tasks as reading by the following examples (Kirman, 1973). A page of print is a purely spatial display. When reading visually, we scan the page and receive a series of spatial displays of information. If a braille reader were to use the same method of reading that a sighted individual uses, then he would place his hand on a given segment of a braille page and input the information. He would then lift his hand and place it on the next adjacent area and so forth. This method would clearly provide poor reading ability because, in strictly spatial terms, the skin cannot provide the same function as the eyes. The braille reader moves his finger across the raised characters and receives both spatial and temporal information cues.

Likewise, the sighted reader would do poorly if he used the tactile methods of information processing. This would consist of dragging printed material across a stationary field. With the eye fixed, visual input would be blurred and information would be lost. Thus, the methods of input and processing of visual and tactile information are very different and we must consider these differences in designing sensory substitution systems. In visual input of information, movement generally impedes perception, but in tactile input it is the lack of movement that is most restricting.

When the tactile system substitutes for visual information regarding the environment for activities such as mobility or vocational skills, this slightly alters the temporal aspects. During walking, the eyes scan the environment and derive informational cues from both the spatial relationships of objects and the changes in these relationships with time. The tactile system is more suited to this task.

In the previous section, we discussed the need for processing linguistic units larger than single letters in order to achieve reasonable speeds. It is not the perception of individual visual features of letters that provides useful information but the integration of these features into recognizable words. The efficient processing of information is possible only if the individual features lose their identity within a larger organization. Likewise, it is much less important to the user of a sensory aid to identify the height of a curb than it is to recognize that it represents the boundary to a street. It has not been difficult to design sensory aids that convert print (or other visual data) into some kind of tactile or auditory output (Nye, 1968). The major problem has been the construction of a machine with an output that has characteristic patterns that can be rapidly identified by the brain. Bach-y-Rita (1972) presents a detailed description of this problem in terms of brain mechanisms.

The use of tactile substitution for auditory perception of speech presents a different set of problems. Except for localization of sound, the auditory system is strictly temporally oriented. The perception of auditory information using the skin has not proven successful (Kirman, 1973). The major reason for this is that the skin has no effective means of converting sound into meaningful information units; that is, it has no cochlea. With practice, we can identify isolated words, phonemes, or syllables using tactile representations. The difficulty arises when we attempt to perceive connected discourse using the skin. A number of methods have been tried to enhance the temporal aspect of the tactile sense (see Section 6.8).

The only tactile method that has proven successful is the vibration method. It consists of placing the hands on the speaker's face with the thumbs on the lips, index fingers on the sides of the nose, little fingers on the throat, and the other fingers on the cheeks. This approach is used by the deaf–blind and was used by Helen Keller. The success of this method is due to the use of information derived from the kinesthetic movements of the finger joints and muscles as well as from the surface of the skin. The success of this method had led to a theory that the fundamental relationship between speech and perceived information is the movement of the articulators rather than the physical features of the acoustic signal (Leiberman, 1967).

Although no conclusive experiments have been done, it appears that the syllable rather than the phoneme is the perceptual unit in speech (Kirman, 1973). This has profound implications for sensory aids. Systems that provide letter-by-letter input necessarily fail in speed because of the time required to reassemble them into meaningful units. Likewise, systems based on recognition of phonemes are inefficient because the brain is not normally required to carry out the synthesis of phonemes into syllables and words. Only systems that can convey larger linguistic elements such as syllables are able to efficiently input information. This, of course, requires a decoder that provides a syllabic breakdown of words into a form easily processed by the tactile sense.

The skin suffers from another limitation. Input to one skin receptor field invariably affects the input to adjacent fields (Bach-y-Rita, 1972). This effect is called *masking of information.*

**Auditory Substitution.** Use of the auditory system as a substitute for visual information input has been a goal of several sensory aids. The least expensive method is to use complex sound patterns that are easily generated by using relatively simple hardware. It is useful to analyze devices that were not successful in order to understand fundamental limits. One such system is the Mauch Laboratories Sterotoner system (Mauch Labs, Dayton, OH).

The Sterotoner was based on the generation of a series of tones that represented shapes of letters. The camera consisted of a series of slits that allowed reflected light to reach photodetectors located behind each slit. Illumination of the lowest detector generated a corresponding low tone. As slits aligned with letter features located vertically above the first slit, it generated higher tones. These tones created musical chords when activated together. With practice users were able to read at 40–60 words per minute. This reading was possible because of the learned sequence of chords that occurred as the sensor moved across the specific letter.

The Sterotoner is no longer available, and the reasons for this are instructive.

1. The ear is uniquely equipped to recognize speech when it is presented in complete utterances. It is not well suited to slow temporal presentations of data as required by the Sterotoner.

2. The use of a letter-by-letter format always leads to slow reading because of the necessity for the brain to reassemble the letters into words and then to ascribe meaning to those words.

3. It was necessary to scan each letter rather than to perceive an entire letter or word at one time. The visual system takes in a much wider range of information than individual spatial characteristics (e.g., curved lines, horizontal lines, etc.) of each letter.

4. The Sterotoner was tedious for the user because it required so much concentration to distinguish letters. This process is not a part of reading visually and is an impediment to rapid identification of words.

The failure of this direct translation method proved that linguistic units larger than letters must be simultaneously displayed to the user. Thus, speech emerges as the only viable method for an auditory reading aid. Nye (1968) and Allen (1978) present detailed arguments in favor of this approach.

The use of auditory substitution for other than reading offers more promise. Mobility for the blind, for example, is dependent on much more gross cues than is reading. In this case, the problem is one of identification of large objects and potential hazards.

**Visual Substitution.** The use of the visual system for aids for the deaf has some potential advantages. One of the major problems that the deaf have in lip reading is the identification of sounds that do not involve the gross movement of the articulators. Visual cues derived electronically can provide assistance in this regard (Section 6.8).

The major methods of using visual imput as a substitution for auditory processing involve the use of banks of filters that provide an analysis of the speech signal into discrete frequency bands (Elliot, 1978). This is not the manner in which useful information is obtained from speech by the auditory system. The reassembly of frequency spectra into recognizable speech units is a complex process for which the visual system is poorly organized.

## 6.5 READING AIDS FOR THE VISUALLY IMPAIRED

Aids exist for individuals with visual impairment or with total loss of vision. Because a large portion of the information that we obtain is through reading, a great deal of effort has been expended in finding ways for the blind to have access to the printed page.

### Low-Vision Aids for Reading

The most common form of low-vision reading aid is large-print books. Books are available in enlarged print through the American Printing House for the Blind and other sources. These books are printed in type size that can be seen by partially sighted people.

Another commonly available aid for the partially sighted is closed-circuit television. These systems consist of a TV camera mounted over a lighted table. The user places the printed material to be read on the table and the camera sends an image to a TV screen in front of the user. Typical systems provide magnification from 4X to 60X. They have tactile controls and most display a choice of either a positive or negative image. Systems are available both in libraries or other central reading rooms and for personal use. Several manufacturers also provide CRT displays that can be formatted in large print. Visualtek (Santa Monica, CA) and Apollo lasers (Los Angeles, CA) manufacture closed-circuit TV systems.

### Altered Reading-Format Methods for the Blind

The blind use two basic methods to obtain information in written form. These are braille and talking books. Both of these modes of information input suffer from the limited number of materials available in these forms. Because speed is important in

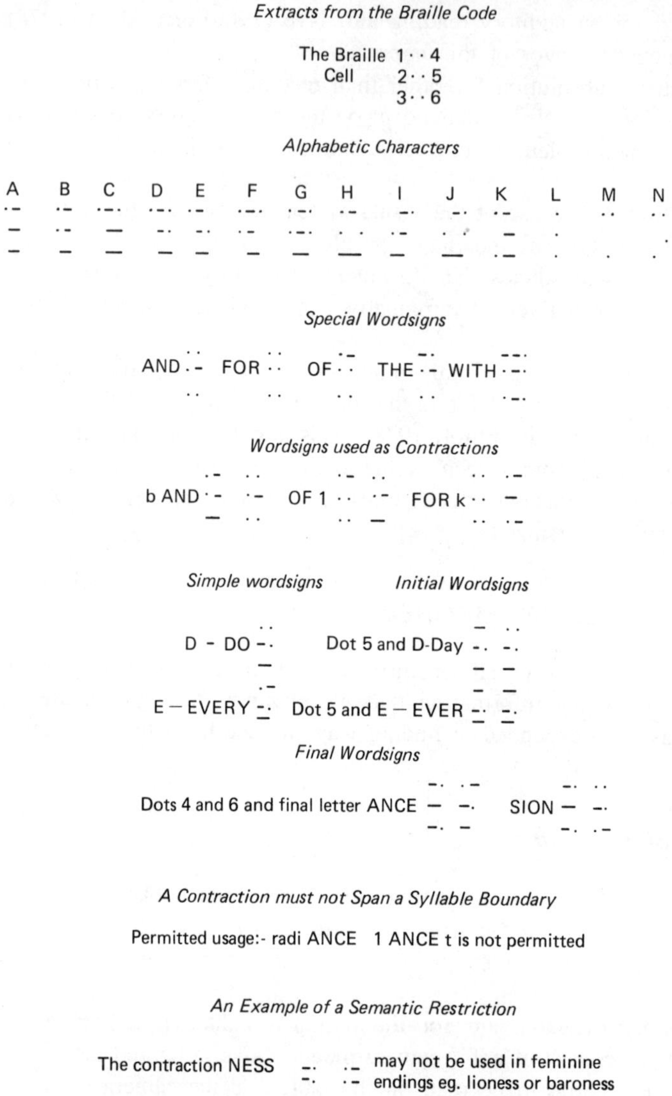

*Extracts from the Braille Code*

The Braille   1 · · 4
    Cell       2 · · 5
                3 · · 6

*Alphabetic Characters*

A   B   C   D   E   F   G   H   I   J   K   L   M   N

*Special Wordsigns*

AND    FOR    OF    THE    WITH

*Wordsigns used as Contractions*

b AND        OF 1        FOR k

*Simple wordsigns*          *Initial Wordsigns*

D - DO           Dot 5 and D-Day

E — EVERY        Dot 5 and E — EVER

*Final Wordsigns*

Dots 4 and 6 and final letter ANCE        SION

*A Contraction must not Span a Syllable Boundary*

Permitted usage:- radi ANCE    1 ANCE t is not permitted

*An Example of a Semantic Restriction*

The contraction NESS        may not be used in feminine
                            endings eg. lioness or baroness

**FIGURE 6.3** Braille uses contractions to signify syllables and whole words. The alphabet is repetitive in groups of 10. Compare A and K (adds dot 3).

reading, several approaches have been used to increase the efficiency of tactile (braille) and auditory (recorded) substitutions for visual reading. When we use only single letters, reading speed is very low (about 30–40 wpm). Figure 6.3 shows an example of contracted braille developed to increase speed. This form uses single symbols for entire words and for affixes, allowing the user to read at a rate of nearly 200 wpm.

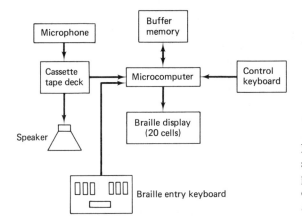

**FIGURE 6.4** Paperless braille systems consist of several components. Both braille input and output and audible output are available.

Speech-compression devices allow recorded messages to be played at faster rates (up to 2.5 times normal speed) without the customary distortion. This greatly increases the rate of information transfer.

One other aspect of reading is important in the design and application of sensory devices. Reading is a symbolic process. The image created from reading a printed page is the result of processing by the central nervous system and is not a direct translation of what is seen. For example, when we read the word "tree," we form an image of this object. This image is the result of a great deal of learning and central nervous system processing. For printed material, the visual system optimizes this process. When we use alternatives, the processing is more difficult and more complex.

### Paperless Braille Systems

There are several major limitations to standard braille materials.

1. The material is embossed on heavy paper that is bulky and that accommodates only a fraction of a normal printed page on one sheet. For example, an imprint text of 400 pages results in four books each the size of a volume of the Encyclopedia Britannica when translated into braille (Mann, 1974).

2. The cost of producing braille material in this form is high.

3. It is not possible to edit material and make corrections once the material is embossed.

4. The systems available for note-taking via braille are bulky and noisy and do not provide any methods of indexing material.

Many of these problems are eliminated in paperless braille systems. Some systems have been developed as computer terminals for the blind (Mann, 1974). Figure 6.4 shows a block diagram of a typical system. This system contains a number of features that overcome the limitations of paper braille. The system accepts cassette tapes that have been previously encoded with digital information

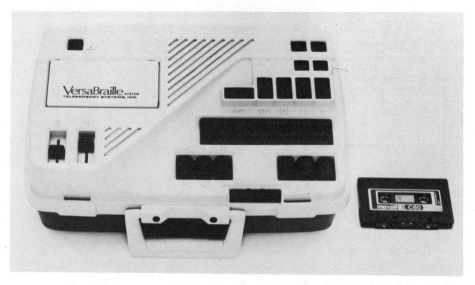

**FIGURE 6.5** A paperless braille system. (Courtesy of Telesensory Systems, Inc., Palo Alto, CA).

sufficient to allow output of braille to the user. The output is via a 20-cell electronically activated braille reading area. The cost of copying and distributing these tapes is very low compared to the costs of reproducing paper braille documents.

The system contains an on-board microcomputer system that facilitiates many other useful features. For example, when reading a prerecorded message, the system presents one line at a time (20 standard 6-dot braille cells). When the user completes that line, he pushes the advance bar and this displays the next line. With practice he can achieve reading rates comparable to those of paper braille. The computer also ensures that no word is split at the end of a line. A single tape cassette can store hundreds of pages of paper braille text.

The system shown in Fig. 6.4 also has provisions for writing material onto tape so that the users can later retrieve it. This feature is based on a 6-button braille entry keyboard similar to that used for mechanical braille writers. There is, however, no noise such as that associated with the mechanical systems. This feature of the device allows the blind user to take notes in class, at meetings, and so on and later review them. He can also use the tape recorder in an audio record-playback mode for recording information.

One of the most powerful features of the paperless braille system is its editing capability. Through the use of a storage buffer and microcomputer control over the tape cassette system, the user can name files and set them up for specific pieces of information. This allows him to easily retrieve the information. The 1,000-character buffer represents one "page" of braille text. Within this page, the user can retrieve any page from memory and delete, add, change, or insert material. Figure 6.5 shows a paperless braille system, manufactured by Telesensory Systems, Inc. (Palo Alto, CA).

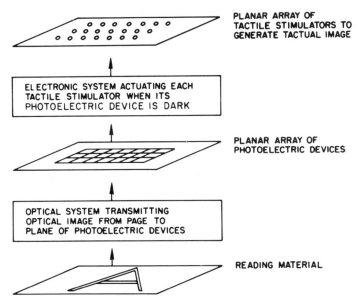

PLANAR ARRAY OF
TACTILE STIMULATORS TO
GENERATE TACTUAL IMAGE

ELECTRONIC SYSTEM ACTUATING EACH
TACTILE STIMULATOR WHEN ITS
PHOTOELECTRIC DEVICE IS DARK

PLANAR ARRAY OF
PHOTOELECTRIC DEVICES

OPTICAL SYSTEM TRANSMITTING
OPTICAL IMAGE FROM PAGE TO
PLANE OF PHOTOELECTRIC DEVICES

READING MATERIAL

**FIGURE 6.6** The optacon uses a phototransistor array to form an image of printed material. This material is converted to a tactile display using piezoelectric crystals. (From Clynes and Milsum, *Biomedical Engineering Systems,* New York: McGraw-Hill, 1969 with permission.)

## Sensory Aids that Provide Access to Printed Materials

All of the currently available reading aids for the blind use an alternative sensory pathway. We may group these devices into two categories: direct translation and speech output. The earliest devices were all direct translation, and developers tried both auditory and tactile devices. Nye and Bliss (1970) and Allen (1971) have reviewed early approaches to direct translation devices.

**Direct Translation Devices Using Tactile Facsimile.** The most widely used reading aid for the blind is the Optacon manufactured by Telesensory Systems, Inc. (Bliss, 1968). Figure 6.6 shows the overall system functions of the Optacon. The environmental sensor is a $6 \times 24$ monolithic array of phototransistors. The user passes a small probe containing this array over the printed material to be read. The probe also contains a lens system, light source, and filter that provide a reflected image from the printed page (Brugler et al., 1969). The lens system provides for varying sizes of print with a range of magnification of 2.5 to 1. The filter prevents reflected light in the near infrared region from reaching the sensor.

Figure 6.7 shows a simplified block diagram of the Optacon. When the probe is placed over a letter, the phototransistor array detects a facsimile image of light and dark regions. The rows of the photoarray are spaced 0.127 mm apart and the columns 0.254 mm apart. This spacing allows for the imaging of pica type. The phototransistors are operated in a charge storage or integration mode. Each is interrogated by applying a pulse to the emitter. During this pulse, the collector

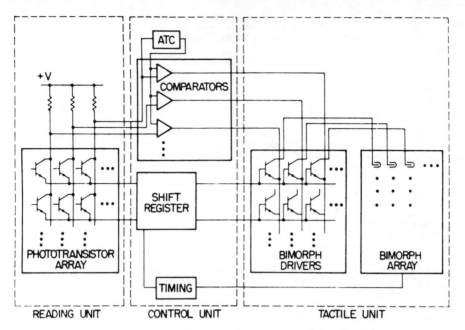

**FIGURE 6.7** The optacon has three major electronic components: reading unit, control unit and tactile unit. See text for explanation of the function of each. (From Brugler, et al., *IEEE J. Solid State Circ.* SC-4, 304-312, 1969.)

current will rise if the transistor is illuminated. The collector voltage pulse is detected by a comparator circuit. The interface consists of an array of lead zirconate piezoelectric crystals arranged in a 6 × 24 array. A one-to-one correspondence exists between the phototransistor elements and the crystals. Figure 6.8 shows one element of this array. An ac voltage applied to the crystal vibrates a nickel stimulator pin that projects through a small hole in the finger rest plate. The comparator circuit disables any crystal whose corresponding phototransistor element is illuminated. An automatic threshold circuit (ATC) compensates for different contrast ratios. The spacing of the stimulator pins is 0.127 (rows) × 0.254 (columns) cm or 100 × the area of the detector array. All 144 stimulators fit on the tip of one finger.

The control unit provides the scanning of both the phototransistor array and the tactile display elements. The emitters of the phototransistors and the transistor switches driving the crystals (bimorphs) are enabled sequentially by a shift register. The threshold circuit (comparator) provides drive current to crystals not illuminated to create an image of the letter. Timing is required to set the frame speed (200 Hz) and the scanning rate of the elements. Each phototransistor and crystal is activated for 50 $\mu$s (20-kHz clock). This allows enough time for all elements to be scanned in one frame and time for stored charge in the crystal to be depleted. The 200 Hz frame rate is ideally suited to the requirements of the tactile sense in the finger. Brugler et al. (1969) describe the electronics in detail. Power consumption for the

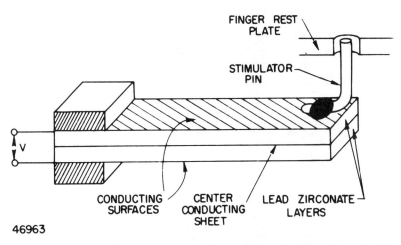

FINGER REST
PLATE

STIMULATOR
PIN

V

CONDUCTING
SURFACES

CENTER
CONDUCTING
SHEET

LEAD ZIRCONATE
LAYERS

46963

**FIGURE 6.8** One element of the optacon tactile display unit. (Reprinted from Sterling, et al., *Visual Prosthesis: the Interdisciplinary dialogue,* NY: Academic Press, 1971 with permission.)

entire unit is under 0.5 W. The batteries (rechargeable NiCd) provide about 12 h of use between charges. The complete unit, shown in Fig. 6.9, weighs about 3.6 kg.

Users require approximately 50 h of practice to effectively use the Optacon, and reading rates achieved are in the range of 20–40 wpm. This slow rate is the major disadvantage of the Optacon. Its principal advantage is that the user can read any printed material without the need for translation into braille or recording onto tape. The device is noisy due to the vibrating reeds, and some users experience difficulty in keeping the probe aligned with the printed material, especially when moving to the next line of text. Braille users also experience some difficulty because the finger receiving the tactile input is stationary in the Optacon with the other hand moving over the page. In braille, the hand receiving the tactile stimulation is the same one that moves over the material. Tactile information is most readily assimilated when the finger is moving over the object, rather than stationary (Kirman, 1973) (see Section 6.4).

**Reading Devices Employing Speech Output.** There are several limitations to these devices. The direct translation devices are slow due to their letter-by-letter facsimile approach. The paperless braille system requires translation of material into digital form. Also, only about 10% of the total blind population is able to use braille (Mann, 1974). Talking books also require translation of the material from written to auditory form. These deficiencies have led designers to search for additional methods that combine speed and ready access to printed material. The most useful of these is a computer that generates spoken output from written material.

Allen (1978) presents the major criteria for successful conversion of printed text to spoken output. He defines four major constraints that must be satisfied.

1. The system must be able to convert all English words to spoken form.

2. The speech output must be intelligible and sound natural.

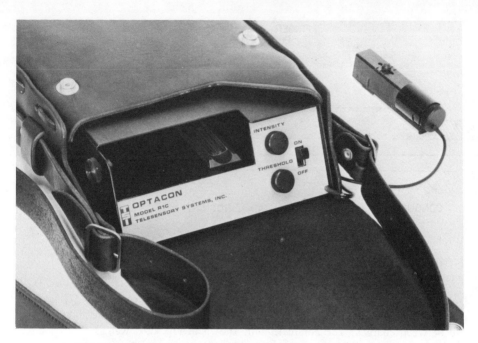

**FIGURE 6.9** The optacon camera is shown to the right of the main electronic unit. The case contains the electronics and tactile stimulator array. (Courtesy Telesensory Systems, Inc., Palo Alto, CA).

3. The system must not cause fatigue for the listener and it must be easily learned.

4. The hardware must be low-cost and require little space and power.

With the availability of microcomputer systems and large-scale integrated (LSI) circuits, we can meet these goals.

Figure 6.10 shows a total system for text-to-speech conversion. Any system designed for this purpose must contain all of the components shown. However, the specific implementation may vary. There are three primary elements included in the print-to-speech system: an optical character-recognition (OCR) transducer, a computer for processing and control, and a speech synthesizer.

The OCR includes a camera that optically scans the page under the control of the computer. The OCR must also interpret the optical image as text characters with recognition of variable type fonts and correction for broken characters or characters that are run together. This process of correction need not be perfect because the blind user can generally interpret the output from context. However, the error rate must be low enough so that the user can depend on the OCR to provide correct interpretation most of the time. There are two basic types of camera systems. In one, the user controls the camera and moves it across the page by hand. The camera associated with the Optacon is an example of this type. For rapid reading (up to 200 wpm), automatic scanning of an entire printed page is necessary. An

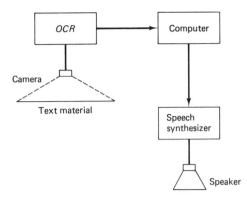

**FIGURE 6.10** A speech output reading aid consists of an optical character recognition system (OCR), computer and speech synthesizer. Various versions may implement each component in different ways.

example of the latter approach is the Kurzweil Reading machine (KRM) available from Kurzweil Computer Products, Cambridge, MA.

The remainder of the OCR must be programmed to recognize features of characters that allow proper identification. For example, the existence of curved lines, horizontal lines, and a broken area on the right side helps to identify a character as an *e*. The OCR system must also compare the geometric features with stored examples of various letters and deal with ambiguities such as broken or connected letters, use contextual information to help identify unknown letters, and separate characters into meaningful units (words). Then the actual synthesis of spoken output is carried out using an on-board microcomputer system.

Allen (1978) has defined the major steps necessary for text-to-speech conversion. These are: lexical analysis; parsing; letter-to-sound, lexical stress, and morphophonemic rules; timing control; pitch control; and phonemic speech synthesis. The lexical analysis uses a lexicon of about 12,000 root words and affixes stored in computer memory. Algorithms analyze words from the OCR into a set of morphs. This leads naturally to a phonetic transcription of the word. At the end of this process, the pronunciation of most of the words imaged is available because 12,000 root words can generate about 10 times that many utterances. Also, the OCR has computed a part of speech set for each word. The parsing algorithms are necessary in order to determine the timing and pitch structure of the synthesized version of the identified word. This part of the program determines the syntactic relationship of the input sentences. Even though it is not possible to completely parse arbitrary English sentences, it is possible to recognize units such as noun and verb phrases quickly with low memory requirements. The result of these first two steps is a data structure that contains most of the linguistic structure necessary to begin the synthesis process.

Because not all words or roots are included in the lexicon, there must be provisions for dealing with unrecognized fragments. The system accomplishes this by converting the letters to phonemes (letter-to-sound rules). These rules do not always work well for common words such as *have* and *behave*. They do work well for nonsense words and misspellings. The output of this stage is a phonetic representation of the words not in the lexicon. The computer can also calculate stress contours for words at this stage. For example, the stress contour of vowels may change based on the word (compare *human* and *humanity*). Some words also change stress depending on their meaning. (e.g., *refuse, invalid*). Also, when we join some roots together, this changes the stress. Allen cites the examples of "inform + ate + ion = information." Morphophonemic rules predict these changes in stress. At this point, the system has completely converted the input sentence to the required phonemic content necessary for speech synthesis.

Timing and pitch control contribute significantly to the intelligibility of the final spoken output. Timing control must determine the correct temporal sequence of the utterance and provide proper pauses in the spoken output. The OCR uses pitch control to provide the proper emphasis to the sentence as a whole as well as to individual words. For example, the inflections normally associated with questions differ from those of declarative sentences. These two aspects of the total system must be capable of providing speech, with proper inflections, that is easy to listen to and understand.

The final step in the process is phonemic synthesis according to a set of algorithmic rules. Sherwood (1979) has reviewed the basic approaches to speech synthesis. Basically, the system must model the human speech mechanism. A time-varying vocal tract model that mimics the function of the articulators, vocal folds, and air supply must be incorporated into a computer system. The OCR then digitally synthesizes phonemic structure, converts it to analog form, and drives a speaker. The set of rules is complicated and is constantly under development. Allen (1976) has discussed the computer algorithms for these processes.

The KRM is the only print-to-speech system currently available commercially. However, Telesensory Systems, Inc., will soon have a modular system available that will allow use of the Optacon imaging system with OCR and text-to-speech modules (Groner and Savoie, 1979). They will also have a complete automatic scanning system available. Jurgen (1980) discusses this system in some detail. IBM has a typewriter attachment that uses a microprocessor to control a speech synthesizer (Jurgen, 1980). This system has 44 kbytes of memory that generate spoken output for keys pressed. Text-editing utilizes rules similar to those for the KRM system to produce spoken output of whole words.

## 6.6 MOBILITY AIDS FOR THE BLIND

Mobility presents significant problems for the blind. Lack of information input via reading is inconvenient, but lack of sight for moving in the environment can be both frustrating and frightening. The blind traveler uses many methods to orient himself to his environment and to move safely within it (American Foundation for the Blind, 1978). By being alert to sensory inputs of smell, sound, air currents, and surface texture, the blind person can orient himself to the terrain and environment and can learn to pick up cues regarding objects. Sound cues provide input via reflections, sound shadows, and echo location. Touch includes the perception of small currents of air or changes in temperature. Temperature changes may occur under a canopy on a warm day or in front of a window on a winter day. Characteristic odors of bakery and restaurants also provide information. Kinesthetic sense helps in the detection of gradients, estimation of distances, and awareness of position. The blind also use travel aids, some of which we discuss in this section.

## Reading versus Mobility

Mann (1974) points out that there are several important differences between reading and mobility aids for the blind. In reading aids, the input is constrained by the printed text. This is not the case for environmental cues that the blind traveler must sense. An error in reading results only in misinformation. An error in mobility could lead to embarrassment or injury. The anxiety associated with such errors places extreme reliability and accuracy requirements on mobility aids.

These requirements and the need to avoid obstacles in the travel path have led to some very different approaches to mobility aids than those taken for reading aids. Nye and Bliss (1970) state that the obstacles of most concern to blind travelers are bicycles, streets, posts, toys, ladders, scaffolding, overhanging branches, and awnings. Most of these are either small or present a small cross-sectional area to the blind traveler. They are also movable and the blind cannot predict their location.

## Canes

The most commonly employed (perhaps 40,000 users) mobility aid for the blind is the long cane consisting of four parts: the crook, the grip, the shaft, and the tip (Farmer, 1978). The crook forms the handle or hood portion. The grip enhances grasping by the addition of leather, plastic, rubber, or some other material and maximizes the tactile information transmitted to the user. The shaft possesses enough rigidity to enable the user to accurately sense distance and position of objects. It must maintain its shape under conditions of stress, such as wind. The periplotogist (orientation and mobility specialist) prescribes the long cane based on the blind user's height, length of stride, and comfort.

Folding canes are also available for the blind. These have additional requirements of a minimum of 5,000 fold-extend cycles (1 year of use), collapsible size to fit into a pocket, and weight under 2.5 kg. They must also be close mechanical equivalents to long canes. Farmer (1978) discusses both of these types of cane in some detail.

The major advantages of the cane are the low cost and simplicity of use. Its major limitations are the inability to detect overhangs and limited range. The user moves the cane in an arc as he walks, and the useful range is approximately one full step in front of the user.

## Electronic Travel Aids

Despite its widespread use, the long cane does not completely solve the problems faced by the blind traveler. Electronic travel aids (ETAs) provide some additional capability. An ETA is a device that sends out signals to sense the environment,

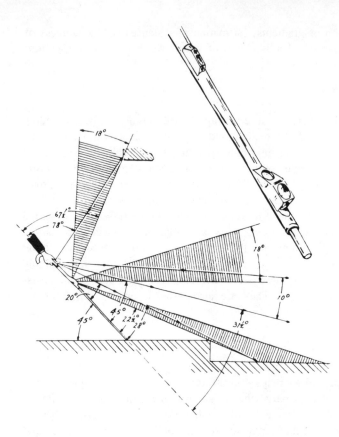

**FIGURE 6.11** The optical triangulation system in the laser cane uses three lasers and three receivers. The reflected beams are shown stripped. (From Nye and Bliss, *Proc. IEEE*, 58, 1878-1898, 1970 with permission).

processes the return data, and provides the user with information about the environment (Farmer, 1978). The major advantage of the ETA is that it can scan an enhanced range and detect overhangs.

Farmer (1978) summarizes the design goals for ETAs. An ETA must detect obstacles and indicate their approximate size and distance. It should also detect downsteps and holes as well as upsteps and low obstacles. The device should be lightweight and easily stored. The user should be able to integrate the output of the device with other sensory input and should easily interpret the output without extensive training. The aid should not interfere with any of the normal sensory channels and should provide both auditory and tactile outputs. No one aid meets all of these specifications, but several embody many of these features.

The laser cane is an ETA that overcomes two deficiencies of the long cane. Figure 6.11 shows the basic principle of the laser cane, which uses optical triangulation ranging (Allen, 1971). Three gallium arsenide lasers illuminate the forward path, an upward path for overhangs and a downward path for drop-offs. Each beam is 2.54 cm wide at 2.5 m, giving resolution of small objects. The gallium arsenide lasers emit a pulse every 40 ms at 900 mm. Figure 6.12 shows the three receivers located below the laser beams. Each of the three channels has a separate output for the user. The downward channel warns via a 200 Hz tone for any drop-off of more than 22 cm (9 in.) that appears two paces in front of the traveler. The upward beam

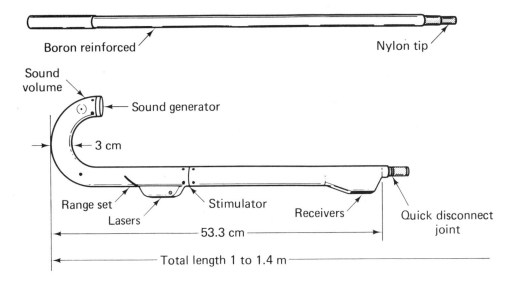

Boron reinforced

Nylon tip

Sound volume

Sound generator

3 cm

Range set

Lasers

Stimulator

Receivers

Quick disconnect joint

53.3 cm

Total length 1 to 1.4 m

Laser Cane Closeup

**FIGURE 6.12** The laser cane receivers and transmitting lasers are located in the handle. The tactile and auditory feedback transducers are also shown. (From Nye and Bliss, *Proc. IEEE,* 58: 1878-1898, 1970).

detects obstacles at head height that appear directly above the cane tip. This channel generates a 2,600-Hz warning sound when it encounters an obstacle. The forward-looking channel has a variable range from 1.8–3.7 m (5–12 ft) and provides an output via tactile stimulators located in the grip or a 1,600-Hz tone that may be turned off. This beam is about 70 cm above the ground. The upward and downward channels also provide tactile stimulation to indicate the presence of objects. The user can increase the effective field of the cane by scanning in an arc as is done for the long cane. A 6-V rechargeable battery provides the needed 600 mW of power.

The device weighs about 3.9 kg (8.6 lb) as compared to the long cane weight of 0.15–0.225 kg (6–8 oz). Tactile feedback from the cane tip in comparison to the long cane is not as good due to the extra weight and additional components, and the price is, of course, much higher. The laser cane is manufactured by Nurion, Inc., King of Prussia, PA.

### Ultrasonic Binaural Sensing Aid

Because the long cane is so effective in aiding mobility, several ETAs augment rather than replace it. We discuss those that use ultrasonic echo-ranging techniques. Figure 6.13 shows the binaural ultrasonic sensing eyeglasses developed by Kay. Allen (1971), Nye and Bliss (1970), and Mann (1974) describe this device.

There is a transmitter located over the nosepiece and two receivers located

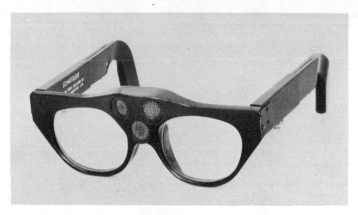

**FIGURE 6.13** The binaural sensing glasses have two receivers and one transmitter located over the nosepiece. The auditory signal is fed to the ears through small tubes. (Courtesy Wormald International Sensory Aids Corp., Bensenville, IL).

below the transmitter on each side. User input is via tubes placed in each ear so as not to interfere with the perception of ambient auditory cues. Processing electronics together with the necessary batteries are in a small package worn at the waist. The hands are completely free for using a cane. Scanning of the environment is possible by head movement from side to side.

Figure 6.14 shows the major components of the system (Rowell, 1974). A transmitter emits 230-ms pulses of ultrasound power swept from 85–45 kHz. This FM signal may be represented by

$$s(t) = A(t)\cos(\omega_o t + \tfrac{1}{2}mt^2) \qquad 0 < t < T \tag{6.1}$$

where  $A(t) = $ a modulation function that inhibits $s(t)$ during the 20-ms reset period

  $\omega_o(t) = $ initial angular frequency

  $m \qquad = $ rate of change in angular frequency

$s(t)$ is repetitive with a period $T = 250$ ms. An idealized scattering object will generate a received signal, $r(t)$, given by

$$r(t) = ks(t-\lambda) \qquad 0 < t < T \tag{6.2}$$

where  $k = $ an attenuation factor

  $\lambda = $ round-trip propagation delay

Thus, $r(t)$ is an attenuated, delayed replica of $s(t)$.

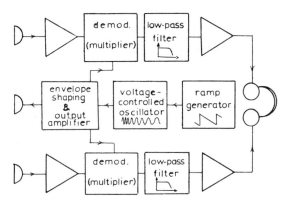

**FIGURE 6.14** The binaural sensing aid consists of a generating system and two receiver/demodulators. Each channel is separately decoded and the audible tone fed to the ear. (From Rowell, 1974 Conference on Engineering Devices in Rehabilitation, Boston, MA).

We can demodulate the return signal by multiplying it by $s(t)$ and using a low-pass filter to remove all but the difference frequency component.

$$f(t) = r(t)s(t) \qquad\qquad 0<t<T \qquad\qquad (6.3)$$

$$f(t) = KA(t-\lambda)A(t)\cos[mt\lambda+\phi(\lambda)] \qquad 0<t<T \qquad (6.4)$$

where  $K$ = amplification constant

$\phi$ = a phase term

$f(t)$ = auditory stimulus presented to user

We obtain equation 6.4 by expanding equation 6.3 and eliminating the high-frequency harmonics. The frequency of the auditory stimulus is $m\lambda$, which is directly proportional to the distance to the reflecting object from the receiver. An object located 25 cm in front of the user produces a frequency, $f(t)$, corresponding to middle $C$. The frequency rises one octave for each doubling of the distance (Jurgen, 1975). Equation 6.4 also shows that objects moving toward the user will generate smaller time delays, $\lambda$, and lower frequencies.

Figure 6.15 shows that azimuthal information (angular location of an object relative to the head) is encoded through the geometry of the two sensors (Rowell, 1974). The user will perceive the true position of an object if the relative amplitudes of stimuli at the two ears is given by

$$\frac{I_r(\theta)}{I_1(\theta)} = e^{k\theta} \qquad\qquad (6.5)$$

where $I_r(\theta)$, $I_1(\theta)$ are defined in Fig. 6.15 and $k$ is a decay constant.

Equation 6.5 shows that the relative intensity of the signal at the two ears is directly proportional to the object azimuth. We can meet this design condition by transducers that have a Gaussian angular response (Rowell, 1974). In actual use, the reflected sound wave is a complex composite of many frequencies. This feature allows the user to distinguish subtle cues such as texture.

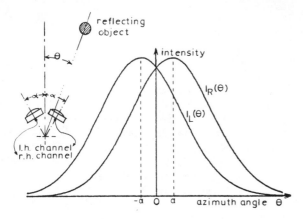

FIGURE 6.15 Azimuth information is decoded in the binaural sensing aid through the relative intensities at the left and right ears. The location of an object is correctly perceived if the curves shown are implemented. (From Rowell, 1974 Conference on Engineering Devices in Rehabilitation, Boston, MA).

The ultrasonic binaural aid is commercially available as the Sonicguide, manufactured by Wormald International Sensory Aids, Ltd., Christchurch, New Zealand.

## Travel Pathsounder

Some designers have been concerned that the Sonicguide user input is so rich in information as to be confusing. The Travel Pathsounder offers an alternative approach. Lke the Sonicguide, the Travel Pathsounder uses an ultrasound echo-ranging technique and is a supplement to the long cane. The major difference is in the form of the feedback to the user. The major goal of this system is to tell the user that the doorway-sized area directly in front of him is unobstructed (Mann, 1974). It does not detect hazards located below the waist.

The user wears the device around the neck at chest height. Two ultrasonic transmitters illuminate a field that is approximately 50 to 60 cm (20 to 24 in.) in diameter at a distance of 18.2 m (6 ft) (Farmer, 1978). The transmitting crystals are similar to those employed in remote television channel selectors. They emit a 40-kHz pulse at a repetition rate of 15 pps. The resolution of the system is such that it detects a clothesline-sized object.

The system provides only three discrete signals to the user. For objects at a distance greater than 182 cm, the device is silent. For objects in the range of 79–182 cm, the device provides an auditory click and a vibration that is felt on the chest. As objects get closer within this range, the device increases the amplitude of the feedback. The user may select either auditory, tactile, or both outputs. When the device detects an obstacle within 79 cm, it changes the auditory tone to a beeping sound and transfers the tactile stimulation to the neck strap.

This device may be particularly useful to older blind individuals who wish to avoid obstacles in the direct travel path and who cannot utilize the complex auditory feedback of the Sonicguide. Users in wheelchairs may also benefit from this approach.

### Mowat Sensor

The blind may use both the Sonicguide and Travel Pathsounder as supplements to the long cane. The Mowat Sensor provides a different function. This device is a small (15 × 15 × 25 cm) aid weighing 185 g (Farmer, 1978). It is hand-held with an ultrasonic transmitter and receiver located at one end of the unit. It is a secondary aid with the long cane or dog guide to locate specific objects such as bus signs, benches, doorways, and other landmarks. The unit emits an elliptical beam that is 15° wide and 30° high (about the size of an adult).

Feedback to the user is via a tactile vibration of the entire aid. Two ranges are available, 4 m and 1 m. When the aid detects an object, it vibrates at a rate that is inversely proportional to the distance from the object. At a target distance of 4 m, the aid vibrates at a rate of 10 pps and increases to 40 pps at 1 m. The Mowat Sensor is also manufactured by Wormald.

## 6.7 VOCATIONAL AND RECREATIONAL AIDS FOR THE BLIND

Reading aids require a specific format for input. Mobility aids are generally low-resolution systems. Neither of these is flexible enough to meet the many varied vocational and recreational needs of the blind. The American Foundation for the Blind (New York, NY) and the Sensory Aids Foundation (Palo Alto, CA) publish catalogs containing many aids for low-vision and blind persons. We present many examples in order to illustrate the range of devices and to stimulate thought regarding new aids.

### Recreational Devices

Games are available for both low-vision and blind use. There are large-print playing cards and boards for common games. There are braille versions of many games such as *Monopoly*, backgammon, *Parcheesi*, checkers, chess, dominoes, and solitaire. Tactile playing cards and dice are also available.

### Household Items

Tactile watches and clocks are available. There are also adapted electrical appliances such as skillets, blenders, and coffee makers. An electric stove lighter is a safe alternative to matches for the blind. Raised and enlarged print telephone dials provide access and light sensors indicate when warning or message lights are illuminated. Other tactile adaptions include compasses, barometers, kitchen timers, and "talking" thermometers and alarm clocks.

### Tools

Many tools have been adapted to provide tactile equivalents to visual cues. There is a carpenter's level with a large steel ball and center tab. An adjustment screw at one end is calibrated with ½° of tilt corresponding to one turn. When level, the ball rolls to the center. Tactile rulers have one raised dot at each ¼ in., two dots at each ½ in., and one dot at each inch. Braille numbers are used also. A tactile tape measure and carpenter's square use a similar approach. Calipers have raised dots indicating each ⅛ in., two dots at ½ in., and three at each inch. There is also a protractor and saw guide with single dots at every 5°, double dots at 30° and 60°, and triple dots at 0°. A standard Starrett micrometer has added raised dots and deepened gradations on the thimble. This device is accurate to 0.001 in. By deepening the grooves in a tire-gage plunger, the blind can use it. There are also guides for chiseling, dovetailing, and drilling.

Audible devices include an electronic level and a position indicator. Machinists can use the position indicator to set depths or align material in a lathe. It measures position or displacement from a preset reference position. The user can set braille-encoded dials for absolute depth and ± tolerances. It generates a tone when it reaches any of the preset values. The tone increases in pitch until the value is reached.

## Instruments

A number of electronic test instruments are available for the blind. Most employ audible and tactile output. An audible multimeter uses a nulling method in which the user turns a dial until a tone is nulled. When null occurs, the reading may be made by tactually reading a raised scale. It includes a 100,000 Ω/V dc voltmeter, precision-nulling ohmmeter, and dc milliammeter.

An audible oscilloscope converts cursor position on the CRT screen to an audible tone whose frequency varies with vertical position. As the vertical height of the CRT signal rises, the tone rises. The user obtains horizontal information by moving a slide that is attached to a linear potentiometer. Users learn the characteristic sounds made by sine waves, square waves, and other periodic signals.

One version of a multimeter provides a speech output as well as audible tone varying with input voltage level. The instrument connects to any multimeter that has a meter-movement output. There are 100 distinct tones ranging from 40–5,000 Hz and giving an accuracy of 1%.

A modified Simpson multimeter provides an audible tone when the meter is off scale. When the unit is on the correct scale, no tone occurs and the user can read the meter by feeling the position of the needle in relation to raised dots on the faceplate.

Both frequency counters and impedance bridges are available with tactile and auditory controls. The counter measures frequencies from 20–100 MHz. The counter automatically locks to the input signal. When the user presses the press-to-talk button, the unit presents the digits in order. The bridge measures ac and dc resistance, capacitance, inductance, and storage and dissipation factors. A tone permits nulling. Then the user reads the dials tactually.

Other devices available include power meters, continuity testers, stopwatches with braille markings, and liquid-level detectors. The latter use electrodes suspended in the solution and give an audible alarm when the liquid reaches a preset level.

### Computer Access and Mathematics

Braille output and talking computer terminals are available. A punchcard reader converts the 12-hole format to a series of 12 pins whose position indicates the presence of a punch. "Talking" terminals use spelled speech outputs to indicate the information present on a CRT. An adaption of the Optacon is also available to read CRT information.

Several types of talking calculators are available. The output is spoken numbers and $+$, $-$, $\times$, $\div$, and $=$. An adaption of existing calculators converts them to braille output.

### Medical

Insulin injections are often needed by the blind because blindness is more common among diabetics. Specially adapted insulin syringes and holders for bottles are available. The holder guides the needle into the bottle. Several syringes can be preset for a specific dosage and then used independently by a blind patient. A "talking" clinical thermometer provides spoken numeric output of temperature using an electronic thermometer. An adapted sphygmomanometer uses raised dots on the meter faceplate.

### Low-Vision Aids

Many magnifying systems are available for specific tasks. Prism glasses, which correct for a decrease in the visual field (tunnel vision), are available from the National Institute for Rehabilitation Engineering, Pompton Lakes, NJ. This organization also has glasses that can be utilized by individuals blind in one eye. These clip onto most spectacle frames and provide crossover of light information to the good eye.

## 6.8 DEVICES FOR AURAL REHABILITATION

Auditory dysfunction presents two major problems. The absence of effective monitoring of speech via hearing leads to diminished oral communication skills. Assistive devices for both sensory input and oral output for the hearing-impaired exist.

Although the problems of auditory impairment are as severe to the victim as those of visual impairment (Schiller, 1974), there has been much less development in this area than in the area of visual substitutes. Mann (1974) points out that the deaf are less visible and it is not therefore as much of a social problem. Also, there are disparities, such as the IRS deduction for blindness but not for deafness. These discrepancies do not limit the impact of deafness, not do they justify the smaller amount of effort applied to the problems of the deaf and hearing-impaired.

## *Hearing Aids*

Hearing loss is often conceived of as a simple loss in amplitude that can be compensated for by an amplifier. Although hearing aids do contain amplifiers, this approach is oversimplified in several ways. First, hearing loss is seldom "flat" at all frequencies. Section 6.3 shows a typical audiogram that illustrates this point. Second, the small size of hearing aids makes it very difficult to obtain high fidelity from the two most crucial components: the microphone and the earphone (referred to as the *receiver* by hearing aid manufactuers). Third, it is difficult to match the acoustic output of a hearing aid to the acoustic properties of the ear.

The three basic types of hearing aids are defined by their location on the body. The oldest type is the body aid currently used for extremely severe hearing loss requiring large gains and/or broad frequency response or for binaural aids. The most common hearing aid is the ear-level type, generally worn behind the ear or in a pair of eyeglass frames. Berger et al. (1977) state that over 88% of the hearing aids sold in the U.S. are ear-level types. The third style is the in-the-ear type in which the entire unit is made small enough to fit into the auditory canal. Hearing aids are also classified as air- or bone-conduction and binaural or monaural. Binaural aids have a separate aid for each ear. Pseudobinaural types provide an acoustic path (tube) to each ear, but they have only one microphone.

**Design Goals and Standards.**   The major design goal for hearing aids is to amplify speech. The speech signal contains not only specific frequencies but also meaningful units of language (see Section 6.4). For this reason, we concentrate on intelligibility of speech rather than on improving the pure tone audiometry results for the user (Section 6.3). Berger et al. (1977) state that 60% of the acoustic power of the speech signal is at frequencies below 500 Hz. This would indicate that low frequencies should be preferentially amplified if we were to use a strict pure tone threshold incrcase as a design criteria. However, 95% of the intelligibility of the speech signal is associated with frequencies above 500 Hz. This is due to the complex frequency relationships that comprise phonemes (Section 6.4) and their organization into syllables.

Hearing aids have two parameters that are normally specified. The output of the aid is given in decibels referred to 20 $\mu$Pa (0.0002 dynes/cm$^2$) and is given as dB SPL (sound pressure level). Hearing thresholds are measured in accordance with the ISO standard of Fig. 6.1. For example, an average hearing threshold of 25 dB at 1,000 Hz is 33 dB SPL. The second parameter is the acoustic gain of the aid, normally specified for a particular SPL input. The maximum acoustic gain of the aid regardless of input is termed the *full-on gain*.

When a hearing aid is fitted, the gain is not set to equal the pure tone hearing level. Rather, a reserve gain of approximately 10 dB is included to account for low-level or distant speech, decrement in the user's hearing over time, and because distortion is maximum at the maximum gain setting of the amplifier. Speech has

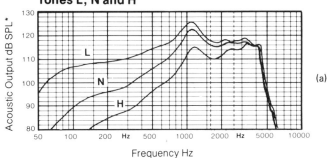

**Saturated Output
SSPL 90/Full-on Gain
Tones L, N and H**

(a)

Acoustic Output dB SPL *

Frequency Hz

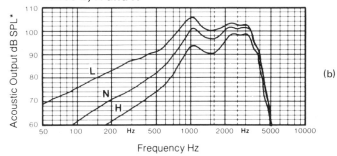

**Frequency Response
50 dB SPL Input/Full-on Gain
Tones L, N and H**

(b)

Acoustic Output dB SPL *

Frequency Hz

**FIGURE 6.16** Frequency response curves for an ear level hearing aid. Three ranges are low (L), high (H) and normal (N). (Courtesy H-C Electronics, Mill Valley, CA).

SPLs in the range of 42 (softest) to 87 (loudest) dB. Normal speech is in the range of 52 to 67 dB (Berger et al., 1977). The maximum SPL that can be applied to the ear without pain and/or acoustic damage is 130–140 dB. The upper limit of output for an aid is specified as the saturation SPL (SSPL) and is usually given at 90-dB SPL input. The gain of hearing aids for speech varies from 50 (ear level) to 70 dB (body level). They are typically specified at 60-dB SPL input. Thus the output of an aid at full gain varies from 110–130 dB SPL.

The frequency response of hearing aids is not flat. Sounds below 500 Hz are sharply attenuated (Fig. 6.16). There is little intelligibility gained from frequencies above 4,000 Hz because these sounds are relatively weak (Berger et al. 1977). The response between 100 and 1,000 Hz rises at approximately 6 dB/octave. Most aids have several frequency ranges that attenuate the lower frequencies to various degrees (Fig. 6.16). Gain is nonlinear with increasing input. Figure 6.16 also illustrates the SSPL response for an ear-level aid. Body-level aids generally have higher gains and wider frequency response. Hearing aid manufacturers conform to American National Standards Institute (ANSI) standard S3.22–1976. This standard specifies test conditions, frequency-response limits and SSPL, gain, 60-dB average full-on gain, distortion, and automatic gain-control parameters (see following).

**Functional Components of Hearing Aids.** Figure 6.17 shows the major

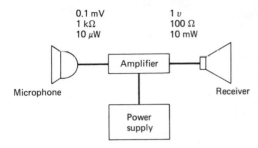

0.1 mV        1 υ
1 kΩ         100 Ω
10 μW       10 mW

Microphone

Amplifier

Receiver

Power supply

**FIGURE 6.17** The major components of a hearing aid are the microphone, amplifier, receiver (earphone) and battery. Signal levels shown are for the input and output of the amplifier.

components of a hearing aid. Body aids contain the microphone, amplifier, and battery in a package worn on the chest. The remaining components are located at ear level. Ear-level and in-the-ear aids have all components at the ear.

The microphone and receiver are the two most important acoustic elements of the hearing aid. Both limit the frequency response and are the major limitations to miniaturization. Current hearing aids usually have electret capacitor microphones (Staab, 1978). The electret consists of two capacitor plates that are charged through a dc power supply. The top plate is a piece of foil coated with gold. When the diaphragm moves, it causes the foil to move and changes the electric field stored in the capacitor. This change in the field is detected by a thick-film FET amplifier built into the case of the microphone. These microphones are rugged and small and have a flat frequency response characteristic up to about 2 kHz. The high-frequency response is peaked near 5 kHz to acoustically compensate for the loss in amplification resulting from blocking the ear canal with an earmold.

The output transducer for hearing aids is called the receiver. Current devices use either an air-conduction or a bone-conduction receiver. Air-conduction receivers are electromagnetic transducers that convert the electrical energy of the amplifier to an acoustic signal that is fed directly into the ear canal. The amplifier output voltage causes a current to flow in a coil. The current sets up a magnetic field in an iron bar and the movement of the bar causes pressure changes against an overlaying diaphragm. A major disadvantage of the magnetic receiver is limited high-frequency response.

Bone-conduction receivers are also magnetic devices. They are designed to cause vibration of the case of the receiver. The receiver case is designed to fit against the head on the mastoid bone posterior to the auricle. When the unit vibrates, it transmits through the skin and bone to the inner ear where it produces the sensation of sound.

Hearing-aid amplifiers serve two basic purposes. These are amplification of the microphone signal with a frequency response matched to speech signals and limitation of signals to prevent distortion or damage to the ear from large acoustic inputs. Figure 6.17 shows typical signal levels of a hearing-aid amplifier. Getreu and McGregor (1971) give the specifications for an integrated-circuit hearing-aid amplifier (Fig. 6.18). These specifications call for an overall acoustic gain of the hearing aid of 40–60 dB at 1 kHz. The slope should increase at 3–6 dB/octave from 400–4000 Hz. When we include the response of the microphone and receiver, the maximum voltage gain of the amplifier is 70–80 dB at 1 kHz. The combined

| | |
|---|---|
| Voltage gain | 70 to 80 dB |
| Volume-control range | ~40 dB |
| Frequency response | constant from 400 Hz to 4kHz |
| Maximum output power | ~0.5 mW peak |
| Battery | single cell |
| Noise at input | ≤1 μV rms |
| Electrical distortion | ≤5% |

**FIGURE 6.18** These specifications were developed by Gettru and McGregor (1971) for an integrated circuit hearing aid amplifier.

response of the microphone and receiver can be used to provide the 3–6 dB/octave gain characteristic, and the amplifier is essentially flat from 400–4000 Hz. Volume-control adjustment of 40 dB is also required. Output power specification depends on the load resistance of the receiver. A voltage swing of 1-V p-p is required. For a 1-k-Ω load, this is 1.0 mW. For a 100-Ω load, it is 10 mW. Getreu and McGregor (1971) present a detailed discussion of the design and implementation of a class B hearing-aid amplifier that meets these specifications.

The limitations of large signals and distortion is referred to as *compression*. We can use two basic types of compression: peak clipping and automatic gain control (AGC) (Staab, 1978). The maximum tolerable acoustic signal at the ear is 130–140 dB SPL. Peak clipping clamps the saturated amplifier output at a value that results in an SPL of less than this at the ear. Because we normally design hearing-aid amplifiers with push–pull outputs, the clipping is symmetrical. Although peak clipping may result in severe distortion of the intensity ratio between vowels and consonants, the quality of the speech output is remarkably good and there is little effect on speech discrimination.

We may also limit the sound pressure output of hearing aids by using feedback either around the output stage or the entire amplifier (AGC). AGC circuits sense the output, rectify and filter it, and feed it back to cause a decrease in gain when the output exceeds a predetermined level. The sensing and filter circuits introduce time delays that can affect speech discrimination. Two time delays are important in AGC circuits for hearing aids. The time from the onset of a signal exceeding the preset limit until the amplifier compensates with reduced gain is called the *attack time* (Fig. 6.19). Speech is typically composed of syllables uttered at a rate of 1 per 100–150 ms with periods of 100 ms between syllables. An attack time exceeding 50 ms results in a loss of information. Good-quality commercial hearing aids have attack times in the range of 2–10 ms. Recovery times must be longer than attack times to avoid AGC flutter, the severe waveform distortion resulting from an AGC circuit that follows every cycle of the input signal. Typical recovery times are in the range of 50–150 ms. During the attack time, the signal instantaneously exceeds the desired threshold before the AGC takes effect. Because this signal could be damaging, additional peak clipping may be used. All compression circuits are nonlinear, and it is very difficult to evaluate their performance except by user evaluation. The intelligibility of speech under conditions of wide dynamic range in the input is the only valid criterion for determining the quality of a compression circuit. Staab (1978) provides a detailed description of compression methods and their effectiveness.

**Acoustic Coupling.** The acoustic output of an air-conduction receiver is fed

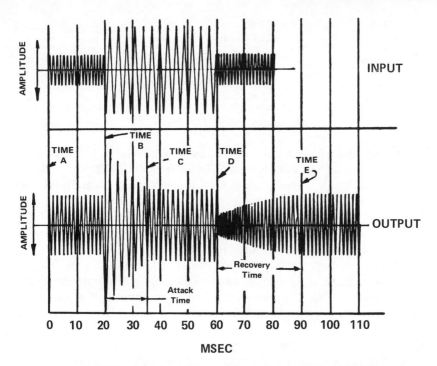

**FIGURE 6.19** Automatic gain control compression circuits for hearing aids have two time delays—attack time and recovery time. See text for explanation. (Reprinted from Staab, *Hearing Aid Handbook*, Blue Ridge Summit, PA: TAB Books, with permission.)

to the ear canal via an acoustic coupler. The design of this coupler is crucial for the effective performance of the hearing aid. For body-level aids, the receiver is attached directly to the ear mold, which is placed in the canal. For ear-level aids, the ear mold is connected to a piece of tubing from the receiver located inside the case of the aid. Both the ear mold and the tubing can drastically affect the acoustical response of the aid.

Ear molds of many designs are available (Staab, 1978). The overall design provides for a 2-ml air volume between the end of the mold and the tympanic membrane. Evaluation of ear molds and overall hearing aid performance is typically carried out using a device known as a *coupler*, which consists of a chamber in the shape of the external ear canal, a 2-ml volume, and a microphone. Staab (1978) discusses its limitations in detail.

Using this coupler, we can determine the effects of tubing diameter and length, vents, and obstructions in the tubing due to ear wax (cerumen) or kinks on overall acoustic response. If we increase the inside diameter of the tubing, the peak response in the 1- to 4-kHz range is increased. Increasing tube length has the opposite effect and results in a shift of response peak downward in frequency. Blockage of the tube with cerumen results in severely decreased high-frequency response. A kink in the tubing will cause a large decrease in low-frequency

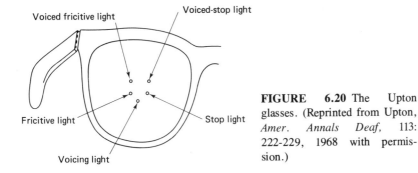

**FIGURE 6.20** The Upton glasses. (Reprinted from Upton, *Amer. Annals Deaf,* 113: 222-229, 1968 with permission.)

response (see problem 6.15). Staab (1978) discusses ear mold design and its effect on overall performance in some detail.

### Aids for the Deaf

The lack of feedback in the deaf or severely hearing-impaired to monitor speech results in severe disabilities in speech production as well as reception of speech. Thus, aids have been developed to help overcome both of these problems. As discussed in Section 6.4, auditory signals have a temporal component not found in reading. This places a severe additional constraint on sensory aids for the deaf not found in aids for the blind (Elliott, 1978).

The type of hearing loss plays an important role in the design of auditory substitution aids. If the person is congenitally deaf and has used sign language for a prolonged period of time, then he may not appreciate the characteristics of normal speech. A person recently hearing-impaired may find the lack of information in the prosthesis to be unacceptable. Older persons may not be able to learn to use a sensory aid due to diminished short- and long-term memory. In general, we know less about hearing loss than we do about visual deficits. This lack of basic information is the most limiting factor in designing sensory aids for the deaf. Despite all of these drawbacks, some aids do exist.

**Lip-Reading Aid.** A major problem experienced by the deaf when attempting to lip read is that many sounds to not appear on the lips. Examples of nonvisible sounds are the letters *T, D, K, G, N, L, J, S,* and *Z* and the sounds *th* and *ts*. Upton (1968) designed a system for aiding in lipreading. His major design goals were to provide additional information that would allow a person to utilize lip-reading cues together with a display of additional sounds. He considered the best method for presenting information so as to require little further concentration or attention to additional displays. The method he chose is based on the processing of the speech information to present an indication of certain sounds. He chose five sounds for display: stop sounds, fricitive sounds, voiced sounds, and combinations of voiced and stop and voiced and fricitive. Figure 6.20 shows the arrangement of four LEDs on the surface of an eyeglass frame. The system uses filters to detect sounds falling into one of the five categories. When a sound occurs, the LED corresponding to it lights.

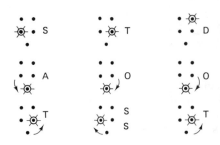

FIGURE 6.21 The Upton glasses lights have specified patterns for unique word groups. The illuminated lights are shown with larger circles. The arrows indicate a transition from one light to another. (Reprinted from Upton, *Amer. Annals Deaf*, 113: 222-229, 1968 with permission.)

The lights are not seen next to the eye, but rather they are projected into space. By orienting the head, the user can cause the lights to appear over the speaker's face. When properly positioned, the lower light of the display appears over the speaker's throat with the others over the lip. Figure 6.21 shows several patterns as they would appear for simple words. Upton, himself hard of hearing, wore the glasses for a period of six months. His evaluation was that the glasses make some errors in recognizing phonemes and ignore others, but they provide a significant improvement in the user's ability to lip read. The system also provides feedback to the user because it detects his speech as well as that of the other person. This provides an important feature, which is fed back via the same channel that the user receives other auditory information. Upton felt that using the glasses did not require additional concentration or attention over that required for lip reading. Several other workers have also designed lip-reading aids similar to the Upton glasses (see problem 6.14).

**Telephone Communications for the Deaf.** Probably the most common auditory aid next to hearing aids is the telephone communication system. With the advent of computer access systems using telephone lines, modems (modulator/demodulators) were developed. These devices convert keyboard entries to a serial code that is acoustically coupled into the telephone receiver. Return data from the computer is coupled into the terminal via a coupler attached to the telephone mouthpiece. A standard code (Baudot) is used. Early versions adapted for the deaf used obsolete teletype units (TTYs). For this reason, many people refer to current electronic devices as TTYs.

Current devices consist of a keyboard, alphanumeric display, and acoustic coupler. They include the necessary electronics for encoding the data for transmission and decoding it for display. Devices vary in size from desk-top to hand-held. They allow any deaf person to communicate with anyone having a similar device. Many police, fire, and hospital departments have TTY equipment for emergency communication by the deaf.

The Tele-ear is an alternative approach that allows a hearing-impaired person to communicate with a hearing individual (Jurgen, 1980). The hearing person uses only a standard touch-tone telephone. The hearing-impaired person has a microcomputer-based decoder that displays up to eight characters as they are received. The hearing person enters letters using the touch-tone keypad. There are multiple letters on each key (e.g., *ABC*) so the user must press this key once for "A", twice for "B" and three times for "C." After a letter is entered, the "*" key is pressed for end of letter. This key is pressed twice for end of word. The decoder then interprets the tones and displays the results on a eight-character display. The system costs about half as much as a TTY, and it can be used with any touch-tone telephone.

**Vocoders.** Many attempts have been made to provide speech information via the tactile or visual senses. The most common approach is to use vocoders. These are devices that analyze the acoustic speech information, break it into frequency ranges and present the relative amplitude of these ranges to the user via tactile or visual displays. Researchers have attempted to provide tactile or visual vocoders since the 1920s, but all have shown only limited success as yet.

Tactile vocoders typically use a bank of filters to break the speech signal down into fundamental ranges (Kirman, 1973). The relative amplitude of the signal in each range is presented to the user via stimulators. The frequency and amplitude of the stimulus can be varied to provide both pitch and loudness information. By selecting about seven filter ranges, we can provide a unique tactile pattern for each phoneme of English. Using this type of system, subjects can identify some words and syllables, but the performance is slow and inaccurate. Error rates approaching 50% are common because of the reasons presented in Section 6.4. Although it is impossible to uniquely define the phonemes of an utterance using a vocoder system, this does not necessarily make it possible to use this information in an auditory substitution system.

Visual vocoders are similar to tactile types except for the display (Pickett, 1972). Displays may be a series of lights, each of which is related to a single frequency range or a CRT display with the frequency ranges displayed as adjacent bars. In either case, the user is presented with a series of patterns that represent portions of the speech signal. Success with visual vocoders has been poor. The major difficulty is the temporal aspect of the speech signal. Displays that are presented in real time are difficult to recognize. Again, the visual system is organized for the input of printed language information, not the presentation of acoustic information in visual form.

Visual systems are useful as training aids. The spectral pattern can be stored on a CRT screen and held there while an instructor points out the major features. Deaf individuals can use such systems to develop their own speech pattern for the same utterance. In this approach, the slow speed and difficulties in interpretation are less important. Other visual aids have related the display pattern to the position of the articulators. An example of this type of system is visual display in which a single spot on a CRT is used to indicate the position of the tongue (Pickett, 1972). By presenting the display to a deaf user, a teacher can help the student to use the tongue properly.

## 6.9 AUGMENTATIVE COMMUNICATION AND CONTROL SYSTEMS

Many individuals suffer from severe motor impairments that prevent them from writing, speaking, and interacting with their immediate environment. Loss of motor ability may be due to neuromuscular disease (e.g., stroke, cerebral palsy) or injury (e.g., head trauma, spinal cord injury). Loss of speech may also be due to damage to the speech mechanism (e.g., cancer of the larynx). Various devices that provide alternative modes of communication or control may aid these individuals. Motor impairment may be accompanied by cognitive disability. Individuals may not have the ability to organize language into meaningful utterances or to understand complex control schemes.

When cognitive and language function is intact but the output modes are impaired, the problem of providing an assistive device are relatively straightforward, and many commercial devices exist for these needs. When there is an impairment of cognitive or language function, then the problems become much more difficult. If the individual cannot read or spell or lacks the ability to organize a symbol set into meaningful communication, it is difficult to provide alternatives. In some cases alternative symbol systems are useful (e.g., pictures instead of words or spelling). In general, there is little that technology can currently offer to language-impaired individuals. In control systems, we can make the schemes of control very simple, but this compromises speed and the number of control signals available.

Morasso et al. (1979) have proposed the general communication/control (c/c) scheme shown in Fig. 6.22. Both motor output for communication and/or control and feedback to monitor the results are important. In the normal person, both of these systems are intact. In the motor-impaired person, there may be deficiencies in either or both of these processes. We must design the augmentative c/c system to compensate for these deficiencies. Command sensors interface the residual motor capability of the person with the c/c system. The controller utilizes these input commands to provide feedback to the user and generate the desired outputs. This control scheme is based on input from the environment and stored control algorithms. Vanderheiden (1978) provides information on specific implementation of this scheme for communication in a yearly updated book. Morasso et al. (1979) review control applications.

## Input Commands–the Interface

The interface is the means by which the user accesses the vocabulary or commands of the aid. This access includes selection of language elements and the organization of them into meaningful utterances as well as selection of items to be controlled. We can classify four major interfaces based on the type of biological energy used to activate the interface. These are biomechanical, bioelectrical, biopneumatic, and biothermal.

Most interfaces are sensitive to movement of a body part and we therefore refer to them as *biomechanical*. This class includes simple switches, keyboards, joysticks, mircoswitches, and many others. The user may activate them with the hand and fingers, with a head pointer, with a sideward movement of the head, movement of the eyes, or many other movements. Most are simple normally open switches that provide a contact closure when pressed. Vanderheiden and Grilley (1975) describe many types of switches intended for use as interfaces.

Bioelectric interfaces sense electric currents associated with physiological events. Examples include electromyographic (EMG), electroencephalographic

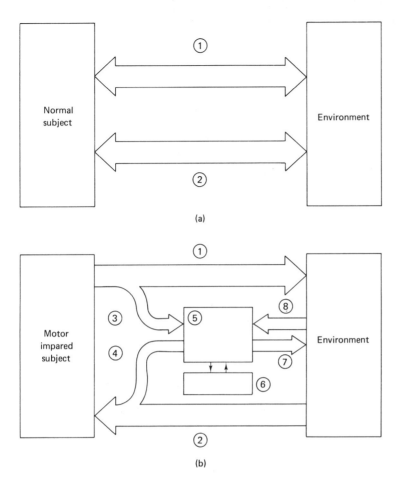

**FIGURE 6.22** A communication and control system consists of several key components. (1) motor output of subject, (2) sensory input to subject. (a) normal subject. (b) motor-impaired subject. Device functions are: commands (3) feedback (4) controller (5) storage (6) output (7) and sensors (8) (Reprinted from Morasso, et al. (1979) with permission).

(EEG) electrodes, and so-called contact switches, which are triggered by displacement currents on the surface of the body. Bioelectric interfaces require the use of a biopotential amplifer and electrodes. Webster (1978) describes both of these components. After amplification and rectification, the signal typically enters a comparator circuit that provides an output if the electrical activity reaches a preset threshold.

Biopneumatic switches use pressure transducers that detect small puffs or sips of air. These puff-and-sip switches often control powered wheelchairs for quadriplegics (see Chapter 8). Biothermal switches sense the difference between the temperature of the skin and that of the ambient environment.

## Output Modes

The output mode of a c/c aid may replace many motor functions. Environmental controllers turn appliances or lights on or off. Page turners and eating aids replace hand function (Chapter 8), and communication aids replace speech or writing. There are two types of outputs used on communication aids: visual and auditory.

**Visual Output.** Visual output may be either transient or permanent (hard copy). One form of transient output is a light (incandescent or LED), which forms an element of an array. When the user turns the light on, the listener knows that he has selected the element in that array position. The elements may be letters, words, pictures, or special symbols (e.g., Bliss symbols). The display is active only until the user makes the next selection. Thus, the listener must be present when the message is generated.

Another form of transient display uses LED or LCD alphanumeric displays. These may be either 16-segment or 5 × 7 dot-matrix arrays, which are grouped as 4, 8, 16, or 32 characters. These displays can present any letter or number and many special symbols for punctuation or shorthand (e.g., @, #, $, %). The display is illuminated for the receiver only until it is full. Then one character is dropped off each time a new one is entered.

Hard copy displays are small thermal or electrostatic printers that provide a typed output of selected elements. The output is strictly alphanumeric (requires reading or spelling) because pictures and special symbols require much more complex printing electronics. Hard copy displays allow the user to generate a message at his own pace and then have it read at a later time. This is important in classroom use, where nonspeaking children must complete spelling tests and written assignments. However, many of the needs of the nonspeaking population are for conversational interaction, and this advantage of hard copy may not be used.

**Auditory Output.** Auditory output devices may be simple sound generators that provide an alarm function or a coded output such as Morse code. Because communication aids replace speech, there is a great deal of interest in aids that provide spoken output. There are two approaches that provide this capability: synthesized speech and prerecorded messages.

The synthesized speech output is very similar to that for reading aids (Section 6.5). The synthesizer and the methods of generating the phoneme strings utilize the same computer algorithms and both require a computer and synthesizer. The major difference lies in the way in which the user selects the language elements. The reading aid must convert text to recognizable words or letters and then generate the phoneme string. This is an unconstrained input domain and is one of the major challenges in reading aids. Communication aids take advantage of the user's language ability and the device does not need to provide syntactic rules or character recognition. Speech synthesis devices for communication store phoneme strings for 500–900 common words and phrases that the user can access through the interface. The computer supplies the proper codes to the synthesizer that "speaks" the words or phrase. For words not in the vocabulary, the user may either assemble a phoneme string or spell the word. The Handivoice models 110 and 120 (H C Electronics, Troy, MI) utilize speech synthesis for output.

Speech synthesis offers flexibility and speed of access. However, current synthesizers do not sound natural and are hard to understand. An alternative approach uses prerecorded messages (words or phrases) accessed by the user. A continous tape loop uses two channels of information. One contains stored messages and the other a digital code for that message. When the user selects an element, the device converts the input to a digital code and scans the tape until it finds the code. When it locates the start bit for the message, it activates the recorder electronics and plays the message through a speaker. The access time is 5 s for a 128-element vocabulary. The major advantage of this approach is the natural speech and the availability of children's and women's voices. The slow speed and limited vocabulary are the major disadvantages. Vocabulary can be altered by changing tape cassettes, but this is not under the control of the physically disabled user. Scitronics (Bethlehem, PA) manufactures a prerecorded message communication aid.

**Human Factors.** Communication aids must be used in many environments. When we design the output, we must consider several factors. Displays and hard copy output must be large enough to be read easily and lens systems can enlarge small display or print characters. Many environments have large amounts of ambient light or sound, and the output must function in these places. LEDs are hard to read in bright light and synthesized speech may be difficult to understand in noisy locations. Thermal printer outputs tend to fade with time and the blue printing is hard for some people to read.

The output format is also important. Strip printers are small and inexpensive. This format is not conducive to long messages or written assignments, however. To maximize feedback, the print head should not cover the printed characters. Some printers, for example, have print heads that are so large that a character is not visible until two more characters have been entered.

The intelligibility of the output to strangers is also important. Speech synthesis may only be understandable with practice. This is limiting in new environments. Visible displays of words are not usable by children or others who cannot read. The output should allow the user and listener to face each other and have eye contact. Many devices require the listener to be either at the side of or behind the user. We must carefully consider these and other human factor concepts when designing the output of a communication aid.

## Controller Features

The heart of a c/c system is the controller. We can usually trace the flexibility or inflexibility of any specific aid to the methods employed in the controller design. The controller provides the method for interpreting the interface signal and relating this to a desired output command. Morasso et al. (1979) describe this process as a mapping from an input (interface) domain to a command (output) domain. We can accomplish this mapping either through hardware or a microcomputer program. Morasso et al. (1979) define three schemes that we can use to select output commands; random access, sequential access, and encoding access.

**Random Access.** When the number of commands available is equal to or less than the number of input signals available, then we call the random access scheme direct selection. For control, a direct selection scheme has one interface for each item to be controlled. For communication, each element in the user's vocabulary has a separate interface. The keyboard is the most common interface for direct selection systems. We can use either standard typewriter or CRT keyboards or specially designed (e.g., enlarged) versions. In direct selection devices, the controller is either hardwired digital electronics or a microcomputer system. Examples of communication aids in this category include the Canon Communicator and Autocom (both Telesensory Systems, Palo Alto, CA), the Handivoice 110 and the VIP (Prentke-Romich, Shreve, OH). The Canon and VIP are calculator-sized devices that have keyboards for alphanumeric entry. The Canon has a thermal strip printer output, and the VIP uses an eight-character LED. We discuss the Autocom later.

Random access devices may also be used when there are more command than input signals. In this case, we divide the command domain into "pages" (memory locations), where each page is as large as the number of input signals. The user accesses the command elements on each page in a direct selection mode. An additional input signal allows the user to change pages. In a general purpose c/c aid, one page may contain control commands for appliances and lights, another commands for a powered wheelchair, a third system commands (editing, mode selection) and the rest words, letters, phrases, etc. (Vanderheiden, 1979).

We can most easily implement a random access scheme by using a microcomputer. The Autocom (Tompkins and Webster, 1981) uses an RCA 1802 microcomputer to detect which one of an $8 \times 16$ array of magnetic reed switches has been activated by a magnet. The reed switches are located beneath a lap tray that fits on a wheelchair. The microcomputer has a programmed time delay to account for random movement of the user. Several levels (pages) of commands are available, and the user may select them through one element of the input matrix. One page contains control characters (e.g., enable display) and the full alphanumeric ASCII keyboard. Other pages may contain control commands for a powered wheelchair, an environmental controller, or stored vocabulary.

The Autocom output is also flexible. A 32-character LED display, thermal printer, or CRT can be used. A second LED display facing the listener is also available. An RS232 output can be interfaced to environmental control devices such as those intended for home use (Ciarcia, 1980). These systems use ultrasonic coupling of commands from the computer to a receiver plugged into a wall outlet. The receiver provides control signals through the house wiring to any device plugged into any other outlet. Using such systems, we can control lights, appliances, or door openers.

We can enhance the random access approach for communication by using low-power random access memories (RAMs) for vocabulary storage. If we provide a separate supply to the RAMs, the stored information is not lost when the aid is turned off, and the user may tailor the vocabulary to his needs by storing elements in the RAM. This greatly increases the flexibility of the aid and is incorporated into the Autocom. As a child develops new vocabulary, he can store the elements in RAM and the aid can grow with him.

We can also program a random access aid to provide different selection modes. The Autocom may be used as a sequential or encoding device through user commands. The random access mode may be altered also. Software can vary the array of active sensors to be in the form of an arc for use with a head pointer, to be only on one-half of the tray for individuals who cannot cross the midline of the body, or to increase the size of each active area for someone with very limited motor control.

**Sequential Access.** Sequential access schemes employ a cursor. They are used when only a few (1 to 5) input commands are available due to severe impairment. In these systems, command elements are displayed to the user in sequence and the user selects the desired element by activating the interface. One type of sequential access system is a scanning controller in which the elements are displayed in a fixed array. Typically, the arrays have a series of rows and columns that contain command elements. They employ several types of scanning. Automatic scanning sequentially steps the device through each element of the array at a user-adjustable rate. When the device illuminates the desired array element, the user must stop the scan by activating the interface. A second activation either continues the scan or returns to the beginning of the array. For arrays with less than 20 elements, the device sequentially scans each element. For large arrays of 100 elements or more, it usually turns on an entire row at one time. When the user activates the interface once, the scan proceeds across the selected row. A second activation stops the scan at the desired element, and a third returns the scan to the first row.

Self-scanning is also available. In this mode, the user causes each increment of the scan by activating the interface. The device uses from one to four input commands to provide control over left, right, up, and down scans. A fifth command may be used for element selection. We may implement the four directions with a joystick if the person has sufficient control.

Scanning aids are available from several manufacturers: Dufco (Cambria, CA), Prentke-Romich, and Zygo (Portland, OR) are the most common. Some have communication and control features. The major advantage of this type of aid is the simplicity of control, which makes it available to individuals with very little motor control. The major disadvantage is the extremely slow speed of message generation. This approach is only useful when physical or cognitive limitations prevent encoding or random access.

Another sequential access system is the microcomputer-based TS-100 (Computers for the Physically Handicapped, Huntington Beach, CA). This aid contains an 8080 microcomputer, video monitor, and a single switch. Ten modes provide a menu approach. All selections are displayed at the bottom of the screen. In the spelling mode, the top of the display contains the letters of the alphabet organized in order of occurrence in English based on previous entries. The letters scroll from right to left at a user-controlled speed. The user stops the scroll when the letter desired appears at the far left. After a selection, a new alphabet begins to scroll. If spelling is not selected, then the user sees a series of 120 word groups. Each group is alphabetical and identified by the first and last words in the group. If the user selects a group, the device sequentially presents words in the same manner as for spelling. The edit mode allows the user to backspace, erase the last word, space, tab, go to the next line, erase the last line, and escape to another mode. Additional modes are control (graphics), numbers, phrases, cursor control, call, and remote control. The last mode allows the user to control external devices.

**Encoding Access.** This mode of operation requires the user to enter a code corresponding to the element desired. The controller must interpret this code and convert it to the signals necessary to output the desired language element. Often a two- or three-digit code corresponds to a word, letter, or phoneme. Alternative symbol systems are not usually available in encoding devices. Encoding systems may use either one or two interface switches. One interface switch sequentially steps through the number codes until the user activates the switch. The user implements this technique, called *scrolling*, using either one digit at a time or two- or three-digit numbers. If the user has additional switches, then one may correspond to each of the hundreds, tens, and ones digits. If there is sufficient motor control, then the user can operate a keyboard to directly enter the number codes. This approach also requires that the user be able to relate codes to desired language or control command. This skill is sometimes lacking in multiply-handicapped individuals. The Liberator (Mulholland), Handivoice Model 120, and Scitronics aids all utilize an encoding method.

## The Artificial Larynx

In contrast to the total loss of the ability to produce speech, some individuals suffer loss of only the larynx. The surgical procedure removes the epiglottis and larynx. The trachea is repositioned to align with a small hole in the neck called a tracheostoma. This loss is usually due to cancer, and it results in an inability to produce the vibrating sound necessary for speech. Because the articulators, central nervous control, and language are intact, we can provide an artificial source of sound vibration that enables speech. Devices that do this are called *artificial larynges*. There are two types of devices: pneumatic and electronic (Salmon and Goldstein, 1978).

**Pneumatic Types.** The pneumatic artificial larynx consists of a cup that fits tightly over the trachcostoma. Air forced through the cup is fed to a vibrating reed or membrane. The vibration is then sent to the mouth via a flexible tube. By moving the articulators of the mouth, the user can form the vibrations into intelligible speech sounds. Tension on the membrane or breath pressure varies the pitch. The cost of pneumatic-type devices is under $50. Salmon and Goldstein (1978) describe several commercial types.

**Electronic Types.** Electronic artificial larynges are battery-powered pulse generators that cause a vibration of either a diaphragm or membrane. Two types are available: mouth and neck. In mouth types, the vibration from the unit is coupled to a flexible tube that is placed into the user's mouth. Operation is similar to that of the pneumatic types, with the user forming the speech sounds by altering the position of the articulators in the mouth.

Although several types are available, the most common is the Cooper-Rand instrument (Salmon and Goldstein, 1978). This device has a small battery pack with pulse generator, separate hand-held tone generator (vibrator), and a small mouth tube attached to the tone generator. It sells for about $175.

Neck-type units are similar in design except that the vibrations are applied to the resonant tract by placing the vibrating surface against the neck or face. Placement may be between the neck and the floor of the mouth, the anterolateral aspect of the neck, or the side of the face. The user can modify the vibrations set up by the artificial larynx by varying the positions of the articulating structures of the mouth. Western Electric makes the most commonly used unit. It sells for about $40. These devices allow users to carry on conversations and speak over the telephone. The speech is understandable, but sounds artificial.

## 6.10 RESEARCH DIRECTIONS

All of these sensory aids will continue to undergo development and improvement. In this section we describe some of the longer-range possibilities. Two major goals have been prevalent in sensory aids research. Direct interaction with the cortex appears to offer promise as a universal visual or auditory substitute. However, lack of understanding of the function of the sensory systems in sufficient detail has made this goal very difficult to achieve. We discuss the major problems below. The second area of interest is in replacing the sensor itself. For the eye, this is not even feasible at this time. However, there is a great deal of work in the development of an artificial cochlea, which we describe in this section.

### Direct Interaction with the Cortex

Direct cortical stimulation of the visual centers of the cortex has shown that such stimulation elicits flashes of light called phosphenes. By implanting arrays of electrodes, researchers have mapped the regions of the visual cortex that are responsive to stimulation (Dobelle et al., 1974). Such mapping indicates that phosphene patterns are distributed throughout the visual areas. Stimulation of a straight line of electrodes, for example, does not yield a straight line of phosphenes but, rather, a widely spaced random pattern. In addition, the map differs from patient to patient, with different electrode positions in the same patient and with eye movements. In the case of eye movements, the entire pattern appears to move with the relative spacing between various phosphenes remaining the same. Sensation is the same even when varying pulse duration, frequency, and pulse train length, although the threshold to stimulation varies. Blind patients can recognize certain patterns when appropriate electrodes are stimulated.

These experimental results have created interest in the development of a visual prosthesis in which the output is direct cortical stimulation (Sterling et al., 1971). Stimulation requires currents up to 8 mA (variable from patient to patient and from electrode to electrode in the same patient) with a net resistance of about 3 $k\Omega$. Thus, the required stimulus voltages range up to 24 V. In order to avoid a net charge transfer to the cortex and associated damage, bipolar pulses are used with a zero dc component (see Chapter 5). Much signal processing takes place in the visual system prior to arrival of the impulses at the cortex. Likewise, the prosthesis must preprocess the optical data from the sensor (Staff of Neuroprothesis Program, 1974). We require three types of preprocessing:

1. Enhancement of both the edges of images and contrast.
2. A correlation between the image and the spatial arrangement of the phosphenes.
3. Linearization of the relationship between brightness of the image on the sensor and the perceived brightness of the phosphenes.

The first of these is probably similar for all patients, and the last two probably vary from patient to patient. It is theoretically possible to determine the effect of the phosphene pattern in different patients and store this information in a read-only memory (ROM).

Using preprocessing means that the camera can use more image-sensing areas than the electrodes. For example, 4–10,000 discrete sensing elements can serve 256 electrodes. We can process the inputs from several adjacent sensors to provide one electrode with the signal that produces the best phosphene brightness for that image. In addition, variable-camera scanning rates can function as a variable iris by compensating for light levels.

A similar approach has been taken to auditory prostheses for the deaf (Mladejovsky et al., 1976). In this case, the sensation is a click when the auditory cortex is stimulated. The signal-processing requirements for the auditory prosthesis are as severe as those for the visual device. Our biggest design challenge is to determine which parameters of the speech signals are crucial inputs to the cortex to provide recognition of words in real time.

## Cochlear Implants

Hearing deficiencies resulting from injuries or disease affecting the middle or outer ear can be repaired by otolaryngologists using prosthetic bone implants or other "spare parts." Damage to the cochlea cannot be treated surgically, and a great deal of effort has been expended in replacing its function. The cochlea is tonotopically organized; that is, low-frequency tones stimulate nerves at the distal end and high-frequency tones at the proximal end. This tonotopic localization carries over into the auditory nerve. Electrical stimulation of either the cochlea (basilar membrane) or auditory nerve results in a sensation of sound (e.g., clicks) (White et al., 1979). Two basic approaches have been taken to electrical stimulation for replacement of cochlear function: direct cochlear stimulation and auditory stimulation. For speech perception, a bandwidth of 3 kHz is adequate, and this requires 8–10 electrodes. Most approaches also take the signal-processing capabilities of the auditory nerve and higher centers into account and use a phase-locking approach. The overall system has three major components: an electrode array, implantable electronics including stimulator, and a speech processor to convert speech information to a stimulus pattern.

May et al. (1979a) describe the requirements for microelectrode arrays that include selective stimulation of the auditory nerve, biocompatibility, a dimensional precision of 0.1 mm, and a charge delivery capability of 10 nC per pulse. An integrated-circuit fabrication process is used for making the tantalum-on-sapphire microelectrode arrays. For eight channels, the overall electrode array is 1.25 cm long with an electrode active area of 5 mm. The electrode active areas are staggered to prevent crosstalk, and the entire array is designed for easy insertion into the auditory nerve. This array has replaced early versions consisting of $SiO_2$ substrates with gold plating, which broke easily on insertion.

The implantable electronics package consists of a series of capacitors that are charged through a CMOS decoding electronics package (May et al., 1979b). The stimulator uses a metered charge delivery approach that sequentially charges one of eight capacitors and then discharges it through the auditory nerve. A major problem with this component is packaging the electronics so as to prevent leaks and insure biocompatibility. The decoding logic signals are coupled through the head using either an RF link, ultrasound (piezoelectric crystals), or optical coupling through the tympanic membrane. The power coupling of the array is designed such that the stored voltage is $2\times$ that needed for stimulation. This means that up to 5 mm misalignment can be tolerated in the auditory nerve.

The major problem in the cochlear implant system is the design of an effective speech processor (Walker et al., 1979). This component must be based on psycholinguistic models of speech perception developed from initial implant studies (Mathews et al., 1979). As we discussed in Section 6.4, the relationship between acoustic cues (e.g., phonemes) and speech recognition has not been demonstrated. The determination of an algorithm to decode the incoming speech signal in real time and convert this information to the necessary stimulation pattern is the major limitation in the application of cochlear implants clinically. Walker et al. (1979) describe one processor approach based on a special purpose microcomputer. They have developed relationships between perceived loudness and charge delivered to the nerve (a linear curve), pitch and pulse rate (highly nonlinear), and frequency discrimination (e.g., ping, buzz, beep, and screech) related to the pulse rate. The overall system functions are: filtering to separate information into broad frequency ranges; smoothing to adjust to loudness levels; estimation for formant (phonemic) content; and determination of appropriate electrode location and pulse rate for stimulation.

# REFERENCES

ALLEN, J. (1971). Electronic aids for the severely visually handicapped. *C.R.C. Crit. Rev. Bioeng.*, 12: 139–66.

ALLEN, J. (1976). Synthesis of speech from unrestricted text. *Proc. IEEE*, 64: 433–42.

ALLEN, J. (1978). An approach to reading machine design. *Human Factors*, 20: 287–94.

AMERICAN FOUNDATION FOR THE BLIND (1978). *How does a blind person get around?* New York: AFB, 15 W. 16th St., 10011.

BACH-Y-RITA, P. (1972). *Brain mechanisms in sensory substitution.* New York: Academic Press.

BERGER, K. W., E. N. HAGBERG, and R. L. RANE (1977). Prescription of hearing aids: Rationale, procedures and results. Kent, OH: Herald Publishing Co.

BLISS J. C. (1968). Sensory aids for the blind, in M. Clynes and J. H. Milsum (eds), *Biomedical engineering systems.* New York: McGraw-Hill.

BRUGLER, J. S., J. D. MEINDL, J. D. PLUMMER, and P. J. SALSBURG (1969). Integrated electronics for a reading aid for the blind. *IEEE J. Solid State Circ.,* SC-4: 304–12.

CIARCIA, S. (1980). Computerize a home. *BYTE,* 5(1): 28–54.

DOBELLE, W. H., M. G. MLADEJOVSKY, and J. P. GIRVIN (1974). Artificial vision for the blind: Electrical stimulation of visual cortex offers hope for a functional prosthesis. *Science,* 183: 440–44.

ELLIOT, L. L. (1978). Development of communication aids for the deaf. *Human Factors,* 20: 295–306.

FARMER, L. W. (1978). Mobility devices. *Bull. Prosth. Res.,* BPRID-30: 47–118.

GERSCHWIND, N. (1972). Language and the brain. *Sci. Amer.,* 226(4): 76–83.

GETREU, I. E., and I. M. McGREGOR (1971). An integrated class-B hearing aid amplifier. *IEEE J. Solid State Circ.,* SC-6: 376–84.

GRONER, G. F., and R. E. SAVOIE (1979). Toward a personal speech-output reading machine for the blind. *Proc. WESCON Prof. Prog.,* Session 6.

JURGEN, R. K. (1975). Technology in health care. *IEEE Spectrum.* 12(1): 70–73.

JURGEN, R. K. (1980). Electronics in medicine. *IEEE Spectrum,* 17(1): 81–86.

KIRMAN, J. H. (1973). Tactile communication of speech: A review and analysis. *Psychol. Bull.,* 80: 54–74.

KLINE, J. (ed) (1976). *Biological foundations of biomedical engineering.* Boston: Little, Brown.

LEIBERMAN, P. (1967). *Intonation, perception and language.* Cambridge, MA: M.I.T. Press.

MANN, R. W. (1974). Technology and human rehabilitation: Prostheses for sensory rehabilitation and/or sensory substitution, in J. H. U. Brown and J. F. Dickson (eds), *Adv. in biomedical engineering.* New York: Academic Press.

MATHEWS, R. G., M. G. WALKER, and M. K. HERNDON (1979). Psychophysical data on human subjects establishing the stimulus-percept data base for an auditory prosthesis. *IEEE Frontiers in Health Care Conf.,* 211.

MAY, G. L., S. SHAMMA, and R. L. WHITE, (1979a). Microelectrode arrays for an implantable auditory prosthesis. *IEEE Frontiers Eng. in Health Care Conf.:* 211.

MAY, G. L., M. SOMA, and R. G. MATHEWS (1979b). The stimulus series implantable multichannel receiver–stimulator units for an auditory prosthesis. *IEEE Frontiers Eng. in Health Care Conf.,* 211.

MLADEJOVSKY, M. G., D. K. EDDINGTON, J. R. EDDINGTON, J. R. EVANS, and W. H. DOBELLE (1976). A computer-based brain stimulation system to investigate sensory prostheses for the blind and deaf. *IEEE Trans. Biomed. Eng.,* BME-23: 286–96.

MORASSO, P., P. PENSO, G. P. SUETTA, and V. TAGLIASCO (1979). Toward standardization of communication and control systems for motor impaired people. *Med. & Biol. Eng. & Comput.,* 17: 481–88.

NYE, P. W. (1968). Research on reading aids for the blind-A dilemma. *Med. Biol. Eng.* 6: 43–51.

NYE, P. W. (1970). Human factors underlying the design of reading aids for the blind. *IEEE Trans. Biomed. Eng.,* BME-17: 97–100.

NYE, P. W., and J. C. BLISS (1970). Sensory aids for the blind: A challenging problem with lessons for the future. *Proc. IEEE,* 58: 1878–98.

PICKETT, J. M. (1972). Status of speech analyzing aids for the deaf. *IEEE Trans. Audio and Electroacoustics,* Au-20: 3–8.

ROWELL, D. (1974). The binaural sensory aid for the blind. *Proc. 1974 Conf. on Eng. Dev. in Rehab.,* Boston, MA.

SALMON, S. J., and L. P. GOLDSTEIN (eds) (1978). *The artificial larynx handbook.* New York: Grune and Stratton.

SCHILLER, R. (1974). The lonely world of silence. *Reader's Digest,* August: 141–45.

SELKURT, E. E. (ed) (1976). *Physiology.* Boston: Little, Brown.

SHERWOOD, B. A. (1979). The computer speaks. *IEEE Spectrum,* 16(8): 18–25.

STAAB, W. J. (1978). *Hearing aid handbook.* Blue Ridge Summit, PA: Tab Books.

STAFF OF THE NEUROPROSTHESIS PROGRAM (1974). Data processing, LSI will help to bring sight to the blind. *Electronics,* January 24: 81–86.

STERLING, T. D., E. A. BERING, S. V. POLLACK, and H. G. VAUGHN (1971). *Visual prosthesis the interdisciplinary dialogue.* New York: Academic Press.

THOMAS, H. E. (1974). *Handbook of biomedical instrumentation and measurement.* Reston, VA: Reston Publishing Co.

TOMPKINS, W., and J. G. WEBSTER (1980). *Microcomputer-based medical instrumentation.* Englewood Cliffs, NJ: Prentice-Hall.

UPTON, H. W. (1968). Wearable eyeglass speech-reading aid. *Amer. Annals Deaf,* 113: 222–29.

VANDERHEIDEN, G. (1978). *Nonvocal communication resource book.* Baltimore: University Park Press.

VANDERHEIDEN, G. (1979). Nonvocal communication/control aids in the classroom and jobsite. *Proceedings WESCON,* Session 6.

VANDERHEIDEN, G., and K. GRILLEY (1975). *Nonvocal communication techniques and aids for the severely physically handicapped.* Baltimore: University Park Press.

WALKER, M. G., R. G. MATHEWS, and M. K. HERNDON (1979). A portable speech processing system for an auditory prosthesis. *IEEE Frontiers in Health Care Conf.,* 212.

WEBSTER, J. G. (ed) (1978). *Medical instrumentation: Application and design.* Boston: Houghton Mifflin.

WHITE, R. L., R. G. MATTHEWS, and G. L. MAY (1979). An implantable cochlear prosthesis for the profoundly deaf: Principles and performance requirements. *IEEE Frontiers in Health Care Conf.:* 211.

## STUDY QUESTIONS

**6.1**   Describe the differences between the use of the tactile and visual systems for the input of printed material. List at least three design constraints that this places on the design of tactile reading aids.

6.2   What is the most important factor that leads to speed in language processing for reading or communication? Describe how this concept has been used in reading and communication aids.

6.3   What is the major limitation in using the tactile sense for perception of auditory information? How can this be overcome?

6.4   Why did the Stereotoner fail, and what design changes might have made it more successful?

6.5   What is the major limitation in using the visual system to substitute for hearing? Design (block diagram or flow chart level) a system that overcomes this problem.

6.6   Read Brugler et al. (1969) on the electronic design for the Optacon. Their Fig. 13 shows the scan electronic control circuit. Describe the operation of this circuit. Why are two clocks used, and why were the two frequencies chosen? Propose an alternative scanning system that retains the essential timing relationships. What method was used to ensure that the vibration amplitude of the crystals did not vary significantly from the top to bottom of one column?

6.7   List the major advantages and disadvantages of the paperless braille systems.

6.8   What are the major advantages and disadvantages of the long cane?

6.9   Verify that the downward beam in the laser cane detects dropoffs about two paces in front of the user. Refer to Fig. 6.11 and estimate the height of the transmitter and the location of the tip of the cane.

6.10  Given the frequency range and pulse width for the binaural sensing aid, calculate the auditory frequency that results from an object 25 cm in front of the user. Repeat for an object located at 50 cm. Compare your results with the specified range display of 1 kHz/m. The velocity of sound in air is 330 m/s.

6.11  What are the requirements for an optical character recognition (OCR) system for speech output reading aids?

6.12  Both reading aids (Section 6.5) and communication aids (Section 6.9) have been designed using synthesized speech as an output. Draw a block diagram of the system components and a flow chart for the control and processing steps required for each application. What are the similarities and differences in the design requirements for these two applications?

6.13  A blind student wishes to major in EE. Design a system that will allow him to complete a basic electrical measurements laboratory course using standard test equipment (meters, oscilloscope, waveform generator). Your "system" should include considerations of alternative instructional modes (such as a "buddy system" with lab partner) as well as hardware. Be sure to define the problem in terms of the learning outcomes for the student rather than in terms of specific tasks to be performed.

6.14  Lowe [Electronics, 52(23): 46–48, 1979] describes a microcomputer-based lip-reading aid. How does this aid differ from the Upton glasses? What functions does the microcomputer perform? How do the displays on the two devices compare?

6.15  Assume that the tubing and ear mold for a hearing aid can be modeled as a simple, R,L,C circuit. Let $L$ = inertance = $\rho l / \pi r^2$, where $l$ = tubing length, $r$ = tubing diameter and $\rho$ = density of air. Let $R$ = resistance = $\triangle P/F$, where $\triangle P$ = pressure difference across any segment and $F$ = flow rate. $C$ = compliance = $V/P$, where $V$ = volume and $P$ = pressure. Derive an equation for the impedance of this system in terms of damping ratio and undamped natural frequency. Use your results to explain the effects of tubing length and diameter, vents, and obstructions in the tubing on frequency response. See Section 6.8.

**6.16** Design a bioelectric interface that uses a single channel EMG to generate eight input commands for a communication and control system. Show major components (e.g., a biopotential amplifier) as a single functional block. What type of access would this system provide for the user? Develop a control scheme using this interface to generate full alphanumeric communication (spelling) and control over a powered wheelchair (left, right, forward, backward).

**6.17** Design a communication and control system to implement a sequential access format with printed output. Assume the user will have only a four-position joystick and an "enter" switch available. Compare the expected speed with that of the system in Problem 6.16.

**6.18** You have been asked to specify a communication and control system for a 20-year-old head-injury patient who has good head movement, no arm movement, normal mental ability, and marginal spelling (first-grade level). She desires to use the system in her community college program. Outline your approach to this problem and specify a system for her. Be sure to carefully list your assumptions.

**6.19** List the features that all communication and control system controllers must have. Contrast random, sequential, and encoding access modes.

**6.20** The Staff of the Neuroprosthesis Program (1974) predicted in 1974 that a complete visual prosthesis would be a reality in five years. Conduct a literature search to determine why this projection was in error. Are the problems mainly electronic, physiological, or a combination of the two?

# 7 Physical Therapy Equipment

*David L. Stoner*
*Terry A. Hull*
*Joseph A. Kleinkort*

## 7.1 LEARNING OBJECTIVES

Upon completing this chapter you will be able to:

- Explain the role of the engineer in physical and rehabilitative medicine.
- Describe the techniques of patient management available to the physical therapist along with the indications and contraindications for each of these techniques.
- Describe traction devices and their therapeutic effects.
- Explain the physical effects of isotonic, isometric, and isokinetic exercise.
- Describe the basic components of a biofeedback system and its therapeutic effects.
- List new trends in the development of physical therapy devices.

## 7.2 PRINCIPLES OF PHYSICAL THERAPY

In recent years, the physical therapy profession has made great strides in broadening its rehabilitative capability. In this broadening trend, the areas of specialization have slowly matured. With this maturity of specialization, a multitude of modalities have flooded the market. We will explain some of these modalities and their uses.

## Philosophy of Physical Therapy

*Physical therapy* can be defined as the treatment of disease or injury by physical means as opposed to treatment with drugs. Such treatments, which contribute totally or partially to the improvement of the patient, include the use of various physical agents such as heat, light, electricity, and mechanical agents such as traction or therapeutic exercise. Krusen et al. (1971) describe the concept of rehabilitation medicine, in which physical therapists play an integral part, as involving "the treatment and training of the patient to the end that he may attain his maximal potential for normal living physically, psychologically, socially, and vocationally."

## Engineering Principles in Rehabilitative Medicine

Rehabilitative engineering involves the application of engineering principles, science, and technology on behalf of the physically disabled, with the goal of improving the quality of life rather than the prolongation or saving of life (Nickel, 1978). There is an increasing awareness that significant economic as well as personal benefits can be derived from investment of time and money into the development of devices, techniques, and training that can free the seriously disabled from dependence on others.

One of the most meaningful contributions engineers can make to the medical profession is the quantification of variables related to patient therapy that have only been described qualitatively in the past. This statement is particularly applicable to rehabilitative medicine.

Both the Veterans Administration and the Department of Education provide support to interdisciplinary groups involved with rehabilitative engineering. The National Institute for Handicapped Research has established 15 Rehabilitation Engineering Centers throughout the country and has charged each with responsibility for a different core research area. Likewise, the Veterans Administration has named two Rehabilitative Engineering Research and Development Centers.

# 7.3 TECHNIQUES OF PATIENT MANAGEMENT

## Therapeutic Heat

A summary of the physiologically produced effects of heat, light, or cold, how they are produced, and how they can be effectively utilized in the management of physically and mentally impaired patients is covered in detail in several texts (Licht, 1967; Krusen et al., 1971; Rusk, 1977). However, with the evolution of even more sophisticated medical and electronic technologies, their concepts of utilization of therapeutic modalities are being updated. We limit ourselves to discussion of what is known about the physiologically produced effects of currently used physical therapy modalities and how these effects are thought to benefit the patient.

## General Physiological Effects of Heat

The overall effects of therapeutically imposed heat are best understood if discussed with reference to all tissues, then redescribed for each of the more popular physical therapy modalities.

On a cellular level, an increase in heat above the cell's normal temperature causes an increase in the cell's metabolic rate (BMR) (Scott, 1972). This increased BMR is due to several events that occur simultaneously within and around the cell. The increased heat causes increased permeability of cellular membranes, which allows for greater exchange of cell cytoplasmic contents with its environment. The increased temperature also increases the rate of cellular chemical reactions, including those that produce and utilize energy. Prolonged exposure to heat can lead to deleterious effects such as protein denaturization and cell death (see Chapter 11) (Fischer and Solomon, 1972; Stillwell, 1971). Increased temperature or even an independent increased BMR of most tissues leads to an increase in blood flow in that area. This increased blood flow can be due to increased metabolic support, such as in exercise, or to an effort by the body's own protective mechanisms to dissipate the heat (Guyton, 1976). Physiologists have known for some time that increased BMR by-products cause increases in local blood flow, and that the hypothalamus can cause massive changes in regional distribution of blood flow in response to changes in the temperature of the blood, especially in the skin. Increased temperature causes increased permeability of vascular capillary membranes, thus allowing greater release of fluids and osmotically active particles into the extravascular spaces. This causes temporary edema within the tissues until the forces acting across the capillary membrane are balanced or the source of heat is removed (Fischer and Solomon, 1972; Guyton, 1976). Increased temperature causes an increase in the elasticity of collagen and elastin fibers that make up the connective tissues of the body. This increased modulus of elasticity allows the connective tissues to be stretched to greater lengths without injury (Stillwell, 1971; Lehmann, 1971).

Mild heat distinctly diminishes the sensation of pain. The pain could be secondary to pressure, ischemia, or excessive muscle tension (Fischer and Solomon, 1972; Stillwell, 1971; Rusk, 1977). Pain and its intensity of perception are modified by heat and many other factors, such as suggestion, attitude, and psychological overlay (Rusk, 1977). Evidence suggests that pain modulation experienced by patients who are receiving a treatment occurs at many levels of the nervous system, not just at the local site of the treatment (see Section 7.7 and Chapter 5). Heat diminishes, and even abolishes in some areas, abnormal states of muscle activity. The vicious cycle of (1) spasm, (2) pain, (3) more spasm, (4) increased pain is broken by the relaxing effects of the heat. With repeated treatments, patients report definite improvement in the level of pain and spasm (Fischer and Solomon, 1972; Stillwell, 1971; Lehmann, 1971).

Thus, the clinical effects of application of heat are many. We might expect a pleasing sensation of warmth of the skin, local increases in blood flow, sweating, decreased skin resistance to passage of electrical current from the sweat, and increased cellular metabolism. Muscle tension may be decreased and connective

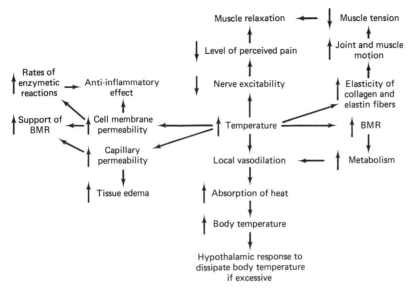

**FIGURE 7.1.** Summary of possible physiologically induced effects of physical therapy heat modalities.

tissue elasticity increased. Ligaments and joint capsules composed of connective tissue gain in elasticity, thus allowing increased motion. Changes occur in nerve excitability and conduction of their impulses, which could lead to moderation of pain. Finally, heat is anti-inflammatory by its effect on capillary permeability and enzymatic chemical reactions (see Fig. 7.1) (Fischer and Solomon, 1972; Guyton, 1976).

### Indications and Contraindications

Heat is indicated for pain modification, musculoskeletal problems, and neuromuscular disorders. These include such problems as sprains, strains, joint loss of motion, chronic joint inflammation, arthritis, muscle spasms dysfunction, and any type of dermal soft tissue trauma. Heat is beneficial in conjunction with and often enhances the physical therapy modalities of exercise, stretching, traction or manipulation, electrical stimulation including trigger point or acupuncture, and ionto- or phonophoresis.

Heat is contraindicated in acute inflammation or trauma, venous obstruction or occlusion, arterial insufficiency, hemorrhage, and coagulation defects (Fischer and Solomon, 1972; Stillwell, 1971; Rusk, 1977; Krusen et al., 1971). The key word here is *acute*. Once some of the conditions stabilize, mild heating may be indicated. Patients with cardiovascular, respiratory, and/or renal failure may be stressed to the point of failure of these systems when exposed to heat. Heat is contraindicated in any acutely active arthritic process with joint inflammation and swelling present. Heat should be used cautiously with persons who have decreased or absent sensation because of the danger of thermal injury. Finally, heat is contraindicated in the presence of active malignancy (Fischer and Solomon, 1972).

### Surface-Heat Modalities

We can divide physical therapy heat modalities into two categories: those that generally heat only superficial structures and those that are capable of heating superficial as well as the deeper structures. Superficial heat sources that can usually be found within the physical therapy clinic are hydrocollator packs, hot liquids such as water or paraffin wax, moist or dry air, whirlpool baths, and infrared radiation. Hydrocollator packs are canvas packs containing a silicone gel paste, which absorbs an amount of water equal to ten times its weight. These packs are placed in 180°F water and following absorption will give off steam heat for 20 min. Thus, the packs are placed against the skin and transfer the heat by conduction (Millard, 1972). Their depth of heat penetration is generally limited to 5 mm because local increases in blood flow secondary to the heat itself carry the energy away before it can affect the temperature of deeper structures (Fischer and Solomon, 1972). Infrared radiation heats by radiation. It has a wavelength of 770–12,000 nm. Its depth of penetration is limited to 10 mm and depends directly on the wavelength of the infrared source (Stoner, 1972). Whirlpool baths not only provide superficial heating but provide the additional benefit of reducing the weight supported by the limb undergoing treatment. To minimize electrical shock hazards, all whirlpool baths should be provided with ground-fault-circuit-interrupters (GFCIs). Most GFCIs interrupt power within 25 ms should leakage current to ground exceed 5 mA. Even though an uncomfortable shock may occur, serious injury and death are prevented.

The physiological effects of surface heat modalities are the same as just described for heat in general. The effects are mostly limited to the skin and underlying fat layers (Millard, 1972). There is some muscle and connective tissue pain modulation, but very little if any effect on BMR or blood flow in deeper tissues. However, these modalities are very effective when used prior to other treatment modalities such as exercise, active and passive assistive joint range of motion, stretching, and manipulation. They can also be used simultaneously with other treatments, such as in the use of hydrocollator packs over electrical stimulation (see Section 7.7 and Chapter 5).

The contraindications for superficial heat are again the same as described earlier for heat in general except that these modalities tend to be somewhat conservative and can be used at times where deeper types of heat cannot. Such a case would be application of heat to a woman directly over her uterus when she is pregnant or during her menstrual flow.

### Diathermy

The term *diathermy* refers to any therapeutic technique capable of producing deep heating. There are only three techniques that penetrate deep enough to be classified as diathermy techniques:

1. Shortwave diathermy utilizes ultrahigh-frequency electrical current between 10 and 100 MHz. The commonly used and FCC-approved frequency is 27 MHz.

2. Microwave diathermy makes use of the fact that electromagnetic waves are absorbed by the human body. The allocated frequency for operation is 2450 MHz.

3. Ultrasonic diathermy is actually a mechanical form of therapy using the propagation and absorption of very-high-frequency (1-MHz) vibrations. Schwan (1972) provides an excellent review of the biophysics of diathermy.

**Ultrasonic Diathermy.** The physics of ultrasound is identical to that of audible sound waves. The only difference is that ultrasound operates at a much higher frequency. Sound waves in both the audible and ultrasonic frequency ranges are longitudinal compression waves. Thus the movement of the molecules in the medium occurs parallel to the direction of wave propagation. This propagation of ultrasound depends on the presence of a medium that can be compressed, because propagation cannot occur in a vacuum.

The ultrasonic intensity, $I$, is given by the following equation:

$$ I = \frac{\rho c}{2} (\omega A)^2 \ \ \text{W/cm}^2 $$

(7.1)

where  $\rho$ = density of the tissues (g/cm³)

$c$ = sound velocity in the tissues (approximately 1500 m/s)

$A$ = amplitude of molecular displacement (cm)

$\omega$ = angular frequency

As sound propagates through the tissues, it is gradually absorbed, thus producing heat. The attenuation in intensity is given by

$$ I = I_0 e^{-\alpha x} $$

(7.2)

where  $I$  = intensity in the tissues at a depth $x$

$I_0$ = surface intensity

$\alpha$ = coefficient of absorption (cm⁻¹)

The depth $x_p$ at which the incident sonic intensity is decreased to a value of $1/e$ is a function of the coefficient of absorption and is called the depth of penetration.

$$ x_p = \frac{1}{\alpha} $$

(7.3)

The depth of penetration for ultrasonic diathermy varies from 0.5–70 mm, depending on the size of the crystal and total output wattage (Lehnam, 1972).

High-frequency electrical energy can be transduced into ultrasound through use of piezoelectric materials. Piezoelectric materials generate an electrical potential when mechanically strained (Peura and Webster, 1978). Piezoelectric materials are of two kinds: naturally occurring materials, such as quartz, and synthetic materials, such as barium titanate and lead zirconate titanate ceramics (Cobbold, 1974).

The piezoelectric effect also works in reverse: A change in potential induced on the crystal surfaces results in a mechanical deformation of the crystal. All therapeutic ultrasonic generators use this piezoelectric effect.

In order to quantitate the physical characteristics of piezoelectric materials, three electromechanical constants are commonly employed: coupling constant $K$, strain constant $d$, and stress constant $g$. Coupling is an expression for the ability of a piezoelectric material to exchange electric energy for mechanical energy or vice versa (Clevite Corp., 1965). Coupling squared ($K^2$) is equal to the transformed energy divided by the total energy input. The same constant is applied for conversion from electrical to mechanical energy and from mechanical to electrical energy. The $d$ constants express the ratio of strain developed along or around a specified axis to the field applied parallel to a specified axis, when all external stresses are constant. Units for the strain constant are pm/V. The $g$ constants express the ratio of field developed along a specified axis to the stress applied along or around a specified axis when all other external stresses are constant. Units for the stress constant are $m \cdot N^{-1}mV^{-1}$.

As an example for a lead zirconate titanate ceramic crystal (PZT-5A), when the electric field is applied in the $z$ direction, and strain is measured in the $z$ direction, $d$ has a value of 374 pm/V. Therefore, if a sinusoidally varying voltage having a peak-to-peak amplitude of 10 V were applied to this crystal, the peak-to-peak displacement would be:

$$374 \text{ pm/V}(10 \text{ V}) = 3.74 \text{ nm}$$

Thus, displacement of piezoelectric crystals is quite small.

Quartz was the most popular piezoelectric material for therapeutic diathermy applications until 1955 (Rogoff, 1972). Since then, manufacturers have tended to use ceramic crystals. Ceramics offer the advantages of ease of fabrication into any desired shape, large piezoelectric constants, and mechanical stability.

Piezoelectric crystals vibrate at their own natural frequency, which is mainly dependent on their thickness. Because the crystal vibrates efficiently at only a single frequency, the high-frequency generator must be tuned to the natural frequency of the crystal. There are two methods for coupling from the high-frequency generator to the crystal: direct coupling through a cable and coupling via a transformer. The transformer offers the advantage that it matches the output impedance of the circuit to the input impedance of the crystal. The most commonly used frequency in therapeutic ultrasound is 1 MHz. The piezoelectric crystal transforms electrical oscillations into longitudinal mechanical vibrations that enter into the body. At high frequencies there is virtually no transmission of ultrasound through air. Thus, the

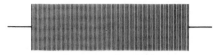

Continuous ultrasound

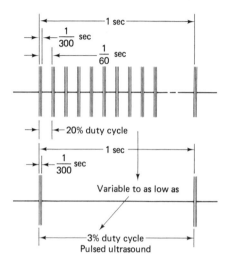

Pulsed ultrasound

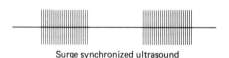

Surge synchronized ultrasound

**FIGURE 7.2.** Continuous, pulsed, and surge synchronized ultrasound.

vibrating surface of the crystal is coupled to the skin surface through use of oil, water, or a gel. The amount of power used in ultrasound diathermy should never exceed 4 W/cm². However, there is general agreement that 1.5 W/cm² should not be exceeded.

Most domestic ultrasound generators are designed to radiate ultrasonic energy continuously. However, many European doctors have proclaimed the advantage of pulsed ultrasound. Pulsed ultrasound is preferred over continuous sound in those cases in which heat is contraindicated or in conditions where it is believed that the beneficial effects are produced by the mechanical action of ultrasound. Figure 7.2 shows the difference between continuous, pulsed, and surge-synchronized ultrasound. The duty cycle of 20% shown may be lowered to the equivalent of from

15% down to 1%. Some investigators feel that a lower rate than 20% duty cycle yields maximum mechanical "micromassage" while lessening the thermal factor ordinarily associated with continuous sound. In some ultrasound units, it is possible to synchronize the pulsed ultrasound with a surged electrical muscle stimulation. The ability to simultaneously apply a synchronized pulse ultrasound and electrical muscle stimulation is thought to offer an additional therapeutic effect in certain cases, because this mode minimizes the thermal effects when exercising a specific muscle.

Ultrasound is indicated for any condition in which the physiological effects of heat are desirable. It is not effective in treating large areas. However, most musculoskeletal problems can be localized to one or several trigger points that are small in size. These areas are easily heated with ultrasound (see Section 7.7). Ultrasound is a very useful treatment modality in joint capsule inflammation or limitations, ligamentous tightness, muscle spasms or inflammation, joint degenerative arthritis, tendonitis, and calcified tendonitis or bursitis. Its contraindications are the same as for any other heat modality, including shortwave and microwave diathermy except when metal implants are present (Lehmann, 1971; Lehnam, 1972). Ultrasound is not contraindicated for use over metal implants as the metal will not concentrate the heat in that area, as is the case with shortwave or microwave diathermy. It should not be applied to the eye in therapeutic dosages, as cavitation (gas formation) may occur within the fluid medium of the eye or the retina could be damaged. It also should not be used over the spinal cord following laminectomy or when the cord is not protected by bone.

**Shortwave Diathermy.** Shortwave heating or conversive heating produces a relatively uniform heat distribution throughout the tissues by the conversion within them of high-frequency current. When electrical current at a frequency above 10 MHz is applied to the skin, it does not cause muscle contraction. However, considerable energy can be safely introduced into the body that will be experienced as deep heat. This is the principle of shortwave diathermy.

In order for tissue temperature to rise, the tissue must absorb and convert electrical energy into heat. Human tissues are energized with high-frequency currents in one of two ways: either electric field coupling or magnetic field induction.

For the electric field technique, electrodes made of sheets of metal are covered with insulation and placed parallel to one another. The air space between the two plates forms a capacitor within which the part of the body to be treated is placed. Thus the patient is actually part of a resonant circuit.

The shape of the heating pattern is dependent upon the shape of the electric field (Scott, 1972). If a uniform field is passed through a homogeneous mass, all parts of that mass should heat simultaneously and to the same degree. However, for heterogeneous human tissues, uniform heating obviously does not occur. Some heating occurs in tissues that have a low fluid content (i.e., fat and bone). However, most heating occurs in tissues with high electrolyte content, such as muscle, liver, kidneys, and blood vessels. These tissues have a lower resistance and thus a greater amount of current flows through them. The heat generated is given by $I^2R$.

Induction (inductothermy) is achieved by sending a high-frequency current

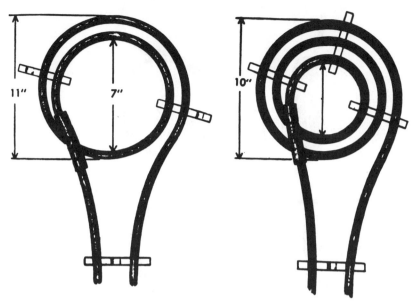

**FIGURE 7.3.** Two patterns for spacing "pancake" coils. (Reprinted from Licht, *Therapeutic Heat and Cold,* Baltimore: Waverly Press with permission.)

through well-insulated flexible heavy wire arranged in coils. These coils may be wound either in a spiral helix about the part to be treated or into a flat spiral "pancake" that has the shape of a watch-spring triptych (Fig. 7.3). Using this method, the tissues are not part of the circuit but are located within the magnetic field produced by the coil (Fig. 7.4). This high-frequency oscillating field induces oscillating currents within the tissues.

The shape of the heating pattern is dependent on the shape of the coil. When wound in a flat spiral, the coil produces a relatively superficial heating pattern

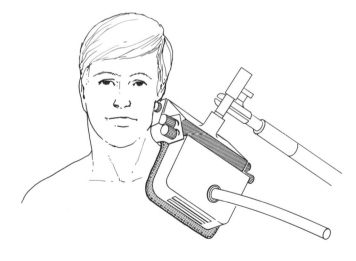

**FIGURE 7.4.** A "molded" electrode with concealed coiled cable. (Reprinted from Licht, *Therapeutic Heat and Cold,* Baltimore: Waverly Press with permission.)

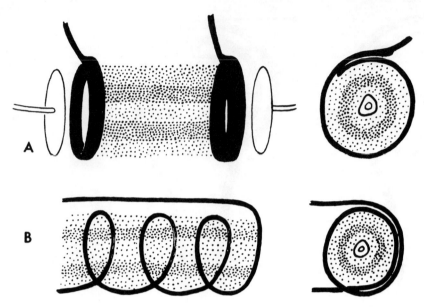

**FIGURE 7.5.** Patterns of heating: a-cuffs, b-coil. (Reprinted from Licht, *Therapeutic Heat and Cold,* Baltimore: Waverly Press with permission.)

(penetration only 30–40 mm). On the other hand, a helix produces a heating pattern like a filled stocking (Fig. 7.5). This pattern is brought about by a combination of capacitive dielectric losses and inductive heat produced by eddy currents induced in the tissue.

**Microwave Diathermy.** The Council on Physical Medicine of the American Medical Association approved a microwave diathermy device for the first time in 1947 (Raytheon, 1947). This form of therapy is used when the production of rather sharply localized deep heat is indicated. The microwave diathermy apparatus generates a beam of high-frequency energy having a frequency of 2450 MHz.

Figure 7.6 shows that four directors are available (Moor, 1972). Directors A and B are 100- and 150-mm diameter hemispheres. Figure 7.7 shows that heat distribution with these directors is not uniform. The maximum temperature is produced at the edge of the radiation field. Director C is a small dihedral right-angled corner reflector. This director gives a maximum temperature in the center of the radiation field (Fig. 7.8). If treatment over a large area is desired, director D is used. Like director C, this director also produces a maximum temperature in a longitudinal area down the center of its rectangular radiation field. These four microwave directors allow the application of microwave diathermy to virtually any body part. The maximum depth of penetration for both shortwave and microwave diathermy is 30 mm. Physiological effects of heat produced by these modalities are the same as discussed previously. Clinically, they are indicated where any of their physiologically produced effects will be beneficial in easing or reversing the diagnosed disease process (Stillwell, 1971; Licht, 1967; Rusk, 1977). They should only be used when the more superficial heat sources, due to their limitation in penetra-

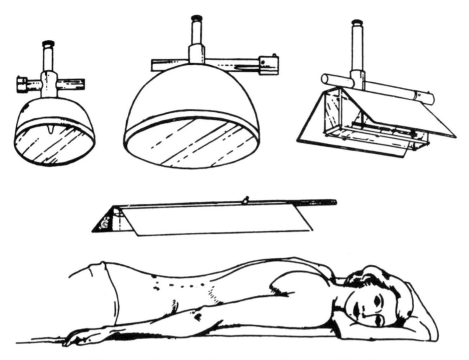

**FIGURE 7.6.** Microwave directors. (Reprinted from Licht, *Therapeutic Heat and Cold,* Baltimore: Waverly Press with permission.)

tion, are of no use. Again, they are excellent modalities to be used for pain modification, muscle relaxation, and any treatment program where increased flexibility of the part or tissue is desirable.

They are contraindicated in any condition in which heat is contraindicated. In addition, because of their depth of penetration, they are not indicated in cases of malignancy, tuberculosis, hemorrhage, deep vascular disease, where pregnancy is present, over areas of decreased or lost sensation, and in cases of metal implants (Lehmann, 1971; Moor, 1972; Lehnam, 1972). In comparing these two units as deep

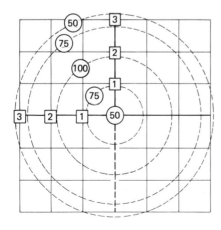

**FIGURE 7.7.** Pattern of heating field with Director A at two inches. (Reprinted from Licht, *Therapeutic Heat and Cold,* Baltimore: Waverly Press with permission.)

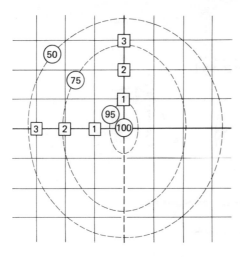

**FIGURE 7.8.** Pattern of heating at three inches from director C. (Reprinted from Licht, *Therapeutic Heat and Cold,* Baltimore: Waverly Press with permission.)

heat modalities, shortwave appears to be more effective than microwave in heating muscle and connective tissues. There is some evidence that heat produced by microwave is concentrated in more of the fatty tissues and associated vasculature (Moor, 1972). This could explain its lowered success rate, as noted in clinical experience when treating problems dealing with muscles or tendons.

### Therapeutic Cold or Cryotherapy

The concepts involved in cryotherapy are basically the same as for therapeutic heat except that the tissues become the source of heat and the modality absorbs the body's heat at a rate dependent on the temperature gradient (Stillwell, 1971; Millard, 1972; Licht, 1972). The loss of body tissue heat is by conduction, convection, or by evaporation depending on the heat-absorbing object or material.

Sources of cryotherapy can be vapor coolants, ice, ice water, and cold packs. The physiological effects of cryotherapy are local vasoconstriction or decreased blood flow, local decreased BMR, local decreases in fluid dynamics, and a general reduction in sweating. It also decreases nerve excitability and nerve conduction velocity, produces local analgesia, and decreases the inflammatory response to tissue trauma (see Fig. 7.9) (Fischer and Solomon, 1972; Rusk, 1977; Krusen et al., 1971). Some potentially harmful effects are frostbite or tissue necrosis secondary to ischemia in severe prolonged cooling.

Clinically, cryotherapy is indicated for any tissue that is in an inflammatory state, for any circumstance involving acute local pain, and for its antispastic effect on muscles. Its physiological effects are the treatment of choice in care of acute soft tissue traumas such as sprains and strains of muscle or tendon. It prevents further trauma caused by excessive edema forming in the area (Licht, 1972; Rusk, 1977; Krusen et al., 1971). Cryotherapy is also the treatment of choice in the initial care of acute burns or abrasions of first or second degree. It slows or prevents the inflammatory response following these injuries, which can destroy more tissue than the injury itself. Cold is also useful in the treatment of local infections because of

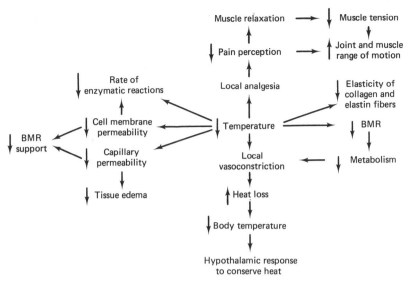

FIGURE 7.9. Summary of possible physiologically induced effects of cryotherapy used in physical therapy.

its anti-inflammatory effect. Because it produces a local decrease in blood flow, it penetrates to cool nerve and muscle, thus slowing chemical reactions necessary for neuromuscular transmission. This has the effect of decreasing the increased tension response of muscle secondary to stretching. Thus, cryotherapy is very effective prior to any treatment designed to stretch muscles or increase joint range of motion limited by muscle shortness or spasticity (Licht, 1972).

Cryotherapy is contraindicated over areas of tissue ischemia, areas of anesthesia, and on patients who have an excessively low tolerance to cold.

Cryotherapy has proven to be very successful, inexpensive, and can be applied both in the clinic and at home. It is the treatment of choice by most therapists for any acute soft tissue injury and often lessens the final degree of pathology when used promptly and correctly.

## Cooling Methods

Tissue temperature can be reduced using the principles of convection (blowing air over the skin), evaporation (spraying with a highly volatile liquid), or conduction (application of solids, liquids, or gases at temperatures lower than skin temperature) (Licht, 1972).

**Convective Cooling.** Convective cooling is rarely used medically. Perhaps the best use of convective cooling is to reduce the highly elevated body temperature associated with heatstroke through the use of manual or electric fans.

Convection (C) is a function of the following: (1) the temperature gradient between the skin and either the ambient air or outer clothing and (2) the rate of air movement past the body surface (Hertig, 1973). Expressed analytically:

$$Q_c = k_e A (T_s - T_a) V^n \qquad (7.4)$$

where  $Q_c$  = convection (W)

$k_e$  = forced convection heat transfer coefficient (W/m²°C)

$V$  = air speed (m/s)

$T_a$  = air temperature (°C)

$T_s$  = skin surface temperature (°C)

$A$  = average surface area of man (1.8 m²)

Colin and Houdas (1967) report a value for $k_e$ of 6.5 W/(m²°C) and a value of $n = 0.67$ for standing cross-flow conditions and 8.7 W/(m²°C) ($n = 0.67$) for reclining, parallel-flow conditions. These coefficients are from measurements on essentially nude men. The reader is referred to Belding (1973) for the influence of clothing.

**Evaporative Cooling.** Evaporative cooling is based on the principle that the evaporation of volatile fluids from a surface requires the consumption of thermal energy and thus results in a lowered temperature. Ethyl chloride has been the volatile fluid of choice for many years. However, Traherne (1962) recommends the use of nonflammable nontoxic chlorofluoromethane. Travell (1952) proposed a standardized procedure for evaporative cooling. A pressurized container of ethyl chloride is fitted with a calibrated nozzle capable of delivering a very fine stream. The jet stream should originate at least 0.5–1 m from the skin surface and be applied at an acute angle to the skin surface. The stream should be swept from a trigger area outward over the reference zone. The sweep speed should be fixed at 100 mm/s and repeated continually with a rhythm of a few seconds on and a few seconds off until all trigger and reference zones have been sprayed. The therapist has to be careful not to chill the skin too much and cause frostbite. Note that ethyl chloride is highly flammable and therefore precautions must be taken to eliminate fire hazards.

We can find the amount of cooling $\Delta T$ provided by evaporation by balancing the heat absorbed by the volatile liquid with the heat given up by the skin.

$$(T_{BP} - T) m_{VL} c_{pVL} + m_{VL} H_{vap} = m_s c_{ps} \Delta T \qquad (7.5)$$

where  $T_{BP}$  = boiling point of the volatile liquid (°C)

$T$  = temperature of volatile liquid as it reaches the skin surface (°C)

$m_{VL}$  = mass of volatile liquid on the skin

$c_{pVL}$  = specific heat capacity of volatile liquid J/(Kg°C)

$m_s$  = tissue mass to be cooled (Kg)

$c_{ps}$  = specific heat capacity of tissue 3600 J/(Kg°C)

$H_{vap}$  = heat of vaporization of volatile liquid (J/kg)

Therefore,

$$\Delta T = \frac{(T_{BP} - T)m_{VLC}c_{pVL} + m_{VL}H_{vap}}{m_sc_{ps}} \qquad (7.6)$$

**Conductive Cooling.** Conductive cooling is the most widely used method of cooling and generally makes use of ice water or melted ice as the refrigerant. Ice can be used in the form of ice packs, ice bags, and ice towels. These are applied for several 10–15-min periods with 5-min breaks for maximum effects. Ice water immersion is used for total tissue coverage and can only be tolerated by most patients for short periods of time. Cold packs—plastic bags filled with special jellies that are still pliable when frozen—are wrapped in a wet towel for more efficient heat absorption and placed in contact with the skin for periods of time up to 1 h. Generally speaking, the time of treatment duration using cold packs lasts about 30 min, at which time the maximum benefits begin to lessen due to a reflex local increase in blood flow (Fischer and Solomon, 1972; Guyton, 1976).

The change in temperature $\Delta T$ brought about by conductive cooling can be calculated from the following equation:

$$\Delta T = \frac{\dfrac{k_c}{\Delta x_c}T_{cf} - \dfrac{k_t}{\Delta x_t}T_B}{\dfrac{k_c}{\Delta x_c} + \dfrac{k_t}{\Delta x_t}} \qquad (7.7)$$

where  $k_t$  = thermal conductivity of tissue (0.47 W/(m°C) )

$\Delta x_t$ = depth of tissue at which body temperature is constant (2.23 cm)

$k_c$  = thermal conductivity of covering material

$\Delta x_c$ = thickness of covering material

$T_B$  = body temperature

$T_{cf}$  = temperature of cooling fluid

### *Therapeutic Light (Ultraviolet Radiation)*

Ultraviolet light (UV) is another naturally occurring modality that can be easily obtained by the patient.

Penetration of UV is only to about 0.1 mm but varies with skin thickness and coloring. The energy-absorbing substances in the skin are the proteins, and the photoinduced chemical reactions are erythema, tanning, epithelialization, bacteriocidal effects, and vitamin $D_3$ synthesis. Erythema is noted after several hours and is secondary to direct or indirect thermal effects or possible release of vasoactive substances such as histamine, serotonin, and bradykinin. Tanning is the result of an increased number of melanin granules in the skin. This is due to an increased number of melanin-producing cells stimulated by exposure to UV. Epithelialization or increased thickness of the outer layers of skin is secondary to accelerated cell division of the epidermis brought about by UV exposure. Bacteriocidal effects are due to altered cell mitosis, which may produce lethal mutations that prevent the bacteria from successfully reproducing. Vitamin $D_3$ is produced in the skin and subcutaneous tissue when the chemical 7-dehydro-cholesterol absorbs the UV light. Vitamin $D_3$ is necessary for proper calcium absorption from the small intestine (Scott, 1972; Stillwell, 1971; Rusk, 1977; Licht, 1967; Krusen et al., 1971).

UV is indicated in any disease condition in which its physiological effects would be useful in controlling or reversing the disease pathology. It is mainly used in the treatment of diseases of the skin, tuberculosis, ulcerations, rheumatic diseases, and some childhood diseases. Skin conditions treated are psoriasis, acne, boils or carbuncles, herpes zoster, lupus vulgaris, eczema, and some types of scar tissue. Its use in treatment of tuberculosis has been replaced with antibiotic therapy. The effect of erythema and epithelialization speeds the healing of the ulcers when used properly. In the treatment of rheumatic diseases, the aims of treatment are the production of vitamin D and an improved psychological condition. At one time, UV radiation was the treatment of choice for rickets in children, as it was caused by vitamin D deficiency. Now, with the advent of calciferol, the need for UV in children has been considerably reduced (Scott, 1972; Stillwell, 1971; Rusk, 1977; Licht, 1967). UV use is declining within the physical therapy field because of the use of topical and systemic antibiotics in addition to vitamin supplements and other pharmacological agents, which produce the same beneficial effects. The greatest use of this modality today is in the treatment of psoriasis and ulceration.

UV is contraindicated in patients who experience toxic photosensitizing effects from foods, diseases, or drugs.

## Ultraviolet Therapy Instrumentation

The entire electromagnetic family of waves (Fig. 7.10) (electromagnetic spectrum) occurs as a result of different frequencies of electromagnetic radiation. Ultraviolet radiation forms a small portion of this spectrum, with wavelengths from 50–400 nm. Because the short wavelength ultraviolet rays are completely absorbed in about 30 mm of air, they are of little interest for therapy. Therapeutic ultraviolet radiation extends from wavelengths of 180 to 400 nm. Sources of UV other than the sun are usually some type of mercury-arc lamp. These lamps are either of the high-pressure, hot-quartz type or the cold-quartz type. The high-pressure lamps produce a broadband spectrum of UV, which produces erythema, pigmentation or tanning, and bacteriocidal effects. The cold-quartz lamps produce a wavelength that is mostly bacteriocidal and are often used for air sterilization in older surgical rooms.

The design and construction of ultraviolet ray sources and the technique of application greatly influence their therapeutic effects (Anderson, 1967). We may classify therapeutic ultraviolet generators into three types (Fig. 7.11): (1) professional, (2) prescription, and (3) solarium. However, all therapeutic lamps have one factor in common: directional radiation control. Directional control concentrates the ultraviolet rays from the source and directs them toward the treatment area.

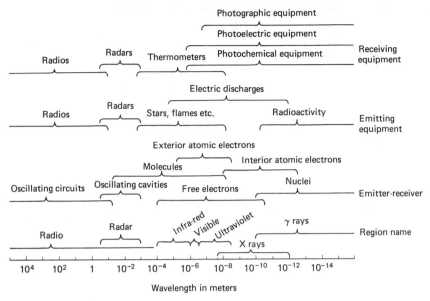

Photographic equipment

Photoelectric equipment

Receiving
equipment

Radios | Radars | Thermometers | Photochemical equipment

Electric discharges

Emitting
equipment

Radios | Radars | Stars, flames etc. | Radioactivity

Exterior atomic electrons

Molecules | Interior atomic electrons

Oscillating circuits | Oscillating cavities | Free electrons | Nuclei | Emitter-receiver

Region name

Radio | Radar | Infra-red | Visible | Ultraviolet | $\gamma$ rays

X rays

$10^4$    $10^2$    $1$    $10^{-2}$    $10^{-4}$    $10^{-6}$    $10^{-8}$    $10^{-10}$    $10^{-12}$    $10^{-14}$

Wavelength in meters

**FIGURE 7.10.** The electromagnetic spectrum. (Reprinted from Fowler and Meyer, *Physics for Engineers and Scientists,* Boston: Allyn and Bacon with permission.)

Two commonly employed methods of directional control are reflection and focusing with lenses. A properly designed reflector can increase the incident ultraviolet radiation on an average treatment area by a factor of five. Figure 7.12 shows some basic reflector designs. Lenses concentrate ultraviolet rays when local applications on small treatment areas are indicated or when very intensive radiation is desired. Note that use of either a reflector or lens modifies the spectral energy distribution. This modification is a function of the reflection or transmission characteristics of the materials used but usually shifts the ultraviolet energy received toward the longer wavelengths (Fig. 7.13).

**Professional Model Lamps.** Professional model lamps are high-powered lamps designed for either general body irradiation (Fig. 7.11a) or local application (Fig. 7.11d). Because of their high-power output, use of these lamps should be strictly monitored while carefully controlling dosage.

The general body irradiation lamp is mobile and has a reflector directional control and adjustable shutters for controlling the radiation area. These lamps are available in a variety of powers and some have adjustable power. In addition to allowing the operator to regulate the light source to bring the dosage within a prescribed range, the power adjustment capability may be used to compensate for radiation source depreciation with usage.

The professional lamp designed for local applications is often called a Kromayer lamp after its inventor, E.L.F. Kromayer of Vienna. This lamp uses a high-pressure mercury-quartz arc as a light source. The source is encased in a housing with a quartz window and is cooled by either water flow or air blast, which makes it possible to use the lamp close to living tissue. Because the arc is very intense, it

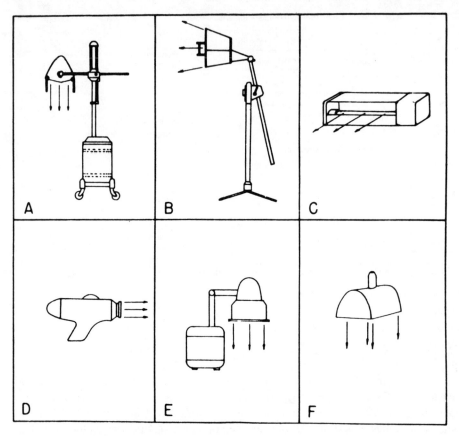

FIGURE 7.11. Schematic diagrams of clinical UV generators. (a) professional model, (b) prescription model, (c) germicidal wall fixture, (d) Kromayer (water or air-cooled), (e) diagnostic lamp, (f) solarium lamp. (Reprinted from Licht, *Therapeutic Electricity and Ultraviolet Radiation,* Baltimore: Waverly Press with permission.)

is suitable for use with either a quartz lens for contact applications or with quartz and metal applicators (Fig. 7.12c and e) to project light into body cavities.

**Prescription Model Lamps.**   Prescription model lamps (Fig. 7.11b) resemble professional model lamps in applicability, spectrum, and coverage but are lower in wattage. They produce ultraviolet rays at a higher intensity than sun lamps but lower intensity than professional lamps. Their primary use is to allow patients to have home treatment; however many physicians use them in their office to supplement professional model lamps.

**Solaria Lamps.**   Solaria lamps are classified as "group" or "individual." Group irradiation (Fig. 7.11f) can be accomplished through the use of a powerful carbon arc with reflectors designed to spread the light over a wide area and ultraviolet-transmitting glass windows to cover the arcing electrode. Transmission of the glass windows is usually such that the ultraviolet spectrum on the short-wavelength side is limited to about 280 nm. Individual solaria lamps are used to

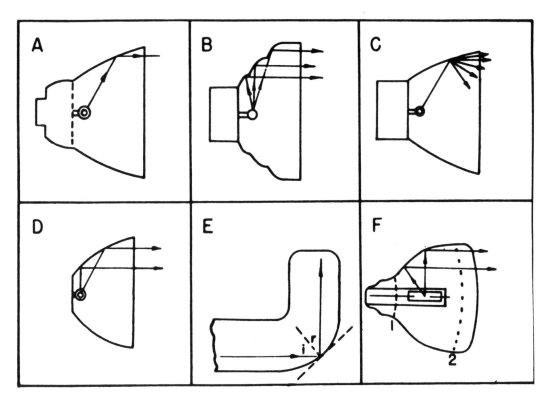

**FIGURE 7.12.** Directional radiation control devices. (a) specular reflection, (b) terrace with specular reflection, (c) diffuse reflection, (d) parabolic specular reflection, (e) internal total reflection in fused quartz, (f) electro deposited aluminum on glass in protective atmosphere. (Reprinted from Licht, *Therapeutic Electricity and Ultraviolet Radiation*, Baltimore: Waverly Press with permission.)

irradiate one or two individuals at a time. These lamps may use high-pressure mercury, carbon arcs, or a bank of four or five 1-m fluorescent ultraviolet lamps.

**Ultraviolet Energy Measurement.** Prescription of ultraviolet radiation includes specification of wavelength, power at the specified wavelength, and duration of the irradiation period. The product of power and duration is the ultraviolet energy in the various wavelengths. However, users of ultraviolet light sources rarely have light-measuring equipment available with which to gather this information. Instead, they must rely upon literature from manufacturers concerning the spectral energy distribution of a particular lamp. This information is usually sufficient except that it cannot predict the rate of deterioration of any specific lamp installation. If deterioration is important, then some form of ultraviolet light measurement must be employed. Anderson (1967) reviews some relatively inexpensive methods for approximating the ultraviolet energy from a specific lamp installation.

Because ultraviolet light dosage depends on several factors (duration, intensity, angle of incidence, and human skin response) it is necessary to skin test every patient before planning and initiating any treatment program. There are several

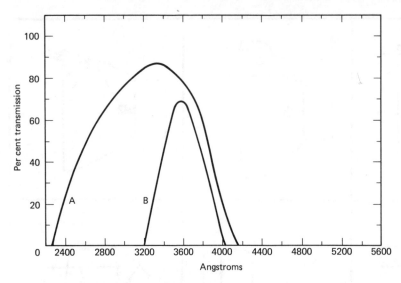

**FIGURE 7.13.** Transmission of UV filters used in fluo-
rescence diagnosis. (a) calcium and aluminum phosphate
glasses with nickel or cobalt oxides, 4 mm thickness, (b)
Wood's nickel oxide-silica glass, 4.5 mm thickness. (Reprinted from Licht, *Therapeutic Electricity and Ultraviolet Radiation,* Baltimore: Waverly Press with permission.)

methods of skin testing UV light, but the one used by most is progressive
irradiation of several small skin areas. This technique involves covering the patient's skin area to be treated for four small openings. A 5 × 7 card will work with
four holes in a series about 2–3 cm apart and 1–2 cm in diameter. The last three
holes are covered and the remaining hole is irradiated. Generally the test should
begin with a small time increment and each increase in exposure time should
double the previous one. A commonly used protocol is to expose the first hole for
120 s, the second hole plus the first for another 60 s, the third plus first and second
for another 30 s, and then all four holes for another 30 s. This gives a total of 240
s for hole 1, 120 s for hole 2, 60 s for hole 3 and 30 s for hole 4. The skin is then
inspected 24 h later and the dosage that just produced a mild reddening of the skin
is termed the minimal erythemic dose or MED. The MED is the basic unit of
treatment and the desired effects of UV are based on progressive increments of the
MED.

## 7.4 PHYSICAL MOBILIZATION AND TRACTION

### *Clinical Uses of Traction*

The use of traction equipment is widespread. It may be found in almost every
hospital and physical therapy department in the United States.

Traction is applied to the cervical or lumbar spine through use of harnesses fastened to the head or pelvic area. The resultant force acts parallel to the axis of the spinal column and thus widens the intervertebral spaces, which relieves nerve root compression by the intervertebral disks. Compression of the nerve roots causes the sensations of pain, burning, and tingling in the neck, shoulders, and arms when the cervical spine is involved. Similar sensations are felt in the back, buttocks, legs, and feet when the lumbar spine is involved.

To better understand the mechanics of traction, we must keep in mind Newton's Third Law of Motion: For every action there is an equal and opposite reaction. The opposite reaction that we must remember in traction of any kind is due to friction (Fig. 7.14). In a horizontal plane, friction is dominant until motion takes place. Stated analytically:

$$\mu = F/R \qquad (7.8)$$

where  $F$ = horizontal frictional force

$R$ = patient's weight

$\mu$ = coefficient of friction

The frictional coefficient of a patient on a couch is about 0.5. This means that ½ the body weight can be pulled before movement takes place. Due to the weight of the body versus the weight of the head, it is far easier to give cervical than lumbar traction. Cervical traction thus requires less weight. For intermittent traction in which the pull is only experienced for a short time (10–30 s), the pull may be significantly more than in static traction, where the force is applied constantly. The majority of traction units on the market have a static capability. However, static traction is usually used in patients who require prolonged bed rest. For cervical traction after 20 lb (9 kg) pull, most authors agree a mild separation of the vertebrae takes place (Harris, 1971; Turner, 1957). Harris (1971) also reports that a lumbar force of 100–200 lb (45–90 kg) can increase vertebral body separation from 1–4 mm. Note that the tractional force applied should be determined by the patient's tolerance and that severe spasm always contraindicates the use of traction. Intermittent traction is quite effective for the cervical lesion if used between 20–40 lb (9–18 kg) pull. However, in lumbar traction, 60–200 lb (27–90 kg) of pull may be indicated. In lumbar traction with a large amount of pull, a device such as a thoracic strap is necessary to stabilize the patient.

Traction should only be given by an experienced physical therapist since the results of improperly applied traction can be very harmful. Traction is contraindicated in: (1) rheumatoid arthritis, (2) pregnancy, (3) spinal infection, (4) malignancy, (5) cord pressure, (6) cardiovascular disease, (7) osteomalacia or osteoporosis, (8) severe muscle spasm, and (9) spinal fracture.

The indications for the use of traction are many. The use of static traction in the acute muscle spasm case where the patient is on bed rest is of questionable benefit due to the small amount of weight used (400 lb maximum). Many physicians merely utilize this method to keep their patients on bed rest.

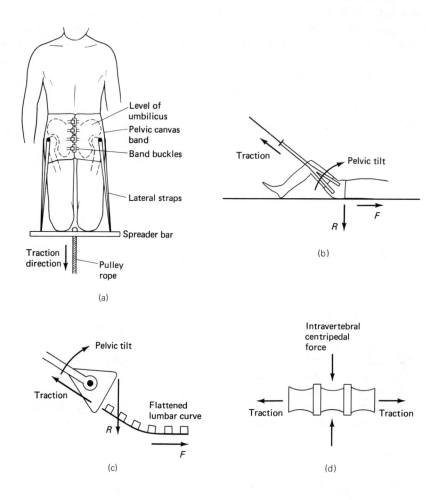

**FIGURE 7.14.** Equipment for pelvic traction. (a) Typical horizontal lumbar traction set up with lumbar harness, (b) and (c) Forces exerted in traction, (d) Centripedal force exerted in the intravertebral disk area when pull is applied to the vertebrae.

Traction can be used successfully in lumbar disk lesions. The greatest proponent of this type of treatment is Cyriax (1974). The force used (10–100 lb) is entirely dependent on each patient and amount of muscle spasm, anxiety, and general physical condition. Lumbar osteoarthritis is an indication for use as long as no osteoporosis is evident. Spondylolisthesis is another condition that indicates use.

Traction can easily be applied to the cervical spine for the treatment of cervical degenerative joint disease, disk prolapse, whiplash, and torticollis. It is advantageous in all cases to reduce spasm of the muscle to a minimum before traction in order to get a better reactive force on the vertebrae involved.

## *Traction Equipment*

Traction was traditionally provided with static weights acting on a harness attached to a patient immobilized in bed. In the 1950s, research demonstrated that considerably more force was required to cause widening of the intervertebral spaces than could be provided with a static system employing weights. However, the required forces were too high to be tolerated for long periods, while intermittent or cycled application of traction of sufficient magnitude proved both effective and relatively comfortable (Health Devices, 1977). Studies also proved that conventional traction applied with a pelvic belt to the lumbar region of a patient lying in a bed was ineffective. All of the linear force was dissipated because of the friction of the lower half of the body against the bed clothing before the force could lengthen the lumbar spine and widen the lumbar intervertebral spaces. Therefore, split beds were developed. The lower half of the bed was free to roll back and forth several inches on a frame to eliminate the friction losses so that traction force could be transmitted directly to the lumbar region.

Several types of intermittent traction devices are in use. One mobile hydraulically powered type of unit can be adjusted to provide traction in either a vertical or horizontal plane. It is therefore suitable for cervical traction in the sitting or supine position and lumbar traction in the supine position. Another type employs a gear motor to drive a cam or crank. A cam-following bearing and lever convert rotary to linear motion. Other types have one to two gear motors to generate and relieve traction force and timers that stop and start the gear motors to maintain or release traction to determine cycling characteristics.

Some traction units contain more elaborate control circuits, ranging from a timer that can set treatment duration and automatically de-energize the machine at the end of the treatment session, to controls that can adjust cycling rate and the ratio of the traction and relaxation portions of the cycle. All such devices provide a method for adjusting the traction force (usually calibrated in pounds) that is applied to the harness.

Original designs employed a fixed-speed gear motor operating at 4–5 rpm. Therefore, a complete traction cycle took 12–15 s. About half the cycle time is expended in increasing or decreasing force to the maximum or minimum level, and the maximum force was applied during the remaining half. This 50% "dwell" period has been determined empirically to be the most comfortable maximum period of toleration for substantial traction for most patients.

Cervical traction units are typically mounted by means of a manufacturer-supplied wallmount made of sheet steel or plate or locally improvised and fabricated mounts and brackets. Others are mounted overhead, on a floor stand, or on standards associated with or integrated into special chairs. Lumbar traction units may be integrated into special beds or tables. Mobile, hydraulically powered units can be used with most beds or special tables. Universal models can be mounted overhead for cervical traction or attached to a bed or special table for either cervical or lumbar traction.

### Extremity Compression

Extremity compression involves the use of elastic materials or pneumatic circumferential bags for tissue compression. It is indicated when there is any type of excessive tissue edema or venous insufficiency (Rusk, 1977; Krusen et al., 1971). The edema can be posttrauma, as in the case of strains or sprains of muscles and ligaments, or it can be postsurgical, as in the case of radical mastectomies or lower-extremity vascular surgery. The physiological effects of extremity compression, by whatever means, are an increased effective venous drainage, a decreased loss of fluids into the extravascular spaces from the capillaries, and an increased lymphatic drainage. The combined physiological effect is reduced and controlled tissue edema of the extremities. Clinically, it is often used successfully in the control of edema associated with varicose veins and postsurgical radical mastectomies. In extremity tissue compression, the pressure should not exceed arterial pressure.

## 7.5 THERAPEUTIC EXERCISE

### Physical Effects

Exercises in involved patients or normal subjects are designed to accomplish several objectives. Usually, they are initiated to correct some muscle or joint dysfunction or to perfect or improve a function that already exists. Properly designed and performed exercises increase muscle power and strength, increase endurance, improve coordination, increase or stabilize joint and muscle range of motion (ROM), and increase speed or movement (Rusk, 1977; Licht, 1967; Krusen et al., 1971). Types of muscle contractions involved in exercises are either isometric or isotonic. Isometric contractions occur when the force of muscle contraction is just equal to the resistance to movement with no change in the muscle length or motion in the involved joint. Isometric or static types of contractions are utilized by the body to provide stability of joint motion and prevent undesirable movement.

If the muscle contraction involves movement of the joint and changes in length of the muscle, it is termed an isotonic contraction. If the isotonic contraction involves a shortening of the muscle length, it is called a concentric type of contraction. If the muscle is lengthened during its contraction, it is called an eccentric contraction. Concentric and eccentric contractions are necessary for joint movements that produce translatory or rotary movement of the body. In physical therapy, most exercise programs are designed to improve muscle and joint dysfunction that is secondary to trauma or disease. The indications for exercise are too numerous to list here. We discuss only the concept of each type of exercise and the general types of equipment used within the physical therapy clinic.

**Isometric Exercise.** Isometric exercise is indicated when it is not desirable or possible for patients to perform exercise with joint movement. Typical cases might include patients with arthritic joints in a state of acute inflammation, patients whose extremities or body is immobilized by casts, or patients with whom joint movement might result in further joint or connective tissue injury. Isometric exercises can be performed by having the patient exert against immovable objects, such as casts or specialized exercise equipment. The advantage to this type of exercise is that it can be performed at just about any place at any time and at the convenience of the patient. Disadvantages are that this exercise increases muscle strength but not endurance, coordination, ROM, or speed. It is also difficult to judge improvement in muscle function by visually monitoring the exercising part.

**Isotonic Exercise.** Isotonic exercise is indicated when the patient requires improvement of dynamic muscle function or increased joint ROM following surgery, trauma, or disease. Most patients who have any musculoskeletal, neurological, or medical disorder lose desired muscle function due to pain involved with movement or to inability to properly exercise. Exercise programs are designed by the physical therapist after he or she has identified loss of muscle function in the evaluation of the patient. Most patients perform isotonic exercises simply by lifting weights against gravity. The weights are progressively increased over a predetermined length of time to the patient's tolerance until the muscle strength and joint ROM are considered normal or reach the desired goals of the exercise program outlined by the therapist. The disadvantage of most isotonic exercise programs in which progressive increases in weight are utilized is that they do not optimally increase the muscle endurance, coordination, or speed of muscle contraction. The advantage is that they can be performed at the patient's convenience using professional or homemade weights or equipment.

## Principles of Exercise

We define several terms that apply to muscular action. *Strength* is the ability to produce tension and is a function of muscle cross-sectional area and the number of motor units that can be activated voluntarily (Darling, 1965). In order for a muscle to do work, motion must occur. Thus external work is determined by the product of force times distance moved. However, internal work also occurs in muscles. Internal work is done in order to overcome frictional and viscous resistance. Note that some of the external work is lost to external friction, wind resistance, and so on. *Power* is work per unit time. The terms *stamina, endurance,* and *work capacity* are often used interchangeably and are defined as the length of the excursion times the number of repetitions times the load (Moffroid and Whipple, 1970). Finally, *skill* is the ability to accurately control muscle in order to achieve a specific physical task.

In developing a therapy program, physical therapists are often concerned with muscular force (strength), work capacity, and skill. We can best explain these three attributes of muscular action and their relation to isotonic and isometric exercise by referring to the work–tension diagram shown in Fig. 7.15. The relationship of external work done per unit time to load is a slightly skewed parabola. At low

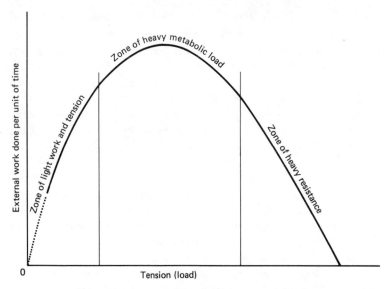

FIGURE 7.15. Schematic diagram of work–tension relationships. (Reprinted from Licht, *Therapeutic Exercise,* Baltimore: Waverly Press with permission.)

loads, work falls off rapidly; likewise, at high loads, muscle movement stops and no work is performed. The maximum capacity for work occurs at a point slightly less than half the maximum load that the muscle can move.

This work–tension diagram demonstrates how we can use both isometric and isotonic exercise to develop strength, working capacity, and skill. Note that exercise in the zone of heavy metabolic load requires the greatest work capacity. Exercise with low loads has less of an effect on muscle but demonstrates skill; exercise at high loads requires strength, but only a small amount of external work is actually done.

It is actually the chronic effects of exercise that are of most interest to the therapist. The adaptation to a long-term exercise program is the improvement of strength or the ability to develop greater tension in applying an effort against a near maximal load. The primary indicator of this adaptation is hypertrophy of the muscle. Darling (1965) presents quantitative evidence suggesting that isometric maximal contractions are more effective in improving strength than are isotonic exercises. In the extreme of exercise to increase strength, the other qualities of work capacity and skill may be only minimally changed.

Another major adaptation of muscles to exercise is in the ability to perform work or an increase in work capacity. In this case, performance is near the top of the work–tension diagram, which rules out the use of isometric exercise. We do not discuss in detail physiological changes that occur in the muscle to increase its working capacity. We can summarize by saying that the adaptation consists of increasing the circulation and building stores of substances used in metabolism, all for the purpose of improving the metabolic capacity of the muscle (Darling, 1965). Common characteristics of exercises designed to achieve maximal work are that the load should be slightly less than half of maximum and that the work duration should be long enough to cause a metabolic stress (at least 5 min).

The third area of muscular adaptation occurs in the area on the left side of the work–tension diagram, where skill is improved. Skill could actually be improved at any load level. However, the key to developing skill is repetition. Because heavy load exercises cannot be repeated in comfort, we usually select low-load exercises.

In Fig. 7.15, we assume that the range of motion was kept constant and that the speed was not allowed to exceed a moderate fixed rate. However, Hellebrandt (1958) found that increasing the speed at which exercise is performed was as effective for increasing the work capacity as increasing the load and that power is the variable on which extension of the limits of performance depends. Others have demonstrated that weight lifting has no effect on a muscle's rate of contraction and that strength and endurance are independent quantities; that is, endurance can vary while strength remains constant (Hill, 1938).

Moffroid and Whipple (1970) further studied the principle that exercise is speed specific and obtained the following results:

1. Low-power (low-speed, high-load) exercise produces greater increases in muscular force only at slow speeds.

2. High-power (high-speed, low-load) exercise produces increases in muscular force at all speeds of contraction at and below the exercise level.

3. High-power exercise increases muscular endurance at high speeds more than does low-power exercise increase muscular endurance at slow speeds.

Thus many exercise programs are based on the use of a constant velocity (isokinetic) exercise device.

**Isokinetic Instrumentation.**   In isotonic exercise, the patient lifts a known weight. We can easily calculate work by knowing the distance the weight was moved. We can then determine power by dividing by the lifting time. Thus, there is no instrumentation requirement for quantifying the results of isotonic exercise.

Isokinetic exercise, on the other hand, does present the engineer with a design problem. A typical isokinetic exercise system consists of three components: (1) the dynamometer, (2) the speed selector, and (3) the recorder.

The dynamometer measures the torque developed by the subject pushing against a moving input attachment. Input attachments provide for torque to be applied to the input shaft of the dynamometer in various manners, such as through flexion–extension of the knee, hip, trunk, shoulder, or elbow and adduction-abduction of the hip or shoulder, or directly at the input shaft as with wrist and ankle flexion–extension and internal–external rotation. The subject is instructed to exert maximal effort against the constantly moving input attachment. The dynamometer can be used to provide a measure of the level of muscular force that can be exerted at each speed of the input attachment. Additionally, through the use of an electrogoniometer (discussed later) and a dual-channel recorder, it is possible to measure torque simultaneously with range of motion.

The speed selector sets a constant speed of rotation of the input shaft. The input shaft cannot be accelerated beyond that speed regardless of input torque. The shaft speed for individual applications can be chosen as a function of the type and condition of the muscle, such as degree of spasticity, and to simulate the mechanical parameters of a specific functional activity, such as its required speed, force, or power.

Dynamometer recorders usually possess two chart speeds in order to optimize data interpretation. The slow speed (1 mm/s) displays the force peaks of individual or repetitive efforts, as in strength and endurance tests. The fast speed (25 mm/s) permits dynamic strength analysis over the subject's entire active range of motion at specific functional speeds. Moreover, the fast speed permits precise measurement of an individual's ability to produce properly controlled force outputs from key muscle groups. Coupled with range-of-motion information, the high chart speed information permits determination of force at specific points in the range of motion (Fig. 7.16).

**Calculations.** We make all strength, power, and endurance calculations from a strip-chart recording of the torque developed parallel to joint angle versus time. Work is the product of force times the distance moved in the direction of the force. For applications using isokinetic exercise equipment, we express the distance in terms of angular displacement. Angular displacement is the change in angular position of the input attachment $\theta$, hence the subject's limb about the axis of rotation. This is equal to the product of speed of rotation $\omega$ and elapsed time $t$.

$$\theta = \omega t \qquad (7.9)$$

Because we calibrate the recorder in terms of torque $\tau$ applied to the input shaft, work is calculated as follows:

$$W = F \times D \qquad (7.10)$$

where   $W$ = work

$F$ = force

$D$ = distance

$$W = \left(\frac{\tau}{L}\right) (2\pi) \left(\frac{\theta}{360}\right) (L) \qquad (7.11)$$

where length $L$ is the distance from the center of the input shaft to the point of force application and $\theta$ must be in degrees. Therefore,

$$W = \frac{2\pi\tau\theta}{360} \qquad (7.12)$$

Because torque is not constant, we must determine work from the area under the torque curve (refer to Fig. 7.16). Finally, power $P$ is the rate of doing work per unit time:

$$P = \tau \times \text{rpm} \qquad (7.13)$$

**Electrogoniometer.** We use electrogoniometry to determine the magnitude and pattern of continuous joint motion for any movement (Johnston and Smidt,

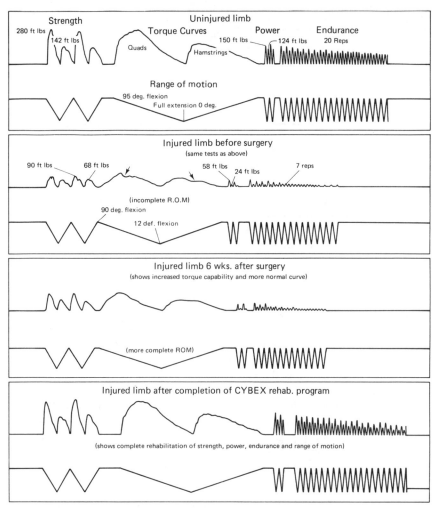

**FIGURE 7.16.** Typical output from isokinetic exercise. (*Courtesy* CYBEX, Bohemia, NY.)

1969). In an electrogoniometer, we substitute a potentiometer for the protractor of a standard goniometer. The device is positioned at the axis of rotation for a joint in any given plane and the arms of the goniometer are attached to the body parts that are proximal and distal to the joint. Thus, movement of these body parts causes rotation in the potentiometer and a concurrent change in the voltage that is recorded. This change in voltage is calibrated in degrees.

## 7.6 BIOFEEDBACK

Biofeedback is beginning to be utilized in physical therapy clinics throughout the United States (Goarder and Montgomery, 1977; Brown, 1975 and 1978; Jones,

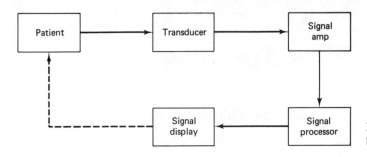

**FIGURE 7.17.** Elements of a biofeedback system.

1973; Whatmore and Kohli, 1974). We can describe the term *biofeedback* as external psychophysiological feedback. It is the utilization of a machine or series of machines to mediate a person's homeostasis by providing external means of monitoring internal body functions. The first use of biofeedback was by Whatmore and Kohli (1974) in the early 1950s by the use of EMG to measure relaxation. However, Kamiya (1969) is usually credited with founding the study of biofeedback in 1958. The basic biofeedback system contains a transducer, amplifier, signal processor, and signal display (Fig. 7.17). The transducer receives the physiological output from the patient and converts that signal into a measurable signal, which is sensed by the amplifier. The amplifier then converts the signal into a manageable quantity, which is sent to the signal processor that filters out unwanted information. The signal display then converts the energy to light, meter movement, or sound to enable the patient to visually or auditorily sense his response psychophysiologically.

The basic psychophysiological loop is as follows: The patient produces the original signal which is picked up, amplified, and displayed by the biofeedback system; he then perceives the feedback to which he must react. Therefore, the subject completes the feedback loop.

We can divide the use of biofeedback in physical therapy into two main areas: neuromuscular reeducation and tension control.

In the area of neuromuscular reeducation, the use of EMG (electromyographical) biofeedback is very effective (Basmajian, 1974). The EMG allows the patient to see or hear how many muscle units are actually firing. He then can alter that activity by mental processes. This type of biofeedback enhances use of any residual capacity a person might have after suffering from a neurological impairment. In the past, the difficulty therapists have encountered with this type of patient is the inability to stimulate the residual or returning neuromuscular capacity available. With EMG biofeedback, the patient can see what capacity he has and can better learn to retrain it by closing the feedback loop. The use of this form of feedback is also helpful in reeducating postoperatively relocated muscle groups, such as those found in joint surgery.

Biofeedback may also be used in stress or tension control in various pain syndromes that patients present at physical therapy departments. In such areas, EMG, GSR, and thermal feedback may be helpful. The GSR (galvanic skin response) is helpful in determining the amount of autonomic nervous system

| For treatment of control of | Biofeedback device | | | | |
|---|---|---|---|---|---|
| | ECG | EEG | EMG | PLETH | THERM |
| Alcohol & drug addiction | | X | | | |
| Arrhythmia | X | | | | |
| Blood pressure | X | | | X | |
| Circulatory disorders | | | | X | X |
| Consciousness state | | X | | | |
| Epilepsy | | X | | | |
| Heart rate | X | | | | |
| Hypertension | | | X | | |
| Insomnia | | X | | | |
| Memory improvement | | X | | | |
| Migraine headache | | | | X | X |
| Muscle relaxation | | | X | | |
| Raynaud's disease | | | | X | X |
| Sexual dysfunction | | | | X | |
| Stress and anxiety | | X | X | | X |

FIGURE 7.18. Selected uses of some biofeedback devices.

activity that is taking place. This is helpful in determining the degree of relaxation. Thermal feedback displays temperature change, which is helpful in certain headache syndromes. If the temperature of the hand is increased, a corresponding change in vascular dilatation takes place, which tends to relieve a majority of headache syndromes. Many headaches are either vascular or tension produced and the use of biofeedback can be beneficial in altering these states. EMG biofeedback is also effective in certain chronic conditions of muscle spasm. There are some cases in which a patient may not be aware of an inordinate amount of muscle spasm. With the EMG, the patient receives information regarding the activity of the muscle in spasm. This allows the patient to learn how to alter the spasm of the muscle.

There are few well-defined contraindications in the use of biofeedback. The most important is that the therapist be comptent in its use and thoroughly screen each candidate before application. The use of biofeedback is not successful in all cases, but the rate of success is highly dependent on the expertise of the practitioner. Figure 7.18 summarizes existing and proposed uses for biofeedback.

## 7.7 NEW DEVICES

### Phonophoresis

Phonophoresis is the utilization of ultrasound to introduce medication through the epidermis without the use of a needle. In the majority of physical therapy clinics, hydrocortisone is applied with phonophoresis. This introduction of steroid with ultrasound is effective in the reduction of tissue inflammation due to tendonitis, bursitis, and arthritic conditions (Kleinkort and Wood, 1975; Griffin et al., 1967). Griffin (1966) feels that both the mechanical and heating effects of ultrasound play a major role in the transfer of hydrocortisone through the tissue. The delivery of hydrocortisone may be accomplished by either a stationary ultrasonic technique or a motile technique. In the stationary application, an intensity of 0.5 W/cm$^2$ must be used and in the motile technique, 1.5 W/cm$^2$ is used. Each method must be applied daily for five days to get the desired results (Kleinkort and Wood, 1975). Physiologically, the combination of the effects of ultrasound on tissue plus the addition of the anti-inflammatory effects of the steroids produces a decrease in tissue inflammation with a subsequent decrease in pain due to inflammation (Azarnoff, 1975).

### Iontophoresis

The term *iontophoresis* has been used since 1908 and is not a new technique (Leduc, 1908). Iontophoresis is the transfer of ions into tissue for therapeutic purposes by means of electricity. The electric current to be used must be direct (galvanic), which causes positive ions to migrate toward the negative pole and negative ions to travel toward the positive pole. The majority of the solution in iontophoresis pools at the sweat glands and hair follicles. However, Mandleco (1978) has shown by radioisotope tagging and core studies that a percentage of a specific solution can penetrate the tissue. The penetration of the solution can be improved by adding propylene glycol or alcohol to the solution. The force that moves the ions is determined by the charge amplitude of each ion and the electric field strength. If the field strength is given as the voltage drop per meter ($E$), and the charge on each particle is given in coulombs ($Q$), then the accelerating force ($f$) is given in newtons and:

$$f = EQ \qquad (7.14)$$

The amount of current used rarely exceeds 4 mA. A reliable ammeter and current regulator must be present. Most standard electrical stimulators found in a physical therapy unit are adequate for conventional iontophoresis. For further details on techniques, either Kahn (1976) or Harris (1967) is an excellent reference.

A new form of iontophoresis developed in 1975 is called *transionic injection* (Kleinkort, 1978). This is a form of pulsed iontophoresis wherein the current generator is a transcutaneous electrical nerve stimulator (TENS) (see Chapter 5). To function properly, the stimulator must have no dc offset.

The main advantage of TENS over a dc generator is the immediate pain relief it renders as it is introducing the medication. This is extremely beneficial in the debilitating conditions of bursitis, tendonitis, and arthritis. A 10%-micronized hydrocortisone solution is used, combined with USP grade petrolatum. The medication is placed under the positive electrode, which is ½ the size of the negative electrode. It is given for two days, the first application for 15 min and the second for 10 min. The majority of patients receiving this technique receive beneficial results of decreased pain and increased motion as long as the area of inflammation is not more than 50 mm under the epidermis. Presently, at Wilford Hall USAF Medical Center (WHMC) in San Antonio, TX, there is an ongoing study to determine the depth of penetration of the ions. An additional physiological benefit to ion injection into the tissue is the reported 15% increase in circulation and an increase in heat production.

## Electrical Stimulation of Trigger Points

The successful use of dc and ac stimulation at specific trigger points in the body with microelectrodes has been used for 20 years. Voll (1975a) has shown that a number of points in the body have decreased skin impedance. These points correspond with classical acupuncture or trigger points (Reichmonis et al., 1976). The superficial stimulation of these loci has been as effective as the use of acupuncture needles without piercing the tissue (Voll, 1975b). The use of superficial electrical stimuli is safer and can be utilized by a physical therapist properly trained in the technique.

Experience at WHMC has shown electrical stimulation of trigger points to be highly beneficial in the treatment of a number of conditions. Its use in chronic and acute pain syndromes as well as postoperative conditions, and pre-, and posttherapeutic exercise programs has been very successful. The utilization of this modality for chronic intractable pain cases has been most encouraging. It has also been found that an initial use of this modality to reduce pain to a certain threshold followed by the use of a specific frequency of TENS has been most beneficial (see Chapter 5).

The theory and physiology involved in the use of this modality is far too complex to cover in detail here. We shall attempt, however, a superficial treatment of this topic and provide references for further study (American Journal of Acupuncture; American Journal of Chinese Medicine; Mann, 1971; Lu, 1974; Tan, 1973; Manaka and Urguhart, 1972).

The majority of units on the market for this form of therapy have an ohmmeter to locate the exact point of impedance depression (Baker, 1971; Hyrarinen and Karlsson, 1977). The use of cathode stimulation causes a microbiological breakdown of tissue in a highly confined area, much the same as an acupuncture needle (Fraden and Gelman, 1979). This tissue stimulation causes a complex neurophysiological process to take place.

In part, the stimulus causes a mobilization of the endogenous opiate system and is holoxone-reversible (Mayer et al., 1977; Pomeranz and Chiu, 1976). The classical gate theory as well as the thalamic neuron theory suggests how this form of stimulation acts (Melzak and Wall, 1965; Lee, 1978).

The use of specific frequencies and waveforms can have varying effects on the outcome of treatment. In general, low frequency (0.1-10 Hz) has been found most effective in body trigger points and high frequency (1-2 kHz) is most effective in auricular trigger points (Voll, 1975b; Frazee, 1975).

This form of stimulation requires an extensive background and knowledge as well as expertise in the area of acupuncture to be effective. However, if the therapist has such a background, this modality can be one of his most useful allies (Dale, 1978).

# REFERENCES

ANDERSON, W. T., JR. (1967). Instrumentation for ultraviolet therapy, in S. Licht (ed), *Therapeutic electricity and ultraviolet radiation*. Baltimore: Waverly Press.

AZARNOFF, D. (1975). *Steroid therapy*. Philadelphia: Saunders.

BAKER, L. E. (1971). Biomedical applications of electrical impedance measurements, in B. W. Watson (ed), *IEE Medical Electronics Monographs*. Piscataway, NJ: INSPEC/IEEE.

BASMAJIAN, J. (1974). *Muscles alive: Their function revealed by electromyography*. Baltimore: Williams and Wilkins.

BELDING, H. S. (1973). Control of exposures to heat and cold, in *The industrial environment – Its evaluation and control*. Washington, DC: DHEW, PHS, Center for Disease Control, NIOSH.

BROWN, B. (1975). *The biofeedback syllabus: A handbook for the psychophysiological study of biofeedback*. Springfield, IL: Thomas.

BROWN, B. (1978). *Stress and the art of biofeedback*. New York: Harper & Row, Pub.

CLEVITE CORP. (1965). *Piezoelectric technology data for designers*. Bedford, OH.

COBBOLD, R. S. C. (1974). *Transducers for biomedical measurements: Principles and applications*. New York: Wiley.

COLIN, J., and Y. HOUDAS (1967). Experimental determination of the coefficient of heat exchange by convection of human body. *J. Appl. Physiol.*, 22: 31.

CYRIAX, J. (1974). *Textbook of orthopedic medicine*, Vol. II. Baltimore: Williams and Wilkins.

DALE, R. (1978). Acupuncture in physical therapy. *Am. J. Acc.*, 6: 63.

DARLING, R. C. (1965). Physiology of exercise and fatigue, in S. Licht (ed), *Therapeutic exercise*. Baltimore: Waverly Press.

FISCHER, E., and S. SOLOMON (1972). Physiological responses to heat and cold, in S. Licht (ed), *Therapeutic heat and cold*. Baltimore: Waverly Press.

FRADEN, J., and S. GELMAN (1979). Investigation of nonlinear effects in surface electroacupuncture. *Am. J. Acc.*, 7: 21.

FRAZEE, J. (1975). Exponential harmonic progression and simultaneous dual frequency stimulation. *Am. J. Acc.*, 3: 315.

GOARDER, K., and P. MONTGOMERY (1977). *Clinical biofeedback: A procedural manual.* Baltimore: Williams and Wilkins.

GRIFFIN, J. (1966). Physiological effects of ultrasonic energy as it is used clinically. *Phys. Ther.,* 46: 18.

GRIFFIN, J., E. ECHTERNACH, and R. PRICE (1967). Patients treated with ultrasonically driven hydrocortisone and with ultrasound alone. *Phys. Ther.,* 47: 595.

GUYTON, A. C. (1976). *Textbook of medical physiology,* 5th ed. Philadelphia: Saunders.

HARRIS, R. (1967). Iontophoresis, in S. Licht (ed), *Therapeutic electricity and ultraviolet radiation.* Baltimore: Waverly Press.

HARRIS, R. (1971). Traction, in S. Licht (ed), *Massage, manipulation, and traction.* Baltimore: Waverly Press.

Health Devices (1977). Inspection and Preventive Maintenance of Intermittent Traction Machines. 6(9): 226.

HELLEBRANDT, F. A. (1958). Methods of muscle training: Influence of pacing. *Phys. Ther. Rev.,* 2: 319.

HERTIG, B. A. (1973). Thermal standards and measurement techniques, in *The industrial environment – Its evaluation and control.* Washington, DC: DHEW, PHS, Center for Disease Control, NIOSH.

HILL, A. V. (1938). The heat of shortening and the dynamic constants of muscle. *Proc. Roy. Soc.,* B126: 136.

HYRARINEN, J., and M. KARLSSON (1977). Low resistance skin points that may coincide with acupuncture. *Loci. Med. Biol.,* 55: 88.

JOHNSTON, R. C., and G. L. SMIDT (1969). Measurement of hip-joint motion during walking. *J. Bone Joint Surg.,* 51A(6): 1083.

JONES, R. W. (1973). *Principles of biological regulation: An introduction to feedback systems.* New York: Academic Press.

KAHN, J. (1976). *Low volt technique.* Hicksville, NY.

KAMIYA, J. (1969). Operant control of the EEG alpha rhythm and some of its reported effects on consciousness, in C. T. Tart (ed), *Altered states of consciousness.* New York: Wiley.

KLEINKORT, J. (1978). *Transionic injection technique.* USAFE Medical Convention, Garmisch, Germany.

KLEINKORT, J. A., and R. WOOD (1975). Phonophoresis with 1% vs. 10% hydrocortisone. *Phys. Ther.,* 55: 1320.

KRUSEN, F. H., F. J. KOTTKE, P. M. ELWOOD (1971). *Handbook of physical medicine and rehabilitation.* Philadelphia: Saunders.

LEDUC, S. (1908). *Electric ions and their use in medicine.* London: Rebman.

LEE, T. (1978). Thalamic neuron therapy and classical acupuncture. *Am. J. Acc.,* 4: 273.

LEHMANN, J. F. (1971). Diathermy, in *Handbook of physical medicine rehabilitation.* Philadelphia: Saunders.

LEHNAM, J. F. (1972). Ultrasound therapy, in S. Licht (ed), *Therapeutic heat and cold.* Baltimore: Waverly Press.

LICHT, S. (1967) *Therapeutic exercise.* Baltimore: Waverly Press.

LICHT, S. (ed) (1972). *Therapeutic heat and cold.* Baltimore: Waverly Press.

Lu, H. (1974). *Complete textbook of auricular acupuncture.* Vancouver, Canada: Academy of Oriental Heritage.

Manaka, Y., and I. Urguhart (1972). *Laymen's guide to acupuncture.* New York: Weatherhill.

Mandleco, C. (1978). *Application of iontophoresis for noninvasive administration of lidocaine hydrochloride in the ionized form.* Univ. of Utah: doctoral dissertation.

Mann, F. (1971). *Acupuncture.* New York: Random House.

Mayer, D. J., D. Price, A. Rafii (1977). Antagonism of acupuncture analgesia in man by the narcotic antagonist noloxone. *Brain Res.,* 121: 368.

Melzak, R., and P. Wall (1965). Pain mechanics: A new theory. *Science,* 150: 971.

Millard, J. B. (1972). Conductive heating, in S. Licht (ed), *Therapeutic heat and cold.* Baltimore: Waverly Press.

Moffroid, M. T., and R. H. Whipple (1970). Specificity of speed of exercise. *Phys. Ther.,* 50: 16.

Moor, F. B. (1972). Microwave diathermy, in S. Licht (ed), *Therapeutic heat and cold.* Baltimore: Waverly Press.

Nickel, V. L. (1978). Rehabilitative engineering — A new era. *Bull. of Prosth. Res.,* BPR 10-30: 1-7.

Peura, R. A., and J. G. Webster (1978). Basic transducers and principles, in J. G. Webster (ed), *Medical instrumentation: Application and design.* Boston: Houghton Mifflin.

Pomeranz, B., and D. Chiu (1976). Naloxone blockade of acupuncture analgesia: Endorphin implicates. *Life Sci.,* 19: 1757.

Raytheon Microtherm Acceptable: Report of the Council on Physical Medicine (1947). *J.A.M.A.,* 135: 956.

Reichmonis, M., A. Marim, and A. Becker (1976). DC skin conductance variation at acupuncture loci. *Am. J. Chinese Medicine,* 4: 69.

Rogoff, J. B. (1972). High-frequency instrumentation, in S. Licht (ed), *Therapeutic heat and cold.* Baltimore: Waverly Press.

Rusk, R. A. (1977). *Rehabilitation medicine.* St. Louis: Mosby.

Schwan, H. P. (1972). Biophysics of diathermy, in S. Licht (ed), *Therapeutic heat and cold.* Baltimore: Waverly Press.

Scott, B. O. (1972). Shortwave diathermy, in S. Licht (ed), *Therapeutic heat and cold.* Baltimore: Waverly Press.

Stillwell, K. G. (1971). Ultraviolet therapy, in *Handbook of physical medicine and rehabilitation.* Philadelphia: Saunders.

Stoner, E. K. (1972). Luminous and infrared heating, in S. Licht (ed), *Therapeutic heat and cold.* Baltimore: Waverly Press.

Tan, L. (1973). *Acupuncture therapy.* Philadelphia: Temple University Press.

Traherne, J. B. (1962). Evaluation of the cold spray technique in the treatment of muscle pain in general practice. *Practitioner,* 189: 210.

Travell, J. (1952). Ethylchloride spray for painful muscle spasm. *Arch. Phys. Med.,* 33: 291.

Turner, D. (1957). New apparatus: A spinal traction treatment table. *Brit. J. Phys. Med.,* 20: 259.

VOLL, R. (1975a). Twenty years of electroacupuncture diagnosis in Germany: A progress report. *Am. J. Acc.,* 3: 7.

VOLL, R. (1975b). Twenty years of electroacupuncture therapy using low-frequency current pulses. *Am. J. Acc.,* 3: 291.

WHATMORE, G. B., and D. R. KOHLI (1974). *The physiopathology and treatment of functional disorders.* New York: Grune and Stratton.

## STUDY QUESTIONS

*Note:* The units given in these problems are typical of those found in actual practice. It is often necessary to make conversions such as those required in these problems.

**7.1** A patient has been referred to physical therapy for heat treatment and exercise of the deep muscles of the hip. What heat modalities might be used? Would it be better to apply heat before or after exercise?

**7.2** Why is it necessary to use a coupling agent between the sound head and the patient when giving ultrasonic therapy?

**7.3** A patient is to be given ultrasonic diathermy at a frequency of 2.25 MHz. A power of 0.4 W/cm$^2$ is desired at a depth of 2 cm. Given that $\alpha$ is 0.15 cm$^{-1}$ at 1 MHz and $\alpha = cf$, where $c$ is a constant and $f$ is frequency, calculate the required input power. Would this be considered a safe power to use?

**7.4** A 160-lb patient with a temperature of 104°F is placed on a bed in front of a fan blowing air at a velocity of 5 mph across his body. If the room temperature is 25°C and the patient's skin temperature is 35°C, how long will it take to reduce his body temperature to 100°F? Assume an effective heat-loss area for convection of 80% of the total body surface area and that the patient is generating heat at a rate of 100 kcal/h. Also assume all other mechanisms for heat loss to be negligible (probably not a good assumption).

**7.5** Through independent study, quantitatively describe other mechanisms for heat loss from the body that should have been considered in problem 7.4.

**7.6** A volatile fluid (ethyl chloride, $C_2H_5Cl$) with the following properties is to be used to provide evaporation cooling:

$$\rho = 0.9 \text{ g/cm}^3$$

$$T_{BP} = 12.6°C$$

$$\text{Mol. Wt.} = 65$$

$$H_{vap} = 92 \text{ cal/g}$$

$$c_{ps} = 0.27 \text{ cal/g°C}$$

If 0.1 ml of this fluid at 10°C is sprayed onto a 25-cm$^2$ area of skin (approximately 2 g), what is the drop in skin temperature?

**7.7** Derive equation 7.7.

**7.8** A patient's leg is wrapped with plastic 0.3 cm thick. In order to cool the leg, ice is placed on the plastic. Calculate the resulting skin temperature given the following:

$$k_t = 0.4 \text{ kcal/(m} \cdot \text{h} \cdot {}^\circ\text{C)}$$

$$\triangle x_t = 2.23 \text{ cm}$$

$$T_B = 98.6{}^\circ\text{F}$$

$$k_c = 0.1 \text{ Btu/ft} \cdot \text{h} \cdot {}^\circ\text{F}$$

**7.9** In the calculation of the minimal erythemal dose (MED) for determination of a patient's initial UV treatment, the first of four exposures is 120 s and the last is 30 s. How long should the second and third exposures be if the range of exposure time is from 30–240 s? If the MED is determined to lie between the second and third exposure times, what first treatment exposure time should be used?

**7.10** A patient weighing 220 lbs requires lumbar traction. At what traction force will a thoracic strap be necessary to stabilize the patient? Assume the traction is applied at an angle of 30° with respect to the bed.

**7.11** Of the three types of exercise described (isometric, isotonic, isokinetic), which type would be best for a patient who requires strengthening of those muscles that straighten the knee but who also complains of marked pain when the knee joint is moved? What would be the exercise of choice for developing muscle power at increased joint speeds?

**7.12** Peak torque generated by the quadriceps muscle group moving at a velocity of 6 rpm is measured to be 280 ft-lb. When this same muscle group is moving at 15 rpm, the peak torque generated is 150 ft-lb. Refer to Fig. 7.16. During generation of each of these torque curves, the electrogoniometer output shows that the leg moves from 90° flexion to full extension (0°). If each of the torque curves can be assumed to be approximated by the function $\sin^2\theta$, calculate the power generated by the quadriceps muscle, in each case. Express the answer in horsepower.

**7.13** Conduct a study to compare and contrast the uses for the following forms of biofeedback:

1. Galvanic skin response

2. EMG

3. Thermal

**7.14** A patient has just undergone a muscle–tendon transfer in which a muscle group that normally functioned to bend the index finger is moved to a position where it now functions to flex or bend the thumb. What types of therapy would best be used to reeducate the patient to bend his thumb?

**7.15** Conduct a study to determine all the factors that might have some effect on the absorption of topically applied medication for iontophoresis.

# Neuromuscular
# 8 Prosthetics
# and Orthotics*

*Eugene F. Murphy*
*Albert M. Cook*
*Richard F. Harvey*

## 8.1 LEARNING OBJECTIVES

Upon completing this chapter you will be able to:

- Describe the major causes and methods of amputation.
- Describe the design goals and tradeoffs for external prosthetic devices.
- List the types of lower-extremity prostheses and describe their major features.
- Describe the major features of upper-extremity prostheses.
- Explain the principles of external orthotic devices and the medical conditions leading to their use.
- List the major medical uses of external orthotic devices.
- Explain the operation of the major orthoses for the upper and lower extremities and spine.
- Describe technical aids available for activities of daily living.
- List the major design requirements for wheelchairs.

*Sections 8.2 to 8.5 were prepared under U.S. Government sponsorship and are in the public domain.

## 8.2 MEDICAL ASPECTS OF EXTERNAL PROSTHESES

### Types and Causes of Losses

External prostheses (artificial limbs) may be needed for a variety of types and causes of losses. The principal causes are congenitally missing or deformed limbs, accidents, or trauma, deliberate surgical amputation because of occlusive peripheral vascular disease, or, occasionally, uncontrolled infection and amputation because of tumors.

**Trauma.** Trauma may lead to direct removal of a limb, as by a power saw, slicing machine, or a railroad wheel. In recent years, there has been some success in *replantation* of such traumatically severed limbs, particularly of hands or below-knee limbs. If the severed portion is promptly packed in ice and brought with the patient to a well-equipped special emergency center, restoration of circulation and reattachments of bone and tendons are often quite feasible. A major problem has been the restoration of nervous sensation and control. There has been increasing progress in microsurgery to reattach the nerves and facilitate the regrowth of the proximal portion of the nerve end into the distal sheath.

Another major occurrence in trauma, usually much less suited to replantation, is crushing of bones or blood vessels so that the limb becomes useless or gangrenous because of damaged blood supply. Osteomyelitis or other infection progression beyond control may also require a surgical amputation, perhaps long after the original trauma.

Reduction of sensation is common with diabetes or Hansen's disease (leprosy), so the patient may not recognize that he has injured himself with a single blow or with prolonged pressure or rubbing, as from an ill-fitting shoe or a wrinkle in the sock. Prolonged pressure or abrasion may lead to breakdown of the skin and an eventual infection, which may ultimately require amputation.

**Medical.** Peripheral vascular disease (PVD) leading to amputation because of gangrene is the most common cause for amputation. There are a variety of efforts to improve circulation by surgical intervention, including the use of arterial grafts (Chapter 4).

**Tumors.** Bone tumors often require surgical amputation, usually disarticulation at the next proximal major joint in order to minimize the risk that a tumor will spread. In some cases, there is also extensive removal of lymph glands, complicating return circulation and increasing the risk of chronic edema.

### Amputation and Postoperative Treatment

**Level Selection.** The most distal level that is medically feasible is generally desirable with only a few exceptions (Fig. 8.1). Increasingly sophisticated instrumentation assists in such selections and allows conservation of more of the limb than was formerly considered prudent.

**Conventional Care.** An elastic Ace bandage is applied over the stump with higher compression distally and decreasing pressure proximally. This supports the

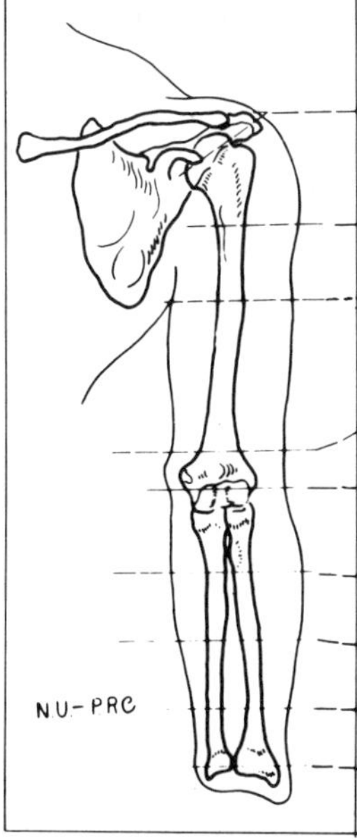

| Prosthesis Type | Functional Loss | Replacement | Main Control Motions |
|---|---|---|---|
| Fore-quarter | No scapular motion | Shoulder plate | Chest expansion |
| Shoulder Disart. | No humeral flexion | Shoulder cap socket | Scapular protraction |
| Short A/E | Poor humeral flexion | Locking elbow with turntable | Scapular protraction and humeral flexion |
| Standard A/E | No humeral rotation control | | Humeral flexion |
| Elbow Disart. | No forearm flexion | Outside elbow lock | Elbow flexion |
| Very Short B/E | Poor forearm flexion | Step-up hinge | |
| Short B/E | No pronation and supination | Manual wrist rotation | |
| Medium B/E | Poor pronation and supination | Step-up pronation and supination | Forearm pronation and supination |
| Long B/E | Fair pronation and supination | Screw-driver fit socket | |
| Wrist Disart. | Hand function, wrist flexion | Terminal device | |

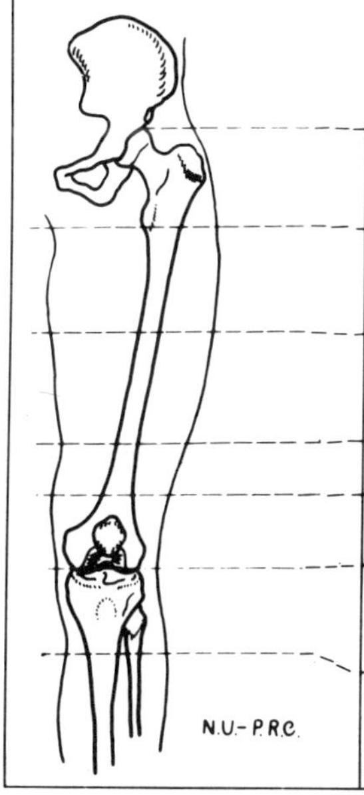

| Type | Suspension Control | Socket | Knee-Shin | Ankle-Foot |
|---|---|---|---|---|
| Hemi-pelvectomy | Plastic pelvic girdle | Plastic with shelf for ischium on sound side. | Standard Bock Variate Navy Hydra-cadence | Standard or SACH soft heel |
| Hip dis. Very short | | Moulded plastic socket | | |
| Short | Pelvic band or suction with Silesian bandage | Quadrilateral Wood | | Standard or SACH medium heel |
| Medium | Pelvic Band or Suction | | | |
| Long | Pelvic band, web belt, or laced socket | Quadrilateral wood, Moulded leather or plastic | Standard / Standard outside joints | |
| Very long & disart. | | | | |
| Very short B/K | High thigh corset, ischial corset, web belt | Wood, Plastic, Moulded leather, Soft liners | Standard steel hinges | Standard or SACH med. or hard heel |
| Short & Medium | Thigh corset, web belt | | Ball-bearing preferred | |

**FIGURE 8.1.** Levels of amputation for upper and lower extremities. Functional loss, type of replacement device and its control are also shown. (From *Orthopedic Appliance Atlas*, Vol. II, Edwards Pub. Co., 1962, with permission.)

stump, reduces edema, and promotes shrinkage of fat and muscles. This bandage must be reapplied several times a day to be effective. Posture and exercises are important to prevent contractures that impose difficulties in fitting and control of an artificial limb.

In some upper-limb amputations a cuff to hold a spoon or other tool can be strapped in place. It is also possible to incorporate a hand or hook (controlled by a cable attached to a shoulder harness) in a plaster socket to reduce the period of reliance upon a single remaining hand to a few weeks.

**Immediate Postoperative Prosthetic (IPPF) Fitting.** In immediate postoperative fitting, a temporary plaster-of-paris rigid dressing or socket is fitted over the stump and usually over the next proximal joint (Berlemont et al., 1969; Weiss, 1967; Burgess et al., 1969). This is done in the operating or the recovery room over a sterile dressing and stump sock. If he or she is in good health and rugged condition, the patient can sometimes walk within the next day or two on a temporary adjustable prosthesis attached to this plaster socket.

In some upper-limb amputations, the rigid plaster dressing includes stainless steel foil electrodes in contact with the skin of the amputation stump. These can be used to pick up myoelectric signals that control an electric hand so that the patient has immediate restoration of function.

**Controlled Environment Treatment (CET).** Instead of a rigid dressing, the stump or residual limb may be enclosed in a transparent plastic chamber supplied with sterile air at a controlled temperature, humidity, and slowly pulsating pressure. A special seal, adapted from the Hovercraft concept, allows slow escape of the air without constricting the proximal portion of the limb. The patient can walk on the other limb with the aid of parallel bars while the transparent chamber remains connected with the air supply through a flexible hose. The surgeon can also observe the wound-healing process.

## 8.3 GENERAL PRINCIPLES IN EXTERNAL PROSTHETICS

Transfer of pressure to tissue is of major importance in the design of external prostheses and orthoses. Devices must fit sufficiently intimately to avoid localized pressure on a few high spots. In turn, the tissue must be trapped sufficiently well to avoid deformity. Shearing of internal tissues is also an important factor. There is an interaction between pressure and time because even small pressure, exerted constantly over very long periods of time, may lead to pressure sores.

### Fit and Alignment

The socket should fit the current shape of the stump, which changes slowly with time as the unused muscles and fat atrophy. The stump may also swell rapidly or shrink almost as rapidly with fluid changes. Fitting is usually done by preparing a plaster-of-paris cast of the stump, pouring a plaster model, and making modifications of the model as it hardens. Plaster is then added or removed from the model. A series of manuals (New York University, 1974–80) describe the series of steps in fitting a prosthesis. These principles are still relatively empirical as yet and they are only partially based on a combination of physiological and bioengineering principles. A transparent socket (e.g., translucent polypropylene) may be used as a check socket or permanent socket. Socket alignment is important to pressure patterns on the stump as well as to the stability and function of any mechanical joints that are present.

## Construction

The two principal types of construction of prostheses are a crustacean load-bearing shell and a skeletal structure.

**Crustacean.** A light-weight shell molded of thermoplastic polypropylene or similar material is used. We form this material either by drape molding of heated material over a plaster model or with the aid of vacuum to permit atmospheric pressure to press the thermoplastic material firmly against the model, even in undercuts. More commonly, shells are carved from light wood such as willow, formed from aluminum or laminated with thermosetting plastics.

**Skeletal.** We use tubular skeletal structures surrounded by an outer foam cover that is either shaped to the outside form or selected from a prefabricated range of sizes. We cover the foam with a flexible plastic "skin-like" sock.

**Weight, Bulk, and Cosmesis.** The prosthesis is normally substantially lighter than the anatomical part that it replaces. Bulkiness beyond the normal dimensions of the human part is undesirable, both because of interference with clothing or with objects and from the standpoint of appearance.

We can make a lower-limb prosthesis natural in appearance because the artificial foot is concealed within the shoe and the ankle and shank are covered with socks or stockings. It is difficult to conceal an artificial limb under direct visual observation, as in bathing clothes or skirts. Dembo and Tane-Baskin (1955) point out that psychological adjustment of the patient to accept a prosthesis is a necessity.

A satisfactory artificial hand with limited motion of the fingers and thumb permits coverage with a plastic cosmetic glove formed to resemble a natural hand. A dozen stock shades are available.

The limitations of motion of other joints of a prosthesis, such as the wrist, elbow, knee, or ankle joint, impose much less restriction on cosmetic appearance under most situations. Typically, a single gross motion is provided that is still adequate to meet most demands of daily life and to permit a unilateral amputee to pass unnoticed while writing, eating, or walking on approximately level ground at a casual walking speed.

## Fundamental Studies

**Locomotion Studies.** Much information is available on straight and level walking at constant speed. There is much less information on starting, stopping, rising, sitting, squatting, walking up or down stairs and ramps, jumping, and running.

Energy consumption during walking at uniform speed on a level surface ideally should be zero because there is no net change in either kinetic or potential energy. Elftman (1955) pointed out that the legs of a normal individual perform remarkably effectively to support the head, arms, and trunk (HAT) on a trajectory approaching a frictionless roller coaster. Potential energy while the body is high during the period of single support over one extended leg converts to kinetic energy while the body is lower during double support, with one leg behind but the other ahead. Then most of the kinetic energy reconverts to potential energy at single support on the other leg. Amputation and neuromuscular disabilities impair this efficient process. Accelerating, decelerating, and stabilizing the limbs consumes energy.

Figure 8.2a shows that energy consumption per unit of body mass per minute has a positive intercept corresponding to quiet standing, somewhat higher than basal metabolism. Consumption increases exponentially with velocity. Figure 8.2b shows that for normal individuals, energy consumption per unit of body mass per meter walked plotted against velocity yields a broad U-shaped curve. Thus, walking speed can vary over a fairly broad range without significant penalty in increased energy consumption for accomplishing a total journey.

In contrast, individuals with handicaps tend to use somewhat higher energy per unit of body mass per meter than the normal individual. Figure 8.2 shows the resulting higher curves at slow speeds.

## 8.4 LOWER-LIMB PROSTHETICS

### Partial Foot and Syme

Partial foot amputation may typically be treated by custom padding or inserts within a conventional shoe to replace the missing portion of the foot. Sometimes a reinforced steel shank in the sole is necessary to prevent sharp bending of the sole beyond the end of the stump of the foot.

We can use the Canadian-type plastic laminate prostheses for the Syme amputation (Wilson, 1961). It eliminates the older steel side bars and mechanical ankle joint but provides a cushion heel of sponge rubber to simulate ankle motion upon heel contact. The VA Prosthetics Center developed a similar prosthesis with medial opening to provide greater section modulus for the plastic laminate shank. This reduces the risk of breakage in the region of the ankle.

### Below-Knee (BK)

**Foot and Ankle.** The foot and ankle participate in vertical support during standing and the stance phase of walking. A peg leg, lacking a foot, allows the center of gravity of the body to drop unduly as it moves ahead of the point of support, whereas a foot (with ankle resisting dorsiflexion) transfers the point of contact with the ground forward as the heel lifts. Because the ground reaction vec-

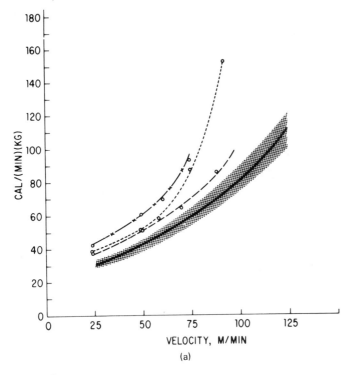

(a)

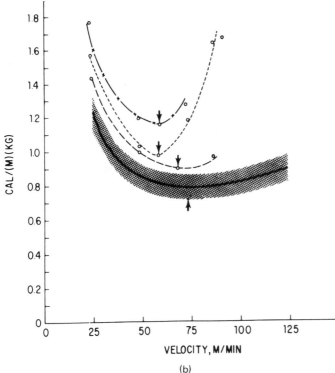

(b)

**FIGURE 8.2.** Comparison of the energy expended during walking by normal subjects, and by amputees using various assistive devices. Solid line: average energy expenditure of normal subjects walking at various speeds. Stippled area: approximately one standard deviation. Broken line: amputee walking with suction-socket prosthesis. Dotted line: amputee walking with pylon. x—x—x—x: amputee using forearm crutches. a) Energy expressed in terms of cal/min kg. b) Energy expressed in terms of cal/m kg. Arrows indicate normal walking speeds. (From *Arch. Phys. Med. Rehabil.*, 40: 415–420, 1959, with permission.)

tor remains ahead of the knee center for a portion of the gait cycle, this improves "alignment stability" of the knee joint.

The "heel lever" from the ground reaction vector to the ankle axis at the initial foot contact (typically, on the latero-posterior edge of the shoe heel in normals and in amputees) is an important factor in determining the rate of plantar flexion and in transmitting bending moment to the knee joint. Inadequate torque to resist plantar flexion allows audible toe slap, for example, with a worn heel bumper or heel cushion (or with paralyzed anterior tibial muscles lacking adequate assistance from an orthosis). Conversely, excessive torque resisting plantar flexion is transmitted through the shank to cause a substantial moment, tending to flex or buckle the knee. Increased torque with greater plantar flexion angle while descending hills (or inadvertently placing the heel upon a pebble) significantly increases the risk of knee buckling.

The Solid Ankle Cushion Heel (SACH) foot–ankle combination (Fig. 8.3) is very widely used. Its present popularity partially arises from low cost, improved materials, better molding techniques, and biomechanical principles for alignment. Because there is no mechanical bearing, the SACH foot is relatively resistant to dust or sand. The "skin" of the molded versions currently used also resists water.

The Mauch Hydraulic Ankle has been successfully worn for years by a small number of test amputees. A hydraulic vane-type piston permits hydraulically damped plantar flexion to eliminate toe slap. Stoppage of further motion in the dorsiflexion direction when the shank is vertical is determined by a small hydraulically damped ceramic ball, at the lowest point of its race, making contact with the hole in the hydraulic piston. Limited amounts of inversion or eversion of the sole of the foot and of internal and external rotation of the foot about the shank are determined by selection of special rubber pieces.

**Shank and Socket.** The socket now is typically made of thermosetting polyester plastic laminate over a modified plaster model, either directly as a hard ,socket or with a thin lining of cellular rubber or plastic.

The Patellar Tendon Bearing (PTB) type of socket combines a variety of ideas and application of biomechanical principles and alignment tools (Radcliffe, 1962). Weight is borne on many areas in addition to the patellar tendon. One of the key features is total contact between the socket bottom and the distal end of the stump. The PTB eliminates the problem of locating the axis of the metal knee joints and the expense of the thigh lacer and metal joints and side bars. More important, the prosthesis is simpler, lighter, more cosmetically acceptable, and more comfortable in warm climates. It also does not create the problems of overtaxing of the cruciate ligaments. The PTB and its variants are by far the most common type of BK prosthesis.

A relatively small proportion of patients are fitted with the University of California Pneumatic Socket (Wilson et al., 1968). This provides a flexible diaphragm in the lower portion of the socket, which can be compressed down into a pneumatic chamber. In other cases, intimate end contact and mild support came from a foam injected into the space between the socket floor and the end of the stump and allowed to polymerize with the stump in place.

**Suspension.** The PTB prosthesis uses the simple "Muley" strap just above

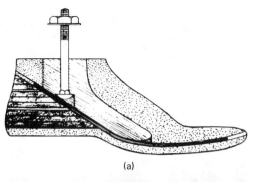

(a)

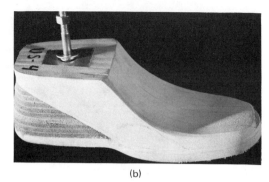

(b)

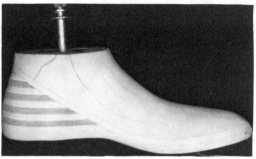

(c)

**FIGURE 8.3.** SACH foot, (a) Sectional drawing showing "keel" for stability, cellular rubber for flexibility; (b) prefabricated blank: (c) shaped foot ready for installation. (From *Orthopedic Appliance Atlas,* Vol. II, Edwards Pub. Co., 1962, with permission.)

the femoral condyles connected with small flexible straps pointing downward and backward on the medial and lateral aspects and pivotally connected to the shank. Initial flexion of the stump axis with respect to the vertical axis of the shank prevents hyperextension of the anatomical knee. A stiff heel wedge encourages further knee flexion after heel contact. The intact quadriceps, unconstricted by a lacer, controls knee flexion.

### Above-Knee (AK)

**Foot, Shank, Thigh, Socket.** The foot and ankle in AK prostheses are similar to those for the below-knee prosthesis. Softer resistance to plantar flexion is provided by either the heel bumper or SACH heel wedge. In the AK case, a greater fraction of ankle joints are the conventional single-axis type than for BK cases.

Above-knee prostheses use a crustacean construction composed of several segments, which are aligned, shaped externally, hollowed internally, and reinforced with plastic laminate. There is an increasing trend to skeletal construction with foam cosmetic covering.

Figure 8.4 shows the suction socket, based on an American Civil War invention by Parmelee in 1863. It eliminates the discomfort due to the pelvic band, problems of initial alignment, and subsequent risk of breakage or wear of the joint. It requires that the amputee control his freedom of motion about the hip joint. Radcliffe (1955) defined biomechanical principles for a quadrilateral socket with high anterior brim to retain the ischial tuberosity on a lower posterior ischial-gluteal seat.

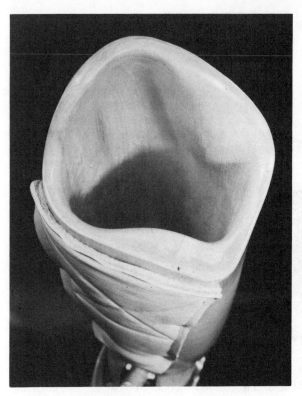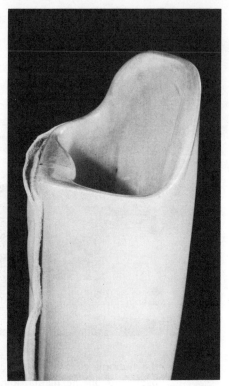

**FIGURE 8.4.** Quadrilateral-type suction socket for above-knee amputation showing weight-supporting contours and absence of mechanical suspension by belts or shoulder straps. (From *Orthopedic Appliance Atlas,* Vol. II, Edwards Pub. Co., 1962, with permission.)

The Total Contact Socket (TCS) for the AK prosthesis provides contact over the distal end of the stump. It reduces edema and improves sensory feedback. The TCS is made from plastic laminate over a modified model from a cast of the stump. Frequently, during casting, metal brim segments define the ischial support, the anterior wall, and the lateral aspect in order to provide support along the lateral side of the stump during weight bearing.

**Stance-Phase Control of Artificial Knees.** Because the knee lacks voluntary muscle control in an AK prosthesis, there is a problem of stance-phase control. In some cases, a simple mechanical knee lock stabilizes the knee at all times during standing but allows manual unlocking for sitting. There are many designs of automatic mechanical or hydraulic knee locks and methods of control. These allow bending during the swing phase of walking but assure knee stability during the stance phase. The most popular controls use weight bearing or the pressure on the heel (or plantar flexion of the ankle). These normally are effective for level and downhill walking but may not cause locking in the event of stumbling.

The increased study of biomechanics of fitting and alignment has led to great improvement in the alignment of artificial limbs. They now provide adequate

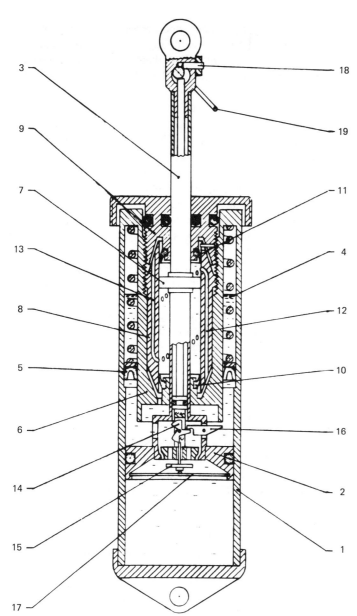

**FIGURE 8.5.** Mauch S-N-S knee lock showing cylinder (1) stance-control piston (2) piston rod (3) hydraulic fluid (4) accumulator piston (5) dashpot (6) swing-control piston (7) control bushing (8) swing adjustment screw (9) check valves (10,11) fluid channels (12,13) pendulum (14) valve (15) counterweight (16) spring (17) stance adjustment screw (18) and selector switch (19). (From *Bull, Pros. Res.*, BPR-10-10, 1968)

stability during stance-phase and smooth transition into flexion late in stance. Hip flexion and inertia forces continue flexion during early swing. The hip extensor muscles can then be used directly following heel contact to help stabilize the knee joint like a toggle, forcing it into full extension against its back stop and preventing knee buckling.

Figure 8.5 (Mauch, 1968) shows the sole survivor of a large number of experimental hydraulic or mechanical knee "locks"—the Mauch Swing and Stance

(S-N-S). Over 8,000 are now in use in this country and abroad. It operates on the hyperextension control principle and is ready to provide high hydraulic resistance to flexion of the knee joint at all times, *except* when there has been prolonged hyperextension movement of the knee, for at least 0.1 s. Normally, bodyweight resting upon the forefoot of the artificial foot automatically provides this unlocking late in the stance phase. The knee can then bend as much as necessary during swing phase, but it is again ready to resist flexion as soon as it begins extension after maximum heel rise and maximum knee flexion. Thus, the knee joint is ready to support the body momentarily in the event of stumbling.

We can manually adjust the resistance to flexion to provide substantially full lock if desired but normally prefer slow yielding to minimize stresses on the stump of the amputee as well as the mechanism. A switch also permits full lock for operating the accelerator pedal of an automobile or for standing at a vise or in a moving vehicle. Conversely, the switch also allows full freedom of motion to permit bicycling.

**Swing-Phase Control of Artificial Knee.**  We can use adjustable mechanical friction to resist motion of the artificial knee joint in either direction. We can adjust this friction, in combination with elastic extension bias, to match a single cadence. This permits comfortable and graceful walking at a single faster speed than would be possible with a pure compound pendulum action of the prosthesis. Any attempt to walk more slowly, however, is likely to cause stubbing of the toe from inadequate knee flexion. Faster walking leads to excessive heel rise and rapid slamming of the shank into full extension about the knee joint just prior to heel contact. Only a few designs make the friction adjustment reasonably accessible through the trouser leg.

A combination pneumatic spring and damper provides a substantial improvement over the single mechanical friction joint. It causes both the elastic extension bias and terminal deceleration from the pneumatic spring by damping with adjustable leakages from the spring to the other side of the piston in either direction (Radcliffe and Lamoreux, 1968). The resultant torque depends on both angle and speed.

Further improvements can be provided with hydraulic dampers supplemented by extension bias as is automatically provided by a reservoir spring maintaining pressure on the oil to react against the unbalanced area of the piston rod. A reservoir is needed because the piston rod displaces fluid as it enters the hydraulic system.

The hydraulic dampers are particularly effective if there is more than a single bypass from one side of the cylinder to the other. The Mauch S-N-S, for example, provides a series of small bypass channels with walls deliberately roughened to assure turbulent flow (Fig. 8.5). As the piston moves, it successively blocks exit holes for the hydraulic fluid from the cylinder into these passages. Thus, the initial swing occurs easily, but the few remaining passages smoothly limit the maximum angle. Conversely, as the returning piston blocks all but the last one or two passages from above the piston, high resistance provides terminal deceleration. The locations of the exit holes determine the resistance patterns.

There are currently experiments on computer control and sometimes on externally powered artificial limbs (Flowers et al., 1979; Radcliffe et al., 1979). Pressure patterns between the socket and the stump convey some degree of feedback to the patient. Transducers can sense these pressure patterns in addition to foot forces, joint positions, and segment accelerations and use them to control swing, stance, or both. The availability of modern methods of carrying out complex calculations on microprocessors has enhanced the popularity of such concepts.

It is unlikely that sufficient external power could be provided or stored in wearable equipment in order to climb more than a curb or a few steps. Note that the swing phase controls described previously deliberately waste mechanical energy; it is not clear how much of this energy could be saved in any practical portable system.

### Feedback of Positions and Forces

Feedback available to the lower-limb amputee is largely indirect. The wearer of a peg leg at least knows more about the location of the lower tip of his pylon than the wearer of a conventional articulated above-knee prosthesis knows about the position of his toe. There may also be minor sounds, vibration, and impacts as the mechanical components of a limb move or make contact. The amputee should learn, formally or informally, to use these cues, but they should not be noticeable to others lest they cause embarrassment to the patient.

### Hip Disarticulation (HD)

The major HD prosthesis is the Canadian hip disarticulation prosthesis (Foort and Radcliffe, 1956). The principal features are a hinged hip joint anterior to and below the normal anatomical hip joint and a substantially hyperextended artificial knee joint.

Radcliffe (1957) describes the biomechanical principles of this type of prosthesis. The patient, in addition to using forward momentum, is typically able to use trunk muscles to tilt the pelvis slightly late in stance phase, press the pelvic socket upon a pad at the top of the thigh behind the mechanical hip joint, and thereby generate a torque causing the knee to begin to flex. The knee should return to its very hyperextended, highly stable position just before heel contact. The Canadian hip disarticulation prosthesis has been successfully applied to hemipelvectomy amputees (Lyquist, 1958).

## 8.5 UPPER-LIMB PROSTHETICS

### General Principles

The upper-limb prosthesis consists of two major parts. The terminal device (hook or hand) provides the functions necessary to replace the normal hand. The rest of the prosthesis is primarily a crane that positions the terminal device in a desired location. Various forces and excursions are needed for independent living. Operation near the head and the body is needed for personal activities (e.g., eating, grooming, dressing, toileting). Functioning away from the body over a table, desk, workbench, and so on, is required for eating and industrial tasks. The amputee should be able to operate the terminal device and to pick up or release objects at the floor, at desk height, or above shoulder level (as in placing objects on shelves or supporting himself by a strap in a public vehicle). The amputee, particularly the bilateral, should also be able to operate behind his back for toileting and dressing purposes.

There are very limited sources of energy and control available, particularly in the bilateral amputee. Therefore, we can establish a hierarchy of functions based on importance to the individual. Daily living activities are most important, followed by vocational and avocational tasks. Taylor (1954) has ranked the functions to be performed by the terminal device as: (1) prehension or grip; (2) elbow flexion; (3) pronation and supination; (4) "turntable" rotation of the elbow axis about the humeral axis; and (5) shoulder extension/flexion and abduction/adduction.

### Terminal Devices

Because of the scarcity of suitable independent sources of power and control, we generally provide only one active motion rather than the very large number of independent motions of which the human hand is capable.

**Hook.** A split mechanical hook can be of any arbitrary shape necessary to provide better function than an artificial hand. The hook is typically made of steel or aluminum. It can often perform tool-like activities that would be impossible or too painful with the normal hand. Various types of hooks are shown in Fig. 8.6. Most hooks have a plane between the two fingers that is inclined or canted with respect to the axis by which one finger opens. The lyre shape is an exception. This shape is used on the APRL and Northrop hooks shown in Fig. 8.6. It is designed to surround cylinders up to 8.25 cm in diameter with at least four contact points. It provides flat grasping of objects near the tip, and the shape of the hook surrounds objects preventing them from being ejected as prehension forces are increased.

Prehension or grasping can be provided in at least two major ways (Fig. 8.7). In the voluntary opening type of hook or hand, a force exerted by the harness and cable pulls on a lever (often called a "thumb"), which pulls the movable finger open against rubber bands or a spring. Relaxation in turn allows the spring to apply the gripping force. In the voluntary closing type the cable tension closes the movable finger (against a relatively weak return spring) to grip the object. To avoid fatigue, the voluntary closing device typically has some form of lock.

**Hand and Cosmetic Glove.** Figure 8.8 shows various types of artificial hands. Mass-produced hands vary considerably in the degree of realism. The APRL hand, for example, has a skin-like glove made from a mold formed from an actual hand.

One of the problems with the present cosmetic glove is the tendency to stain readily. Low content of plasticizer is desirable to reduce the tendency to pick up stains and carry them down into the depths of the material. On the other hand, with

| | Name | Operation | Prehension Force | Hook finger type | Operating lever | Metal type | Style | Application |
|---|---|---|---|---|---|---|---|---|
| | Dorrance | Voluntary opening | Rubber bands Constant | Canted, straight or special | Thumb | Steel (5) Alum. (55) | Many | Many |
| | David | | Springs, constant force | Canted | Thumb | Plated steel | One, several sizes | |
| | Thornton | | Rubber bands | Canted (clip) | Thumb | Plated steel | One | |
| | Trautman | | Springs, constant Locks closed | Straight | Lever | Steel | Sizes | Farm work, Special purpose |
| | Northrop Sierra 2-load | | Clock spring 3½ # & 7 # | Straight, Lyre shaped | Thumb | Alum. | One | Light duty |
| | A P R L | Voluntary closing / Automatic lock | Selective force / Meet load release | Straight finger Lyre shape 3″ or 1½″ | Lever points down | Alum. | One | Light duty |

**FIGURE 8.6.** Types of artificial hooks for upper extremity function. (From *Orthopedic Appliance Atlas,* Vol. II, Edwards Pub. Co., 1962, with permission.)

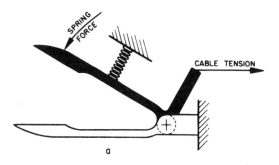

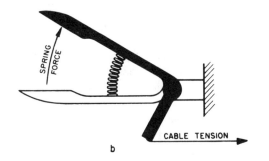

**FIGURE 8.7.** Types of control mechanism for hooks. (a) Voluntarily opening type. (b) voluntarily closing type. (From *Human limbs and their substitutes,* (1968), p. 223 with the permission of the National Academy of Sciences, Washington, D.C.)

| | Name | Operation | Prehension Type | Finger motion | Thumb motion | Cosmetic | Comment |
|---|---|---|---|---|---|---|---|
| 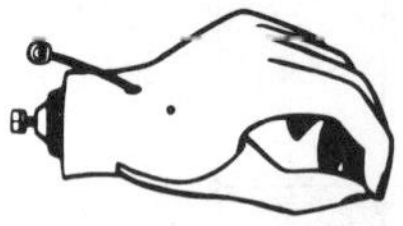 | Trautman | Voluntary opening | Finger tip (no large grasp) | None | Yes<br>Locks closed | Painted wood | Cheap Fair, Cosmetic |
| 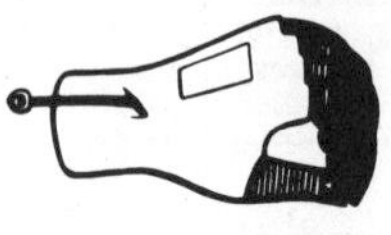 | Becker | Voluntary opening | Finger tip No effective large grasp | Yes Yes<br>Coupled<br>3 fingers | | Leather glove | Heavy and clumsy |
| 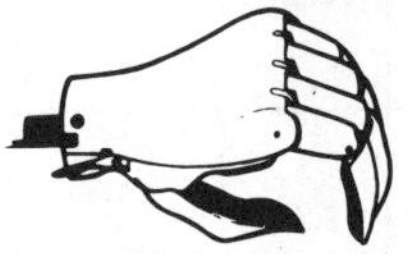 | Pecorella | Voluntary closing<br><br>Ratchet | Large grasp<br><br>Irregular | Single tree Three-position<br>Coupled lever release | | Poor<br>Glove painted metal | Complicated weak grip |
| 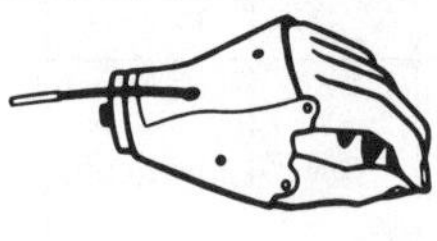 | Miracle | Voluntary closing | Finger tip Ratchet lock Lever release | Coupled<br><br>4, together with thumb | | Painted metal glove | Fair hand for heavy duty. |
| 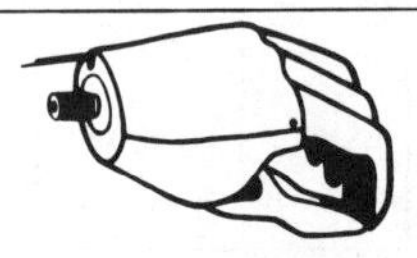 | A P R L 4 C | Voluntary closing Automatic lock Selective force | Finger tip<br><br>3-jaw chuck | Index & middle finger<br><br>Fan | 2-position Alternator 1-¾" & 2-¾" | Plastic glove<br><br>Cosmetic (P V C) | Best all around |

**FIGURE 8.8.** Types of artificial hands for upper extremity prostheses. (From *Orthopedic Appliance Atlas,* Vol. II, Edwards Pub. Co., 1962, with permission.)

the polyvinyl chloride plastic that has been used for cosmetic gloves, considerable plasticizer content has been needed to obtain sufficiently low modulus of elasticity to permit flexibility over the moving joints.

### Power Source

**Muscular.** We can use muscular power from the body, typically by motion of intact joints, to place the prosthesis in the desired position through torques and forces exerted upon the socket and transmitted to the rest of the prosthesis. We can also use muscular power to operate the terminal device and the various joints without dependence upon the other hand.

The harness (Fig. 8.9) is typically used for a number of purposes. It suspends the prosthesis, stabilizes it in place, and retains the prosthesis against external loads. It must fit comfortably and snugly without undue constriction, and straps must be adequately wide to distribute loads comfortably. The harness also transmits small body motions for control (e.g., the small motion and force needed to operate an elbow lock). The harness also transmits large and strong body motions to provide substantial power input as well as control of major functions of the artificial

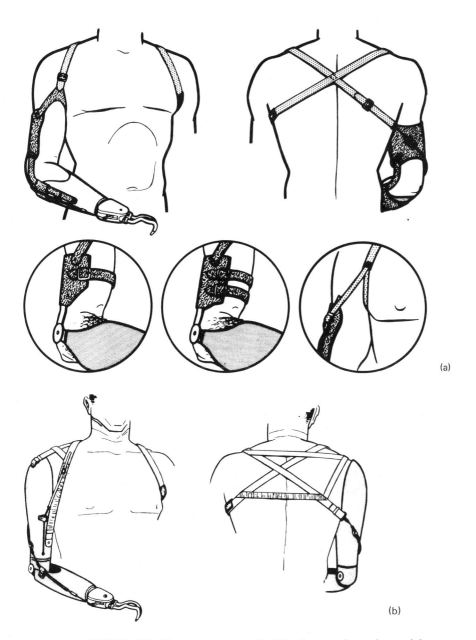

**FIGURE 8.9.** Harness systems. (a) The below elbow figure-eight harness has a simple webbing loop that passes around the sound shoulder. The front portion is used for suspension, and the rear portion is used for attachment of the cable. (b) The above elbow figure-eight harness consists of a loop around the opposite axilla. The front portion supports the arm and the rear portion attaches to the control cable so that arm flexion gives forearm flexion and terminal device operation. (From *Orthopedic Appliance Atlas*, Vol. II, Edwards Pub. Co., 1962, with permission.)

| Operation | Forces (lb.) | Displacements (in.) | Remarks |
|---|---|---|---|
| Forearm flexion (maximum with no load on hook) | 9 | 2 | Full flexion with lever arm fixed at 1 in. from elbow axis |
| Prehension, voluntary-closing hook | 5-35 | 1.5 | APRL hook; prehension force, 2-15 lb. |
| Prehension, voluntary-opening hook | 10,20 | 1.5 | Northrop two-load hook; prehension forces, 4 and 8 lb. |
| Elbow lock | 2 | 0.6 | |

**FIGURE 8.10.** Forces and displacements required for operation of a cable/harness system. (From *Human limbs and their substitutes*, (1968), p. 200, with the permission of the National Academy of Sciences, Washington, D.C.)

arm. Pursley (1960) summarizes the forms of harnesses for a wide variety of upper extremity amputations. For above-elbow prostheses, the forces and displacements needed are shown in Fig. 8.10. These are substantially less than the forces and excursions available from a Bowden cable and arm harness.

The operating cable of the typical hook or hand has approximately a 2:1 mechanical disadvantage compared with the fingertips. One method of improving operation is a two-position thumb. The inner position is used for approximately 90% of tasks requiring less than 38 mm. The thumb can be released by mechanical pressure to open to take objects up to 76 mm, though the fingertips are required to travel no more than the original 38 mm. This arrangement permits a 1:1 ratio of fingertip travel to control-cable travel.

Several versions of force multipliers have been designed (e.g., see Fletcher, 1954). Figure 8.11 shows one type of system. A carriage carrying a compound leverage system moves freely along a track to transmit tension from the harness to the terminal device with a 1:1 displacement ratio. When a resistance is encountered, a spring is stretched, causing a dog to latch at the appropriate point between teeth of a fine rack. Further tension from the harness operates through the compound lever system with a high mechanical advantage. Childress et al. (1974) have described another concept known as the "Synergetic hook" to obtain the same goal.

**Pneumatic.** Pneumatic power has been used occasionally at a few centers in this country and especially in Germany and Scotland for control of artificial arms, particularly for bilateral cases. The most commonly used material is carbon dioxide, typically purchased as a liquid under very high pressure. This is, of course, commercially available for beverage and commercial uses. The organization of systems for providing recharged portable tanks or canisters has offered considerable difficulties.

Compressed air is thermodynamically undesirable because very high pressure would be needed to store any significant quantity of energy. The corresponding thickness and weight of the tank walls and the necessity to throttle the gas wastefully down to a suitable working pressure are undesirable. There have been a few calculations and experiments to explore other sources of operating gas, but none has seemed really promising.

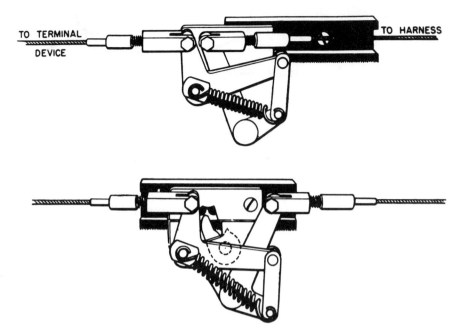

TO TERMINAL DEVICE

TO HARNESS

**FIGURE 8.11.** One type of force multiplier. A high mechanical advantage in the lever system of the terminal device permits large finger travel with small harness-cable travel. When finger tips engage upon an object, the force multiplier increases mechanical advantage in the over-all lever system at the time it is required. (From *Human limbs and their substitutes*, (1968), p. 217, with permission of the National Academy of Sciences, Washington, D.C.)

**Electric.** Electric power from rechargeable portable batteries is relatively simple, inexpensive, and allows convenient recharging. Therefore it has become by far the most widely used system for external power.

Nickel-cadmium storage batteries have been widely used because they can be sealed, operated in any position, and selected for convenient voltages both for control electronics and for operation of motors. Batteries can be safely recharged at least overnight and perhaps more rapidly if necessary.

Small electric motors with gear-reducing trains are readily available but are rather noisy. Alternatively, the heavier torque motor operates at slower speed, requiring less gear reduction but typically requiring somewhat greater weight and bulk.

The Bock and Viennatone electric hands provide simultaneous motion of the index and middle finger and of the thumb. These hands, worn within a tinted rubber or plastic shell and an outer cosmetic glove, look reasonably normal in midranges of motion, though somewhat distorted, particularly when fully opened to surround the largest possible object.

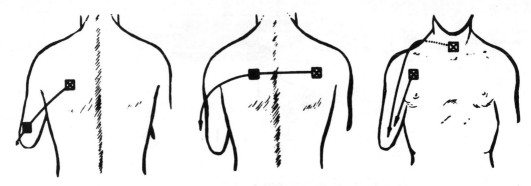

**FIGURE 8.12.** Essentials of harness controls, (a) arm-flexion control: (b) shrug control; (c) arm-extension control; ⊠ stabilization point; ■ attachment point; → control path to prosthesis. (Reprinted from *Human limbs and their substitutes,* (1968), p. 219, with permission of National Academy of Sciences, Washington, D.C.)

## *Control*

**Direct Neuromuscular Control.** The most common mode of control of artificial arms is through the harness system shown in Fig. 8.9. Three types of movements used for control are shown in Fig. 8.12. The forces and displacements for these movements are shown in Fig. 8.13. The harness also provides sensory feedback of both applied force and position attained. The movements shown in Fig. 8.12 are used to operate both the terminal device and an elbow lock in an above-elbow prosthesis.

A very short below-elbow stump can sometimes be used to actuate a terminal device rather than to flex the elbow. A shoulder harness is then used to flex and to lock the artificial elbow, as in an above-elbow prosthesis.

**Proximal Segment Operating Switch or Valve.** A very short stump may be used to control a pneumatic valve, electric switch, or clutch. The movements shown in Fig. 8.12 (e.g., a shoulder shrug) can also control switches. Lucaccini et al. (1966) describe the direct use of bulging and hardening of a muscle as a control signal.

**Myoelectric Control.** Electrical signals accompany muscle contraction. These signals are present in the stump of an amputee (Scott, 1967) and he may voluntarily contract the muscles as if he were opening or closing his hand or

| Control | Forces* (lb.) | Displacements* (in.) |
|---|---|---|
| Arm flexion . . . . . . . . . | 63.0 ± 5.4 | 2.09 ± 0.41 |
| Shrug . . . . . . . . . . . . . | 60.8 ± 23.8 | 2.24 ± 0.59 |
| Arm extension . . . . . . . | 56.5 ± 6.6 | 2.30 ± 0.66 |

*Mean ± standard deviation

**FIGURE 8.13.** Displacements and forces generated by the movements shown in Figure 8.12. (From *Human limbs and their substitutes,* (1968), p. 219, with permission of National Academy of Sciences, Washington, D.C.)

bending his wrist or elbow (Scott, 1968). Stainless steel electrodes built into the socket wall and pressed against the skin at the desired point are used to detect these signals. We must place the biopotential amplifier at or near the electrode site to minimize noise.

The Russian Hand (Kobrinski, 1961) detected flexor and extensor muscle activity in the forearm. The net activity determined the direction in which the motor of the electric hand turned. Bottomley (1966), Scott (1967), Scott et al. (1978), and others have developed a variety of methods using the myoelectric activity of a single muscle compared with fixed or floating levels to provide control of a motor. An example control scheme is off at very low signal levels, on at intermediate levels, off for a narrow buffer range, and on in the reverse direction for the highest signal level.

**Processing of Myoelectric Signals.** Conventionally, myoelectric signals are amplified, integrated, and further amplified. The integration time represents a compromise between the desirable rapid speed of decision, operation, and thus dexterity, versus the necessity to smooth the sharp and random spikes of the myoelectric signal. Voluntary or reflexly obtained patterns from many electrodes have been explored as a means of controlling multiple functions such as elbow, wrist, and hand (Wirta, Finley, and Taylor, 1978).

Multiple muscle signals from a single pair of electrodes, processed with an autoregressive moving average (ARMA) method, have been described by Graupe et al. (1977). This concept is contrary to the usual goal of obtaining a "clean" myoelectric signal from a single muscle, for example, the biceps, and another "clean" signal from another such as the triceps. Graupe has used a single electrode pair on the lateral surface of the humerus, for example, picking up some signals from either muscle group when voluntarily tensed by the amputee. These can then be processed, and both the amputee and the computer trained to discriminate the motion desired.

Another version, using autoregressive integrated moving average (ARIMA), has been studied by Lyman and Freedy (1979). Other than the direct integration and amplification of signals, none of these methods has yet attained significant clinical use.

### Feedback of Position or Force

The amputee receives feedback from a number of sources. The most important is visual observation of the arm and terminal device. The pressure and shear pattern between the socket and stump is a sensitive measure of the forces, moments, and torques being applied to the prosthesis by the body harness, the environment, and gravity. The pressure patterns between the body and the harness afford considerable information about the forces applied to the prosthesis. Proprioception of all remaining body segments also provides a major part of feedback. For example, an above-elbow amputee fitted with a muscle-powered harness can determine the amount of elbow flexion by the amount of motion of his shoulder joint. The elbow will flex in proportion to the tension of the cable, which reduces the gap between the cable housings attached to the upper arm and to the forearm.

Various experimental systems using vibrators or electrocutaneous stimulation have been proposed (Conzelman et al., 1953; Solomonow and Lyman, 1980). These systems are based on the output of a transducer located in the terminal device.

## Prostheses for Various Levels of Amputation

**Wrists.**  The conventional terminal device allows manual preset adjustment of rotation about the longitudinal axis of the forearm. In a wrist disarticulation, or long below-elbow stump (Fig. 8.14a), voluntary wrist rotation is possible under control of the stump. Flexible straps supporting the socket permit rotation of the socket with respect to the humeral cuff of the harness.

For shorter below-elbow stumps (Fig. 8.14b), voluntary rotation devices have an inner socket that rotates within a rigid forearm shell. The prosthesis is supported by single-plane elbow hinges, permitting only flexion and extension. The inner socket can directly drive the wrist and terminal device. A powered wrist drive is available from the Otto Bock Co. of West Germany.

**Below-Elbow.**  The conventional long below-elbow prosthesis typically has a plastic laminate cuff extending well up along the ulnar surface to provide a reaction point for moments due to loads on the terminal device. A cutaway portion over the radial aspect near the proximal brim allows free rotation. The medium below-elbow case, if the stump can rotate through as much as 90°, can be fitted somewhat like the long below-elbow case (Fig. 8.14c). The short below-elbow case is sometimes fitted with a separate socket attached to one element of step-up elbow hinges (Fig. 8.14d) to produce greater flexion of the forearm. The torque is so reduced that an above-elbow type of cable lift is typically needed.

A self-suspended prosthesis reduces dependence on the harness and permits removing and donning the prosthesis without removing clothing. One type has electrodes built into the stump socket for myoelectric control.

**Above Elbow.**  The conventional AE arm is a crustacean plastic laminate. Most AE prostheses have a body-controlled elbow lock (Fig. 8.9b). The amputee locks the elbow and can then use his stump and total body motion to lift large weights.

Electrically operated elbows use either switches or myoelectric control. Some devices (e.g., the Boston Elbow) retain the cable for the terminal device and power only the elbow. Others provide power for both the terminal device and the elbow and possibly a wrist rotator.

A turntable is typically provided between the socket and humeral section of the arm. This device permits voluntary rotation of the forearm about the humeral axis. The terminal device is moved toward the body for personal activities and away for bench or table work.

**Shoulder Disarticulation and Forequarter Prostheses.**  Some very high AE amputees retain a small amount of humerus but not enough for direct control. They may be able to generate control signals for myoelectric or switch control. Complete shoulder disarticulation amputees can use a nudge control (Fletcher and Wilson, 1954) by pressing the chin on a disk located on the anterior shoulder portion of the socket.

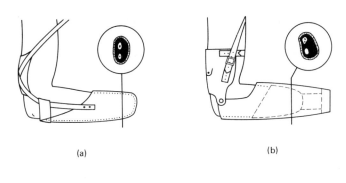

(a)                                    (b)

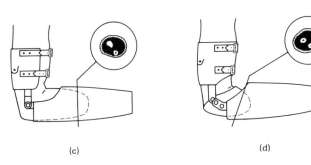

(c)                                    (d)

**FIGURE 8.14.** Schematics of below-elbow prostheses. For each type, an insert gives the cross sectional anatomy 1 in. from the end of the stump. Sections are taken from the normal anatomy of the forearm. Sockets, hinges, cuffs, and suspensions are for (a) single socket; (b) rotation type; (c) double-wall socket; and (d) split socket. (From *Human limbs and their substitutes,* (1968), p. 228, with permission of National Academy of Sciences, Washington, D.C.)

The forequarter or interscapulothoracic case can be fitted with a lightweight shoulder-disarticulation type of prosthesis. External power is usually beneficial, though added weight may be a problem. There are few control sites available in this case. Excursion multipliers may be required. These use unfavorable mechanical advantage through levers and pulleys to produce useful excursions. Seamone and Schmeisser (1974) have fitted both unilateral and bilateral shoulder-disarticulation cases with an electric winch system. Control techniques used include myoelectric, body motion with small excursions, skin motion sensors, small motion transducers, a magnetic diode sensing eyebrow movement, and an accelerometer sensing clicking of the teeth.

### Bilateral Amputees

**Special Problems.** The bilateral problems are not simply double those of the unilateral arm amputee who has one remaining normal arm available. The bilateral amputee completely lacks the dexterity and sensory feedback from a remaining natural arm.

**Independence.**   The bilateral upper-limb amputee desires to be as independent as possible. For many decades, even bilateral above-elbow amputees have been able to be independent in donning and doffing their prostheses, grooming and personal care, dressing, eating, and so on. Velcro, snaps, and "zippers" or slide fasteners will facilitate dressing and undressing. A few simple devices such as button hooks may also be useful. Bilateral amputees must be able to reach the body, often with the aid not only of turntables but of a wrist flexion device on at least one side; but they must also work away from the body on a table and preferably at other levels.

## 8.6 MEDICAL PROBLEMS IN ORTHOTICS

### Definition

An *orthosis* may be defined as an assistive device that, when applied to the exterior of the body, will restrict or enhance motion or reduce the stress on the body part. The objective of an orthotic application is restoration of the body part to as near normal function as possible. The practice of designing, fabricating, fitting, prescribing, and checking of orthoses is called *orthotics* and is commonly practiced by *orthotists*. Increasing involvement of engineers in this field is a result of demands for innovative design, electronic components, and material improvements in these orthotic appliances.

### Medical Uses

Orthoses have been variably called splints or braces and were used to immobilize joints or limbs. Commercially available splints were manufactured by the J. Elwood Lee Company of New York around the turn of the century (Davis, 1973). Medical use of orthoses has increased steadily since the early twentieth century as materials and component design have improved. Orthoses, when designed, fabricated, and fitted properly, are used for one or more of the following purposes: (1) protection of diseased or injured body parts; (2) prevention or correction of deformities; (3) stabilization of structurally unstable joints; and (4) enhancement of motion and function. A major reference in this field, *The Atlas of Orthotics,* was compiled under the auspices of the American Academy of Orthopedic Surgeons (1975). A major feature is a biomechanical analysis system (McCullough and Sarrafian, 1975) which provides a rational basis for prescription.

**Protection of Diseased or Injured Body Parts.**   The use of orthoses for this purpose is quite common. Fracture care may include the use of orthoses to immobilize the injured skeletal parts while healing takes place. Plaster casts combined with other orthotic components are used in immobilization of fractures and their adjacent joints in order to keep the body part at rest. Similar application of orthoses is common to the treatment of sprains, strains, and other soft tissue injuries of the skeletal system. Immobilization not only allows healing to take place but reduces the associated pain. Other common uses of orthoses for protection are in the many types of arthritic disorders seen in medical practice. Rheumatoid arthritis, which is an acute and chronic inflammatory disorder of joints, may be aided in its acute stage by immobilization. The advantage of orthoses over plaster cast immobilization is that the orthoses can be readily removed for exercise to prevent development of scar tissue or contractures that would later limit the use of the joint. Orthoses may also be used in acute traumatic arthritis secondary to injuries and in acute flares of degenerative arthritis, which is one of the most common forms of arthritis seen in adults. Additional rheumatic disorders such as bursitis and tendonitis may on occasion be immobilized with an orthosis. Hemophilia is a bleeding disorder that is inherited and characterized by occurrences of hemorrhages, most commonly in a joint. The immobilization of these joints with an orthosis during these episodes combined with the ability to remove the orthosis for maintenance of range of motion is an important aspect of treatment.

**Prevention or Correction of Deformities.** There are many medical conditions that, if allowed to progress without prevention of deformation of joints, would result in severe handicaps. Some of the previously mentioned joint disorders can, if not properly treated, go on to severe deformities. Therefore, many orthoses are used, not only to protect the joint and body part, but to prevent deformities from occurring about the joint. Once a deformity or contracture is formed about a joint, it is very difficult to correct and surgery is often quite limited in regaining normal range of motion. There are certain medical conditions that, when left to progress without preventive orthoses, may cause significant changes in body alignment. An example is structural scoliosis of childhood that may progress to a very severe deformity. The Milwaukee Brace, developed by Dr. Walter Blount and associates about 1945, is an orthosis that both prevents progression of the scoliosis and aids in correction through encouraging active participation on the part of the patient. Diseases of peripheral nerves or muscles causing weakness may result in an abnormal posture of a joint or limb. This abnormal posture, if left unattended, can result in severe contractures and cause long-lasting deformity even after the primary illness has cleared. An orthosis may be of value in these disorders because it can be used to prevent the contractures and be removed for exercise to preserve range of motion of the involved joints or muscles. Deformities occurring as a result of osteoporosis, a disorder accompanied by increasing thinning of the bone structure of the spine in elderly individuals, may be aided with the use of a spinal orthosis. These orthoses prevent the excessive flexion of the spine and associated potential for compression fractures of vertebrae in these individuals.

**Stabilization of Structurally Unstable Joints.** Certain joints after injury of the soft tissue or paralysis of the musculature about the joints are unstable. This instability may cause difficulty in use of the limb for functional activities. An example would be a severe injury to a knee resulting in ligamentous instability. On occasion, these knees are either not ready for surgery or surgery is incomplete in its restructuring of the knee and an orthosis is required for activity. Occasionally, these orthoses are used only in vigorous activity such as sports, and specially designed knee orthoses have been developed for this purpose. Most other limb joints have had various types of orthoses developed to provide some stability following disease or injury of the joints. Additionally, various types of spinal orthoses have been developed, many of which are soft orthoses or corsets, to aid in the limitation of movement of the vertebral column and, therefore, aid in stabilizing diseased or injured joints within the vertebral column.

**Enhancing Motion and Function.** When, because of a disease or injury, the motion of joints in the limbs or trunk is limited due to structural changes or weakness, an orthosis may be provided to enhance motion or function. Structural changes, such as shortening of limbs, may be aided by length-providing orthoses. Paralysis of various kinds may cause a limb to be limited in its function or nonfunctional. Various congenital muscle deficiencies may cause loss of function and may, on occasion, be limited to single muscles and, on other occasions such as in amyoplasia congenita (arthrogryposis), be more generalized. Orthoses in this latter disorder may be very beneficial in enhancing function while also preventing the severe contractures that these children develop with time. Many types of muscular dystrophy (e.g., Duchenne's type) may also be aided in prevention of deformities and enhancement of movement by the use of orthoses.

Other individuals that benefit from orthoses include those suffering from many types of lower motor neuron disorders. The lower motor neuron includes the nerve cell in the spinal cord and its nerve from the spinal cord out to the muscle. Disorders of the lower motor neuron may cause flaccid paralysis. (Flaccid paralysis refers to the fact that the muscle has lost some or all of its tone.) There are many chronic disorders such as various types of spinal muscular atrophy, including Werdnig-Hoffmann disease. A rather classical acute disorder of the lower motor neuron is poliomyelitis, for which many orthotic devices and components have been developed.

Certain injuries to peripheral nerves and disorders of peripheral nerves also cause flaccid paralysis. When the central nervous system is involved, such as with a brain injury, stroke, or spinal cord injury, a paralysis may also occur, but it often is accompanied by spasticity. This spastic paralysis means that the muscle has an excessive amount of tone, which may be a critical problem in attempting to provide an orthosis because of the marked forces generated by this spasticity. The use of orthoses in spinal cord injury is quite common and the type of orthosis depends upon the level of the injury. Quadriplegics are those who have an injury of the neck with resultant paralysis of the upper extremities as well as the trunk and lower extremities. Paraplegia refers to individuals with paralysis that does not involve the upper extremities. The orthoses for these patients are usually developed both to prevent deformities and to enhance function. In many cases, an altered or additional source of power is required to assist them in function. Brain-injured and stroke patients often have paralysis of one or the other side of the body, although, occasionally, all four extremities may be involved. For these individuals, orthoses are provided to prevent further deformities and to aid in function.

Cerebral palsy is a disorder that is characterized by dysfunction of the brain that persists (but not necessarily unchanged) and is present before the growth and development of the brain is completed. Children with this disability may have variable types of paralyses and abnormal movements. They may have spasticity as a primary problem similar to the brain-injured or spinal-cord-injured but also may have disorders such as athetosis, which is an involuntary movement disorder. The complexities of these children require considerable innovation in the development of orthoses to improve function.

## 8.7 GENERAL PRINCIPLES IN ORTHOTICS

### Terminology in Orthotics

The Committee on Prosthetic-Orthotic Education has aided in clarifying the terminology used in orthotics as summarized by Harris (1973). The effort of this committee was to encourage the use of the term orthosis instead of utilizing variable terms such as brace and splint. They, additionally, recommended that the description of the orthosis be by the joints it includes. This terminology eliminates a term such as short-leg brace or long-leg brace by changing the term to ankle-foot orthosis (AFO) or knee-ankle-foot orthosis (KAFO). They additionally recommended certain functional terms to be used in the description of components such as "free," "assist," "stop," "hold," and "lock." The use of these new terms along with a descriptor of the type of material used in fabrication may aid considerably in the further understanding of orthotic systems.

### Body Mechanics

Basic to the understanding of orthotic devices is an understanding of the body functions or mechanics that they most affect. Many texts have been written on applied anatomy, kinesiology, and functional anatomy. These terms are often used interchangeably. Steindler has defined *kinesiology* as that part of physiology of motion that describes and analyzes locomotor events so far as they reflect the action of mechanical forces (Steindler, 1955). Because bone is the essential stabilizing structure upon which the forces of gravity and muscle work to provide motion, it is necessary to understand some of the physical properties of bone. Bone has two primary properties that are important, elasticity and unit stress resistance. Although it is unlikely that in the development and use of orthoses we would reach the limits of these physical properties of bone, it is important that they be recognized in the development of safe orthotic devices. More care must be exerted when creating deforming forces on abnormal bone or on muscle and its associated tendons and ligaments. The potential strength of compact bone is said to be about 230 times greater than that of muscle for similar cross section (Rasch and Burke, 1967).

In addition to considering the physical properties of bone, muscle, and associated soft tissues, it is important to be able to get the terminal device, that is, the hand or foot, into the proper placement for function. Each joint of the extremity plays a different role in that placement. Each joint may have different types of movement, including gliding, rolling, rocking, and rotational movements. The shape of the articular surface of the joint tends to dictate the freedom of motion of the joint. The freedom of motion of each joint may be defined in terms of degrees with one degree for motion in one plane only, two degrees for motion occurring in two planes perpendicular to each other, and three degrees for motion in amphiarthrotic joints such as the shoulder joint or hip joint (Steindler, 1955). It is important to recognize these different planes of motion available to the joint in order to have the orthotic device move freely or to restrict the joint from movement in any or all planes.

An additional factor involved in the kinesiology of motion is the intensity and direction of force that the muscle creates across the joint. This is especially important when one is attempting to counteract the force of a muscle when that muscle is either spastic or is not counteracted by opposing muscles about the joint. The study of the actions of individual muscles and groups of muscles about a joint is highly complex. Studies of these actions of muscles are well documented by Basmajian (1978) and should be used as a reference when designing orthoses that would include a need to augment or counteract the effects of certain muscles or muscle groups.

Because orthotic systems are often developed to enhance a certain function, kinematic analysis of such functions has been used in the design process. Kinematics is the determination of displacement of the segments of the body, including paths of motion, ranges, velocities, directions, and accelerations. Engen (1970) used a system of kinematics in his design of an upper extremity orthosis. He studied several different functions of the upper extremity, including reaching, writing, and hair grooming. In his kinematic study, he used a movie camera, mirrors, and a time clock to record the sequence of movement. Methods of this type, combined with some basic understanding of physical properties of the locomotor system and the function of joints, is important to the development of successful orthoses.

## Material Properties

Construction of orthoses that are to be used permanently should be designed for strength and durability, thus reducing the risk of mechanical breakdown. They should, likewise, be constructed in as simple a manner as the function permits. The finish of the splint is important from an aesthetic point of view, but the fitting is of much more importance (Murdoch, 1970). Important to meeting these criteria is a selection of the correct material, which depends partially on the understanding of the principles of mechanics and materials, including concepts of forces, deformations and failure of structures under load; improvements of mechanical properties by heat treatments or other means, and concepts of design (Murphy and Burstein, 1975). Today, there is an ever-increasing number of new materials for use in orthoses. The traditional metal and leather bracing is still important in some areas but has been mainly replaced with new metal alloys or plastics. The benefits of some of these new materials are that they may reduce the weight, improve the strength, improve the workability, and reduce cost.

## Design Principles

When the orthosis is designed to stabilize or create a deforming force on the part, a three-point pressure system is used. In order for this system to work most effectively, the middle point of this three-point system should create pressure at the vertex of the deformity. In prevention of motion in spinal orthoses, an irritative focus is often used to attempt to have the individual wearing the orthosis pull away from the irritation and, thus, correct the deformity actively. Another system of stabilization in trunk orthoses is the use of intra-abdominal pressure by use of a thoracoabdominohydropneumatic support mechanism causing containment of the intra-abdominal pressure. This system elevates the intra-abdominal pressure to the point where there is strong support of the vertebral column (Morris and Markolf, 1975).

Additionally, in design of orthoses, it is important that cosmesis be provided to the maximum extent possible within functional limits. In general, patients have a tendency to avoid using any orthosis that is prominent or is irritative either to their skin or their immediate environment. The material should be carefully selected so there are no surface irritants to cause problems with the skin of the individual wearing the orthosis. Excessive tightness of the orthosis must be avoided in order to prevent pressure sores, edema, or painful conditions that will, likewise, limit the use of the orthosis. The orthosis must also be easily donned and removed. Whenever possible, psychological dependence and physical dependence should be avoided by intermittent use of exercises with removal of the orthotic device. Clothing damage from sharp edges or soilage from lubricants should also be reduced as much as possible.

## The Orthotic Team

In order to give the patient the maximum benefit in evaluation and determination of the type of orthosis needed, it is important that a team approach be used. The usual members of this team include a physician who has an active interest in the field of rehabilitation and who has good knowledge of the operative and nonoperative approaches for correction of the disorder in addition to having knowledge of orthotic applications. The orthotist is another important member of the team, having experience and skill in design and development of orthoses. This person's experience can be combined with the experiences of an engineer, who has knowledge and experience in the engineering principles related to the orthosis. The fourth member of the team is either a physical therapist or occupational therapist, depending upon whether the lower extremities or the upper extremities are the primary problem. This person is involved in the development of the orthotic prescriptions so that they might be better prepared to train the patient in the use of the orthosis once the fitting is completed. The patient, too, is a member.

## 8.8 LOWER LIMB ORTHOTICS

In considering the mechanics of the lower extremity, it is important to note that the hip joint has three degrees of freedom of motion, including abduction and adduction in the frontal plane, flexion and extension in the sagittal plane, and internal and external rotation in the transverse plane. At the knee, there are two degrees of motion, flexion and extension in the sagittal plane and axial rotation in the transverse plane. The ankle joint is track-bound and has only one degree of freedom of motion, flexion and extension in the sagittal plane. Joints of the foot allow some additional freedom of motion, primarily inversion and eversion in the frontal plane (Steindler, 1955). In development of a lower-extremity orthosis, it is important to take into consideration these degrees of motion so that they may be preserved or restricted as required. There are many different joint components available for the hip, knee, and ankle that allow a selection of motion at each joint. *The Atlas of Orthotics* (Staros and LeBlanc, 1975) describes several of these joint components with their capabilities outlined.

In addition to understanding the freedom of motion at each joint in the lower extremity, it is important to know the effect of body weight on the function of the joints when standing or walking. Figure 8.15 shows that the reference point utilized in assessing the effect of body weight is called the center of gravity (CG). The center of gravity is that point in the body where the body would be perfectly balanced in any position. In a human, the center of gravity is located within the pelvis just in front of the second sacral vertebra and in the midline. The force reaction from the floor up to the center of gravity creates the line of gravity that affects the forces at each of the joints in the lower extremity. An understanding of the movements of this line of gravity during standing and locomotion is of utmost importance in design of a proper lower-extremity orthosis. It is also important to consider the fact that this body weight can be used as a force to control specific motions at the joint by alteration of the line of gravity.

The gait cycle in locomotion begins with striking of the heel on the floor and is completed when the heel on the same extremity again strikes the floor. During this cycle at ordinary speeds, a given leg is in contact with the floor or in stance phase for approximately 60% of the time. About 40% of the time, that limb is in the swing phase. Due to some overlap, about 25% of the gait cycle consists of both extremities being in contact with the floor or the so-called double support. A well-organized review of human locomotion is provided by Peizer and Wright (1970). Their discussion includes a review of the biomechanics of gait and also an analysis of the kinetics of gait.

Modifications in the freedom of motion at each joint can have a dramatic effect on the forces developed at each of the joints in a limb equipped with an orthosis. If an individual has difficulty in controlling the knee due to weakness of the quadriceps and, additionally, has weakness about the ankle for which bracing is required, several changes can be made at the ankle to alter the flexion and extension force at the knee. For example, if the individual has an ankle–foot orthosis with a rigid ankle allowing no degrees of motion, one can alter the force at the knee by adjusting the plantar or dorsiflexion at the ankle. When the ankle is put

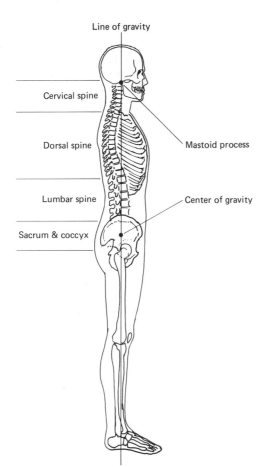

Line of gravity

Cervical spine

Dorsal spine

Lumbar spine

Sacrum & coccyx

Mastoid process

Center of gravity

**FIGURE 8.15.** The line of gravity for standard posture.

into plantar flexion, the foot becomes flat on the floor much earlier and, therefore, creates a stronger and longer extension force at the knee compensating for the weakness of the quadricep or knee extensors. However, if that AFO is placed in dorsiflexion, it takes longer for the foot to be flat on the floor and the extension force at the knee is reduced in time and is much weaker. This would allow the knee to bend more easily and, perhaps, be an additional risk to the individual in walking. The force at the knee in individuals with AFOs can also be affected by cutting off the back edge of the heel or putting a soft cushion in the posterior aspect of the heel (Lehmann, 1979). With these abilities to modify the reaction of the floor to the center of gravity in any individual with an orthosis, it becomes extremely important to understand the biomechanics of locomotion before attempting to design and develop a lower-extremity orthosis for use in standing activities or gait.

In addition to understanding the biomechanics, it is important to recognize that there are changes in energy costs when orthoses are placed on the lower extremity. Studies have shown that in the hemiplegic patient, a provision of an AFO tends to reduce the oxygen consumption or energy cost while walking at normal speeds by up to 20%. Other studies have shown the effect of orthoses in both normal and disabled subjects (Bard and Ralston, 1959). Another consideration to be made when designing and developing lower-extremity orthoses is the sensation of the individual. Sensory feedback as to pressure or pain and also as to limb or joint position is especially important for proper use of the lower extremities. Deficiencies in sensation must be taken into account, both for the safety of the individual and to provide more positive control of joints.

**Lower-Limb Orthoses for Protection of Diseased or Injured Body Parts.** Many types of rigid orthoses have been developed for long-term stabilization of fractures that are slow to heal or for infections of bones such as tuberculosis. Orthoses of this type are usually not very complicated but must conform to the three-point pressure system described under basic principles. The central pressure point must be as close as possible to the point of maximal bending moment of the extremity. These immobilizer orthoses may also be used for certain disorders of childhood. The hip abduction KAFO, used for stabilization of the hip joints in children with Legg-Perthes disease, is a good example. This orthosis stabilizes the hip joints bilaterally at 45° abduction and 20° internal rotation to allow the heads of the femurs to be centered in each acetabulum during the healing time of this self-limited disease, which consists of aseptic necrosis and replacement of the femoral head. A similar type of abduction KAFO is used in congenital dislocation of the hips in children. Many types of orthoses have been developed out of canvas with metal reinforcement to be used to stabilize the knee or knee and ankle after injuries. This type of immobilizer generally functions on a principle of having circumferential pressure on the whole extremity, therefore, controlling movement in all directions.

There have been many recent advances in development of orthoses to immobilize fractures while allowing the individual to walk on this orthosis. These so-called *cast braces* have been developed for both tibial and femoral fractures. These orthoses require three-point pressure systems to prevent movement of the fractures and, additionally, require a redistribution of the axial pressure on the limb to a site proximal to the fracture. The redistribution of pressure in the tibial cast brace is from the foot to the patellar tendon area. In the femoral cast brace, it is redistributed to the pelvis and to the thigh. This pressure on the thigh has been shown to aid in the prevention of shortening of femoral fractures. These orthoses not only provide immobilization of the injured part but provide a functional component for walking (Hardy and Baddeley, 1979). Polypropylene ischial weight-bearing sockets have been included with the lower-extremity orthoses to reduce axial load-bearing on diseased or painful hip joints. Likewise, patellar-tendon-bearing sockets have been developed to reduce pressure on painful feet or ankles following injuries. These types of polypropylene sockets and their associated orthotic components represent, again, an ability to protect a part while preserving function.

**Lower-Extremity Orthoses for Prevention or Correction of Deformity.** Classic types of orthoses have been developed for prevention or correction of deformities in cerebral-palsied children. These children, because of paralysis and associated spasticity, athetosis, or ataxia, become quite vulnerable to the develop-

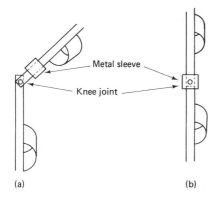

(a)

(b)

**FIGURE 8.16.** The drop lock has a metal sleeve that drops over the metal joint to lock it. (a) flexible joint, (b) locked joint.

ment of deformities of the joints or muscles. The major concern is to allow freedom at the joints for activities while providing an ability to lock the joint in a position to create a preventive or corrective force.

The joints most commonly treated in this manner are the knee joint and the ankle joint. At the knee, it is possible to develop several different types of locking mechanisms as part of the knee joint component. Figure 8.16 shows the most common type—a simple drop lock, which restricts the movement of the levers on each side of the joint. The ankle is more difficult to stabilize with a drop lock and, therefore, the usual procedure is to create stops where the joint cannot progress beyond a certain point. Typical of these stops are plantar flexion stops to eliminate foot drop positions in these children. When spasticity is involved, these stops or locks are very difficult to utilize because stretching of the involved spastic muscles sometimes creates a tremendous force. Careful design and fitting of these orthoses are required to prevent damage to the child's limb. Increased durability and strength of the material is also required so that these orthoses do not wear out rapidly. Many other types of orthoses have been developed to correct the deformation created by muscle or soft tissue contractures about joints. Orthoses of this type include special ratchet-type joints to allow a gradual "cranking out" of the joint, creating a prolonged stretching force. Again, these orthoses must be designed in compliance with a three-point pressure system.

**Lower-Extremity Orthoses for Stabilization of Structurally Unstable Joints.** Common to many injuries of the lower extremity is a resultant instability of the involved joint. The knee is, perhaps, the most commonly involved secondary to severe ligamentous injuries. When these are not fully correctable by surgery or the individual is not ready for surgery, a knee orthosis (KO) may be used. The design of knee orthoses is based on the stability required. Quite commonly, the desire is to provide mediolateral and rotatory stability while allowing full knee flexion and extension. A common knee orthosis used for this purpose is called the Lenox Hill orthosis. When there tends to be a laxity of the soft tissue structures in a knee allowing the knee to hyperextend, a rigid three-point pressure orthosis preventing this instability is used. One orthosis of this type is called a Swedish knee cage. When instability (in the mediolateral direction) occurs at the ankle, a double-upright, single axis ankle–foot orthosis is utilized. Important to any ankle–foot orthosis is the shoe. Various types of shoes are available and should be matched to the needs of the orthotic device and to the pathomechanics of the individual's foot. Alterations in the last, shank, arch, heel, and sole are available to modify the stability and/or biomechanics of the lower extremity. Sometimes an appropriate shoe modification may obviate the need for a conventional orthosis. Inattention to the development of a good shoe and attachment of the orthosis to the shoe (or insert) may result in a grossly inadequate device.

**Lower-Extremity Orthoses for Enhancement of Motion and Function.** Most complex of the lower-extremity orthoses are those designed to maintain stability of paralytic extremities while enhancing function. A good understanding of the biomechanics of gait is needed in order to design, develop, and fit these orthoses. The degrees of freedom of motion at each joint must be determined through analysis of the deficiencies in the extremity and through determination of the functional performance that we would expect of that extremity. Such biomechanical analysis approaches are usually accomplished through the orthotic team. At that time, the individual's deficits are reviewed in depth, the goals or functions of the orthoses are developed, a design and material selection is determined, and, after fabrication, appropriate fitting and training is provided.

With the advent of various plastics, especially laminated-type plastics, the weight of the lower-extremity orthoses has been somewhat reduced and also the cosmesis of the orthoses has been improved. These factors have led to some increased acceptance on the part of individuals with paralysis. When dealing with spinal-cord-injured patients, it has been found that, when the paralysis involves the lower trunk muscles and all of the muscles of the lower extremities, the energy cost for ambulation with the orthosis is three to five times normal. This energy cost has become somewhat of a deterrent for long-term use of these orthoses. If the individual has some ability to flex the hips, the energy cost comes down within a more reasonable limit, and if they are able to extend their knees, they are usually quite successful ambulators with lower-extremity orthoses.

The design of these orthoses must take into consideration stabilization of the hip, knee, and ankle during the various phases of gait. These individuals will often have no sensation, and careful fitting and design of the orthoses is extremely important. Although leather and metal double-upright orthoses are still used, the polypropylene orthosis with a fixed ankle–foot component is becoming more common. These fixed ankle–foot components allow the individual to have interchangeable shoes. The material itself gives some elasticity that resists both plantar flexion and dorsiflexion during the gait phases. When the individual has instability at the hip due to paralysis, the orthosis can be extended above the hip with a pelvic band or corset. This pelvic orthosis is attached to the lower-extremity orthosis through a hip joint that can be developed to allow appropriate degrees of motion. Standing orthoses have been developed for children and adults to allow functional standing and some movement through shifting of the center of gravity. An example of this is the Verlo orthosis (Taylor and Sand, 1975).

## 8.9 SPINAL ORTHOTICS

Figure 8.15 shows that the spinal column in humans is a very complex structure. It consists of 33 individual vertebrae. Twenty-four of these vertebrae are jointed as a flexible column, with the last nine, including the sacrum and coccyx, being fused. The cervical area or neck has seven vertebrae, the thoracic area has twelve vertebrae, and the lumbar area has five vertebrae. In developing a spinal orthosis, the large number of segments involved in addition to the poor pressure-point tolerance on the anterior surface of the body creates some unique problems. In analyzing the biomechanics of the spinal column, it is difficult to individualize each of the joints between the vertebrae. Normally, the spinal column is assessed by area. The cervical spine has, as its normal posture, a curve with the convexity directed anterior (lordosis). The articulation between the skull and the first cervical vertebra allows extensive flexion and extension. The articulation between the first and second cervical vertebrae allows the maximum rotation. The total cervical spine allows a full three degrees of motion, including flexion and extension, lateral bending, and rotation. The dorsal spine has, as its posture, a curve with the convexity directed posterior (kyphosis). Movement in the dorsal spine includes flexion and extension to midpoint but little hyperextension. There is also some limited rotation and lateral bending. The lumbar spine has, as its normal posture, a curve-directed anterior (lordosis). Movement of the lumbar spine is free in flexion but limited in hyperextension. There is very little lateral flexion or rotation in the lumbar spine. Movement between vertebrae is guided by the joints or so-called articular facets. The movement is one of gliding with associated compression and traction of the disks that are between pairs of vertebrae (Rasch and Burke, 1967). The line of gravity in the normal upright posture runs from a point just behind the ear at the mastoid process running slightly ahead of the cervical spine, just in front of the dorsal spine, intersecting the spine at the lumbo–dorsal junction, proceeding behind the lumbar spine to or directly behind the center of the hip joint to slightly in front of the knee joint, passing in front of the ankle joint to a point on the floor between the ball and heel of the foot. Deviation to either side of this line of gravity results in increased muscle activity of the paraspinal muscles and creates a bending moment. Decisions as to the appropriate posture to be maintained with an orthosis should be made based on the pathokinetics of the spine and the functional outcome desired.

Stabilization of the spinal column is usually accomplished through two methods. The first is the application of the three-point pressure system and the second is the utilization of the intra-abdominal contents as a hydraulic mechanism. Additionally, irritative restraints have been developed to attempt to have the individual pull away from the orthosis as a method of active distraction and as a reminder to restrain motion. A problem with spinal braces has been limited control of the movement of the many-segmented column. Many studies have shown that, when rigid orthoses are applied to the spinal column, increased movement occurs at either end of the spinal column restricted by the orthosis. Physical and psychological dependence on spinal orthoses may develop in individuals with resultant muscle-wasting and atrophy. It is important that these be counteracted through appropriate exercise programs.

**Spinal Orthoses for the Protection of Diseased or Injured Body Parts.**   In order to immobilize the spinal column, the orthoses must conform with the previously mentioned principles of a three-point pressure system, an irritative restraint, or a hydraulic system using the abdominal contents. In the cervical area, the usual reason for providing immobilization is fracture of the cervical spine or injuries to the soft tissues. An additional reason is sometimes to support the weight of the head following fusions or other operative procedures about the neck. Cervical orthoses are abbreviated CO. Some difficulties in applying the three-point pressure system have to do with the fact that there are limited areas on the head and neck to apply such pressure. Most of the cervical orthoses that have been used following injury to the neck have included a focus point on the chin or the lower aspect of the mandible. This has created some problems in that the mandible must be mobile for feeding activities and for communication. Long-term use of a pressure point over the mandible has resulted in significant dental problems.

A typical cervical orthosis that prevents flexion and extension is a SOMI orthosis. SOMI stands for Sternal Occipital Mandibular Immobilizer. This orthosis uses a three-point pressure system, including a base from the sternum, clavicle, and shoulder areas up to the mandible in front and to the occiput posteriorly. It is used after spinal-cord injury and fusion but does allow some movement, especially in rotation and lateral bending. Molded cervical orthoses have been developed and incorporate the mandible, occiput, neck, and shoulder to provide limitation of flexion and extension, lateral bending, and rotation.

When greater stabilizing or corrective forces are needed beyond what externally applied orthoses generally provide, Halo traction is considered. Figure 8.17 shows that the Halo traction orthosis is a metal ring secured to the skull with four pins below the maximum diameter of the skull. This ring provides a firm point from which distraction forces can be created with traction over a bed, attachment to a body cast, or through distal skeletal sites such as the femurs or pelvis. Halo orthoses are very effective in immobilizing the cervical spine and are used following fractures of the upper cervical spine, epecially at the first and second cervical vertebrae level. Additionally, they are used effectively in traction prior to the patient having fusions for structural scoliosis. The complications of Halo orthoses are usually due to excessive forces being developed in the distraction process. This excessive force may result in peripheral nerve injuries or actual traction injuries on the spinal cord itself. Another advantage of the Halo orthosis is that, when it is incorporated into a body cast or other distal skeletal fixation, the individual may use a wheelchair or even become ambulatory and, thus, the Halo provides both immobilization and function (DeWald, 1975).

The thoracic spine is often immobilized to prevent forward movement or flexion. A common orthosis used to restrict flexion in this area is called a thoracolumbar sacral orthosis (TLSO). This orthosis is commonly called the Jewett brace and has a three-point pressure point system with pressure anteriorly at the

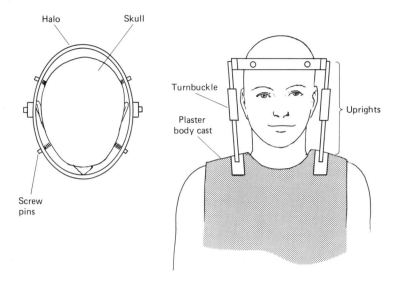

Halo   Skull

Turnbuckle

Plaster
body cast

Uprights

Screw
pins

**FIGURE 8.17.** For neck fractures, the halo orthosis has
screw pins that engage the skull. The uprights contain
turnbuckles that stretch the spine and provide stability.

upper sternum and over the symphysis pubis and posteriorly at the midportion of
the dorsal spine. This orthosis has been used for prevention of further compression
fractures of the dorsal spine in osteoporosis and also to attempt to improve posture
in individuals with progressive kyphosis due to various types of arthritis or infections. In the lumbar area, it is common to use a lumbosacral orthosis (LSO). A
common type of orthosis used in this area is the Knight orthosis, which prevents
flexion, extension, and lateral movement. Other TLSOs include rigid jackets of
polypropylene, which limit movement in all directions.

    **Spinal Orthoses for Prevention or Correction of Deformities.** Most of the
orthoses described in the previous section also provide some prevention or mildly
corrective action. In a cervical spine, the orthoses are essentially the same as for
protection. In the thoracic and lumbar spines, there are flexible LSOs and TLSOs
that are made of cloth reinforced with metal or other synthetic stays. These spinal
orthoses act like a girdle and tend to elevate the intra-abdominal pressure, creating
the hydraulic effect for maintenance of better support of the lumbar spine. They,
additionally, provide a mild three-point pressure system that reminds individuals to
restrict motion but may lack rigid immobilization capacity. These flexible spinal
orthoses can extend from the upper-thoracic area through the sacrum or be limited
to segments of the spinal column.

    A special category of orthosis was developed by Dr. Walter Blount in 1945
and is called a Milwaukee brace. This brace was developed to provide nonoperative
treatment for structural scoliosis (Blount and Moe, 1973). In classifying structural
scoliosis, about 60% are idiopathic, meaning the cause is unknown. Another 20%
are the result of malformation of the vertebrae before birth. The remaining 20% are

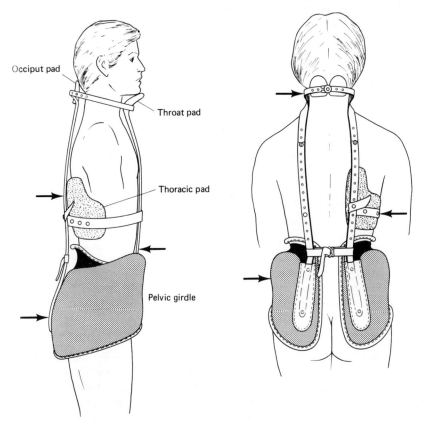

**FIGURE 8.18.** The Milwaukee brace. The side view shows that the abdominal force is balanced by forces on the back and pelvis. The posterior view shows that the thoracic pad force is balanced by forces on the neck and pelvis. The throat and occiput pads encourage the patient to maintain alignment of the spine. Large arrows show forces of the three-point system.

Occiput pad

Throat pad

Thoracic pad

Pelvic girdle

due to secondary involvement of the vertebrae after birth. The Milwaukee brace is a special form of spinal orthosis that provides prevention and a corrective force. Several modifications have been made in the orthosis since its development in 1945 so that it is much more streamlined, easy to wear underneath clothing, and is less of a problem for the long-term use required for correction. Many guidelines have been developed by Dr. Blount and his associates for treatment of individuals utilizing this orthosis.

Figure 8.18 shows that the orthosis comprises a closely fitting pelvic girdle with one anterior metal upright and two posterior metal uprights attached to a cervical ring that has a throat mold anteriorly and occiput pads posteriorly. In addition, a thoracic pad is placed over the prominent side of the rib cage on the side of the convexity of the thoracic curve. This thoracic pad is used partially as a distracting force but primarily as an irritant to have the individual pull away from the pad to help maintain spinal alignment. The early versions of the Milwaukee brace had a chin pad, which caused significant dental problems, but this has now been generally eliminated except in a few instances in which a chin pad is still required for maximum correction. This orthosis is now considered essential in the treatment of scoliosis but requires close observation so that, if the curve progresses beyond safe levels, appropriate intervention with skeletal traction or surgery can be provided. In general, the orthosis is worn full time, day and night, along with an exercise program performed while in the orthosis. The orthosis seems most useful in the child who is too young for surgery or a child near the end of the growth period and for a curve that is cosmetically acceptable if progression can be prevented (Piggot, 1979).

**Spinal Orthoses for Stabilization of Structurally Unstable Joints.** Any of the previously mentioned spinal orthoses can be used for stabilization of unstable joints in the vertebral column. A rather unique thoracolumbar orthosis, however, was described by Siebens et al. (1972). This orthotic device was developed and designed to help halt progression of spinal deformities that occurred in neuromuscular disorders such as myelomeningocele (spina bifida), cerebral palsy, quadriplegia, and other chronic muscle disorders. The principle behind this TLSO is that it is formed in a manner to provide a redistribution of pressure from the buttocks to the anterolateral costal margin of the rib cage. In addition, the orthosis is indented in the upper-abdominal area to provide some hydraulic resistance to diaphragmatic contraction to facilitate chest expansion. This orthosis was developed out of plastic material and suspended from an attachment in a wheelchair. Recent studies of this thoracic suspension orthosis (modified TLSO) have shown good results in supplying trunk support and arresting progressive spinal deformities in mature patients who cannot tolerate surgery, or to postpone surgery in skeletally immature patients or to support patients whose disease process is so well established that spinal surgery will not be in the patient's best interest (Drennan et al., 1979).

**Spinal Orthoses for Enhancement of Motion or Function.** There are few, if any, spinal orthoses that are utilized to improve specific motions or functions of the vertebral column. The complexities of the biomechanics of the spinal column may well limit successful orthoses of this type.

## 8.10 UPPER-EXTREMITY ORTHOSES

The upper extremity is a highly complex unit of the human body. A primary function of the upper extremity is to place the hand and digits in a proper position to perform complex activities. Although strength may be a requirement for certain functions of the upper extremity, the primary requirement is dexterity and versatility. The upper extremity works as an open-ended kinetic chain and has a significant amount of freedom of movement. The shoulder has three degrees of freedom of motion, being an amphiarthrotic joint. The elbow has two degrees of freedom of motion, providing flexion-extension and axial rotation. The wrist also has two degrees of freedom of motion, including flexion-extension and ulnar-radial deviation. The hand shows two degrees of freedom of motion at the metacarpophalangeal joints (knuckles) of flexion-extension and abduction-adduction. The interphalangeal joints each have one degree of motion in flexion and extension to neutral.

When sensation in the extremity is lost, other methods of interpreting function must be incorporated, such as visual contact. The large number of muscles in the upper extremity provide versatility in direction and force of movement. The effect of gravity on function of the upper extremity is quite different than in the lower extremity or the trunk. The center of gravity of the body is only rarely useful in attempting to create a force for joint function. This can only occur when the upper extremity is a closed kinetic chain with the floor, such as in doing a push-up. The majority of activities allow only the weight of the extremity distal to the joint to be useful as a gravity force. Gravity can be especially helpful in extending the elbow or wrist. Gravity must be adjusted for when attempting to bring the hand to the face or in any action taking the hand and arm away from the floor. Unique methods of providing motor power to the upper extremity orthosis have been developed, including: (1) redirection of force of a proximal joint to a distal joint; (2) redirection of force of another bodily movement to a joint of the upper extremity; (3) the use of elastics such as rubber bands and springs; (4) the use of pneumatic systems such as a carbon-dioxide cylinder and a McKibben muscle; and (5) various electrical systems utilizing switches.

Immobilization or stabilization of the upper-extremity joints is accomplished through provision of the three-point pressure system. The elbow joint is the only one that lends itself to long-enough lever arms using the length of the humerus and the forearm to get an effective three-point pressure system. However, the antecubital fossa and the olecranon process of the elbow are extra sensitive to pressure and therefore cannot tolerate pressure to any degree. Functional splints, to be effective, must follow very closely the movements of the joints of the upper extremities to allow for smooth and coordinated functions. A patient who does not have an effective and smooth functioning upper-extremity orthosis will often discard it. The terminal device or hand of the upper extremity is the most critical element of any orthosis. If the hand cannot be functional with the use of the orthosis, it probably will not be used. The functions of the hand are to provide fine sensory feedback, fine motor control, and varying degrees of power. The power system is divided into many different types of grips. Power grips are generally grasps using all or most of the digits. Precision grip is made up primarily of so-called thumb-to-finger tips, or the three-jaw-chuck pinch. This three-jaw-chuck precision pinch makes up about 50% of the precision activities of the upper extremities (Sarrafian, 1975). The thumb-to-side-of-index-finger key grip is a somewhat stronger precision grip but has less fine movement capabilities. Any effective orthosis must allow for use of these grips, depending on the particular function desired. Of utmost importance in design or development of upper-extremity orthoses is the cosmetic effect. Individuals wearing these orthoses exhibit them on a regular basis and demand that they be cosmetically acceptable. The weight and durability of the orthoses are also important because of many fine dexterity functions that require lightweight orthoses with maximum strength for efficiency and effectiveness.

**Upper-Extremity Orthoses for Protection of Diseased or Injured Body Parts.**   The literature includes many different designs of upper-extremity orthoses for protection of joints. Rheumatoid arthritis is a major disease of the joints of the upper extremity and may cause severe deformities of any or all of the joints. Many different rigid and protective orthoses have been developed for the upper extremities of these individuals. The use of rest orthoses at night to protect the digits, wrist, and elbow from trauma is most common. The use of orthoses to prevent deviation of the wrist to the ulnar side in rheumatoid arthritis is also common. In addition to orthoses for acute arthritis problems, there are many types of orthoses utilized for protection of injured joints, such as those sprained or strained in sports. Orthoses range from very simple finger-type splints for stabilization of finger joints to more complex immobilizers for the elbow and shoulder. An important requirement of any upper-extremity orthosis for protection is to keep the orthosis simple and leave as much of the upper extremity as possible free for function.

**Upper-Extremity Orthoses for Prevention or Correction of Deformity.**   Many of the previously mentioned orthoses for protection of joints are also used to prevent the development of contractures or deformities of the joints in the arthritic and otherwise diseased or injured upper extremity. Many orthoses have been developed for prevention of deformities in weak upper extremities due to muscular dystrophies or myopathies, peripheral nerve injuries, and the previously mentioned lower motor neuron and upper motor neuron diseases, including poliomyelitis, spinal-cord injury, and brain injury. When the muscles of the upper extremity are weakened so that gravity may influence the position of the limb or when spasticity is present to cause an imbalance, orthoses are used in order to prevent deformity due to contractures. Typical of these orthoses are rest orthoses, which keep the joint in a position of function during rest periods such as a night's sleep. Many varieties are available commercially and they are also fabricated by occupational therapists and orthotists in their respective departments. A large group of dynamic orthoses have been developed using rubber bands or springs as a deformation force. An example of this type of splint is a hand orthosis (HO) that provides interphalangeal extension to prevent a flexion deformity of the joint of a finger. This is accomplished through providing a three-point pressure system with the central pressure point over the dorsum of the joint of the finger and rubber bands pulling the distal ends together as the corrective force.

Another type of orthosis may be used when an individual has a radial nerve palsy and is unable to extend the wrist. Figure 8.19 shows that this wrist–hand orthosis (WHO) provides elastic or rubber bands over the dorsum of the wrist, pulling the distal part of the orthosis in the hand towards the proximal part of the orthosis in the forearm and causing a bending moment to extend the wrist and fingers. This orthosis allows the individual to use the functioning muscles to flex the fingers and wrist effectively.

**Upper-Extremity Orthoses for Stabilization of Structurally Unstable Joints.**   Most of the orthoses used for protection or prevention in the upper extremity can also be provided for stabilization. Many soft fabric orthoses provide some limited stabilization of the wrist and elbow, which reduces the full range of

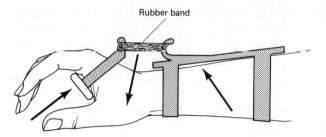

Rubber band

**FIGURE 8.19.** Wrist-hand orthosis for radial nerve palsy. The rubber band tension extends the wrist. The patient flexes the wrist against the tension of the rubber band. Large arrows show forces of the three-point system.

motion of these joints. Commonly used orthoses for minor sports injuries generally conform to a total contact principle, restricting motion in all directions.

**Upper-Extremity Orthoses for Enhancement of Motion and Function.** Orthoses that enhance motion or function of the upper extremity may be very complex. Some of the dynamic orthoses mentioned in the previous sections, such as the radial nerve WHO, may be used as functional orthoses to aid in motion and function. The majority of these orthoses substitute motor power for limited or absent muscle function. When there is limited muscle function, it has been very difficult to match a supplementary motor power with the residual function. Often, the substituted auxiliary motor function is either inadequate or overly active. When there is no muscle function, a variety of systems have been used. A very successful functional orthosis is the tenodesis splint (Fig. 8.20a) for individuals with paralysis primarily of the forearm, wrist, and hand. The purpose of the tenodesis splint is to allow finger and thumb flexion to create a precision grip through redirection of the force of wrist extension. Early developers of this tenodesis splint determined that the three-jaw-chuck type of pinch is the most effective and is the basis for most of these tenodesis splints (Engel et al., 1967). When an individual with a spinal-cord injury has residual function so that extension of the wrist can take place voluntarily, the use of the tenodesis splints is fairly good. An absence of sensation may create a problem and future development of sensory transducers is going to be important.

When, however, the individual does not have voluntary wrist extension, an external source of power must be identified. A harness that allows for transfer of power from shoulder flexion, biscapular abduction, or chest expansion through a cable to create a wrist extension force causes tenodesis pinch to occur. Other sources of power may be a carbon-dioxide or other pneumatic system operating the McKibben muscle. Figure 8.20b shows that the principle behind this system is that gas flows through tubing into an expandable cylinder enclosed in a diagonally braided covering. The assembly is closed at the distal end. The gas expands the cylinder, which shortens the length of the cylinder and creates a force to extend the wrist. This system has been fairly effective; however, the weight of the carbon dioxide cylinder limits mobility. External electric power sources have also been used. However some difficulties have been encountered with these units because of the low efficiency of the motor and gearing, unless the motor is large. Further design improvements may help increase this orthosis' efficiency. Other methods of electrical stimulation of the individual's own muscles, directly or via the intrinsic

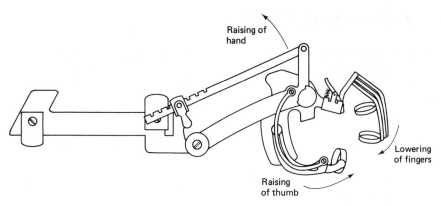

**FIGURE 8.20(a).** The tenodesis splint helps quadriplegics who can raise the hand but have no control over the digits. Raising the hand transmits forces through lever systems. This lowers the fingers, raises the thumb, and causes thumb-finger pinch.

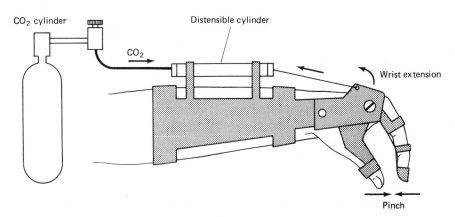

**FIGURE 8.20(b).** McKibben muscle attached to a tenodesis splint. The gas pressure expands the distensible cylinder, which is woven and is called a McKibben muscle. Its length shortens. This pulls the wrist back and the flexor tendons pull the fingers together. A three-jaw pinch of the thumb and fingers results.

nervous system, have been in an experimental or research stage for many years and are not for general use.

The basic principles of functional orthoses for the upper extremity require that the orthosis be designed based on the kinematics of the functions that the orthosis is to perform. After an orthosis has been designed to meet these functional goals, it is important that fitting be done carefully to support the fine activities required in the upper extremity. Training in the use of these orthoses is also a major concern and is usually done with the assistance of occupational therapists. A rather complete listing of forearm and hand orthoses is provided by Guilford and Perry (1975).

## 8.11 TECHNICAL AIDS, ASSISTIVE DEVICES

The devices discussed in the previous sections of this chapter all provide general replacement of function regardless of the task to be carried out. In this section, we discuss devices intended for very specialized functions. We also discuss general purpose devices not connected to the body directly—manipulators. Assistive devices are generally grouped by the function to be aided. One large group is called *aids to daily living* (ADL), which we discuss in this section. General references describing all of these devices are Robinault (1973), Lawton (1956), and Rosenberg (1968). Adams et al. (1975) discuss devices for recreation. General suppliers of these aids are Cleo Living Aids (Cleveland, OH), Be-OK Self Help Aids (Brookfield, IL), Abbey Medical Equipment (Los Angeles, CA), and others listed in the Green Pages Rehab Source Book (P.O. Box 1586, Winter Park, FL 32790) or Accent on Living Buyer's Guide (Cheever Pub. Co., P.O. Box 700, Bloomington, IL 61701).

### Aids to Daily Living

Most aids to daily living are addressed to the problems of restricted manipulative or mobility capability. Some others are for individuals suffering impaired gastrointestinal function. Some categories of aids are: eating, grooming, dressing, writing, and recreation. We can categorize manipulative devices by the type of handle used for enhanced function. Seven types of handles are typically used (Fig. 8.21): extended and expanded, oversized, functional slip-on grip, swivel, suction, bent or offset, and Velcro. These handles are used on devices in all subcategories of ADLs.

**Eating Aids.** Utensils (knife, fork, and spoon) are available with all of the special handles. Most are intended to compensate for lack of finger strength, lack of reach, or available use of only one hand. Oversized utensils also can accommodate for decreased fine-motor ability. Handles may be attached at either an angle to the utensil or in line with the utensil handles, depending on the residual control possible by the individual. Swivel handles (Fig. 8.21) provide greater flexibility. Combinations of knife and fork or fork and spoon are also available for one-handed individuals.

There are also powered feeders that allow someone with no limb function to eat by activating an interface (see Chapter 6) and causing the fork to scrape the food off the plate, bring it to mouth height, and hold it. The individual may control the device with head movement, puff/sip switches, or chin movement. Once the spoon is positioned, the individual can lean forward and take the food. Most devices also have a provision for rotating the plate to bring all food into range of the spoon.

Ramey et al. (1979) describe a microcomputer-controlled eating system for individuals with limited or absent upper-extremity function. Figure 8.22 shows the feeding cycle. The powered manipulator holds the utensils in a rest position ($P_1$) until the user sends a signal to the computer via a shoulder, chin, neck, or head movement. The manipulator then executes a preprogrammed path ($P_2$) from the rest position to the plate. A search pattern follows until the utensil position coincides with the morsel desired. The user then activates the switch again and a prepro-

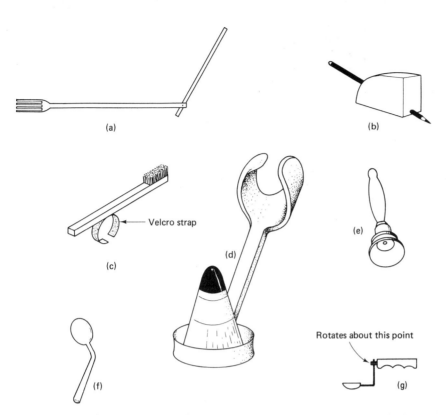

**FIGURE 8.21.** Types of handles used on aids to daily living. (a) fork with extended handle, (b) oversize pencil holder, (c) toothbrush with velcro handle strap, (d) badmitten serving tray for amputee with slip-on handle, (e) buttoner with suction handle, (f) spoon with bent handle, (g) spoon with swivel handle.

grammed path ($P_3$) from the plate to the mouth is executed. Once the user has removed the food from the utensil by leaning forward, a switch signal instructs the manipulator to return to the rest position. Ramey et al. describe the detailed electronic, mechanical, and software design for this system.

Food preparation aids of all types are also available. These include rounded knives that can be used with a rotating rather than sliding motion, food-holding boards for one-handed individuals, and powered appliances adapted to use by the disabled. Can openers, knife sharpeners, food processors, ovens, and blenders are among the many adapted appliances available.

Reachers are available in a variety of styles. These devices have a terminal clamp that is closed by the user by pressing a handle or squeezing a grip. They are useful for people in wheelchairs or others who can't reach shelves or the floor due to limited range of motion.

**Dressing Aids.**   Dressing aids serve two basic purposes: extended reach and improved or one-handed grasp. Devices that allow a shirt or blouse to be buttoned with one hand (called buttoners) are available with all of the special handles. A

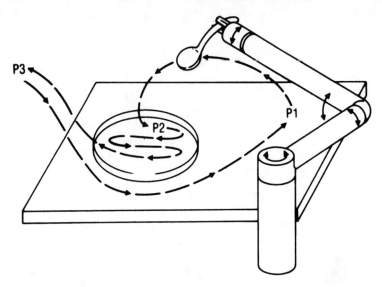

**FIGURE 8.22.** The feeding cycle for a microcomputer controlled feeder. $P_1$ is rest position. $P_2$ and $P_3$ are preprogrammed paths from the plate to the mouth and from the mouth to the rest position. (From *Computer*, January, 1979, pp. 55, with permission of IEEE.)

suction cup buttoner is shown in Fig. 8.21. The device is pushed through the button hole, the button is grasped in the hook end and the button is pulled through the button hole. By pushing on the buttoner, it can be freed from the button. The thickness of cloth, size of the button, and degree of motor impairment all affect success.

Extended-handle shoe horns, sock pullers, and zipper pullers are designed for individuals with limited range of motion. The longer handle makes it possible to complete tasks requiring a long reach.

**Grooming Aids.** Brushes (hair and tooth), combs, razors, mirrors, and soap holders are all available with the handles shown in Fig. 8.21. These allow a disabled person to care for himself and can be very important in developing independence.

Modified bathtubs, toilets, faucets, and showers also allow more independent activities by the disabled. Raised toilet seats or seats that lift up can help a person with lower-limb weakness. Bags and catheters are available for individuals with paralysis affecting elimination.

Some aids are designed to convert two-handed tasks to one-handed ones. For example, mirrors with a ring that goes around the neck allow people to comb or brush their own hair without holding the mirror. Most grooming aids are very simple adaptions of standard items.

**Writing and Reading Aids.** Holders for pencils with enlarged grips or bent handles are available (Fig. 8.21). These are useful when an individual has limited finger or finger/thumb movement. Weighted hold-downs are available for keeping

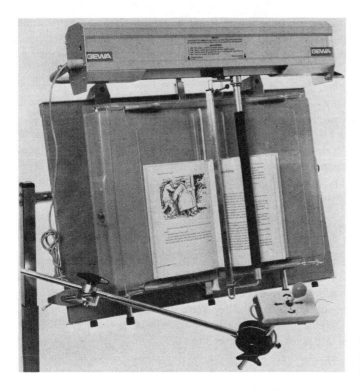

**FIGURE 8.23.** Gewa page turner feature four step control. (Courtesy Zygo Industries, Portland, OR)

the wrist in position in cases of tremor. Paper holding systems help one-handed individuals position the paper while writing. There are also one-handed typewriters available. These have the most-used keys grouped in the center of the keyboard.

Book holders and page turners may aid a person with upper-limb disability. Page turners may be simple sticks held in the mouth or mounted to the head. There is usually a rubber tip that is used to turn the pages by moving the head. Powered page turners rely on a moving lever to accomplish the turning, with the person using an interface similar to those for eating aids. Both methods are only partially successful. Multiple pages tend to turn, and it is difficult to keep the book open to the current page.

A recently introduced page turner, made by Gewa in Sweden (available from Zygo Industries, Portland, OR), overcomes most of these problems. This device is shown in Fig. 8.23. It uses a four-step process to ensure accurate page turning. Step 1 causes a roller to move across the page. Once positioned at the middle of the next page (Fig. 8.23), the roller is rotated (step 2). This causes the page to move to the left and to fold up. The third movement causes the roller to rotate in the opposite direction to flip the page over the top of the roller. The final step is to move the roller (and the new page) to the left. The roller can be positioned at the centerfold of the book or magazine when the page turn is completed. Each step requires a separate signal from the interface (see Chapter 6). This system may be much more reliable than single-movement page-turner designs.

Book holders may be used to position reading material. In some cases, these devices may be used as writing aids when an individual cannot lean over a table. For example, in arthritis of the spine, it is necessary for the person to remain erect at all times. By placing the writing materials on a book holder, this may be accomplished.

**Recreational Aids.** Many adapted games and sports have been developed for the disabled. In many cases, these adapted activities require special equipment. Wheelchair sports are gaining popularity and we discuss special design considerations for sports wheelchairs in the next section. Other games may need adapted equipment as well. Figure 8.21 shows an adapted holder for a badminton shuttlecock to allow an amputee to serve. Similar aids exist in archery, bowling, riflery, and table games. Adams et al. (1975) describe many adapted recreational activities and the equipment necessary for the disabled to enjoy them.

### Driving Aids and Modified Vehicles

Independence in vocational and recreational activities for the disabled depends heavily on the ability to operate automobiles independently. Most cities provide special public transportation for the physically disabled, but these systems are often unreliable, have infrequent schedules, and require a great deal of preplanning. If a physically disabled individual can independently operate an automobile, then his freedom and choice of activities is greatly enhanced.

We can design manual controls for operating brakes and accelerator when an individual has normal upper-body strength and mobility. Specially powered driving aids are also available for quadriplegics and others with weakened upper-extremity function. Typical modern systems depend on the use of a vehicle equipped with power brakes, power steering, and automatic transmission.

We can categorize manual hand controls for braking and acceleration into four groups (Reichenberger and Newell, 1975): push-pull, push-right-angle-pull, push-twist, and crank. In each of these systems, the individual operates the brakes and accelerator with one hand and steers with the other. Generally the steering is done with the right hand and the other controls use the left hand. Each system consists of a mechanical linkage, control handle, and associated connecting hardware with the push-pull system. The user activates the brakes by applying a force to the control handle in a direction away from the body and parallel to the steering column. He accelerates by pulling the control handle back. With the push-right-angle-pull, the user controls the brakes in the same manner as the push-pull type. He accelerates by pulling toward the lap in a downward direction. The push-twist control requires the same braking movement as the other two. The user accelerates by twisting the control handle. The crank control requires clockwise rotation for braking (away from the driver) and counterclockwise rotation for acceleration. *The Atlas of Orthotics* (Reichenberger and Newell, 1975) contains a list of manufacturers of manual driving aids. Steering assists are also available to facilitate one-handed steering. These "spinners" rotate as the wheel is turned, and feature modified handle types.

For quadriplegics and others with weak upper extremities, we can design power-assisted driving aids. These usually require extensive modifications of vehi-

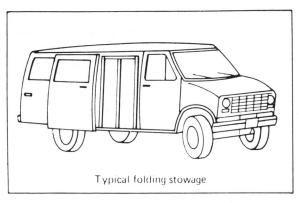

Typical folding stowage

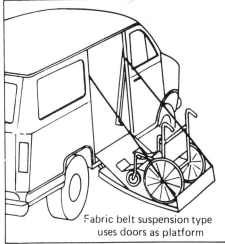

Fabric belt suspension type uses doors as platform

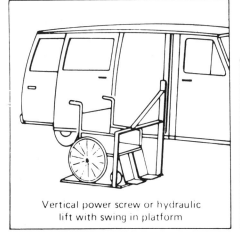

Vertical power screw or hydraulic lift with swing in platform

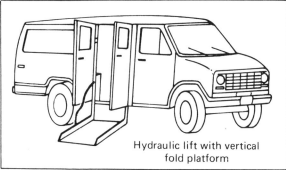

Hydraulic lift with vertical fold platform

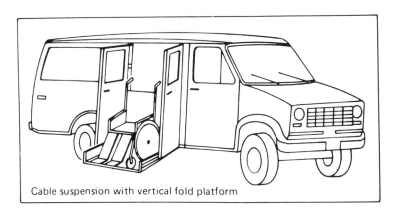

Cable suspension with vertical fold platform

**FIGURE 8.24.** Powered lifts for wheelchair entry into a van. (Reprinted with permission from *Clinical engineering: principles and practices*, Prentice-Hall, 1979.)

cles (usually vans) to accommodate powered lifts for entry (Fig. 8.24), tie-downs for stabilizing the wheelchair in position for driving (Fig. 8.25), and special low-activation force servo systems for steering and braking. The Veterans Administration has standards for driving aids and lifts and is developing one for tie-downs purchased for their patients (Veterans Administration, 1975 and 1977). The lifts shown in Fig. 8.24 have controls usable by the handicapped driver that raise and lower the lift, open the door, and stow the lift. Rear entry is also often used. An individual in a powered wheelchair can control these features independently and achieve maximum independence. Individuals with modified vehicles are required to pass the same driving tests as able-bodied drivers.

## 8.12 WHEELCHAIRS

A wheelchair is an orthotic device. It is more than a chair with wheels, and its proper prescription depends on many factors, including the type of disability of the individual. Proper fitting of a wheelchair can be therapeutic, especially for children with neuromuscular disabilities (Trefler et al., 1978). Wheelchairs have two major subcomponents: the supporting structure and the propelling structure.

### *Supporting Structure*

The supporting structure of a wheelchair consists of a frame, seat, back support, arm rests, and foot rests. Additional components that may be included are inserts for positioning, clothing guards, and a folding mechanism.

**Frame.** We define wheelchair frames by their strength. The standard chair will accommodate individuals up to 90 kg (200 lbs). The frame is made of cold rolled steel tubing, and a typical chair weighs about 20 kg. A heavy-duty chair will handle weights in excess of 90 kg with seat widths up to 61 cm (24 in.). It is also made of cold-rolled steel and weighs about 25 kg. Lightweight chairs are made of a special chrome-alloy thin-walled steel tubing. They will accommodate children and small adults and weigh about 13–19 kg. There are five frame sizes typically available: small child, large child, junior, adult, and oversize. These vary in seat width (30–61 cm), and height (40–50 cm). Most manufacturers provide a variety of width, weight, and height combinations. Special chairs are available for young children or children who require a great deal of special trunk support.

**Seats.** The wheelchair seat is the most important part of the structure. We must design seats to distribute the patient's weight over the largest possible area. This reduces pressure at localized points such as the bony prominences. The seat design should reduce pressure on the buttocks and transfer some to the thigh area to reduce the possibility of decubitus ulcers (pressure sores). Our design objective is to assure that the patient is provided with the smallest total seat area consistent with size, disability, and clothing (Peizer, 1975). If the seat is too wide, the patient may experience difficulties in maintaining trunk alignment or in reaching the hand rims. Increasing the width of the chair also makes it more difficult to turn and go through doors. If the seat is too narrow, the patient may develop skin abrasions or pressure

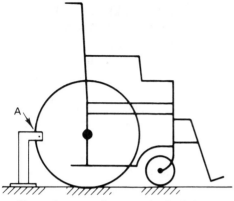

Pin or clamp attaches to each wheel rim at Point A (floor or wall-mounted)

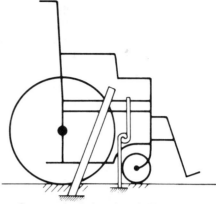

Occupant lap belt and vertically-acting over-center toggle on each side

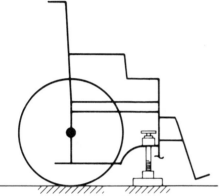

Lateral bar across lower frame members, attached with a single vertical wing-bolt to floor fitting

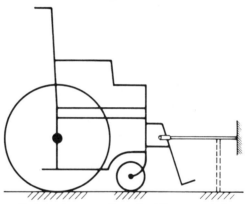

Dash, engine cover, firewall, or floor-mounted clamp, attaches to one footrest frame

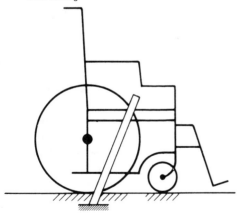

Occupant lap belt only

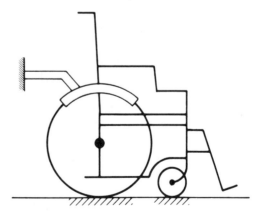

Tightly-fitting "fender" over one or two wheels

**FIGURE 8.25.** Tie downs for stabilizing wheelchairs in vans. (Reprinted with permission from *Clinical engineering: principles and practices*, Prentice-Hall, 1979.)

sores on thighs or hips. If the seat is too shallow (front to back) the weight bearing area is reduced and the unit pressure on the buttocks is increased. A seat that is too deep increases pressure on the popliteal area behind the knee.

The hammock seat is not appropriate for individuals with weakness that tends toward internal rotation of the hips or spasticity of the thigh adductors. This type of seat may actually contribute to improper alignment of the legs. For this reason, many individuals require other types of seats. When designing these seat types, we must consider many factors. The type of disability is the most important factor. Persons with spinal cord lesions may have a loss of sensation below the waist and decreased pelvic and trunk control. With higher lesions, there may be total loss of trunk support and loss of upper-extremity function. In neurological diseases (e.g., cerebral palsy, multiple sclerosis), the sensation may be intact but the muscular control is absent. Insensitive patients usually require pads or inserts to distribute the pressure during prolonged loading of tissue (Freeman et al., 1979).

Trefler et al. (1978) have defined the seating needs of children and adults with neuromuscular disorders other than spinal-cord injury. They define three broad classes of patients based on the severity of their disability. Mild cases are those with fair trunk control, no contractures or pelvic problems, no spinal curves, and good midline, head, and hand control. This individual requires only inserts to stabilize the hips and possibly a seat belt to provide safety. Moderate disabilities include some hip problems, moderate extensor thrust, a need for midline support, a need for minimal head support, and limited arm/hand control present. These individuals need more substantial seating and positioning support.

Severe disabilities include fixed hips, scoliosis, kyphosis, poor trunk support, and no hand function. These individuals need custom-fitted seating systems.

Seating systems for the moderate or severe patient are based on a careful consideration of each of the anatomic regions needing support. These are: pelvis, hips, trunk, shoulder girdle and arms, head, knees, and feet. For moderate disabilities, modular inserts are used at each of the anatomic regions needing support (Trefler et al., 1977; Daher et al., 1977). In each of these systems, a series of modular inserts is available in a range of sizes. Modules are selected for each level of support needed by the patient. They are inserted into standard wheelchairs or attached to special wheeled bases. For the severely disabled patient, more complex seating systems are required. These may be molded from plaster casts similar to orthotic devices, cut from plastic or foam pieces on a "cut-and-try" basis, or mold-formed using a plastic bag filled with beads. In the latter approach, the bag is evacuated after the patient's contour has been taken. This bag is then used as a mold for forming the foam insert. Hobson et al. (1978) describe an alternative approach known as "foam-in-place" seating. This method uses a foaming plate into which modular seat and back molds can be inserted. The molds are fabricated from polyethylene plastic closed on all sides except one. A sheet of thin latex is stretched over the open side and this side is in contact with the patient. Once the patient is seated in the chair, a two-part foam is injected into the back of the foaming mold. The reaction of the two foam components causes the foam to rise and force the latex sheet to form around the shape of the patient. In about ten minutes, the foam hardens and the mold is complete. The completed insert can then be attached to a wheelchair. This technique reduces the fine cutting and fitting necessary in other techniques.

**Back Rest.** The back-rest height is determined by the level of trunk support required. All of the inserts and custom seats described previously include back and trunk support. For most individuals in the mild category, the back is a cloth structure that merely provides low-back support. The height is determined by the degree of support necessary. For support of the trunk, a three-point system (see Section 8.8) is used, with pads or inserts at a midscapular, midcervical, or midhead level, depending on the needed support. Care must be taken to insure that pads do not stimulate primitive reflexes (e.g., by contact with the occipital area).

Reclining backs are also available in either semi- or full-reclining models. The semi-reclining types have a maximum of 30° tilt and are intended for persons who cannot sit vertically (e.g., hip extension contractures, spine deformity, etc.). Full reclining types are for patients who must rest frequently, who cannot relieve pressure by a change in position while upright, or who need the added leverage to propel the chair.

**Arm Rests.** Arm rests provide support for the arms and hands as well as serving as a basis of support for changes in position and transferring from the chair to cars or other chairs. If the arm height is too low, there is a tendency for the patient to slump forward and lose trunk stability. If it is too high, the shoulders are forced up and it is difficult to sit for prolonged periods of time. Two types of arm rests are available. The standard or full-length type is the same length as the seat. The desk type is reduced by 25 cm at the front to allow the chair to be moved close to tables. Either type may be removable to facilitate transfer into or out of the chair.

**Foot and Leg Rests.** The foot-rest support angles down and in front of the chair at about 20° from seat level. Some types are detachable and others reduce direct foot contact to reduce contractures stimulated by contact with the ball of the foot (e.g., in some cerebral palsied children). The standard footplate is 15 cm deep.

### Propelling Structure

**Patient-Powered.** Two basic types of propulsion are available: patient-powered (manual) or externally powered. The manual types have large wheel rims that the patient uses to turn the wheel. One-handed versions provide two rims on one side with an axle linking one rim to the opposite wheel. Attachments to hand rims include knobs to increase grasping ability. Wheels are either hard rubber (gray to reduce marks on floors) or pneumatic. The latter reduce the power expenditure required, but they also require more maintenance. Power expenditures have been determined from patient-powered wheelchair use by healthy paraplegic college students (Kamenetz, 1969). For normal propulsion on a smooth surface at 1.9 km/hr, the power expended is about 170W. This is typical of daily activities such as dressing (140–210W), washing hands and face (170W), or walking at 4 km/hr (170W). The normal pace for the college-age paraplegics was 3–5 km/hr with pneumatic tires over a course of 0.3 km with ramps, inclines, and so on. The hard pace was 6–8 km/hr. Energy expenditure at the slow pace was 340W and at the hard pace 690W.

**Externally Powered.** The power expenditures required for patient-powered wheelchairs are too high for some individuals. Electric motors attached to each drive wheel allow persons with upper limb weakness due to high spinal cord lesion or neuromuscular disease to move independently. The design criteria that we must meet are: adjustable speed with a minimum of at least 1.6 km/hr; capability to negotiate at least a 2.5 cm obstacle; enough power to ascend a 10% (6°) slope and descend safely; a turning radius of less than 76 cm; removable battery and motor (i.e., not riveted to frame); and energy sufficient to operate one full day without recharging and to fully recharge over night (Peizer, 1975). Current systems employ two motors, one on each drive wheel. Both motors are reversible. Turning is accomplished by turning one motor on in the forward direction and the other in the reverse direction. To move forward, both motors are turned on. We can use either on/off or proportional control systems. The most common and simplest control system is a relay that turns either or both motors full on as required (on/off control). Proportional control, though more complex electronically, provides smoother control and higher motor speed as the control is engaged further. Most power systems attach to standard wheelchairs. Various methods are used to provide power to the wheels. Some systems use a friction wheel in contact with normal drive wheels. Others provide separate drive sheaves attached to the shafts of the motors and connected by belts to pulleys on or connected to the wheels.

Controls are similar to the interfaces used for control and communication systems (Section 6.8). A joystick operated by the hand, chin, mouth, or head is common. A tongue switch provides up to seven double-throw switches (four for wheelchair control, the rest for other functions such as feeder or page turner). These switches are manipulated with the tip of the tongue. The VA and others have developed a puff/sip switch. This interface has two air switches that respond to positive air pressure (puff). These activate relays for forward movement of the wheelchair. Two other switches require negative pressure (sip). They activate relays that drive the motors in the reverse direction for backward movement. By turning on only one forward motor, the user can turn the chair. A proportional drive system is available with these switches in which a constant light breath pressure must be maintained. Voice-activated switches have also been used experimentally. As more microcomputer control systems for the disabled (see Chapter 6) become available, this mode of control, requiring pattern recognition of certain words, will become more common.

There are also special wheelchairs for stair climbing and curb climbing. Some of these are described in the *Atlas of Orthotics* (Peizer, 1975). Two recent conferences provided detailed design goals for improvement in both manual and powered wheelchairs (Moss Rehab. Hosp., 1978 and 1979).

## Wheelchair Sports

Many individuals confined to wheelchairs actively participate in sports activities such as basketball, track, archery, bowling, riflery, and many other sports (Adams et al., 1975). The National Wheelchair Athletic Association (Woodside, NY) coordinates activities in this country. Most sports wheelchairs are custom designed by the athletes themselves. Special features depend on the sport. For example, in track, the chair must be lightweight, have a low center of gravity, and have small hand rims for maximum speed. In basketball, we must design for maximum maneuverability, provide some protection for both the chair and user due to contact, and have a higher center of gravity to facilitate shooting. Special hubs, wheels, frames, and push rims are available. Some standards do exist for international competition (Adams et al., 1975). We can enhance the stability of the chair by providing a camber in the wheel/axle mechanism. The standards provide a great deal of flexibility for creativity and innovation, and wheelchair athletes exercise large amounts of both.

International competition is based on a ranking system that takes into account the degree of disability of the user. International Disabled Olympic games are held every four years in the same year as the able-bodied Olympics. Accomplishments by athletes in these competitions represent the same type of world-class performance as that found in able-bodied sports. There is a continual refinement of technique and equipment based on experience and the availability of new materials. Many of these advances are reported in the journal *Spokes and Sports* (5201 N. 19th Avenue, Phoenix, AZ 85015).

## REFERENCES

ADAMS, R. C., A. N. DANIEL, and L. RULLMAN (1975). *Games, sports, and exercises for the physically handicapped*. Philadelphia: Lea & Febiger.

AMERICAN ACADEMY OF ORTHOPAEDIC SURGEONS (1975). *Atlas of orthotics*. St. Louis: C. V. Mosby.

BARD, G., and H. RALSTON (1959). Measurement of energy expenditure during ambulation with special reference to evaluation of assistive devices. *Arch. Physical Med. Rehab.*, 40: 415–20.

BASMAJIAN, J. V. (1974). *Muscles alive, their functions revealed by electromyography*. Baltimore: Williams and Wilkins.

BERLEMONT, M., R. WEBER, and J. P. WILLOT (1969). Ten years of experience with the immediate application of prosthetic devices to amputees of the lower extremities on the operating table. *Prosth. Inter.*, 3(8): 8–18.

BLOUNT, W. P., and J. H. MOE (1973). *The Milwaukee brace*. Baltimore: Williams and Wilkins.

BOTTOMLEY, A. H. (1966). Signal processing in a practical electromyographically controlled prosthesis. *Committee on prosthetics research and development: The control of external power in upper-extremity rehabilitation*. Nat. Acad. Sci.—Nat. Res. Counc. Pub. 1352: 271–73.

BURGESS, E. M., R. L. ROMANO, and J. H. ZETTL (1969). *The management of lower-extremity amputations: Surgery, immediate postsurgical prosthetic fitting, patient care*. Washington, D. C.: Vet. Admin. Dept. Med. Surg., Prosth. Sens. Aids. Ser., TR 10-6.

CHILDRESS, D. S., N. BILLOCK, and R. S. THOMPSON (1974). A search for better limbs: Prosthetics research at Northwestern Univ. *Bull. Prosth. Res.*, BPR 10-22: 200–12.

CONZELMAN, J. E., H. B. ELLIS, and C. W. O'BRIEN (1953). Prosthetic device sensory attachment, U. S. Patent 2, 656, 545.

CORKER, K., J. LYMAN, and S. SHEREDOS (1979). A preliminary evaluation of remote medical manipulators. *Bull. Prosth. Res.*, BPR-10: 107–34.

DAHER, R. L., R. N. HOLTE, and I. T. PAUL (1977). Progress report: A complete system for meeting the seating requirements for the multiply handicapped. *Proc. 4th Ann. Conf. Sys. Dev. Disabled,* Seattle, WA: 44–47.

DAVIS, A. B. (1973). *Triumph over disability: The development of rehabilitation medicine in the U.S.A.* Washington, DC: Smithsonian Institution.

DEMBO, T., and E. TANE-BASKIN (1955). The noticeability of the cosmetic glove. *Artif. Limbs,* 2(2): 47–56.

DEWALD, R. (1975). in *Atlas of orthotics, biomechanical principles and application,* 407–17. American Academy of Orthopaedic Surgeons. St. Louis: C. V. Mosby.

DRENNAN, J. C., T. S. RENSHAW, and B. H. CURTIS (1979). The thoracic suspension orthoses. *Clin. Orthopedics,* 139: 33–39.

ELFTMAN, H. (1955). Knee action and locomotion. *Bull. Hosp. for Joint Diseases,* 16(2): 103–10.

ENGEL, W. H., M. A. KMIOTEK, J. P. HOHF, J. FRENCH, M. J. BARNERIAS, and A. A. SIEBENS (1967). A functional splint for grasp driven by wrist extension. *Arch. Physical Med. Rehab.,* 48: 43.

ENGEN, T. J. (1970). Development of upper extremity orthotics. *Orthotics and prosthetics,* March, 24: 12–29.

FLETCHER, M. J. (1954). New developments in hands and hooks, in P. E. Klopsteg and P. D. Wilson (eds), *Human limbs and their substitutes.* New York: McGraw-Hill (reprinted with new bibliography, New York: Hafner, 1968).

FLETCHER, M. J., and A. B. WILSON, JR. (1954). New developments in artificial arms, in P. E. Klopsteg and P. D. Wilson (eds), *Human limbs and their substitutes.* New York: McGraw-Hill (reprinted with new bibliography, New York: Hafner, 1968).

FLOWERS, W., R. W. MANN, S. R. SINSON, and D. ROWELL (1979). Clinical evaluation of a computer-interactive above-knee prosthesis. *Bull. Prosth. Res.,* 10-32: 229–31.

FOORT, J., and C. W. RADCLIFFE (1956). The Canadian type hip disarticulation prosthesis. Berkeley, CA: University of California, Berkeley. Institute of Engineering Research, Prosthetic Devices Research Project Series 11, issue 28.

FREEMAN, J. J., D. L. STONER, J. B. SMATHERS, D. E. CLAPP, and D. D. DUNCAN (1979). Safety program, in J. G. Webster and A. M. Cook (eds), *Clinical engineering: Principles and practices.* Englewood Cliffs, NJ: Prentice-Hall.

GRAUPE, D., A. A. M. BEEX, W. J. MONLUX, and I. MAGNUSSON (1977). A multifunctional prosthesis control system based on time series identification of EMG signals using microprocessors. *Bull. Prosth. Res.,* BPR 10-27: 4–16.

GUILFORD, A., and J. PERRY (1975). *Atlas of orthotics, biomechanical principles and application,* 81–104. American Academy of Orthopaedic Surgeons. St. Louis: C. V. Mosby.

HARDY, A. E., and A. S. BADDELEY (1979). Pressures generated in the thigh muscles and under the thigh cast of an uninjured subject wearing a cast brace. *J. Bone Joint Surg.*, 61: 362–64.

HARRIS, E. E. (1973). A new orthotics terminology—A guide to its use for prescription and fee schedules. *Orthotics and Prosthetics*, 27: 6–19.

HOBSON, D., K. D. DRIVER, and S. HANKS (1978). Foam-in-place seating for the severely disabled. *Proc. 5th Ann. Conf. Sys. Dev. Disabled*, Houston, TX: 153–56.

KAMENETZ, H. L. (1969). *The wheelchair book*. Springfield, IL: Charles C Thomas.

KOBRINSKI, A. E. (1961). Problems of bioelectric control, in *Automatic and remote control*. (Proc. of 1st Inter. Fed. Auto. Contr. Inter. Cong. Moscow, 1960, 2: 619–23). London: Butterworths.

LAWTON, E. B. (1956). *A.D.L. activities of daily living, testing, training, equipment*. New York: N.Y. Univ. Inst. Rehab. Med.

LEHMANN, J. F. (1979). Biomechanics of ankle-foot-orthoses: Prescription and design. *Arch. Physical Med. Rehab.*, 60: 200–207.

LONG, C. (1966). Upper-limb bracing. in S. Licht (ed), *Orthotics, Etcetera*. E. Licht: New Haven, CN.

LUCACCINI, L. F., P. K. KAISER, and J. LYMAN (1966). The French electric hand: Some observations and conclusions. *Bull. Prosth. Res.*, BPR 10-6: 30–51.

LYMAN, J., and A. FREEDY (1979). Fundamental and applied research related to the design and development of upper-limb externally powered prostheses (progress report). *Bull. Prosth. Res.*, BPR 10-31: 70–71.

LYQUIST, E. (1958). Canadian-type plastic socket for a hemipelvectomy. *Artif. Limbs.*, 5(2): 130–32.

MAUCH, H. A. (1968). Stance control for above-knee artificial legs—Design considerations in the S-N-S knee. *Bull. Prosth. Res.*, BPR 10-10: 61.

MCCULLOUGH, N. C. III, and S. K. SARRAFIAN (1975). in *Atlas of orthotics, biomechanical principles and application*, 65–80. American Academy of Orthopaedic Surgeons. St. Louis: C. V. Mosby.

MORRIS, J., and K. MARKOLF (1975). in *Atlas of orthotics, biomechanical principles and application*, 312–31. American Academy of Orthopaedic Surgeons. St. Louis: C. V. Mosby.

MOSS REHABILITATION HOSPITAL (1978). *Wheelchair-I, report of a workshop*. Philadelphia: Rehab. Engr. Center.

MOSS REHABILITATION HOSPITAL (1979). *Wheelchair-II, report of a workshop*. Philadelphia: Rehab. Engr. Center.

MURDOCH, G. (ed) (1970). *Prosthetic and orthotic practice*. London: Edward Arnold.

MURPHY, E., and A. BURSTEIN (1975). in *Atlas of orthotics, biomechanical principles and application*, 3–30. American Academy of Orthopaedic Surgeons. St. Louis: C. V. Mosby.

NEW YORK UNIVERSITY Prosthetics and Orthotics (1974–80). Post Grad. Med. Sch. series of manuals: Lower limb prosthetics, upper limb prosthetics, lower limb orthotics, spinal orthotics, upper limb orthotics. New York: N. Y. Univ.

PEIZER, E. (1975). in *Atlas of orthotics, biomechanical principles and application*, 431–53. American Academy of Orthopaedic Surgeons. St. Louis: C. V. Mosby.

PEIZER, E., and D. W. WRIGHT (1970). Human locomotion. in Murdoch, G. (ed), *Prosthetic and Orthotic Practice.* London: Edward Arnold.

PIGGOT, H. (1979). Management of structural scoliosis. *Surg. Annual,* 11: 267–94.

PURSLEY, R. J. (1960). Harness patterns for upper-extremity prostheses, in *American Academy of Orthopaedic Surgeons, Orthopaedic Appliances Atlas,* Vol. 2, "Artificial limbs," 105–28. Ann Arbor, MI: J. W. Edwards.

RADCLIFFE, C. W. (1954). Mechanical aids for alignment of lower extremity prostheses. *Artif. Limbs,* 1(2): 20–28.

RADCLIFFE, C. W. (1955). Functional considerations in the fitting of above-knee prostheses. *Artif. Limbs,* 2(1): 35–60.

RADCLIFFE, C. W. (1957). Biomechanics of the Canadian-type hip disarticulation prosthesis. *Artif. Limbs.,* 4(2): 29–38.

RADCLIFFE, C. W. (1962). Biomechanics of below-knee prostheses in normal level, bipedal walking. *Artif. Limbs,* 6(2): 16–74.

RADCLIFFE, C. W., D. M. CUNNINGHAM, J. M. MORRIS, and L. LAMOREUX (1979). Design of prosthetic and orthotic devices and biomechanical studies of locomotion. *Bull. Prosth. Res.,* 10-31: 88–94.

RADCLIFFE, C. W., and L. LAMOREUX (1968). UC-BL Pneumatic swing-control unit for above-knee prostheses—design, adjustment, and installation, *Bull. Prosth. Res.,* BPR 10-10: 73–89.

RAMEY, R. L., J. H. AYLOR, and R. D. WILLIAMS (1979). Microcomputer-aided eating for the severely handicapped. *Computer,* 12(1): 54–61.

RASCH, P. J., and R. K. BURKE (1967). *Kinesiology and applied anatomy.* Philadelphia: Lea & Febiger.

REICHENBERGER, A. J., and P. H. NEWELL, Jr. (1975). in *Atlas of orthotics, biomechanical principles and application,* 462–78. American Academy of Orthopaedic Surgeons, St. Louis: C. V. Mosby.

ROBINAULT, I. P. (ed) (1973). *Functional aids for the multiply handicapped.* United Cerebral Palsy Associations, Inc., Hagerstown, MD: Harper & Row.

ROSENBERG, C. (1968). *Assistive devices for the handicapped.* Minneapolis: Amer. Rehab. Fnd.

SARRAFIAN, S. (1975). in *Atlas of orthotics, biomechanical principles and application,* 33–56. American Academy of Orthopaedic Surgeons. St. Louis: C. V. Mosby.

SCOTT, R. N. (1967). Myoelectric control of prostheses and orthoses. *Bull. Prosth. Res.,* BPR 10-7: 93–114.

SCOTT, R. N. (1968). Myoelectric control systems. *Adv. Biomed. Engr. Med. Phys.,* 2: 45–72.

SCOTT, R. N., J. E. PACIGA, and P. A. PARKER (1978). Operator error in multistate myoelectric controls systems. *Med. Biol. Eng. Comput.,* 16(3): 296–301.

SEAMONE, W., and G. SCHMEISSER, JR. (1974). Status of the Johns Hopkins research program on upper-limb prosthesis-orthosis power and control system. *Bull. Prosth. Res.,* BPR 10-22: 237–43.

SIEBENS, A. A., J. P. HOHF, W. E. ENGEL, and N. SCRIBNER (1972). Suspension of certain patients from their ribs. *Johns Hopkins Med. J.,* 130: 26–36.

SOLOMONOW, M., and J. LYMAN (1980). Electrotactile stimulation relevant to sensory-motor rehabilitation. *Bull. Prosth. Res.*, BPR 10-33: 63–72.

STAROS, A., and M. LeBLANC (1975). in *Atlas of orthotics, biomechanical principals and application*, 184–234. American Academy of Orthopaedic Surgeons, St. Louis: C. V. Mosby.

STEINDLER, A. (1955). *Kinesiology of the human body*. Springfield, IL: Charles C Thomas.

TAYLOR, C. L. (1954). The biomechanics of the normal and of the amputated upper extremity, in P. E. Klopsteg and P. D. Wilson (eds), *Human limbs and their substitutes*. New York: McGraw-Hill (reprint edition with new bibliography, New York: Hafner, 1968).

TAYLOR, N., and P. SAND (1975). Verlo orthosis: Experience with different developmental levels in normal children. *Arch. Physical Med. Rehab.*, 56(3): 120–22.

TREFLER, E., P. HUGGINS, D. HOBSON, S. HANKS, and S. CHIARIZZIO (1977). A modular seating system for physically handicapped children. *Proc. 4th Ann. Conf. Sys. Dev. Disabled*, Seattle, WA: 41–43.

TREFLER, E., R. E. TOOMS, and D. A. HOBSON (1978). Seating for cerebral palsied children. *Inter-clinic Infor. Bull.*, 17(1): 1–8.

VETERANS ADMINISTRATION (1975). *VA standard design and test criteria for safety and quality for special automotive driving aids for standard passenger automobiles*, VAPC-A-7505-8. New York: VA Prosthetics Center.

VETERANS ADMINISTRATION (1977). *VA standard design and test criteria for safety and quality of automatic wheelchair lift systems for passenger motor vehicles*, VAPC-A-7703-2T. New York: VA Prosthetics Center.

WEISS, M. (1967). Myoplasty—immediate fitting of artificial leg—Ambulation. *ISRD-Proc. 10th World Congress, Indus. Soc. Rehab.–Prob. & Sol.* New York: Inter. Soc. Rehab. Disab. (now Rehab. Inter.), 101–4.

WILSON, A. BENNETT, JR. (1961). Prostheses for Syme's Amputation, *Artificial Limbs*, 6(1): 52–75.

WILSON, L. A., E. LYQUIST, and C. W. RADCLIFFE (1968). Air-cushion socket for patellar-tendon-bearing below-knee prosthesis—Principles and fabrication procedures, *Bull. Prosth. Res.*, BPR 10-10: 5–34.

WIRTA, R. W., F. R. FINLEY, and D. R. TAYLOR (1978). Pattern-recognition arm prosthesis: A historical perspective—A final report. *Bull. Prosth. Res.*, BPR 10-30: 8–35.

## STUDY QUESTIONS

**8.1** What are the basic differences between upper- and lower-prosthetic and orthotic devices in terms of desired output and control system design?

**8.2** A major problem in both prosthetic and orthotic devices is the need to find enough control sites for operation of the device. What are the major approaches taken to this problem, and how do they depend on type of power (including muscular) and control?

**8.3** Figure 8.2 shows that there are significantly higher energy expenditures for pylons than for lower-extremity prostheses equipped with those using an artificial foot. Explain this in terms of the biomechanics of walking.

**8.4** Contrast the design requirement for swing and stance phase control in above-knee prosthetic legs. What design tradeoffs must be made to accommodate for both functions?

**8.5** List the advantages and disadvantages of the artificial hook and artificial hand. Which system would you prefer to have? Why?

**8.6** Describe the major types of feedback that the user has for both lower- and upper-extremity devices. How do these differ, and what is the significance of poor feedback for each case?

**8.7** Childress (1974) describes an electrical approach to force multiplication in an upper-extremity prosthesis. List the design goals for this system and describe this system. Compare its operation with the mechanical system shown in Fig. 8.11. List the disadvantages and advantages of each system. Which system is "better"? Explain why you chose it.

**8.8** Conduct a literature search on processing methods for myoelectrically controlled upper-extremity prostheses (the references in Section 8.5 will get you started). Define the major approaches at the block diagram and flowchart level. Which offers the most promise? Explain why in terms of number of control sites required, user training required, amount of signal processing needed, and overall complexity and cost.

**8.9** The Mauch hydraulic ankle is an alternative to the SACH foot. Find a reference describing this system and compare it to the SACH foot. Why do you think that the SACH foot is much more popular than the hydraulic ankle? List the design goals and the method of implementation for each system.

**8.10** What is the three-point system? How is it applied in orthotic design?

**8.11** Draw a force diagram describing the role of the center of gravity in lower-limb orthoses. What is meant by the "line of gravity" and how is it usable in lower-limb orthotics? How are these concepts altered for upper-extremity orthotics. Why?

**8.12** What are the effects of lower extremity orthoses on energy expenditure? What factors affect this?

**8.13** Define the terms *lordosis* and *kyphosis* and relate each to the normal and abnormal spine. What is scoliosis and how is it treated using orthotics?

**8.14** List the methods and devices used for cervical stabilization. What are the advantages and disadvantages of each approach?

**8.15** How does the Milwaukee brace differ from other spinal orthoses?

**8.16** What are the major functions of the hand, and how are they aided by orthoses?

**8.17** List at least five simple aids to daily living. Propose and design at least one aid not mentioned in the text.

**8.18** Contrast the use of a microprocessor-controlled eating aid such as that discussed in Section 8.11 with able-bodied eating. What changes in motor planning are required to use this device?

**8.19** List the major aspects of wheelchair prescription. How are problems of seating and positioning solved, and what differences would you expect between a spinal cord injury and cerebral-palsied patients in terms of seating needs?

**8.20** All modern wheelchairs have limitations in terms of stability (especially going downhill), energy expenditure, maneuverability, and moving over rough (as little as 1 in.) surfaces. Pick one of these problems and conduct a literature search to determine what current approaches to solutions are. Also include a study of sports wheelchairs. Design a modification of a wheelchair to solve one or more of these problems.

# 9 Internal Prosthetics and Orthotics

*Harry B. Skinner*

## 9.1 LEARNING OBJECTIVES

Upon completing this chapter you will be able to:

- Define the types of materials used for implants and describe their properties.
- Describe the biological response to foreign materials.
- List the major mechanical and biological requirements for implanted materials.
- Describe the major approaches to replacement of joints.
- Describe the design and application of internal orthotic devices.

## 9.2 INTRODUCTION

The types of devices used for internal prosthetics and orthotics have evolved over a period of several hundred years (Williams and Roaf, 1973). They have been developed to replace a damaged, diseased, or worn part of the anatomy or to repair or assist in the reparative process of tissue. Orthopedics has been the field that stimulated the earliest work.

Metals, polymers, and ceramics in that order have been developed for biomaterials use. Stainless steel was introduced for prosthetic use in the 1920s because of its corrosion resistance. Subsequently, Vitallium, a cobalt-chromium-based alloy, and tantalum were found to be relatively well tolerated by tissues. Titanium and its alloys have been developed as biomaterials since 1950.

Polymers came into use in the 1950s for applications requiring their different properties. Since then, many polymeric materials have been tested for clinical usefulness. Among these are polymethylmethacrylate, polyethylene, polyethylene terephthalate (nylon), polytetrafluoroethylene (Teflon), polydimethylsiloxane (silicone), and polyacrylonitrile. Some of these are in clinical trials and some of these have achieved a place, at least for the present, among standard implant materials.

Ceramics have been used as implant materials on a very limited basis. They have largely been disregarded in the past for use in the body due to their characteristic brittleness and low flexural strength. Recent work, however, has indicated that they are quite compatible in the physiological environment. Aluminum oxide and carbon have found application as prosthetic components.

ASTM Committee F-4 on medical and surgical materials and devices has been organized to provide standards of composition for materials, standard specifications for constructing devices, and standards for testing them. These standards are tabulated in the Annual Book of ASTM Standards (ASTM, 1978). Thus, listed standards range from specifications for acrylic bone cements to wrought cobalt-nickel-chromium-molybdenum-tungsten-iron alloy for surgical implant applications. These specifications provide compositions and strength requirements for materials. They provide dimensions and thread sizes of the various pins, rods, and plates. Also included are surface finish standards and standards for care and handling of implants. These standards are not uniformly helpful, however, because they are "consensus" standards derived from committees with balanced representation from producers, users, and interested parties. Thus, in some cases, the standards are vague and not terribly restrictive. They do, however, provide a starting point in providing standards to be followed in production and testing so that valid comparisons can be made between products. Standards are added and revised periodically to keep them current.

## 9.3 BIOCOMPATIBILITY OF MATERIALS

### Requirements of Prosthetic Materials

**Mechanical Requirements.** The subject of requirements for implants includes two major considerations: the effect of the physiologic environment on the material and the effect of the material and its degradation products on the fluids and tissues of the body. The requirements for implants have been tabulated by several investigators (Morral, 1966; Levine, 1968; Crimmens, 1969; Williams and Roaf, 1973). The requirements on prosthetic materials from the material viewpoint are: (1) sufficient mechanical properties to withstand the stress states while in use [(a) strengths that are sufficient at implantation and do not diminish upon contact with the physiologic environment; (b) cyclic or static fatigue resistance; (c) time-dependent deformation resistance; (d) stress corrosion resistance; (e) elastic properties compatible with tissue; (f) friction and wear properties compatible with tissue application; (g) hardness values similar to the tissue of implantation]; (2) chemical behavior such that physical or mechanical degradation is not significant [(a) chemical and electrolytic corrosion resistance; (b) resistance to solution and swelling]; (3) mechanical design such that fabrication is both possible and not detrimental to strength; and (4) durability, to give reliable performance for the lifetime of the prosthesis even under attack by the physiologic environment.

Materials used as biomaterials fall into the three main categories of solid materials: metals, ceramics, and polymers. These biomaterials differ from other materials of the same category only in being biocompatible. Metals are either elements or solutions (alloys) of elements with a crystalline structure that provides free electrons for electrical conductivity. Their structure is composed of atoms with similar electrical charge, which allows one atom to slide on another, accounting for their properties of ductility and strength. Most ceramic materials are crystalline also but differ in that they are usually compounds of ionic materials. Glasses and some elements are also classed as ceramics. The ionic nature of the constituent elements in ceramics accounts for the reluctance of these atoms to slide across each other. Hence, deformation is difficult to achieve, and, although strength tends to be high, failure occurs catastrophically because of flaws usually introduced in manufacture. Polymers differ in structure from metals and ceramics in that they are one-dimensional (chains) in structure rather than three-dimensional, as are ceramics and metals. Polymers are chains of smaller molecular units (mers) that are based either on carbon bonds or on silicon–oxygen bonds. Because the bonding between chains is weak, polymers tend to be weaker, fairly ductile, and exhibit time-dependent deformation, as chains slide by each other relatively readily.

The term *medical-grade* refers primarily to polymers that have undergone special precautions in manufacture to prevent residual toxic materials.

Properties of materials are very structure-sensitive. Much more detailed information can be obtained from the very readable texts on materials by Van Vlaak (1970) and Moffatt et al. (1965).

**Biological Requirements.** It is required that materials demonstrate minimal biological response. Materials should not induce a toxic response, an immune response, a carcinogenic response (cancer), a chronic inflammatory response, abscess formation, or a breeding place for future infection. Materials must demonstrate tissue union or attachment to aid in the permanence of the implant where required. Strength and durability are required to withstand applied stresses. Mechanical properties, such as the modulus of elasticity, are also important. Design flexibility to allow operating room alterations and design such that implementation can be accomplished with a minimal of trauma to tissue is also important. Above all, an implant must have the ability to be sterilized.

The primary factor in choices of materials for implantation as protheses is the *biocompatibility*. This term refers to the biological response that a material evokes. All other factors are secondary in the evaluation of a material for implantation.

The body responds to implants in numerous ways. Phagocytosis or the ingestion of foreign matter by a cell is one means of removal. The process is performed by several types of white blood cells and other mobile cells called *macrophages* that surround the piece of debris and isolate it inside the cell in order to try to digest it. Organic and inorganic foreign material of sufficiently small size can be phagocytized. If the material cannot be digested, the cell holds it until it dies, at which time another cell picks it up (Anderson, 1971).

An inflammatory response is a natural occurrence of wound healing. The initial acute inflammation is characterized by a dilation of blood vessels, edema, and an increased concentration of white blood cells in the inflamed area. It usually subsides in a few days to a few weeks. Longer or chronic inflammations are a serious consideration if caused by the implant. These result in continuous pain and loss of function with little or no healing.

An implant may cause mechanical irritation of the surrounding tissue by simple abrasion, thus causing the tissue to die. An abscess, which is a localized cavity of pus containing macrophages and leukocytes that have died from engulfing necrotic tissue, may then form. The presence of the prosthesis usually prolongs or prevents the healing of an abscess. Although local irritation can cause a sterile abscess, that is, without the presence of a pathogenic organism, one of the major problems with implants today is the possibility of blood-born bacteria from an infection elsewhere in the body starting an infection at the implant site. Eradication of the infection usually, but not always, requires removal of the implant.

The toxicity of an implant is very important with regard to its compatibility with the surrounding tissues (Autian, 1967). Materials that cause illness or death by chemical interaction with tissue are referred to as poisons. Concentration, method of action on tissue, and the vulnerability of tissue all play a part in determining the effect of a poison. Although high concentrations of such substances as salt and sugar are necessary for toxicity, other substances such as arsenic, mercury, lead, and cyanide can be injurious in small quantities. Larger concentrations of iron, copper, tin, zinc, cobalt, silver, vanadium, aluminum, and yttrium are necessary to produce a toxic response (Robbins, 1967). Ferguson et al. (1962) point out that ions of all alloys presently in use in humans are found in the tissues around implants in rabbits. The toxicity of a particular element depends a great deal on its dissolution rate and rate of removal. That is, the degradation rate of the implant controls the toxicity to some extent. Corrosion is the degradation and loss of substance from a solid material through chemical interaction with its environment. Corrosion of implant metals is reduced by passivation, which is the formation of an adherent metal oxide (Dumbleton and Black, 1975). Corrosion is not an important clinical problem with implants. Although some of the constituents of metallic alloy implants can be toxic, the low corrosion rate of prosthetic metals minimizes the adverse effects. The various tissues of the body, bone, muscle, blood, and so on are affected by particular poisons in different ways and to different extent merely because of the nature of the tissue (Robbins, 1967; Anderson, 1971).

Encapsulation of an implant by the body is another factor in the biological response to an implant. In an attempt to phagocytize an implant of large size, cells may coalesce to form giant cells, which then surround an implant. These cells, each unable to engulf the implant, together form a fibrous encapsulation with healthy tissue separating the implant from the body. Even the most nontoxic impervious orthopedic implants are often found to be walled off from the body with this fibrous tissue (Laing et al., 1967) (see Fig. 9.1). Mechanical trauma due to moving muscles in soft tissue has been found to accentuate the fibrous encapsulation reaction to implants (Davila et al., 1968).

Another biological response that might result from an implant is the formation of neoplasms. A *neoplasm* is a new growth of an abnormal collection of cells whose growth exceeds and is uncoordinated with that of normal tissue and may be malignant, benign, or undefined. The possible formation of these growths is a very serious concern of the surgeon (Harrison et al., 1976).

A necessity in the use of materials for applications in the musculoskeletal system is attachment. Many applications require only short-term attachment that is readily, and in most cases acceptably, achieved with screw fixation. Other implants require long-term fixation to accomplish their function. Present technology is such that polymeric materials are used as space-filling agents to diffusely transfer the stress of prostheses to bone as a means of attachment.

Other techniques of attachment are under study, although still in the experimental stage. One possibility is the use of porous material either as a prosthetic material or as a coating for a solid prosthesis or orthosis. The concept that is being exploited is that bone surrounding the implant will grow into small holes or pores in the surface of the implant, thereby providing fixation. Studies in animals have shown that ingrowth of bone occurs if the pore size is greater than 100 $\mu$m (Klawitter and Hulbert, 1971). Some of the types of materials being considered are porous coatings of titanium balls on the surface of implants, sintered fiber–metal composites, porous polyethylene, and porous polysulfone coatings. These are at present at the stage of clinical trials in animals and limited trials in humans.

Because biological systems seldom have consistent sizes and shapes, a certain amount of flexibility in implants is necessary to allow operating room alterations. This, of course, can compromise strength and durability not only by changing design but by changing the internal stress states in the material. Designs are required that can be implanted with a minimum of trauma and tissue dissection, which would delay healing and increase morbidity.

Sterilization is, of course, an absolute requirement and can be accomplished by three main techniques. These are heat, chemical, or radiation. It is possible to change properties and designs by sterilization, so the choice is important. Heat or gas cannot be used for polyethylene because of residual effects such as warping or absorption of gas. All techniques can be used for metals (Webster and Cook, 1979).

## Materials Used for Implantation

**Metals.** Three metals are in common usage as implant materials. These three are stainless steels, cobalt-based alloys, and titanium and its alloys. None of these is clearly superior to the other but each provides advantages for certain applications.

Stainless steels used for implants are iron-based alloys (solutions) of multiple other elements that enhance and maintain the stability of the structure, the strength, and the corrosion resistance of the alloy. The crystalline structure of stainless steels

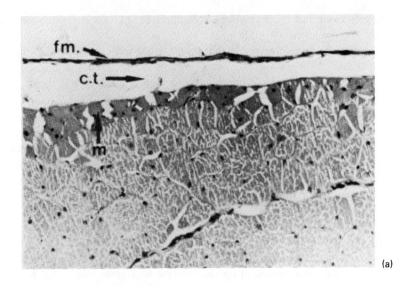

(a)

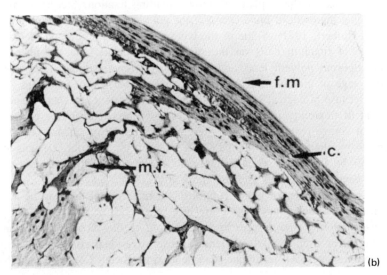

(b)

**FIGURE 9.1.** Examples of tissue response to various materials. Zircalloy is a zirconium alloy. Vespel SP-21 is a polyimide. Pyroceram is a ceramic material produced by crystallization of glass. (From Escalas et al., *J. Biomed. Mater. Res.* 10: 175–195, 1976 with permission of John Wiley and Sons.) (a) Microphotograph of the tissues in contact with a solid 316L stainless steel control sample. A very thin fibrous membrane (f.m.) adjacent to the implant is shown, separated from muscle fibers (m) by a very poorly cellular connective tissue layer (c.t.). The fissuring apparent in the muscle is a fixation artifact. (b) Microphotograph of the fibrous membrane (f.m.) and ad-

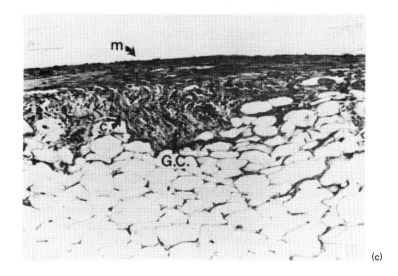

(c)

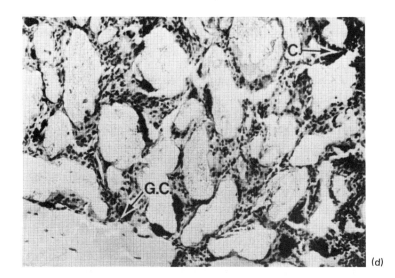

(d)

jacent tissues in a solid sample of Zircalloy. The membrane appears extremely thick and moderate cellularity is present in its basal layers. Muscle fibers (m.f.) show centrally located nuclei. (c) This photomicrograph of the fibrous membrane (m) around a solid specimen of 9608 Pyroceram, shows a very abundant underlying fibrous and small round cells proliferation (c) with occasional giant cells (g.c.). (d) Clusters of inflammatory small round cells (c) are abundant in the tissue proliferation between particles of Vespel SP-21. Conventional foreign body giant cells (g.c.) are abundant in this microphotograph.

used for implants is face-centered cubic and this structure is called *austenite*. The designation of this steel by the American Iron and Steel Institute is AISI 316LVM. The composition is shown in Fig. 9.2. Each element performs a particular function in the alloy. Molybdenum raises the resistance to chloride environment but cannot be used in excess because it causes embrittlement of the steel. Chromium causes the production of chromium oxides, which form the stable, protective oxide surface film. Carbon is a detrimental element, which is removed partially by vacuum melting. Its removal improves corrosion resistance because its presence reduces the chromium oxide stable surface film by forming chromium carbide. Nickel and chromium both stabilize the austenitic crystal structure of the steel, preventing the transformation to other structures that have inferior properties. These other structures of stainless steel are commonly magnetic and, thus, magnetic implants should not be used. The physical properties are somewhat variable depending on the treatment history but typically have a yield strength of between $2.4–7.9 \times 10^8$ N/$m^2$ depending on the amount of cold working, a modulus of $2.0 \times 10^{11}$ N/$m^2$, and a tensile strength of $5.5–9.6 \times 10^8$ N/$m^2$ depending on the amount of cold work. These are standards specified by the ASTM (1978). Strength is also dependent on grain size or average size of the crystal in the steel, surface finish, and inclusions. A larger grain size reduces the strength. A surface finish that is rough predisposes to fatigue or corrosion failure. Inclusions can cause much the same problem and can greatly increase corrosion rates if on the surface.

The cobalt-based alloys are primarily made up of cobalt-chromium with lesser quantities of several other elements. The compositions (see Fig. 9.2) vary somewhat depending on whether the alloy is for casting or for implants that need subsequent shaping. The cobalt-chromium alloy in the face-centered cubic crystal structure provides a better corrosion resistance. The cobalt-chromium alloys are cast into shapes as accurately as possible for finishing by grinding because the hardness prevents the use of conventional metal-cutting tools. Slight composition changes allow some cold working (wrought alloy). In the cast condition, the cobalt-chromium alloys have an ultimate tensile strength of $6.5–7.2 \times 10^8$ N/$m^2$ with a 0.2% yield strength of $4.5 \times 10^8$ N/$m^2$. The wrought alloy has a cold-worked ultimate tensile strength of $10^9$ N/$m^2$. The modulus of elasticity of these alloys is $2.4–2.5 \times 10^{11}$ N/$m^2$, which is stiffer than steel (ASTM, 1978).

Pure titanium and its alloy of 6% aluminum and 4% vanadium have been found to be well tolerated by tissue and to be extremely inert from a corrosion viewpoint (see Fig. 9.2). This is because the very stable oxide of titanium that forms on the surface is extremely tenacious and readily reforms if damaged. Titanium has a lower elastic modulus of $1.03 \times 10^{11}$ N/$m^2$ and has a yield strength of about $5.5 \times 10^8$ N/$m^2$ with an ultimate strength of about $6.2 \times 10^8$ N/$m^2$, which increases somewhat with the alloying effects of the aluminum and vanadium. Titanium in the pure form is hexagonal close-packed in crystal structure. The addition of the vanadium alters the structure to body-centered cubic, while aluminum stabilizes the hexagonal structure. Combinations of the two structures from the addition of both elements have better mechanical properties without loss of the corrosion resistance.

| Element | Stainless steel | Cobalt chromium (wrought) | Cobalt chromium (cast) | Titanium (grade 1) | Titanium 6Al-4V |
|---|---|---|---|---|---|
| Iron | 59-70 | 3.0 Max | 0.75 Max | 0.20 Max | 0.25 Max |
| Cobalt | — | 49-58 | 57.5-67 | — | — |
| Chromium | 17-20 | 19.0-21.0 | 27.0-30.0 | — | — |
| Nickel | 12-14 | 9.0-11.0 | 2.5 Max | — | — |
| Titanium | — | — | — | Balance | Balance |
| Aluminum | — | — | — | — | 5.5-6.50 |
| Vanadium | — | — | — | — | 3.5-4.5 |
| Carbon | 0.08 Max | 0.05-0.15 | 0.35 Max | 0.10 Max | 0.08 Max |
| Manganese | 2.00 Max | 2.00 Max | 1.00 Max | — | — |
| Phosphorus | 0.030 Max | — | — | — | — |
| Sulfur | 0.030 Max | — | — | — | — |
| Silicon | 0.75 Max | 0-1.00 Max | 1.00 Max | — | — |
| Molybdenum | 2.00-4.00 | — | 5.0-7.0 | — | — |
| Tungsten | — | 14.0-16.0 | — | — | — |
| Nitrogen | — | — | — | 0.03 Max | 0.05 Max |
| Hydrogen | — | — | — | 0.015 Max | 0.0125 Max |
| Oxygen | — | — | — | 0.18 Max | 0.13 Max |
| Other | — | — | — | — | 0.40 Total |

**FIGURE 9.2.** Summary of ASTM composition of implant materials. (Compiled from ASTM (1978), part 46, pp. 477, 480, 483, 487 and 500.)

These three materials are all now presently on the market as implants in various applications. From a tissue acceptance and corrosion viewpoint, each of the materials in their cast or wrought forms are very similar. Mechanically, there is very little to separate the different metals. Perhaps the most important future concern mechanically will be the low modulus of elasticity of titanium and its alloys because of the possibility of more closely matching the properties of bone. Differences in ultimate strength and maximum strain are really not too important because the design of the prosthesis or orthosis should prevent utilization above the yield strength. Stainless steel is perhaps somewhat more corrosion susceptible because its preimplant passivation treatment can be compromised by physical damage.

**Polymers.** Four main types are used as implant materials for internal prosthetics and orthotics. These are ultrahigh-molecular-weight polyethylene (UHM-WPE), polymethylmethacrylate (PMMA) and its copolymers, polytetrafluoroethylene (Teflon), and the silicones. Other polymers are used as suture materials but these are not discussed. Each of the three polymers finds particular application depending on its special properties.

Polymers are materials made of long-chain molecules with repeating units that number into the millions (Mark, 1967). These long-chain molecules are formed from single units by a chemical reaction initiated by various additives. Exact control of the reaction is somewhat difficult and results in variations in samples from batch to batch. The molecular weight, the amount of branching or side chains on the main chain of molecules, and the amount of crystallization all have considerable bearing on the properties of the polymer.

Ultrahigh-molecular-weight polyethylene (RCH-1000, Hifax 1900) has become indispensable as one-half of the total joint system for any of the successful total joints on the market today (see Fig 9.3). In contact with stainless steel or the cobalt-chromium alloys, it exhibits excellent wear behavior and frictional properties (Galante et al., 1975). UHMWPE is the product of polymerization of ethylene ($H_2C = CH_2$) a two-carbon hydrocarbon. Molecular weight has been found to have a significant effect on the properties in that higher molecular weight results in a denser, stronger, and less ductile material with little change in biological properties. Side branching from the main chain of the molecular structure results in decreased strength and crystallization because side chains hinder molecular alignment. The degree of crystallization is expressed as a percentage because there are "islands" of crystallization from the random alignment of chains during the freezing process. Ultrahigh-molecular-weight polyethylene has a crystallinity of as much as 90% because there is little side branching. Because it is a thermoplastic compound in which temperature increases cause softening and eventual melting, it requires cold sterilization techniques to avoid distortion.

Polymethylmethacrylate (PMMA) is the base polymer for a commercial polymer sold under the brand name of Simplex P used for fixation of prostheses to bone. The structure of polymethylmethacrylate is based on the repetitive unit of methylmethacrylate, an organic compound with a carbon double bond such as found in ethylene (see Fig. 9.3). This commercial PMMA is provided as a powder and a liquid. The powder consists of PMMA and a PMMA polystyrene copolymer with

| Polymer | Structure of repetitive unit | Tensile strength $(10^4\,\mathrm{Pa})$ | Reference |
|---|---|---|---|
| Polyethylene | 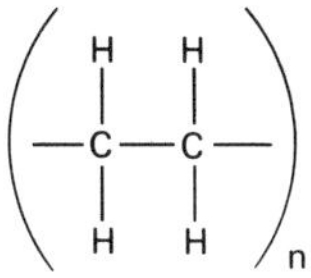 | 4.4 | Dumbleton and Black (1975) |
| Polymethylmethacrylate | 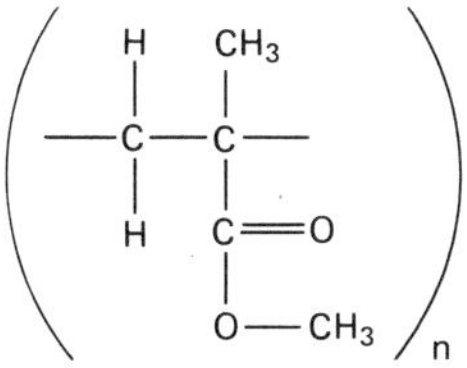 | 4.8–7.5 | Dumbleton and Black (1975) |
| Simplex P | 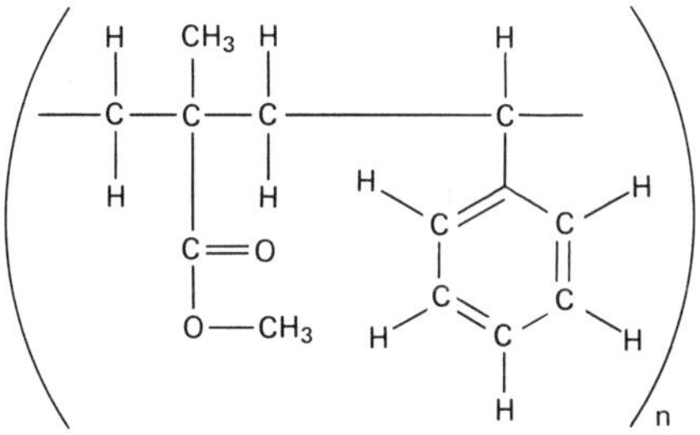 | 4.5 | Dumbleton and Black (1975) |
| Silicones | 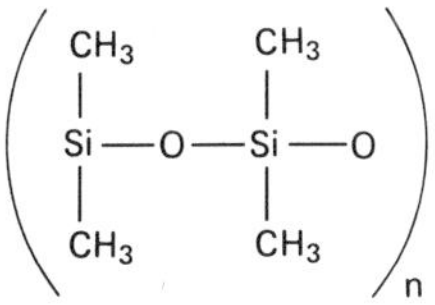 | Very variable | |
| Polytetrafluoroethylene | 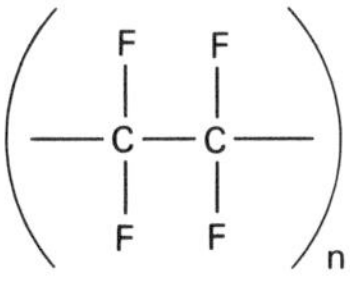 | 1.7–3.1 | Billmeyer (1966) |

Polyethylene repetitive unit:

$$\left(\begin{array}{c} \overset{\displaystyle H}{\underset{\displaystyle H}{|}}\ \overset{\displaystyle H}{\underset{\displaystyle H}{|}} \\ -C-C- \end{array}\right)_n$$

Polymethylmethacrylate repetitive unit: backbone —C—C— with H, H on one carbon and CH$_3$, C=O, O—CH$_3$ on the other.

Simplex P repetitive unit: —C—C—C— ... —C— with CH$_3$, C=O, O—CH$_3$ groups and a benzene ring (styrene unit).

Silicones repetitive unit:

$$\left(\begin{array}{c} CH_3 \quad\; CH_3 \\ Si-O-Si-O \\ CH_3 \quad\; CH_3 \end{array}\right)_n$$

Polytetrafluoroethylene repetitive unit:

$$\left(\begin{array}{c} F \;\; F \\ -C-C- \\ F \;\; F \end{array}\right)_n$$

**FIGURE 9.3.** Structures of polymeric biomaterials shown with tensile strengths.

barium sulfate added for radiopacity. A vial of monomer is also provided with stabilizers, accelerators, and catalysts distributed between the two components. A combination of these two, solid and liquid, causes polymerization of the monomer to bond the spherical particles of copolymers together with a polymethylmethacrylate matrix. These are provided in a sterile condition to the surgeon who mixes them at the operating table, inserts the material into the cavity for the prosthesis, and places the prosthesis into the cement and waits for polymerization to occur (about 10 min) to provide rigid fixation of the prosthesis to the bone.

Considerable investigation of the properties and kinetics of the PMMA system have been undertaken in the interest of providing the strongest, safest grouting material for fixing prostheses to bone (Charnley, 1970). Because the process of polymerization is so exothermic, bone-cement temperatures have been measured as high as 60°C. The rate of the reaction is of considerable interest to the surgeon because placement of the cement in bone at the appropriate stage is a crucial portion of the operation. Many variables affect this, including room temperature, body temperature, and so forth. Mechanical properties of the cured poly-methylmethacrylate are poor. The elastic modulus is $1.4-3.4 \times 10^9$ N/m² and the tensile and compressive strength are $4.5 \times 10^7$ and $8.9 \times 10^7$ N/m² respectively. These properties may be reduced even further by various additives, which may be added preoperatively or intraoperatively. For example, antibiotics such as gen-tamicin have been incorporated in the acrylic to improve infection resistance. This has given mixed results and probably lowers the strength of the acrylic. Similarly, during the placement of the cement in the bone, blood almost invariably becomes laminated into the acrylic and thereby weakens the acrylic. Overall, poly-methylmethacrylate is the best attachment technique for prostheses to bone yet available but leaves much to be desired.

The silicones are a type of polymer based on a silicon–oxygen–silicon repeti-tive unit (see Fig. 9.3) with the name polydimethylsiloxane, which can be made in varying molecular weights. Properties vary with molecular weight and cross-linking from fluids to a class of materials called silicone rubbers. The silicone rubbers are used in plastic and reconstructive surgery and in orthopedic surgery in low-stress applications. The consistency of the silicone rubber is such that it "feels" like cartilaginous structures. The silicone rubbers have poor mechanical properties and tear easily without fillers such as silica to strengthen them. They are tolerated by tissue and do not seem to be degraded by the body environment.

Polytetrafluoroethylene (Teflon) is similar to polyethylene in structure (see Fig. 9.3) and properties. It is affected by crystallization and temperature in a similar fashion to polyethylene. Its low coefficient of friction promoted its use in early total joint replacement but its tendency to flow under stress caused it to be abandoned. It is now used as one of the components in a material called Proplast used for plastic and reconstructive procedures.

**Ceramics.** Ceramics are a class of materials that are either compounds of at least one metal and one nonmetal or a single nonmetallic element. Examples are metal oxides and glasses. Most of the ceramics that have been tested in vivo for compatibility have been found to be biocompatible with tissue if dissolution of a toxic substance does not occur. Because most ceramics are insoluble in water, they are generally biocompatible. The only ceramic that at the present time is finding clinical application in a commercial product is aluminum oxide. It is being used in the bearing surface components of total hip prostheses. Aluminum oxide is very hard and quite strong in compression, although less so in tension. The strength (Semlitsch et al., 1977) of commercial $Al_2O_3$ is $4 \times 10^9$ N/m² in compression and

$3.5 \times 10^8$ N/m$^2$ in tension, both minimum values. Carbon, in several of its forms, is finding use as a biomaterial. Its crystal structure is either amorphous or hexagonal depending on the method of manufacture. It can be applied as an amorphous coating on other materials, or can have a glassy structure and appearance as well as fiber and fabric configurations. It is well tolerated by tissue and is insoluble and thus does not degrade in vivo. Mechanical properties vary markedly with form (Benson, 1971). It is being used in fiber form to strengthen Proplast, a porous Teflon–carbon fiber composite. Although ceramic materials are very good from a compatibility viewpoint, their mechanical properties, particularly their tendency to fail catastrophically at relatively low stress, have made their application as biomaterials unattractive.

**Tissue Response to Implant Materials.** The response of tissue to metals depends primarily on chemical and mechanical factors. We have already mentioned toxic response to corrosion products. Of the three primary implant metals, only stainless steel corrodes significantly. Corrosion is seldom clinically important except perhaps in some patients who complain of pain until the implant is removed. Corrosion of stainless steel primarily occurs where two metal surfaces are in contact, for example at a screw-plate interface. Titanium is found in tissues in relatively high concentrations adjacent to implants but provokes very little tissue response. Stainless steel and the cobalt-chromium alloys tend to develop an encapsulating fibrous capsule, much more so than titanium. Titanium and its alloys are indicated for patients who have demonstrated an allergic dermatitis reaction to nickel, which is present in both of the other implant alloys.

The tissue response elicited by any of the common implant materials is quite dependent on the size, shape, and surface morphology. Implantation of powders of metals and polymers produces varying reactions that are particle-size dependent (or surface-area dependent) and perhaps material dependent (Galante et al., 1975). Coarse powders of stainless steel produce minimal reaction while fine powders produce marked fibrosis and inflammation. Powders are important because they are generated as wear particles in joint replacements.

Tumors have been formed in experimental animals but these have not been material dependent but more dependent on the chemistry, morphology, and size of the implant. Larger implants or those with large impervious surfaces tend to cause more tissue reaction, probably because of mechanical trauma caused by soft tissue movement around the implant. Porous materials constructed of any biocompatible material generally provoke much more favorable tissue reactions. Malignant tumor formation from implants of any of the common materials in humans has never been demonstrated.

Evaluation of the tissue response of polymers must be made only on medical grade polymers to be meaningful. Commercial polymers are produced with numerous additives, catalysts, colorants, accelerators, fillers, and so on. For example, the use of a catalyst other than stannous octate for crosslinking silicone rubber polymers makes them unsafe for implantation because toxic catalysts are not removed during curing. When the common medical-grade polymers, polyethylene and polymethylmethacrylate, are tested, the tissue response is relatively benign. Remember, however, that except for the silicones, polymers have the same bonds as are found in biological systems. Thus, radioactive tracer studies have shown exchange of labeled carbon from implant to host.

Polymethylmethacrylate has two features that cause additional problems. The first is that in vivo polymerization produces a high local temperature that causes thermal damage to at least some of the cells in the adjacent area. Also, at the time of polymerization, excess monomer is given off, collected by the bloodstream, and can cause hypotension at the time of polymerization.

In summary, PMMA, UHMWPE, and silicone preparations cause only a minimal foreign-body reaction, with a thin fibrous tissue capsule, unless the physical form of the implant is altered.

In cases of wear particles, such as might occur with UHMWPE as a component in joint arthroplasty, a more inflammatory response is observed with deposition in lymph nodes. When the low-molecular-weight fluid form of silicone rubber is injected, fibrosis and cyst formation and mild chronic inflammatory reactions are observed.

The tissue response to the mechanical aspects of prosthetics and orthotics has long been neglected. The moduli of elasticity in conjunction with the appropriate geometric factor cause a difference in the flexural rigidity, torsional rigidity, and axial rigidity of implants in relation to bone. This difference is probably one of the major causes of loosening of prostheses at the attachment interface with bone. Because of the relative unloading of bone by prosthetic and orthotic components firmly attached to bone, a disuse osteoporosis occurs. This osteoporosis results from resorption of bone because of the lack of stress upon it.

## 9.4 PROSTHETICS

### Introduction

Prostheses have been developed primarily for the replacement of a joint in one of the extremities. Arthroplasty is the surgical treatment of joint diseases to relieve pain and improve motion (Williams and Roaf, 1973). The hip joint, the articulation between the femur and the pelvis, enjoyed most of the earliest work. This was probably due in part to the severe disability caused by problems with the weight-bearing joints at the hip and the knee.

Total joint arthroplasty is indicated (is appropriate as a medical treatment) in patients with severe destruction of the joint such that pain and limitation of motion are disabling. Usually, total joint arthroplasty is not indicated until conservative (nonsurgical) methods have failed in controlling the pain and disability. Destruction of joints occurs from a number of causes. Probably the most common cause is arthritis, a general term that refers to a vast number of diseases but that primarily refers to two or possibly three diseases (Turek, 1967). The most disabling of the arthritides is rheumatoid arthritis, which is an inflammatory disease of the soft tissues of unknown cause that causes severe destruction of the joint surfaces. The second main type of arthritis is osteoarthritis, which is a type of wear-and-tear arthritis that nearly everyone develops if they live long enough because of use of the joint. An increasingly frequent type of arthritis, similar to osteoarthritis, is traumatic arthritis. This arises from traumatically produced irregularities in the normally smooth surfaces of joints.

Although severe disabling arthritis is the main indication for arthroplasty surgery, individual joints have other indications. For example, nonunion of fractures around the femoral neck, aseptic necrosis of the femoral head (death of the bone of the femoral head due to a variety of causes), and fractures of the femoral neck in patients too old to tolerate the long periods necessary for healing of the fracture are relative indications for total hip replacement. The sequellae of childhood diseases such as congenital dislocated hip and other diseases that result in deformed femoral heads can cause severe arthritis, which requires arthroplasty.

The alternatives to total joint arthroplasty are very limited. The only alternative that provides as much pain relief is fusion, or causing bony union across the joint. For young patients with disabling arthritis of the hip or knee who need to be able to carry on heavy labor, fusion is a viable alternative in that it gives a painless, rugged replacement for the joint. Of course, it is not suitable for a patient who requires that he have motion at his hip or his knee. Fusion does not eliminate the possibility of future arthroplasties so that fusion may be accomplished early in life and later on converted to total joint arthroplasty. This may be an excellent idea when considering the state of the present art of total joint arthroplasty.

### Hip Prostheses

In the early 1960s, Charnley (1970) developed a total hip replacement to essentially its present state by using a high-density polyethylene acetabular component articulating with a metal femoral component, which were both cemented in place. This provided a "low-friction" arthroplasty that was firmly attached on both sides to bone. This is approximately where total joint replacement is now. Since that time, total knee replacement, total elbow replacement, total ankle replacements, and other joints have been designed. The total hip replacement has met with the greatest success because of its great success in relieving pain and providing motion. The total knee and other joints have been less successful.

The hip joint is a ball-and-socket joint for which the pelvis forms the socket for the femoral ball. It is a stable joint in that more than half of the head of the femur is contained within the socket or acetabulum. The anatomy allows free movement in all planes while being stabilized for weight transmission by the powerful muscles surrounding it (See Fig. 9.4).

Hip prostheses replace the function of the hip and thereby relieve the symptoms of arthritis in the hip. These symptoms are typically anterior thigh pain and groin pain, particularly with motion of the hip, accompanied by decreased motion due to destruction of the joint surfaces of the hip. The hip tends to have stiffness, particularly after rest, and the patient develops a limp due to muscle spasm around the hip. The diagnosis is obvious from the physical examination of the patient and from the x rays of the hip. Nonoperative treatment consists of cane or crutches to reduce weight-bearing stresses on the hip, accompanied by mild anti-inflammatory and analgesic drugs.

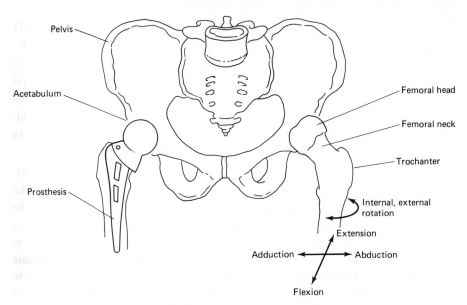

Pelvis

Acetabulum

Prosthesis

Femoral head

Femoral neck

Trochanter

Internal, external
rotation

Extension

Adduction ← → Abduction

Flexion

**FIGURE 9.4.** Austin-Moore type of prosthesis used for hemi-arthroplasty for femoral neck fractures and aseptic necrosis. The prosthesis is placed into a reamed cavity in the femoral shaft after excision of the femoral head.

When nonoperative treatment fails to relieve the symptoms of hip pain and decreased motion, operative treatment is considered. Three possibilities exist. One of these is hemiarthroplasty of the Austin-Moore or Thompson endoprosthesis type in which the femoral head is replaced by a ball identical in size to the femoral head connected to a stem that goes down the intramedullary shaft of the femur (see Fig. 9.4). The second possibility is total hip replacement (THR) in which an acetabular component and a femoral component similar to the Austin-Moore prosthesis combine to renew both joint surfaces. Both components are cemented in place with PMMA. This is currently the standard procedure for severe arthritis of the hip (Fig. 9.5). The third technique is surface replacement arthroplasty, which has an acetabular component similar to the total hip component but only has a cup that fits over the femoral head after a small amount of sculpturing of the femoral head (Fig. 9.6). These components are cemented in place in a manner similar to the two components of the total hip replacement (see Fig. 9.7).

The hemiarthroplasty of the Thompson or Austin-Moore type is indicated for fractures of the femoral neck in people over 60, in some cases of aseptic necrosis of the femoral head in which the acetabulum and its cartilage are in good condition, and in nonunions of the femoral neck. Its advantage is that, by an operation of less than one hour, the patient can be gotten out of bed and ambulated in a very few days with nearly full weight bearing. The prosthesis does not provide total pain relief and has problems with loosening in the femoral shaft and with migration of the metal ball into the pelvis. The Thompson prosthesis can be cemented into the femoral shaft to avoid the femoral loosening problem.

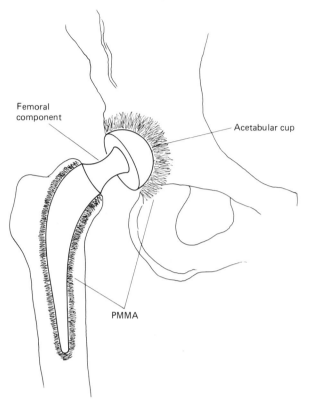

Femoral
component

Acetabular cup

PMMA

**FIGURE** **9.5.** "Low-friction arthroplasty." Drawing illustrates the components of total hip replacement. The femoral component is metallic, the acetabular cup is UHMWPE, and the shaded material is PMMA used as a grout to obtain fixation of the implants.

Surface replacement arthroplasty is a compromise between hemiarthroplasty and total hip replacement (Freeman, 1978). It is a relatively new technique, having been developed in the last few years. It can be used in cases in which there is severe arthritis in the hip and the acetabulum but in which the bone stock of the femoral head is normal. It has been used in younger patients because it is a smaller operation that preserves the possibility of either conversion into a THR at a later date if failure should occur or of conversion to a fusion of the hip if a complication such as infection should occur. Surface replacement anthroplasty cannot be used in cases of aseptic necrosis or other diseases in which the femoral head and neck are severely distorted.

Total hip replacement (THR) has been remarkably successful in alleviating the pain and disability experienced by patients with hip arthritis. There are many brands of THR, which are named after various prominent orthopedists who have had a hand in developing them. Basically, however, they all consist of a high-density polyethylene cup with ridges on the outer surface to allow cement fixation to the acetabulum and a metal femoral component that is placed into the femoral shaft after amputating the femoral head at the base of the femoral neck (see Fig. 9.5). Prior to implantation, the metal components are sterilized by steam and the high-density polyethylene components are radiation sterilized. Various sizes and shapes are usually available prior to surgery to allow for individual variations in the

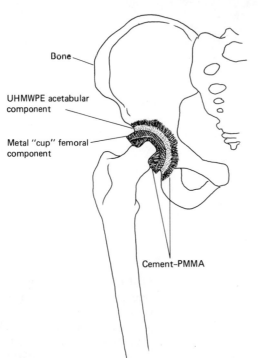

Bone

UHMWPE acetabular
component

Metal "cup" femoral
component

Cement–PMMA

**FIGURE 9.6.** Surface replacement arthroplasty. A thin metal cup is cemented to the head of the femur and a thin MW cup is cemented to the acetabulum. Note that much more bone stock is saved than in Fig. 9.5.

patient. The placement of the two components is crucial to providing a long-term good result. Incorrect placement of the polyethylene cup can result in dislocation of the femoral component. Placement of the femoral component such that the distal end (towards the foot) is against the lateral cortex of the femur increases the bending moment on the prosthesis and can hasten fatigue failure and loosening. The coefficient of sliding friction of the femoral head and the acetabulum lubricated with normal synovial fluid is roughly 0.002, while that of cobalt-chromium alloy on ultrahigh-molecular-weight polyethylene is approximately 100 times greater unlubricated. This is important because the frictional torque tends to loosen the two components. Wear of the prosthesis has been a matter of concern but has not proven to be a problem. Wear rates have been on the order of 0.15 mm per year. The primary causes of failure are infection, loosening, recurrent dislocation, and component breakage (Charnley, 1975). Problems with loosening, wear, dislocation, and failure can be relatively easily managed by replacement of components. The problem of infection, however, cannot be disposed of so easily. Careful precautions are taken to avoid infection in the dangerous stage of implantation. Laminar airflow filtration in the operating room to remove bacteria and extra precautions in preparations for surgery in terms of extra drapes for the patient and garb for the surgical team are used in addition to preoperative, intraoperative, and postoperative antibiotics (Brady et al., 1975). These precautions are taken because eradication of an infection that becomes seeded in and around a prosthesis can seldom be achieved without taking the prosthesis out. Furthermore, the infection may progress to

| Prosthesis | Indication | Components femoral | Material acetabular | Fixation |
|---|---|---|---|---|
| Hemi-endoprosthesis (Austin-Moore, Thompson) | Femoral neck/head pathology | Femoral head intramedullary stem/stainless steel or Co-Cr alloy | — | Impaction into intramedullary canal |
| Total hip replacement (Charnley, C.A.D.) | Femoral head, neck Acetabular pathology | Smaller femoral head, stem/stainless steel, Co-Cr alloy or titanium | Thick UHMWPE cup | Simplex P cement fixation to both intramedullary canal and acetabulum |
| Surface replacement arthroplasty (Wagner, THARIES) | Femoral head, acetabular pathology Neck should be normal | Thin femoral head shell/ stainless steel, or Co-Cr alloy | Thin concentric polymeric cup/ UHMWPE | Simplex P cement fixation acetabulum and to top of femoral head |

**FIGURE 9.7.** Summary of presently available prosthetic components for the hip. Names in parenthesis refer to the surgeon who first introduced the prosthesis.

osteomyelitis (bone infection) and become extremely difficult if not impossible to cure, leaving the patient with open draining wounds for the rest of his life. Even if the infection is controlled, placement of a second prosthetic arthroplasty has a high likelihood of recurrence of infection. Thus, after removal of the prosthesis and eradication of infection the patient is left with a hip joint with no articulating surfaces, which is called a Girdlestone operation. The patient then walks with a lurching gait because of the instability at his hip.

### Total Knee Replacement

**Design Considerations.** The success of the total hip prosthesis stimulated attempts to achieve the same success with the total knee prosthesis. The basic approach has been to employ the same concept of a metal component articulating with a plastic component, with the two components cemented into the tibia and femur. The motions of the normal knee are, in addition to flexion and extension, rotation about the long axis of the leg and lateral rotation. This differs from the hip because its ball-and-socket does not restrict motion in any direction.

The knee in its normal motion of flexion and extension has a complicated motion, including sliding and rotation, because the radius of curvature of the femoral condyles is not constant (see Fig. 9.8). The hip's position in relation to the acetabulum is maintained by the anatomy while the knee is anatomically unstable. In the normal knee, medial and lateral ligaments and two central ligaments (the cruciate ligaments) stabilize the knee with the assistance of the muscles acting across the knee. We must account for these ligaments in some manner in total knee replacement, either by preserving them or accounting for their function in prosthesis design (Sonstegard et al., 1978). Tremendous forces are applied to the knee, as they are to the hip, in some cases approaching six times body weight. The design goals are to produce a prosthesis that will provide normal knee function, withstand the stresses applied to it, and function without complications for the life of the patient. Minimal bone resection is desirable.

The indications for performing total knee replacement (TKR) are to relieve pain, restore stability, and permit a functional range of motion in cases of disabling arthritis of the knee. The indications for TKR are essentially the same as for knee fusion except for motion restoration. The state of the art of TKR is such that it only started in the early 1970s. Thus, long-term follow-up data are not available. The operation at this time should only be performed on the patient over 55 years of age with severe disabling symptoms, younger persons with relatively short life expectancy, or other mitigating factors, because proof of reliability has not been demonstrated for more than ten years.

Loosening of the implant, fracture of the tibia under the implant, and infection are the early problems with a total complication rate of perhaps 10%.

Again, careful precautions are taken to prevent infection, which can result in removal of the implant. Salvage procedures for the patient who has had total knee replacement prostheses removed include knee fusion and amputation. At this point, the type of prosthesis used becomes very important because a prosthesis that required removal of a great deal of bone stock is going to make knee fusion more difficult and result in a much shorter limb for the patient. Some shortening is desirable, although 3.5–5.0 cm, as might result from some types of TKR, is too much. Amputation may be a late sequela of an osteomyelitis that cannot be eradicated and a knee fusion that cannot be obtained.

Loosening and fracture under the implant are problems related to design. Failure to take into account that the dense bone in the tibia is very close to the joint can result in the placement of the prosthesis such that the weak trabeculae of bone readily fail. Similarly, designing a prosthesis shaft to be placed in either the femoral or tibial medullary canal without consideration of the torque that either of these shafts would have to transmit to the bone can readily result in loosening problems (Walker, 1977). In addition to allowing for the anatomy in terms of the motion that occurs at the knee, we also have to consider the moment arm each muscle group anteriorly and posteriorly has in relation to the center of rotation in flexion and extension. Moving the axis too far forward, for example, could drastically reduce the effectiveness of the quadriceps on the anterior of the thigh, weakening it to the point of instability of the knee. Functional range of motion of the knee is from essentially 0° of flexion to 100–110° of flexion. A smaller range of motion in flexion can drastically hinder such a function as rising from a chair. The problem of wear, which is unlikely to be of concern in total hip replacement, is of considerable concern in total knee replacement because of the difference in design. The design of many total knee replacement tibial components includes grooves that can readily collect wear debris and accelerate wear.

**Total Knee Replacement Design.** There are 200 or 300 total knee replacement prosthetic designs. Many of these are very similar and are named after a particular orthopedist or engineer who made a small modification to another design or had some idea that he felt would improve the function or the ease in insertion or attachment. Fortunately, these can be separated into three groups, based on whether the stability of the knee after TKR is dependent on the prosthesis, the ligamentous structures, or both. This concept is termed the *constraint of the prosthesis,* in that a fully constrained prosthesis needs no ligaments for a stable joint (see Fig. 9.9). The first group is the resurfacing type of prosthesis that replaces the surface of the femoral condyles. These are unconstrained in that they provide minimal stability to the knee. They are designed for knees that basically have a destroyed articulating surface without ligamentous instability. The prosthesis in some cases can be put in unilaterally, that is, on one of the condyles or on both condyles. The femoral shape is curved, either with a constant radius of curvature or with one that varies in a manner similar to the anatomy of the femoral condyle. Examples of this are the polycentric and the Marmor prostheses (Laskin, 1976). Little bone is removed.

The second type is the condylar type, which is an unconstrained, partially stabilizing prosthesis. In this type of prosthesis, the tibial component conforms very closely, in most cases, to the contour of the femoral condyle, providing stabilization. These prostheses tend to require removal of more bone for implantation. The artificial femoral condyles are designed to move in grooved, conforming polyethylene runners of the tibia. These are intended for patients with less ligamentous stability than in the resurfacing types. Examples of this are the U.C. Irvine and the geometric total knee replacements. The third type of prosthesis is the constrained

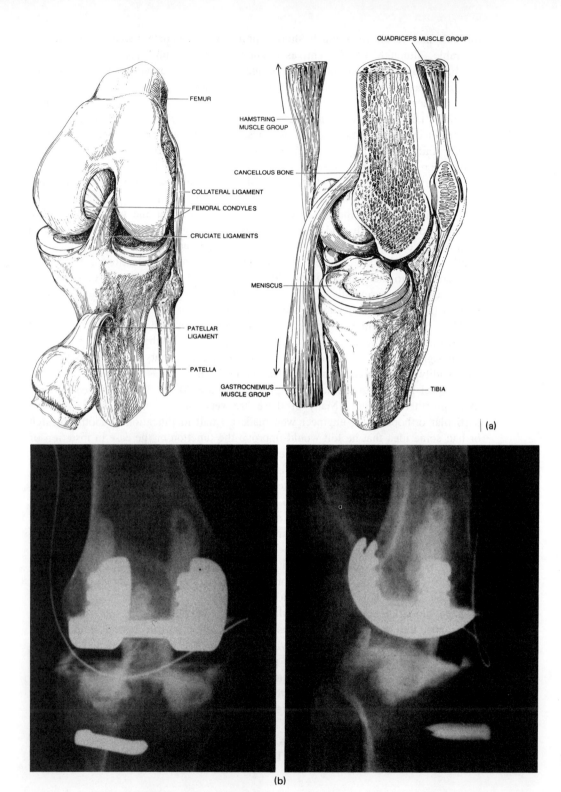

FEMUR

QUADRICEPS MUSCLE GROUP

HAMSTRING MUSCLE GROUP

COLLATERAL LIGAMENT

CANCELLOUS BONE

FEMORAL CONDYLES

CRUCIATE LIGAMENTS

MENISCUS

PATELLAR LIGAMENT

PATELLA

GASTROCNEMIUS MUSCLE GROUP

TIBIA

(a)

(b)

type, which is subdivided into hinges and ball-and-socket types. These prostheses are constrained because the femoral component is connected to the tibial component. This is indicated for the severely destroyed unstable knee often with severe angular deformity. This type, unfortunately, removes the most bone in order to provide the greatest stability. These prostheses have a greater tendency to loosening problems because their greater constraint transmits more of the forces to the interface between prosthesis and bone. Examples of this are the Spherocentric, which is the ball-and-socket condyle type, and the Guepar and the Walldius, which are two hinge-type prostheses.

**Problems.** There are many designs that have been tested in short-term studies. None have long-term follow-up (five years or greater) in any one disease entity. There are variations in the patient population and severity of disease in each patient. There are variations in surgical techniques. All of these problems lead to difficulty in interpreting the value of total knee arthroplasty and of particular designs. Total knee replacement prosthetic failure modes are loosening of the bone–cement interface, the cement–UHMWPE interface, and dislocation. Dislocation has been a rare complication associated with inaccurate prosthetic placement in unconstrained models. Loosening of the UHMWPE in the cement is a result of deformation of the tibial component from high stress levels.

Another problem in total knee arthroplasty and in total hip arthroplasty is cost. Each type of total arthroplasty design has a different set of instrumentation for implantation. This instrumentation tends to be stainless steel, tends to be produced in relatively low quantities, and has a very high cost. Further, to stock a prosthesis, for example, for a total knee, requires stocking two to three femoral sizes, two to three tibial sizes in width, and perhaps two to three different heights of tibial component in addition to having high medial sides and high lateral sides in the tibial component. Because of the high cost of a prosthesis (several hundred dollars) this results in a large investment for equipment for insertion and for stocking prostheses. This places a very large burden on a hospital to keep more than one type of prosthesis available for implantation. Most hospitals, therefore, stock only one model of prosthesis.

---

**FIGURE 9.8.** Facing page. (a) Normal left knee is depicted in views from the front and side. In the front view the knee is bent somewhat, exposing the interior of the knee and the arrangement of the ligaments. The side view portrays the main muscle groups that control the knee. Bending is done by the hamstring and gastrocnemius groups, straightening by the quadriceps group. Part of the femur has been cut away in the side view. (From Sonstegard, D. A. et al., Surgical replacement of the human knee joint, © Copyright (1978) by *Scientific American, Inc.* All rights reserved.) (b) Anteroposterior and lateral roentgenographic views of total knee replacement. The postoperative films show the Bechtol type of TKR in place. The bony notch in the center of the AP film shows that the cruciate ligaments have been preserved. Thus, the prosthesis is unconstrained. The lateral view shows that the prosthesis conforms to the shape of the condyles and, thus, is condylar.

| Prosthesis | Characteristics | Advantages | Disadvantages | Examples |
|---|---|---|---|---|
| Unconstrained | Resurfacing of femur. Nonconforming tibial component | Minimal bone resection. May be used for unilateral replacement. Ligaments retained may be difficult to insert | No contribution to stability. Can correct only mild deformity | Marmor Polycentric |
| Unconstrained partially stabilized | Resurfacing of femur. Tibial component conforms to femoral component | More bone resection. Conforming components more stable. May correct moderate deformity. Some provide patellar replacement | Greater potential for loosening. Ligaments sacrificed in some types. Collects wear particles | U.C. Irvine Geometric Total condylar |
| Constrained | (a) Hinge | Can correct marked deformity. Stable | Ligaments sacrificed. Large bone resection. Great potential for loosening | Guepar Walldius |
| | (b) Ball-and-socket types | Can correct marked deformity. Stable | Ligaments sacrificed. Large bone resection. Great potential for loosening | Spherocentric Stabilocondylar |

**FIGURE 9.9.** Summary of total knee replacement designs.

## Other Joints

The weight-bearing hip and knee joints are particularly prone to traumatic and degenerative arthritis. In addition, they are often involved in the other major crippling arthritis, rheumatoid arthritis. Perhaps because they are not weight-bearing, most of the other joints of the body are not nearly as involved with traumatic and degenerative arthritis. Rheumatoid arthritis, however, is a major cause of joint destruction in other joints. The number of joints other than the hip and knee with arthritis severe enough to require total joint arthroplasty is considerably smaller. Whereas in 1976 the number of total hips and knees implanted was on the order of 140,000–150,000, the total number of other joints was estimated to be around 10,000 (Hori et al., 1978). Arthroplasty of these other joints is performed primarily to relieve pain and secondarily to provide a functional range of motion.

**Metacarpal, Phalangeal, and Proximal Interphalangeal Joints.** The joints between the phalanges of the fingers and the metacarpals of the hand are nearly pure hinge joints. Ligaments stabilize the medial and lateral sides of the joints, while anteriorly and posteriorly, tendons maintain joint alignment (see Fig. 9.10).

Prior to implant arthroplasty of these joints, resection arthroplasty, or fusion were the only alternatives. Resection arthroplasty merely removed the joint, allowing the space to fill in with fibrous tissue, which provided a false joint. Fusion, of course, provided stability and relief of pain but no motion. In the last 15–20 years, two concepts of joint replacement have evolved. The first and most popular is the polymeric implant popularized by Swanson (1972a) and Niebauer et al. (1969) independently. This is actually only an improvement on the resection arthroplasty. The Swanson or Niebauer prosthesis is implanted to provide initial stability such that early motion of the joint can occur and encourage the formation of a stable fibrous capsule. They are relatively easy to implant and relatively easy to remove in case of failure. No cement is used. Fairly good results are obtained. The Swanson prosthesis differs from the Niebauer in that the Niebauer has a Dacron mesh to allow some tissue attachment to the stems.

The next level of sophistication in implant design for these joints is the mechanical metal–plastic type. Because these are relatively constrained types of prostheses, the complexities of motion and the multiple forces in these joints have to be considered in more detail. Some design considerations are discussed by Williams and Roaf (1973). Very important are stability, motion, and minimal wear debris. Joint axis of motion (of each joint), alignment of motion of all prosthetic joints, and strength are factors that deserve careful attention because of the fine function of the hand.

The mechanical metal-on-plastic hinge designs, including the Steffee, the St. Georg, the Schultz, and the Walker-Vari-axle, are in clinical trials with some early good results.

**Metatarsal Phalangeal Joint of the Great Toe.** This joint is a hinge joint similar to those in the hand. An elastomeric prosthesis of silicone rubber designed by Swanson (1972b) is available for use in conjunction with bunionectomies of the great toe. Pain relief and cosmesis are important, while motion is less important. It has been reported to improve on the results of resection arthroplasty. One consid-

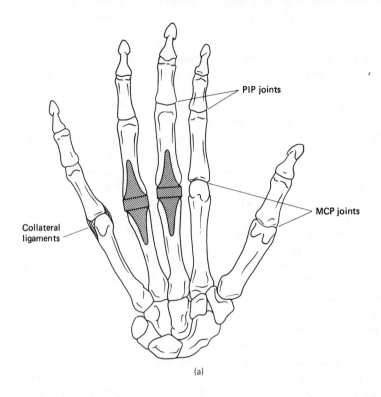

(a)

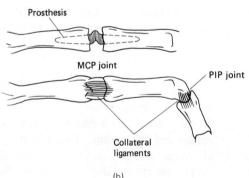

(b)

**FIGURE 9.10.** (a) Position of placement of Swanson-type silicone rubber flexible implants. Normal joint anatomy is demonstrated. They are often used to replace all four metacarpophalangeal joints. (b) Cross-sectional drawing of implant in position. Lateral view of typical metacarpal phalangeal joint and proximal interphalangeal joint (PIP) is shown.

eration that has to be borne in mind in metatarsal phalangeal joint replacement is the circulatory status of the foot. Poor circulation can greatly increase the risk of infection.

**Glenohumeral Joint.**    Total shoulder replacement (glenohumeral joint) has received relatively less attention than the hip and knee joint, perhaps because it is not a weight-bearing joint and, thus, arthritic pain is not as disabling. The glenohumeral joint is the articulation between the humerus (arm) and the scapula. It is a ball-and-socket joint with the humerus constituting the ball and the scapula, providing a very shallow socket (glenoid) against which only about one third of the humeral head can rest. This provides a wide range of motion but necessitates

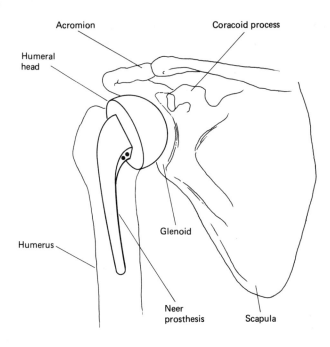

Acromion

Coracoid process

Humeral
head

Humerus

Glenoid

Neer
prosthesis

Scapula

**FIGURE 9.11.** The Neer prosthesis articulates with the glenoid. The prosthesis is analogous to the Austin-Moore for the hip in that it has a polished hemispherical joint surface with a stem that is placed in the intramedullary cavity.

muscle tension to provide stability. The scapula has a wide range of motion in relation to the rib cage to further increase the motion possible by the humerus. Total joint arthroplasty of the shoulder replaces the glenohumeral joint and is indicated for pain and loss of motion of the shoulder. The shoulder joint also can be fused to obtain a pain-free result that is quite functional because of scapulothoracic motion. The results of total joint arthroplasty of the shoulder have to compare favorably with those of fusion to be indicated. Hemiarthroplasty has been reported since about 1955 using a metal surface replacement similar to the Austin-Moore hip prosthesis with a stem design by Neer (1955) (see Fig. 9.11). A number of types of total shoulder arthroplasty prostheses have since evolved. The most popular one is the extension of Neer's prosthesis, in which a ultrahigh-molecular-weight polyethylene (UHMWPE) glenoid component similar to the anatomical glenoid is cemented to the scapula to articulate with the humeral component. Designs are now under study with ball and socket, which are self-retaining to improve stability and nonretaining in which the ball is on either the glenoid side or on the humeral side (Walker, 1977). The important considerations in the design are maintenance of the appropriate moment arms for the muscle acting around the joint to improve stability and, of course, the trade-off of stability against motion of the joint. The normal human joint has a tremendous range of motion and depends on the muscles around the joint for stability. A second major problem in total shoulder joint arthroplasty is the attachment of the glenoid component. In marked contrast to the hip, the scapula has minimal bone stock available for attachment of a prosthetic component.

**Ankle Joint.** The ankle is a hinge joint of the talus in the mortise formed by the tibia and fibula. The dome shape of the talus allows hinge motion in only the anteroposterior plane.

Total ankle replacement is available for patients with severe arthrosis of the tibiotalar joint. Designs mimic total hip replacement designs with a metal on UHMWPE bearing surface that resembles the anatomy of the ankle. These designs have been available for less than ten years and are in the clinical trial stage of testing. Early results are promising but have to be compared to the results obtained with ankle fusion (Manes et al., 1977; Evansky and Waugh, 1977).

**Elbow Joint.** The elbow joint is an articulation between the humerus and the two forearm bones, the radius and the ulna. Flexion and extension, and rotation of the radius around the ulna (pronation and supination) are the motions of the elbow joint. Trauma, degenerative arthritis, or rheumatoid arthritis may cause destruction of the elbow such that even the unsupported weight of the forearm and hand may cause severe pain. Previous alternatives have been resection arthroplasty and interpositional arthroplasty in which soft tissue is interposed between the bone of the elbow articulation. Arthrodesis or fusion of the joint is a possible alternative to total joint arthroplasty but is very difficult to accomplish. Soft tissue interpositional type of arthroplasty has produced mixed results. To be successful, total joint arthroplasty must relieve pain caused by flexion and extension motion between the humerus and ulna and allow radio-ulnar motion, that is, pronation and supination. The proximal end of the radius is often resected to permit this.

The total elbow has been approached from two viewpoints, that of the anatomic type of replacement and the hinge type of replacement. The forerunner of the anatomic elbow is the hemiarthroplasty of the humeral condyle, which duplicates the natural joint surface. This prosthesis gave satisfactory results. Ewald (1975) modified this prosthesis and constructed a polyethylene ulnar articulation and reported it to have encouraging early results. The hinge type of total arthroplasty was pioneered by Dee (1973) and now several other hinge types are available (Garrett et al., 1977). All of these are cemented into place between the ulna and the humerus (Fig. 9.12). A major problem faced by these prostheses is that the angle between the humerus and the ulna changes during flexion and extension and the radius transmits the forces from the hand to the ulna before they are transmitted to the humerus. This causes a loosening torque at the bone cement interface in the humeral component. Total elbow replacement is still in an early stage of development.

**Penile Implants.** Neurological problems, vascular disease, medications, and trauma can cause impotence (the inability to maintain a functional erection), but approximately 90% of patients have impotence from psychogenic problems. After the failure of treatment, including sex counseling and psychiatric therapy where necessary, consideration can be given to placement of a penile prosthesis. Attempts at prosthetic replacement for the treatment of impotence are perhaps 25 years old. In the last four or five years, the prosthetic replacement designed by Small et al. (1975) (SMALL-CARRION) has become the most popular prosthesis. The name of the prosthesis, taken from the names of its developers, is somewhat unfortunate, because patients seldom want the small prosthesis. The prosthesis consists of paired sponge-filled silicone prostheses that are placed into the corpora cavernosa of the penis. These have given excellent results, although some difficulty is encountered because the penis is in the erect position at all times. Variations on this have

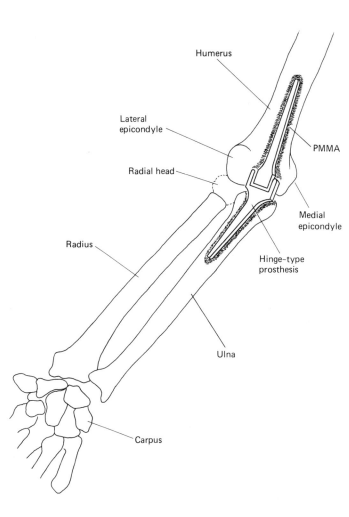

Humerus

Lateral
epicondyle

Radial head

PMMA

Medial
epicondyle

Hinge-type
prosthesis

Radius

Ulna

Carpus

**FIGURE 9.12.** A hinge-type elbow prosthesis is cemented in the ulna and humerus. The fore-arm anatomy is such that the radius is large in size near the hand while the ulna is large at the elbow. Both bones are small at their other ends. This means that stress must be transmitted between the two bones through ligaments. Forces on the hand, therefore, cause a large moment to be applied to the ulna because of its offset position. This contributes to the loosening of the constrained prosthesis.

evolved with a rigid shaft and a soft hinge at the base (Finney, 1977). Another approach to this same problem has been the inflatable prosthesis, which employs a reservoir implanted in the abdomen and a pump placed in the right hemiscrotum (Furlow, 1979). The main problem encountered with prosthetic replacement for the penis are pain when too large a prosthesis is implanted and infection, which occasionally requires the removal of the prosthesis.

**Augmentation Mammoplasty.** The augmentation mammoplasty utilizing implants became popular in the 1960s (Grossman, 1976; Georgiade, 1976). The breast today is looked on as a symbol of femininity and, as such, women with "deficient" breasts are apt to feel inadequate. Breast augmentation is performed for deficiency in bulk (micromastia), marked asymmetry, or atrophy, which commonly occurs after several pregnancies. The common implants in use today are the silicone gel implants manufactured with a thin silicone membrane, and the inflatable implant, also of silicone, but filled with normal saline.

Mentioned only to be condemned is silicone injection mammoplasty. Injection of silicone liquid was practiced in the late 1960s by both ethical and unethical practitioners, using medical grade and industrial grade silicone. Problems with injection of silicone liquids have developed, although sometimes several years after injection. Mastectomy was the usual treatment, although systemic effects have been reported.

The silicone bag implants are implanted beneath the breast tissue but above the chest-wall muscle. They have given satisfactory results in many cases. Recently, however, problems with fibrous encapsulation with gradual shrinking have been encountered. The shrinking tends to force the gel-filled membrane into a sphere, which distorts the breast contour. Research is now directed at preventing the fibrous capsule and breaking it up after formation. Infection is a constant danger with these implants and erosion of the implant through the skin can occur.

**Unsolved Problems.** Many of the total joint replacements just described have unsolved problems. In all fairness, we must state that only limited experience has been accumulated on some of the prosthetic designs. Therefore, the high rate of failure of some of the prosthetic joints will undoubtedly be improved as clinical experience is accumulated. One of the problems in prosthetic joint design has been the lack of suitable experimental models to test the prosthetic designs and while, admittedly, many poor design concepts have gone directly into human trials, trials in various experimental animals would probably have not yielded the information necessary to prevent these problems.

Wear is another problem that needs to be considered. A metal-on-polyethylene low-friction surface has a very low wear rate. Walker (1977) has estimated from a wear rate of 0.1 mm per year in total hips that the number of wear particles is above three billion. Wear rates, of course, are affected by the type of wear that is occurring and the presence of polymethylmethacrylate, which could conceivably become trapped between the metal polyethylene joint; particularly, in some knee prostheses in which the polyethylene joint would allow gravity collection, wear rates could be very high from gouging. In addition to high wear rates that might cause the prostheses to eventually fail, the wear particles are a problem as they are collected by the reticuloendothelial system and deposited in lymph nodes.

The problem of loosening of the attachments of prostheses from bone is a serious consideration in the long-term success of joint arthroplasty. There has been some work on polymer cements similar to PMMA that are biodegradable, but these have not been too promising. Reports of attachment of total hip arthroplasties with porous materials are preliminary but promising (Judet et al., 1978). Some concern has been expressed about the delay necessary to get bone growth into pores and about the difficulty in removing the prosthesis in the event of failure.

Dislocation of prostheses is a relatively uncommon problem but does occur in hips and knees (Etienne et al., 1978). It is largely a technique problem and is rare if components are installed correctly. Fatigue failure is encountered in total hip prosthetics but is only serious in heavy individuals.

Infection is a major cause of failure of prosthetic joint replacements. It is a devastating cause also because in many cases it means prosthesis removal and severe loss of function. The best approach is prevention with the use of antibiotics whenever a bacteremia is suspected. This would mean that procedures such as dental extractions, cleaning of teeth, or bladder instrumentation should be preceded by antibiotic coverage. The only suggestion that the problem may be reduced in the future is that porous materials have been reported to have increased resistance to infection over nonporous materials after tissue ingrowth is established (Merritt et al., 1979).

## 9.5 ORTHOTICS

### Introduction.

Internal implants began with fracture-fixation orthotics and this is still important today. The reasons for putting metal devices into the body to fix a fracture have to be weighed against the disadvantages. The disadvantages are many. Probably the most important risk is that of infection. This can often result in a situation much worse than the original fracture if the fracture had healed without any intervention at all. Application of some fracture fixation devices can actually prevent healing of the fracture by maintaining a separation between the fracture fragments. Further, placing a fixation device internally usually means that it has to be removed at a second operation. Also, surgery to place and remove the implant is usually much more expensive than the treatment of fractures without surgery. Often, although not always, internal fixation of fractures results in a longer time for the fracture to heal. Despite this, return to function often occurs much sooner with operative treatment of fractures.

One of the main proponents of internal fixation of fractures is a Swiss group called the Association for the Study of Internal Fixation (ASIF) (Muller et al., 1970). They maintain that it is much easier to treat the complications of internal fixation, namely infection and nonunion, than it is to treat the "fracture disease," which is joint stiffness and osteoporosis. The objective of the ASIF is to achieve early return to function of the injured limb and allow pain-free mobilization of the muscles and joints prior to healing of the fractures. The ASIF group is perhaps more aggressive in treating fractures with open technique than are physicians in the United States. Certain indications for surgery, however, are generally accepted. In most cases of joint incongruity from a fracture, internal fixation is indicated because treatment without internal fixation usually results in early traumatic arthritis of the joint and destruction of the cartilagenous surfaces. In other cases internal fixation is necessary to mobilize the patient to prevent or treat pulmonary problems because the patient is old and will not tolerate prolonged bed rest or because young patients have multiple organ system injuries. Often patients with fractures of multiple extremities can have their convalescent period drastically reduced by internal fixation of one or two fractures to allow ambulation of the patient. Ambulation can be permitted because upper-extremity internal fixation can allow crutch walking or lower-extremity internal fixation can allow partial weight bearing on other fractures treated by closed methods. Economic indications are becoming more and more prevalent. Treatment of a particular fracture with an in-hospital stay of eight weeks compared with a hospital stay of one week after an operation, thereby allowing the patient to return to work at one month postinjury rather than three months postinjury, becomes very important economically. Further, the public is demanding more and more surgery for internal fixation. A small amount of deformity that might result from closed treatment of a fracture becomes larger and larger in the mind of the public as time goes on. Internal fixation is also used for reconstructive procedures to correct angular deformities in a bone that has healed previously in an unacceptable position.

## Types of Hardware

Because of human frailties and human activities, people tend to injure themselves in much the same way, again and again. Many devices carrying the name of their inventor have been developed to treat these same types of fractures that occur over and over. The materials used for these fracture-fixation devices are stainless steel or sometimes one of the cobalt-chromium alloys. The ASIF group has manufactured a complete set of fracture fixation devices for small bone fractures, large bone fractures, and external fixation devices. Many other companies have produced similar devices. This can cause safety problems in a number of ways. Because of differences in composition between batches of stainless steel and differences that result from different mechanical working, the chemical activities of a plate and screw are likely to be such that electrochemical corrosion is thermodynamically possible. Thus, it is mandatory not to mix devices between manufacturers and particularly undesirable to mix stainless steel products with cobalt-chromium alloys. It is important to remember that materials replacing or augmenting function of the musculoskeletal system are going to undergo cyclic bending and torsional stresses that, depending on design, may be very high. The number of cycles on the hip or knee approaches $10^7$ in less than ten years for a patient who walks only two or three miles per day. Bone and soft tissue can remodel to accommodate stress; implants cannot and, therefore, must be designed to keep cyclic stress levels below the endurance limit for implants intended for long-term use. Surface scratches from handling can be points of fatigue crack propagation. Also, because the human body rarely has bony surfaces that are smooth and flat or canals in the center of bones that are straight, devices for bending plates and other fracture fixation devices are available. This also weakens the device by local increase of work hardening in addition to any surface damage that might be done. These are causes of device failure that must be avoided whenever possible.

**Long-Bone Fracture Fixation.** Long-bone fixation has primarily gone in two directions. The first of these is through the use of intramedullary rods that go down the center of a bone and thereby provide stability after fracture. These are primarily used for fractures near mid-shaft. Three nails or rods, the Kuntscher-type clover leaf nail (Kuntscher, 1967) the Hansen-Street diamond cross-section, and the Sampson-type (Allen et al., 1978) fluted nail are used for femur fractures, as shown in Fig. 9.13. These types of nails are used in tibias also. The Rush pins are probably used most for radius and ulna fractures but can be used for humerus fractures, fibula fractures, and various other bone fixations. The Sage nails are

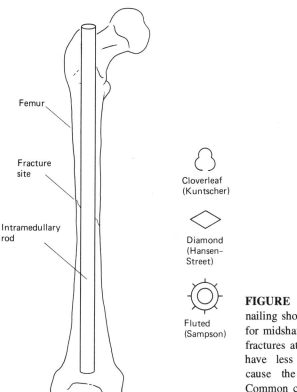

Femur

Fracture
site

Intramedullary
rod

Cloverleaf
(Kuntscher)

Diamond
(Hansen-
Street)

Fluted
(Sampson)

**FIGURE 9.13.** Intramedullary nailing showing optimal fixation for midshaft fractures. Note that fractures at the distal end would have less secure fixation because the bone widens out. Common cross sections of nails are shown.

designed specifically for use in the radius and ulna. Lottes nail is specially designed for placement in the tibia (Crenshaw, 1971). One more pin deserves mention here and that is the Steinman pin. This pin is used for traction treatment of many bones but especially the long bones of the leg, the femur and tibia, by placement transversely to apply traction.

Occasionally, long-bone fracture fixation can be obtained with screws if the fracture is an appropriate long spiral or oblique fracture, but usually screw fixation has to be supplemented with bone plates to provide adequate stability (Fig. 9.14). The rate of healing of long-bone fractures is optimized when compression is applied at the interface between the bone fragments. This is accomplished by screw fixation, by application of plates under compression with additional compression devices, and by the use of plates that have oval holes in which the screw is placed eccentrically, causing compression as the screw is tightened. Most bone plates are quite sturdy to resist the bending and torsional stress. Semitubular plates are used to best effect on fractures of bones that will be under minimal stress and have quite curved surfaces.

The biomechanics of long-bone fixation is quite important. Intramedullary rods, for instance, can often allow full use of the limb without external support because of their central location. Plates, however, even when applied to the proper

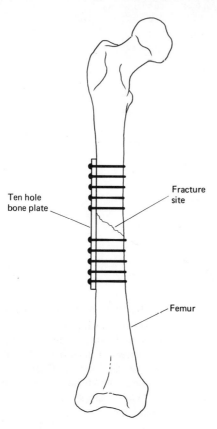

Ten hole
bone plate

Fracture
site

Femur

**FIGURE 9.14.** Diagram of use of a bone plate to fix a femur fracture. Notice that the screws go through ten cortices on each side of the fracture.

surface of the bone so that they are primarily under tension, will generally not be adequate to allow weight-bearing if applied to a tibia or femur without external support. Empirical evidence indicates that tibia fractures require screw fixation with at least six cortices of fixation on each side of the fracture, a much larger number than that for femur fractures. Lesser amounts of fixation provide inadequate stabilization of the fracture. Intramedullary rods, although very good for midshaft fractures, tend to be less effective for fractures at either end of the bone because their fixation in the short end is much less. In these cases, fractures need additional external support.

**Small Long Bones.** Internal fixation is used in fractures of the long bones of the hand and foot to allow healing to occur with a minimum of deformity and to allow maximal motion while healing is occurring. Fixation is not usually required to achieve healing. Most fractures of the hand and foot are fixed with Kirschner wires (Fig. 9.15), which are manufactured as smooth or threaded rods in various sizes up to about 1.5 mm in diameter. Fixation achieved with these wires is generally fair.

**Spinal Fractures.** The use of internal metallic orthoses to assist in obtaining spinal fusion in the thoracic and lumbar regions is a relatively new innovation. Previously, unstable fractures and scoliosis (curvature of the spine) were treated

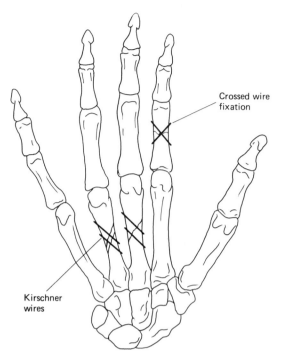

Crossed wire
fixation

Kirschner
wires

**FIGURE 9.15.** Kirschner wire fixation of oblique metacarpal fractures and crossed wire technique for transverse fractures of the phalanx.

with long-term plaster cast immobilization and bed rest to achieve stability through fusion of the spine. Internal stability is now achieved with the use of Harrington rods. These are essentially .64 cm diameter steel rods connected to hooks on each end that are placed beneath the lamina of a vertebra above and below the area to be fused (see Fig. 9.16). These can be placed either in compression or in tension, although they are usually used in applying tension to the spine. These are placed posteriorly on the spine and, because of the normal curve of the spine, this tends to straighten it. Harrington rods have been quite successful in achieving spinal fusion. Although quite useful in treating thoracolumbar spine fractures, their main use is in obtaining correction and fusion in cases of severe scoliosis. Scoliosis is lateral curvature of the spine. Cervical spine fusion requires little in the way of orthotic implant materials. Usually 18- or 20-gage wire is all that is necessary to achieve adequate fixation.

    **Fractures about the Hip.** Fractures of the proximal femur in the vicinity of the hip joint are problems encountered primarily in older people. Because this type of patient tolerates bed rest very poorly, there is a strong tendency to operate on these fractures to enable ambulation. These fractures can be divided into essentially two types; trochanteric fractures and femoral neck fractures (see Figs. 9.17 and 9.18). Femoral neck fractures typically present less of a mechanical problem than trochanteric fractures and are often treated with some sort of pin device, either a Knowles pin, Deyerle pin, or Hagie pin (Crenshaw, 1971), although they can be treated with a compression plate and nail as we describe for intertrochanteric fractures.

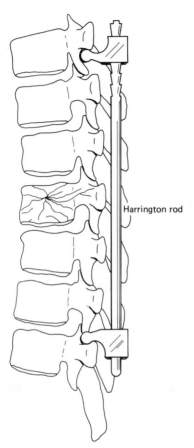

Harrington rod

**FIGURE 9.16.** Harrington rod fixation of a lumbar vertebra fracture. The hooks at the top and bottom are placed in the posterior elements and the rod is used to distract the fracture fragments. For fractures, usually two rods are used, one on each side of the spine.

Intertrochanteric fractures are often comminuted. Comminution of the intertrochanteric fracture usually means that the medial cortex of the femur has been disrupted in such a way that stable bony contact of the fracture fragments will not occur. This means that weight-bearing forces would have to be borne by the fracture-fixation device. This imposes large bending moments on the device with extreme fiber stresses approaching the elastic limit and certainly above the endurance limit for fatigue. Therefore, the strength of the device has to be very high. The devices that are used for intertrochanteric hip fractures are many but they are primarily an outgrowth of the Smith-Peterson nail with a Thornton side-plate, which is an outmoded device. One of the most popular similar devices is the Richards screw (see Fig. 9.18). The Ken nail and the Jewett nail are similar. The advantage that the Richards screw and the Ken nail type of device have is that the component placed in the proximal fragment, the femoral head, is able to slide through a barrel in the other component. This permits apposition of the fracture fragments as a function of time without having the device enter the hip-joint surface by cutting through the femoral head. Figure 9.19 shows fixation using Enders nails.

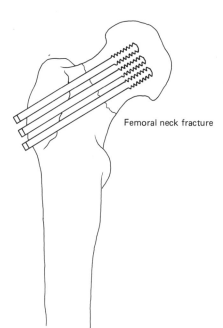

Femoral neck fracture

**FIGURE 9.17.** Femoral neck fracture fixation is shown with the use of Knowles pins. This technique is valuable for many femoral neck fractures. The pins are introduced from the side under x-ray visualization.

**Knee Fractures.** Intra-articular fractures of the knee can be particularly disabling. Treatment of distal intra-articular femur fractures requires anatomic alignment of the joint surfaces to achieve functional results. This can often be obtained with cancellous bone screws, which have large threads to grip the spongy (cancellous) bone in the knee area. Often, a blade plate is necessary when the femur is fractured proximal to the joint. A blade plate is a bone plate with a 90° bend in it, which forms a blade that goes into the condyle of the femur while the plate is attached to the side of the femur. On the other side of the joint, the tibial condylar fractures are quite common. These often require surgery, again with screws and sometimes with T-shaped buttress plates to provide a congruent joint surface.

**Ankle Fractures.** These require anatomic alignment of the joint surfaces such that even 2 mm of displacement can result in severe early traumatic arthritis of the ankle joint. Screws, pins, plates, and occasionally wires are used to reduce and hold these fractures in position to allow motion of the joint.

### Unsolved Problems

The primary problem encountered in internal fixation of fractures is the inability to obtain adequate fixation to allow motion of the adjacent joints. Comminuted fractures of almost any bone are examples of this problem. Examples of fractures that are commonly problems are elbow intercondylar and supracondylar fractures of the humerus and subtrochanteric fractures. The elbow becomes stiff and loses motion

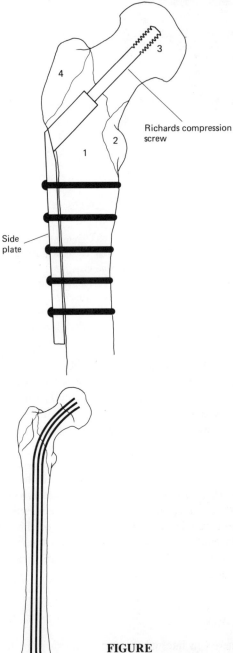

Richards compression
screw

Side
plate

**FIGURE 9.18.** Comminuted intertrochanteric fractures with 4 fragments present a challenge to obtain fixation because of the many pieces. Weight bearing places a large bending moment on the fracture fixation device. The Richard's type compression screw in the head of the femur slides in a barrel in the plate, allowing the fracture fragments to approximate.

**FIGURE 9.19.** Intertrochanteric fracture fixation with the use of Ender's nails. These are introduced at the knee and driven across the fracture at the hip with x-ray visualization.

easily after an injury. Movement of the joint after a fracture without causing motion of the fracture (which would encourage nonunion) is very important. Because the fracture occurs at or slightly above the condyles, there is little place to attach plates or other devices, even with wide exposure. Subtrochanteric fractures of the femur are usually comminuted and they are difficult because of comminution and are too high to be fixed with intramedullary nails. Other fractures present similar problems. Osteoporosis or the loss of bone mineral leaves bones with strengths that are too poor to achieve adequate fixation with screws. Patients with osteoporosis (including many postmenopausal women) have the same pulmonary problems and so on that require fracture fixation in normal patients. A better, different way of treating these patients is necessary.

Metal removal is a costly problem. It is recommended that most patients have their fracture fixation devices removed. This reduces the risk of osteoporosis beneath the device. One possibility would be biodegradable plates and screws. Metal removal is expensive from a hospital utilization point of view and from a patient work-loss viewpoint.

# REFERENCES

ALLEN, W. C., K. G. HEIPLE, and A. H. BURSTEIN (1978). A fluted femoral intramedullary rod: Biomechanical analysis and preliminary clinical results. *J. Bone Joint Surg.*, 60-A: 506–15.

AMERICAN SOCIETY OF TESTING AND MATERIALS (1978). *Annual book of ASTM standards,* Part 48: 181–82.

ANDERSON, W. A. D. (1971). *Pathology.* St. Louis: C. V. Mosby.

AUTIAN, J. (1967). Toxicological aspects of implants. *J. Biomed. Mater. Res.*, 1: 433–49.

BENSON, J. (1971). Elemental carbon as a biomaterial. *J. Biomed. Mater. Res. Symp.*, 2: 41–47.

BILLMEYER, F. W. (1966). *Textbook of polymer science.* New York: Interscience.

BRADY, L. P., W. F. ENNEKING, and J. A. FRANCO (1975). The effect of operating room environment on the infection rate after Charnley low-friction total hip replacement. *J. Bone Joint Surg.*, 60-A: 80–83.

CHARNLEY, J. (1970). Total hip replacement by low friction arthroplasty. *Clin. Ortho. Rel. Res.*, 72: 7–21.

CHARNLEY, J. (1975). Fracture of femoral prosthesis in total hip replacement: A clinical study. *Clin. Ortho. Rel. Res.*, 111: 105–20.

CRENSHAW, A. H. (ed) (1971). *Campbell's operative orthopaedics.* St. Louis: C. V. Mosby.

CRIMMENS, D. S. (1969). The selection and use of materials for surgical implants. *J. Metals,* 21(1): 38–45.

DAVILA, J. C., E. V. LAUTSCH, and T. E. PALMER (1968). Some physical factors affecting the acceptance of synthetic materials as tissue implants. *Ann. N.Y. Acad. Sci.*, 146: 138–45.

DEE, R. (1973). Total replacement of the elbow joint. *Ortho. Clin. N.A.*, 4: 415–33.

DUMBLETON, J. H., and J. BLACK (1975). *An introduction to orthopaedic materials.* Springfield, IL: Charles C Thomas.

ESCALAS, F., J. GALANTE, and W. ROSTOKER (1976). Biocompatibility of materials for total joint replacement. *J. Biomed. Mater. Res.*, 10: 175–95.

ETIENNE, A., C. CUPIC, and J. CHARNLEY (1978). Post-operative dislocation after Charnley low-friction arthroplasty. *Clin. Ortho. Rel. Res.*, 132: 19.

EVANSKY, P. M., and T. R. WAUGH (1977). Management of arthritis of the ankle. *Clin. Ortho. Rel. Res.*, 122: 110.

EWALD, F. C. (1975). Total elbow arthroplasty. *Ortho. Clin. N.A.*, 6: 685.

FERGUSON, A. B., JR., Y. AKAHOSHI, P. G. LAING, and E. S. HODGE (1962). Trace metal concentration in the liver, kidney, spleen and lung of normal rabbits. *J. Bone Joint Surg.*, 44-A: 317–22.

FINNEY, R. P. (1977). New hinged silicone penile implant. *J. Urol.*, 118: 585–87.

FREEMAN, M. A. R. (ed) (1978). U.C. symposium: Total surface replacement of hip arthroplasty. *Clin. Ortho. Rel. Res.*, 134: 2–102.

FURLOW, W. L. (1979). Inflatable penile prosthesis: Mayo Clinic experience with 175 patients. *Urol.*, 13: 166–71.

GALANTE, J. O., P. G. LAING, and E. LAUTENSCHLAGER (1975). Biomaterials, *Amer. Acad. of Orthoped. Surg. instructional course lectures*, 24: 1.

GARRETT, J. C., F. C. EWALD, W. H. THOMAS, and C. B. SLEDGE (1977). Loosening associated with G.S.B. hinge total elbow replacement in patients with rheumatoid arthritis. *Clin. Ortho. Rel. Res.*, 127: 170.

GEORGIADE, N. G. (1976). *Reconstructive breast surgery*. St. Louis: C. V. Mosby.

GROSSMAN, A. R. (1976). *Augmentation mammoplasty*. Springfield, IL: Charles C. Thomas.

HARRISON, J. W., D. L. McLAIN, R. B. HOHN, G. P. WILSON, J. E. CHALMAN, and K. N. MacGOWAN (1976). Osteosarcoma associated with metallic implants—Report of two cases in dogs. *Clin. Ortho. Rel. Res.*, 116: 253–57.

HORI, R. Y., J. L. LEWIS, J. R. ZIMMERMAN, and C. L. COMPERE (1978). The number of total joint replacements in the United States. *Clin. Ortho. Rel. Res.*, 132: 46–52.

JUDET, R., M. SIGUIER, B. BRUMPT, and T. JUDET (1978). A non-cemented total hip prosthesis. *Clin. Ortho. Rel. Res.*, 137: 76–95.

KLAWITTER, J. J. and S. F. HULBERT (1971). Application of porous ceramics for the attachment of load bearing internal orthopedic applications. *J. Biomed. Mater. Res. Symp. #2*, Part 1: 161–229.

KUNTSCHER, G. (1967). *Practice of intramedullary nailing*. Springfield, IL: Charles C. Thomas.

LAING, P. G., A. B. FERGUSON, and E. S. HODGE (1967). Tissue reaction in rabbit muscle exposed to metallic implants. *J. Biomed. Mater. Res.*, 1: 135–49.

LASKIN, R. S. (1976). Modular total knee replacement arthroplasty. *J. Bone Joint Surg.*, 58-A: 766-73.

LEVINE, S. N. (ed) (1968). Materials in biomedical engineering. *Ann. N.Y. Acad. Sci.*, 146: 1–359.

MANES, H. R., E. ALVAREZ, and L. ASLAVINE (1977). Preliminary report on total ankle arthroplasty for osteonecrosis of the talus. *Clin. Ortho. Rel. Res.*, 127: 200.

MARK, H. F. (1967). The nature of polymeric materials. *Sci. Amer.*, 217(3): 148–59.

Merritt, K., J. W. Shafer, and S. A. Brown (1979). Implant site infection rate with porous and dense materials. *J. Biomed. Mater. Res.,* 13: 101–8.

Moffatt, W. G., G. W. Pearsall, J. Wulff, and H. W. Hayden (1965). *The structure and properties of materials,* Vol. I, III. New York: Wiley.

Morral, F. R. (1966). Cobalt alloys as implants in humans. *J. Mater.,* 1: 384.

Muller, M. E., M. Allgower, and H. Willenegger (translated by J. Schatzker) (1970). *Manual of internal fixation.* New York: Springer-Verlag.

Neer, C. S. (1955). Articular replacement for the humeral head. *J. Bone Joint Surg.,* 37-A: 215–28.

Niebauer, J. J., J. L. Shaw, and W. W. Doren (1969). Silicone-dacron hinge prosthesis design evaluation and application. *Ann. Rheum. Dis.,* 28: 56.

Robbins, S. L. (1967). *Pathology.* Philadelphia: W. B. Saunders.

Semlitsch, M., M. Lehmann, H. Weber, E. Doerre, and H. G. Willert (1977). New prospects for a functional life-span of artificial hip joints by using the material combination polyethylene/aluminum oxide ceramic/metal. *J. Biomed. Mater. Res.,* 11: 537–52.

Small, M. P., H. M. Carrion, and J. A. Gordon (1975). Small-Carrion penile prosthesis: New implant for management of impotence. *Urol.,* 5: 479–86.

Sonstegard, D. A., L. S. Matthews, and H. Kaufer (1978). The surgical replacement of the human knee joint. *Sci. Amer.,* 238(1): 44–51.

Sullivan, B. A., C. A. Holmsey, and G. W. Woods (1978). Stabilization of Thompson femoral head prosthesis with a porous stem coating—A case report. *Clin. Ortho. Rel. Res.,* 137: 132–36.

Swanson, A. B. (1972a). Flexible implant arthroplasty for arthritic finger joints: Rationale technique and results of treatment. *J. Bone Joint Surg.,* 54-A: 435.

Swanson, A. B. (1972b). Implant arthroplasty for the great toe. *Clin. Ortho. Rel. Res.,* 85: 75–81.

Turek, S. L. (1967). *Orthopedics principles and their application.* Philadelphia: J. B. Lippincott.

Van Vlaak, L. H. (1970). *Material science for engineers.* Reading, MA: Addison-Wesley.

Walker, P. S. (1977). *Human joints and their artificial replacements.* Springfield, IL: Charles C. Thomas.

Webster, J. G., and A. M. Cook (eds) (1979). *Clinical engineering: Principles and practices.* Englewood Cliffs, NJ: Prentice-Hall.

Williams, D. F., and R. Roaf (1973). *Implants in surgery.* London: W. B. Saunders.

## STUDY QUESTIONS

**9.1**   What are the three major types of materials used in implants and what are the advantages and disadvantages of each?

**9.2**   Describe the response of the body to a foreign body.

**9.3**   Which metals are commonly used for implants? Why are they desirable?

**9.4** What are the three polymers commonly used as implants and what typical applications does each find?

**9.5** What problems can be encountered with the use of industrial-grade polymers for implant materials?

**9.6** What is the primary alternative to total joint arthroplasty?

**9.7** What advantages does surface replacement arthroplasty offer over THR?

**9.8** What are the complications (or failure modes) of THR? What possible methods can be used to correct these problems?

**9.9** Why was metal-on-UHMWPE an advance over previous metal-on-metal bearing surfaces for joint replacement?

**9.10** What is the constraint of a prosthesis?

**9.11** What are the types of TKR?

**9.12** How could the differences in design between TKR and THR account for the greater incidence of loosening of prosthesis in TKR?

# Electro-surgical Equipment

# 10

G. Guy Knickerbocker
John J. Skreenock

## 10.1 LEARNING OBJECTIVES

Upon completing this chapter you will be able to:

- Describe the therapeutic effects resulting from electrosurgery.
- Describe the means by which electrosurgical currents are generated, controlled, and applied.
- Describe the hazards associated with these devices.
- Evaluate the various factors that affect performance and safety of these devices.
- Enumerate the guidelines and standards applicable to this class of instruments.
- Set up a preventive maintenance program specific to these devices.
- Formulate a program for user education.

## 10.2 INTRODUCTION

Near the turn of the century, the use of electric current for lighting and motive force had been well established. High-frequency currents generated with spark-gap devices were just beginning to be used for long-distance communications (Marconi, in Newfoundland, received the first overseas radio message from England in 1901). But even by this time, first steps in electrosurgery had been taken. Thompson in

1889 and d'Arsonval in 1891 had demonstrated that high-frequency currents could be passed through the body with heat generated but without shock and muscular stimulation (Elliott, 1966).

In the first decade of the twentieth century, spark-gap currents were used to treat lesions. Step-by-step progress was made, and well within the first quarter of this century virtually all of the electrosurgical techniques we know today—fulguration, desiccation, cutting with a sinusoidal current—had been explored and used clinically. In 1928, Cushing and Bovie, (1928) advanced the use of electrosurgery by bloodlessly removing brain tumors using equipment designed by W. T. Bovie, a physicist. An era began then, so notable that, to this day, Bovie's name is still widely applied as essentially synonymous with the term "electrosurgical unit" despite the fact that it, rightfully, is the trademark of only one manufacturer.

Today, hardly an area of the healing arts does not use electrosurgical devices in one way or another. They are used to create essentially bloodless entry into the body for general surgery, to excise tissue masses from virtually every organ of the body, to treat and remove lesions from the skin, to remove unwanted hair, and to control bleeding. They are found in surgical suites, emergency rooms, physicians' offices, dental offices, and even in the practice of veterinary medicine.

This chapter explores the several technical aspects of these devices that are related to their performance and safety. This subject matter deals with techniques that use high-frequency currents to achieve surgical effect and for which we use the commonly accepted term *electrosurgery*. *Surgical diathermy* is another term that is frequently, and correctly, used synonymously. The inappropriate use of the term *electrocautery*—which refers to the application of instruments heated by the passage of electric current through the instruments themselves—in place of "electrosurgery" should be avoided. Electrocautery is covered in Chapter 11.

## 10.3 MECHANISMS OF THERAPEUTIC EFFECT

In electrosurgery, current from the generator usually flows through the patient's body to cause a therapeutic effect. Figure 10.1 shows that at the surgical site, an electrode couples current from the delivery cable to the body. The current density at that point is sufficiently high that adequate local heating creates controlled tissue destruction. The electrosurgical effect is governed principally by the geometry of the electrode, the amplitude and waveshape of the electrosurgical current, and the duration of the application. Commonly recognized electrosurgical therapeutic effects are cutting and coagulation.

### Cutting

The leading edge of an electrosurgical electrode has a relatively small surface area and is of negligible frontal area. When it contacts tissue, current from the electrode passes to the tissue at very high density. The tissue offers an electrical resistance whereby a limited zone at the edge of the electrode is heated rapidly and intensely

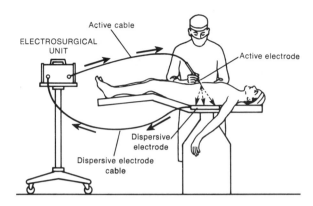

**FIGURE 10.1.** An electrosurgical unit in use. Arrows indicate flow of electrosurgical current in a complete circuit. (Adapted from *Health Devices,* Vol. 6 (3–4), 1977, ECRI, Plymouth Meeting, PA.)

by Joule heating. As a result, the cellular water in that area is rapidly volatilized. Tissue is cleanly cut and the effect is as if a very sharp knife had been drawn through the tissue.

Undamped, continous sinusoidal currents characteristically yield clean electrosurgical cuts. There is, however, little or no control of bleeding accompanying the cutting action when such a continuous wave is used.

### Coagulation

The cells adjacent to the electrode during cutting volatilize rapidly. The tissue falls away and does not increase in temperature sufficiently to achieve denaturation of the protein in the tissue. Coagulation to seal tissue and overcome oozing and bleeding is accomplished by one of two techniques. One is *desiccation*—and the other is *fulguration*. In both cases, the heat flows into the tissue from the site of application of the current. The temperature rises sufficiently in a finite band of tissue near the electrode to attain drying or tissue destruction without volatilization.

Desiccation occurs when the electrode is in intimate contact with the tissue. Current spreads into the tissue with adequate current density to raise the temperature sufficiently to destroy cellular components. The waveshape of the current is of relatively little importance in determining the effectiveness of desiccation. The area of contact of the electrode must be sufficient, and the current or power level low enough, to avoid volatilization of cellular fluids in the surface tissue layers.

Coagulation is also achieved by the technique of fulguration. The generator supplies a high open-circuit voltage with the electrode held a short distance above the tissue to be coagulated. Effective fulguration results with a waveform of high crest factor [ratio of peak (crest) voltage to effective (rms) voltage] and short duty cycle. The high voltage (often several thousand volts) ionizes the air gap between electrode and tissue and creates a spark. The spark is quickly quenched and the energy delivered to the tissue at the foot of the spark diffuses into the tissue before the next spark. The sparks tend to dance over the tissue and no one spot is bombarded repeatedly. This spreads superficial coagulation over an area with little penetration and without any excavation as would occur during cutting.

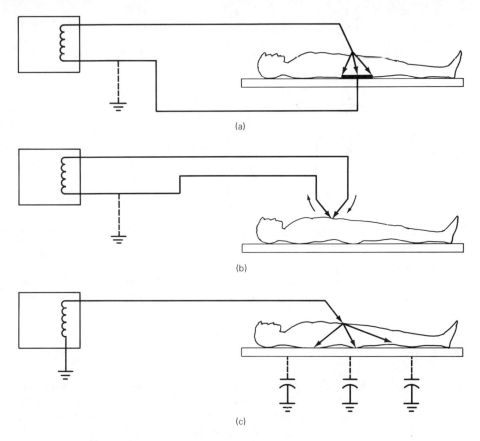

**FIGURE 10.2.** Functional circuit for electrosurgery. (a) Diterminal-unipolar. (b) Diterminal-bipolar. (c) Monoterminal.

## 10.4 MODES OF OPERATION

A generator of radio-frequency energy causes current to flow in the region to be treated to achieve the electrosurgical effect. At least one electrode, together with the conductor that connects it to the generator, is involved in the circuit. Terminology that describes the rest of the circuit has not been consistent. We use the terms *monoterminal* and *diterminal* (usually called *biterminal*) to denote whether a single conductor, or two conductors, complete the circuit between generator and patient. The more conventional terms—*unipolar* and *bipolar*—describe the configuration of the electrode applied to the surgical site as shown in Fig. 10.2.

### *Diterminal Mode*

In the diterminal mode, cables are provided for the entire circuit from the generator to the electrodes. A unipolar electrode configuration uses a single electrode connected through a cable to one of the output terminals of the electrosurgical genera-

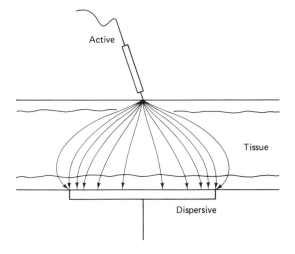

**FIGURE 10.3.** Current is concentrated at the smaller active electrode site to create therapeutic effect, while it is diffused at the larger dispersive electrode, thus minimizing heating at this site.

tor. We usually call this electrode the *active electrode* and obtain a therapeutic effect because current density at the site where this electrode contacts tissue is high enough for heating to occur. We apply a second electrode to a second site on the patient in an area uninvolved in the surgical procedure. The area of this second electrode is large. This reduces the current density in the tissue lying immediately beneath the electrode to a low value. Thus the temperature rise at this site is negligible (Fig. 10.3). This second electrode has been commonly called the *ground* electrode but, because many electrosurgical generators have an ungrounded or isolated output, such a term is frequently inappropriate. Because its function is to disperse current safely at this site of contact to avoid burns, it is appropriate to call it the *dispersive electrode* and we will do so throughout this chapter. It has also been referred to as the return, inactive, or neutral electrode.

In certain cases, we can avoid the use of a dispersive electrode by bringing a second electrode into the immediate region of the active electrode and restricting the current pathway through the patient to the electrosurgical site. Figure 10.4 shows this bipolar (occasionally called biactive) electrode. It is widely applied in neurosurgery when each of the blades of a pair of special forceps is connected to

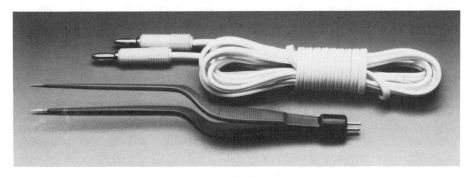

**FIGURE 10.4.** A bipolar electrode with cable. (Courtesy of Aspen Labs, Inc., Littleton, CO.)

respective output terminals of the generator and used to coagulate bleeding vessels during surgical procedures on the brain. Bipolar forceps, used through an endoscope, are also increasingly used as one means for female sterilizations in which the fallopian tubes are coagulated, and sometimes severed, to prevent pregnancy.

There are risks inherent in the use of unipolar electrodes and these are reduced when the bipolar electrode assembly is used. However, the future awaits the development of acceptable active bipolar electrodes for general surgical use, particularly those intended for cutting applications.

### Monoterminal Mode

At the radio frequencies of electrosurgical currents, the capacitance between the patient and the surrounding space and grounded surfaces presents a low impedance. Thus, it is possible to carry out electrosurgical procedures without the use of the dispersive electrode and its associated cable. This is the monoterminal mode. (Fig. 10.2).

The technique is usually restricted to those procedures that require low power and it can only be accomplished with generators in which one of the output terminals is grounded or ground-referenced. It is more effective in those generators that have a high operating frequency or are rich in harmonic output. However, the monoterminal mode suffers at least two significant disadvantages that restrict it from more widespread use and, in fact, suggest that the use of diterminal mode is to be preferred. First, the capacitive coupling between patient and ground is a variable that depends on the patient's position in the room, size, and other factors that can lead to inconsistent electrosurgery. The second is a most important disadvantage. Because the electrosurgical generator is of the grounded type, if the patient has an inadvertent conductive contact with a grounded object, this contact can become the preferred pathway for the electrosurgical current. If the contact involves only a small area of the patient's body, a burn can occur at the contact.

## 10.5 ELECTROSURGICAL CURRENT WAVEFORMS AND GENERATORS

The electrosurgical generator generates the necessary waveforms, amplifies them, controls them, and delivers them to the patient. In this section, we discuss the ensemble of waveforms that are commonly used for electrosurgery and the output configurations that deliver them.

### Waveform

The principal electrosurgical effects, cutting and coagulation (particularly, fulguration), are achieved with radio-frequency currents that have different waveforms. Cutting currents are most effective if sinusoidal in form with little or no modulation. Effective fulguration currents are highly modulated with high ratios of peak-to-effective current (crest factor). Although crest factor is widely regarded as a prominent descriptor by which the relative cutting or coagulating properties of a given electrosurgical current can be predicted, it is probably not the sole determining factor.

Figure 10.5 shows various electrosurgical currents. The continuous wave (CW) or unmodulated sinusoidal current (Fig. 10.5a) is used for its clean cutting characteristic with virtually total absence of any coagulating or hemostatic capability. It is equally well generated by vacuum-tube technology and the solid-state technology that has rapidly taken a place of prominence in electrosurgery. Frequency of this waveform ranges from approximately 250 kHz to 4 MHz.

The spark-gap waveform shown in Fig. 10.5b has spanned the entire history of electrosurgery and continues to be supplied by several electrosurgical device manufacturers. It is generated by the cyclic discharge of the energy supplied to, and stored in, an inductive coil and occurs when the voltage across a series of air gaps exceeds the breakdown strength of the air in the gaps (Fig. 10.6). The resulting discharge causes the system to oscillate at a frequency determined by the coil's inductance and the capacitance connected across the terminals of the coil, a discharge that decays in accordance with the well-known behavior of damped oscillatory systems. Because the coil is normally energized at line frequency, a random burst of cyclic discharges occur around each peak of line voltage or at twice line frequency. Typically, the frequency of the damped oscillations is of the order of 500 kHz. The waveform is rich in harmonic content.

Waveforms such as those in Fig. 10.5c, in which a carrier is modulated by a 60-Hz signal, unrectified, half- or full-wave rectified, have been widely used for practical reasons. They provide characteristics that are a blend of cutting and coagulating characteristics. These characteristics can be generated by tube or solid-state technology with stable performance, and the generators do not require the frequent adjustment typical of many spark-gap units.

Many generators can combine two waveforms, one with a predominant cutting characteristic, the other coagulating. This provides simultaneous cutting and hemostatic control. Hence the designation of this mode called *blend*.

The ease with which solid-state technology can be employed to generate a vast spectrum of pulsed and shaped waveforms has led to its widespread use in electrosurgery. A block diagram of a typical solid-state generator is shown in Fig. 10.7. Figures 10.5d and e also show examples of electrosurgical currents generated in solid-state units. For some time, solid-state electrosurgical units could not duplicate the coagulation characteristic that the spark-gap generators enjoyed. As a result, urologists, who relied upon the unique characteristics of the spark-gap, stuck tenaciously to the use of this type of generator for transurethral prostatectomies in which hemostatic control is of utmost importance. Newer solid-state devices increasingly permit improvement and units made with them challenge the supremacy of the spark-gap capability for coagulation.

### Output Configuration

Figure 10.8 shows the three broad classes of output circuits. Two of them are grounded configurations. In the directly grounded configuration of Fig. 10.8a, one end of the output coil is directly connected to ground. In the ground-referenced

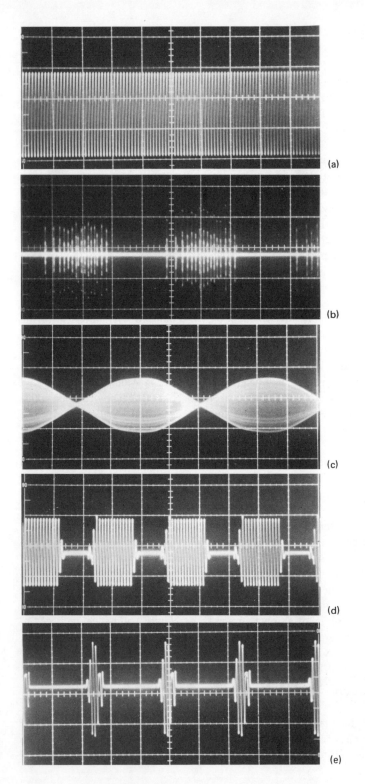

**FIGURE 10.5.** Electrosurgical current waveforms. (a) Continuous wave used for cutting (20 μs/div). (b) Spark-gap generated waves with coagulating characteristics (2 ms/div). (c) Modulated wave with cutting and coagulating characteristics (2 ms/div). (d) Solid-state-generated blended waveform with moderate hemostatic characteristics (20 μs/div). (e) Solid-state-generated waveform for coagulation (20 μs/div).

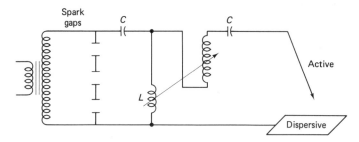

**FIGURE 10.6.** Spark-gap circuit.

configuration of Fig. 10.8b, grounding is accomplished with a frequency-dependent impedance, normally a capacitor.

At electrosurgical frequencies, there is no essential difference in performance of these two configurations. A disadvantage of the former, sufficient to cause it to fall into disuse, is that the grounded terminal, normally connected to the dispersive electrode, serves to ground the patient directly. Consequently, the patient is placed in an unfavorable situation. Should he be contacted by another electrically operated device, he would provide a good grounding pathway for any fault currents from that device. With the use of a ground-referenced electrosurgical unit, the current that passes through the patient from faulty equipment, at least at power-line frequencies, is limited.

Both forms of grounded devices share a common shortcoming, which leads to the third type of output. Should the dispersive electrode cable become open-circuited during use of a grounded-output electrosurgical unit, any other grounded object that may be in contact with the patient can serve as a return pathway for electrosurgical currents. This problem is mitigated if the output circuit is not directly or indirectly grounded (to the extent that it is possible given the parasitic capacitances associated with any electrical circuit) and the isolated output circuit of Fig. 10.8c results. We discuss other factors that affect the selection and application of output configuration later in this chapter.

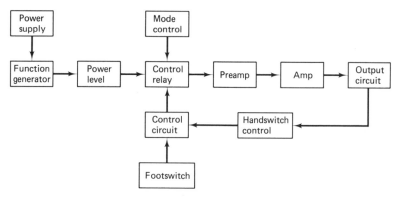

**FIGURE 10.7.** Block diagram of a typical solid-state generator.

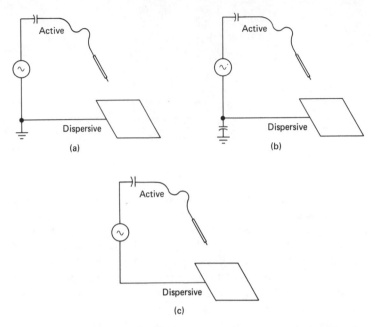

**FIGURE 10.8.** Characterization of output circuits of electrosurgical units. (a) Directly grounded. (b) Ground referenced. (c) Isolated.

Figure 10.8 also shows a capacitor in series with the active cable. This passes all the desired RF current that produces electrosurgical heating but blocks all the low-frequency currents that might be generated in the output circuit and lead to a risk of shock and neuromuscular stimulation.

## 10.6 ELECTRODES AND ACTIVATION CONTROLS

Electrodes and the means by which the electrosurgical generator is switched on are important in assuring both safety and performance of the electrosurgical treatment.

### Active Electrodes

The shape of the active electrode is an important factor in determining performance. A small electrode produces a high current density in the tissue and results in cutting. A large electrode spreads the current over a greater area of tissue and results in desiccation or coagulation. Figure 10.9 shows a sample of the variety of electrode shapes that have evolved to meet a range of specialized needs.

The flat elongated blade 2–3 mm wide and 1.5–2 cm long, with relatively sharp edges and tip, is commonly used in general surgical procedures. The blade serves the dual function of a cutting instrument when held so that the edge of the electrode faces in the direction of movement through the tissue and as a desiccating

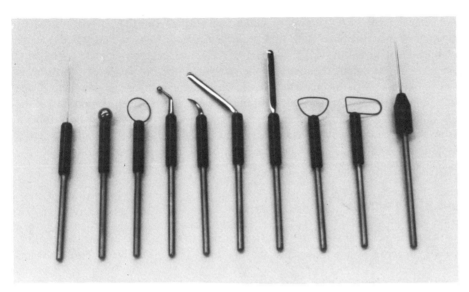

**FIGURE 10.9.** A variety of electrosurgical electrodes. (Courtesy Greenwald Surgical Co., Inc., East Gary, IN.)

electrode when one of the flat sides of the blade is held against the tissue and activated for the control of bleeding.

Loops, fashioned from fine wire, are used frequently for the removal of tissue masses and readily permit excavatory procedures. Such electrodes are commonly used, for example, in the delicate sculpting of gingival tissue that is necessary during dental electrosurgery or the removal of a conical portion of tissue from the cervix in gynecological electrosurgery. The urologist makes use of the loop through a resectoscope, within the urethra, to literally carve away the interior of the prostate and relieve problems associated with hypertropy of that gland. Needle-shaped electrodes are particularly effective for desiccation when plunged into the tissue to be treated. Skin lesions such as warts are frequently treated by this means. A cone of desiccated tissue is created around the imbedded portion of the needle and the core of the lesion is readily destroyed and removed.

Ball- and disk-shaped electrodes are effective for desiccation and fulguration because of their greater area and are in common use to achieve coagulation. In vascular areas such as tonsil beds and during neurosurgery, it has been found practical to combine the electrosurgical coagulation electrode with the tip of a suction catheter. The suction device, insulated except at the tip, is used to clear the area of blood. Then the bleeding site can be more readily identified and controlled by a brief application of current while touched by the suction tip.

It is common practice for surgeons to gain hemostatic control by touching the active electrode to the body of hemostatic clamps that had previously been used to clamp off bleeders and left in place. In effect, the hemostatic clamp becomes the electrode.

Tissue-grasping forceps are usually insulated except for their tips and are provided with a cable for connection to the electrosurgical generator. These provide a convenient means for grasping bleeding sites, which can then be coagulated by activation of the generator. Both tips can be energized from the single active cable to form a unipolar electrode. Or each tip of the forceps can be separately energized from each of the output terminals of the generator, the bipolar forceps previously discussed (Fig. 10.4). In this latter mode, coagulating currents are confined to the tissue immediately adjacent to the grasping site and other tissues or portions of the body are relatively uninvolved in the electrosurgical circuit. Long-shafted forceps can be introduced through a laparoscope and used to desiccate the fallopian tubes for the purpose of female sterilization. These can also be implemented in either the unipolar or bipolar mode.

## Activation Controls

The electrosurgical generator is usually activated by foot-operated switches. Alternatively, fingertip-operated switches may be built into the active electrode assembly.

Foot-operated switching permits simpler construction of the active electrode handle and generally results in a lighter handle and more flexible cable for this active electrode. Although foot switches are extensively used, they suffer some practical disadvantages. They are prone to being stepped on inadvertently with resultant activation of the generator and possible risk to the patient and attending personnel. They are also subjected to additional physical abuse including exposure to hostile environments, particularly moisture. Generators that can supply both cutting and desiccating (coagulation) outputs usually have multifunction foot-switches, generally with two switching pedals. Commonly, the left-most pedal activates cutting and the right-most activates coagulation to avoid confusion. Unless the surgeon is quite familiar with the feel of the foot switch, he can inadvertently activate the wrong function. Furthermore, he can delegate control of the foot switch to an associate, but with the disadvantage that he loses full control.

In some electrosurgical units, the surgeon can obtain blended output (the simultaneous combination of cutting and coagulating waveforms) by simultaneously closing both foot-controlled switches. However, it is far more common to make that an option controlled by a front-panel selector switch on the generator. Because the blended output is generally used to perform primarily a cutting function, the blended output, for such operation, is supplied in place of the continuous sinewave when the surgeon pushes the "Cut" pedal.

Hand-switched active electrode assemblies are widely available, both in reusable and single-use styles. They have the obvious advantages that unintentional activations are diminished as control is placed in the hands of the operator, and the foot switch is not exposed to be inadvertently stepped on. Hand switches avoid hand–foot coordination problems and reduce the tendency for some operators to stand on the coagulation activation pedal. This latter operation provides sustained activation for a sequence of coagulation manuevers but is a questionable technique.

Hand-switched active handles are usually provided with two switches, which may be of push-button, slide, or rocker style, that allow selection of either the cut (or blended) or coagulation modes by fingertip control.

As the complexity of surgical procedures has increased, so have electrosurgical demands. Multiple uses of a single electrosurgical unit have become increasingly common. It may be the surgeon who needs two different styles of active electrode and has a hand-switched active handle and a handle under foot-switch control, both plugged into the unit at the same time. Or it may be a cardiovascular procedure in which two surgical areas are being prepared simultaneously, one surgeon working in the thoracic region with a hand-controlled electrode, the other elsewhere with a foot-switch-controlled electrode, and both instruments fed from the same electrosurgical generator. In such cases, the surgeon must find out whether activation of, for example, the hand-controlled electrode simultaneously energizes the other electrode. Many generators are designed this way, and the surgeon, in using such a unit, must avoid inadvertent burns both to the patient and attending staff and assure that he achieves the proper electrosurgical effect. A simple matter such as the simultaneous application of two paralleled electrodes connected simultaneously to the patient may alter the loading of the generator to the point of changing the performance at one or both of the electrodes.

When the active electrode is not in use, it should be properly shielded to avoid burns from inadvertent activation. This can be accomplished by attaching within the surgical field a holster or quiver made of insulating material (the barrel of a sterile disposable syringe works fine) into which the electrode handle can be placed except when it is being used.

### Dispersive Electrodes

The dispersive electrode leads the electrosurgical current away from the body. Its large area keeps the current density and temperature rise low. Coupling is usually achieved by direct, conductive contact with the body by a metal electrode with or without the use of an intermediary layer of conductive gel to lower the contact resistance. Alternatively, adequate coupling can also be obtained with electrodes that are capacitively coupled to the patient. This may be via metal foil electrodes, with an intervening thin dielectric, applied directly to the patient's skin. However, in dental electrosurgery, for example, a large electrode is often installed just under the upholstery layer of the patient chair. Coupling is adequate and avoids the need for the patient to undress.

Dispersive electrodes may be either reusable or disposable. Plate electrodes, usually several hundred square cm in area, are available in both reusable and disposable form. The disposable plate electrodes are usually of aluminum foil on a moisture-resistant cardboard backing. Reusable plates are usually made of stainless steel. They are usually placed under the buttocks of the patient, where contact with the plate is generally assured by gravity. Quality of the electrical contact is improved by the use of a conducting electrode gel spread liberally over the surface of the electrode before it is placed under the patient.

There are also a variety of self-adhering electrodes, generally of smaller area than the plate-type electrodes. Among the direct-contact type, electrodes may be obtained either pregelled or requiring conductive gel to be applied just prior to application of the electrode. The pregelled electrodes generally have a gel-impreg-

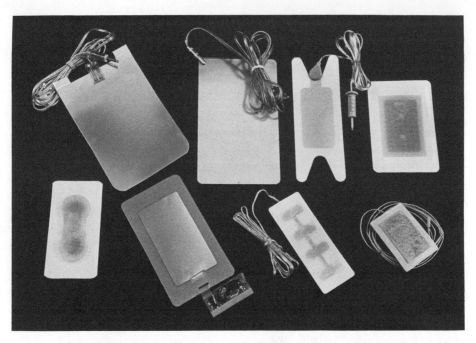

**FIGURE 10.10.** A selection of dispersive electrodes (clockwise from upper left) disposable cardboard plate-type electrode with cable; reusable stainless steel plate; self-adhering capacitively coupled electrode; pregelled self-adhering; pediatric pregelled self-adhering with disposable cable; pregelled self-adhering with disposable cable; self-adhering plate which requires gelling; pregelled self-adhering.

nated foam matrix (pad) that provides the contact between the patient's skin and the metallic electrode. They are packaged to preserve gel wetness over the expected shelf life of the product. Capacitively coupled self-adhering electrodes are also available.

Despite the small size of many of the self-adhering single-use dispersive electrodes, they have proven not only convenient and effective but, in general, have established a satisfactory record of avoidance of burns. For certain surgical procedures, particularly in which the patient may be repositioned during the surgery or where the plate-type electrode cannot be safely or conveniently used, the self-adhering electrodes have proven valuable and offer a somewhat greater flexibility in choice of sites on the body where they may be placed.

Disposable dispersive electrodes were introduced in the early 1970s. To indicate the extent to which this product line has grown, *Health Devices* (ECRI, 1979) published an evaluation of the single-use dispersive electrodes available at that time and included 22 different electrodes supplied by 13 different manufacturers. A selection of dispersive electrodes, both reusable and disposable, is shown in Fig. 10.10.

There are other forms of reusable dispersive electrodes for minor procedures that do not demand high electrosurgical currents. These include metal bracelets (similar to expansion watchbands), conductive fabric straps that can be placed on an extremity, and small flexible plates that can be wrapped around an arm or a thigh and held in place with an elastic strap. Circulation in the limb may be adversely compromised unless strict attention to the tightness of the straps is observed.

## 10.7 VARIABLES AFFECTING THE ELECTROSURGICAL CURRENT

Many variables affect the performance of an electrosurgical unit. We have already discussed current waveform and electrode size and geometry. This section briefly covers other important variables associated both with the generator and the patient. We must take these into account either in the design of new equipment or the assessment of an existing device. We cover: electrosurgical power and current, open-circuit voltage and crest factor, generator output impedance, frequency, and contributions of impedances at the active and dispersive electrode sites to the total circuit impedance.

### Power and Current Requirements

The expenditure of power at the active electrode requires that the generator be capable of supplying adequate current. This passes through the conductive tissue underlying the active electrode and must develop a power density sufficient to achieve the desired therapeutic effect. The generator must deliver power into a load, which includes impedance at the active electrode site together with other circuit impedances (the remainder of the patient's body beyond the site of electrosurgical activity, the dispersive electrode–patient interface, lead impedances, etc.).

The power needs for electrosurgery vary widely. Delicate neuromicrosurgery, retinal repair in ophthalmic surgery, or gingival reconstruction in dental surgery require low power of the order of a very few tens of watts. In general surgery, power needs for cutting tasks typically range from 30–100 W, and coagulation requires somewhat less, say 25–50 W. Underwater procedures, such as the transurethral prostatic resection, are the most power demanding with a need for 250 W or more to perform cutting functions and 150 W or more for coagulation. Load impedances vary markedly in the range of a few hundred ohms and load currents generally range from 100 mA to 1.5 A.

### Frequency

The fundamental frequency of the electrosurgical current is not a primary determinant of the performance of the waveform. It should be higher than the range at which shock or neuromuscular stimulation can occur. A frequency above 100 kHz is usually satisfactory, with most commercial units operating either around 500 kHz or in the range from 1.8 to 3 MHz.

Practical technical considerations place limitations on how high the frequency can be. As frequency increases, the effects of parasitic reactances (inductance of leads, capacitance of leads to ground, etc.), become more significant. For example, with increasing frequency, the loading effect of line capacitance to ground reduces output voltage, lead inductance decreases load currents, the degree of isolation of units with an ungrounded output is degraded, and the possibility of resonance in parasitic pathways lowers stability of the delivered output.

## Load Impedance Associated with the Patient

During electrosurgical procedures, the load impedance is typically of the order of 300 $\Omega$ but it varies, depending on several factors. Though that portion of the load impedance that is associated with the patient involves all tissue in the current pathway within the patient, the greater contribution to the total impedance comes from the tissue immediately under the active electrode. Consequently, changes in impedance largely reflect events going on at the active electrode. Load impedances tend to be higher during cutting procedures than during coagulation, particularly when the coagulation is accomplished by desiccation with an electrode of broad area of contact with the tissue. The nature of the electrode plays a significant role. Electrodes of larger area result in lower impedances. The load impedance changes during the duration of application of the electrosurgical current. This reflects the changes in hydration of the underlying tissue or the degree of carbonization that has taken place. The component of impedance associated with the patient is largely resistive in nature.

The contribution of the impedance at the interface of the dispersive electrode and the patient to the total load impedance is normally small—usually much less than 10% of the total impedance. With any effective dispersive electrode that is in direct contact with the patient and with which a conductive gel is used, the electrode impedance is usually of the order of 1 or 2 $\Omega$ resistive. Dispersive electrodes that are capacitively coupled to the patient present a higher impedance, 25 $\Omega$ or so, which is, nevertheless, still a small portion of the total impedance. Though not associated with the patient, the contribution of lead inductance to the total impedance is frequently overlooked. For example, a dispersive electrode cable, with inductance typically of 5 $\mu H$, can contribute as much as 50 $\Omega$ to the total impedance—considerably more if someone, who is compulsively neat, coils up the excess cable length.

## Open-Circuit Voltage and Crest Factor

Fulguration and cutting require an adequate open-circuit voltage. Fulguration is normally carried out with the active electrode about 3 mm above the surface of the tissue. The open-circuit voltage must be adequate to break down the air gap. The breakdown strength of air is approximately 1 kV/mm. Thus, typical waveforms for fulguration require open-circuit voltages of the order of 3 kV. Cutting uses a smaller gap of about 0.3 mm. Thus, the open-circuit voltage is about 300 V rather than 3 kV (Harris, 1978). As the blade is passed through tissue and cells are volatilized, a gap is created across which breakdown must be continually re-

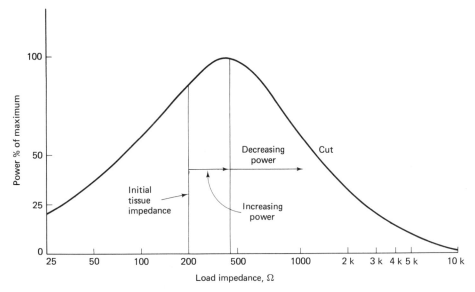

**FIGURE 10.11.** Output power (%) as a function of load impedance for a typical electrosurgical generator.

established in order for cutting to proceed smoothly. The insulation on cables and handles must be adequate to withstand the peak open-circuit voltage.

A high crest factor is required for hemostatic (fulgurating) ability. The waveforms of high crest factor have short duty cycles (i.e., long off-periods between the times when large pulses of energy are delivered to the tissue), which favor the flow of heat to surrounding tissue necessary to achieve coagulation without the volatilization of tissue immediately under the electrode. Solid-state generators with moderately good coagulation characteristics have crest factors of the order of 6–8. The crest factor of spark-gap units generally exceeds 10 (ECRI, 1977).

## Output Impedance

The performance of an electrosurgical unit is strongly affected by its output impedance. The effect of output impedance is reflected in the output power versus load impedance curve, a typical plot of which is shown in Fig. 10.11). The subject is complex and only briefly presented here. Harris (1978) has presented a discussion of some of the pertinent factors but little on this subject appears in the literature.

Figure 10.11 shows that there is an intentional rolling off of the power-versus-load-impedance curve at higher impedances. Thus, the coagulation process tends to be somewhat self-limiting as increasing tissue impedance with coagulation prevents the output current from rising without limit. The curve is also rolled off toward lower load impedances.

If the curve has a rising slope at the value of load impedance when contact is

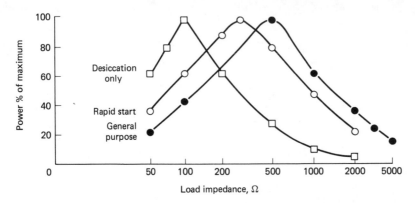

**FIGURE 10.12.** Output characteristics for various electrosurgical purposes. (Adapted from Harris FW paper read at 13th Annual meeting of AAMI Wash., D.C. 1978, with permission of Vallelab, Inc., Boulder, CO.)

first made and, as electrosurgical effect proceeds, impedance rises, the power rapidly increases. The magnitude of the slope thus determines the vigor of the onsct that the surgeon perceives.

Figure 10.12 shows that the output curves may be different for the coagulation function than for cutting functions in those units in which each is delivered separately.

## 10.8 HAZARDS AND ADVERSE EFFECTS

There are a number of hazards and adverse effects attributable to the use of electrosurgical devices. We can categorize them into the following broad classes: burns due to radio-frequency (RF) currents, fires, low-frequency shock and dc burns, and radio-frequency or electromagnetic interference to other equipment.

### RF Burns

There is a risk of burns due to the RF currents used in electrosurgery. Most often, they are caused by Joule heating in the underlying tissue at the site of an electrode. If the current density under an electrode is too great, the heat generated cannot be dissipated fast enough, either by convection due to circulation of blood in the underlying tissue or by the thermal heat-sink capabilities of the electrode. The electrode may be the dispersive electrode. It could be another electrode that monitors the patient (i.e., an ECG electrode or temperature probe) and that serves as an inadvertent pathway for the return of electrosurgical currents to ground (Finlay et al., 1974; Spierdijk et al., 1978). Burns may also occur as a result of inadequate insulation or an insulation breakdown on the active cable at a point where it was draped over the patient.

Becker et al. (1973) demonstrated that burns from electrosurgical currents

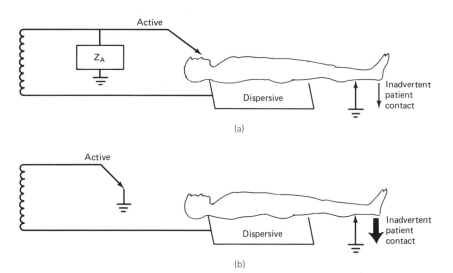

**FIGURE 10.13.** Conditions leading to inadvertent currents to ground using an isolated-output electrosurgical unit. (a) $Z_A$ is an inadvertent low impedance from the active side to ground. (b) The surgeon draws a spark from a grounded surface to test for electrosurgical output.

under electrocardiographic electrodes were possible at current densities of the order of 100 mA/cm$^2$ when these currents passed for at least 10 s. Current densities of this order or greater can occur at the dispersive electrode, particularly under two abnormal conditions. If the patient moves or is moved during a procedure and loses contact with a portion of the plate-type electrode initially placed underneath, the risk of a burn is present. Similarly, if a self-adhering dispersive electrode placed on the patient pulls loose or pressure is placed on the electrode so that uneven contact with the electrode occurs, again the risk of excess current concentration and burn is high. Gel or a saline-soaked towel that is used with the dispersive electrode may dry out and introduce the threat of burns as resistance between the dispersive electrode and patient increases.

A surgeon has received serious burns of the eye when the eyepiece of an endoscope, through which an electrosurgical procedure was being carried out, was inadequately insulated. Burns can also occur if the electrosurgical unit is inadvertently and unexpectedly activated. Attending personnel or the patient can receive a burn under such conditions if the active electrode is not suitably protected from contact.

Figure 10.13 shows that the isolated-output electrosurgical unit presents unique opportunities for burns if activated while the active electrode is not in contact with the patient. The degree of isolation of the output is degraded should an inadvertent low impedance occur from the active side of the output circuit to ground. Then current can flow through any patient contact with ground and cause a burn. A particularly hazardous situation occurs if the surgeon follows an outdated practice of testing for electrosurgical output by attempting to draw a spark from a grounded surface with the active electrode. When the active electrode is grounded, the dispersive electrode, being ungrounded, effectively becomes an active electrode and the full output of the electrosurgical unit is applied to the patient. In this case, the potential for burns at an inadvertent ground contact on the patient is severe.

## Fires

The power from discharge of an electrosurgical unit is more than adequate to ignite flammable agents. Thus, flammable anesthetic agents should not be used. Flammable agents could be used to prepare the patient for surgery (e.g., alcohol or acetone used to clean and degrease the surgical site) and remain pooled around and under the patient. Such materials have been ignited by the application of electrosurgery (Plumlee, 1973). Occasionally, when precautions have not been properly taken, accumulations of flammable gases in body cavities, whether residual flammable anesthetics or by-products of digestive processes (methane and hydrogen) in the bowel, have been ignited with disasterous results (Bond et al., 1976).

## Low-Frequency Shocks and DC Burns

Low-frequency shocks and stimulation of the patient's neuromuscular system can occur if the output circuit is incorrectly designed and can support the flow of low-frequency currents. Such currents can result if the electrosurgical current is modulated with low-frequency components. At the active electrode–tissue interface, rectification and demodulation occur and the low-frequency components are recovered. There are reports that suggest that ventricular fibrillation has been induced by such a mechanism. (Hungerbuhler et al., 1974; Geddes et al., 1975). A capacitor in series with one of the output leads, usually the active lead, effectively reduces the risk.

Burns have occurred when direct currents unintentionally flowed through the patient from monitor circuits within the electrosurgical unit intended to interrogate the continuity of the dispersive electrode cable when a blocking capacitor failed (Leeming et al., 1970). Equipment design must preclude the possibility of direct current through the patient during normal operation and anticipated fault conditions.

## RF and Electromagnetic Interference

Because the electrosurgical unit is an RF generator of significant power, it has been responsible for disruption of function of many other devices in the patient vicinity. For example, it has altered the rate of administration of drugs by susceptible infusion pumps (ECRI, 1972). Unless steps are taken to incorporate appropriate filtering in the input of physiologic monitors used at the time of surgery, recordings of low-level physiologic signals such as the electrocardiogram are routinely obliterated during activation of the electrosurgical unit. It has altered the function of some pacemakers during electrosurgery (O'Donoghue, 1973). This suggests that patients with pacemakers undergoing surgery should either not be subjected to electrosurgery or their cardiac activity should be closely monitored during the procedure.

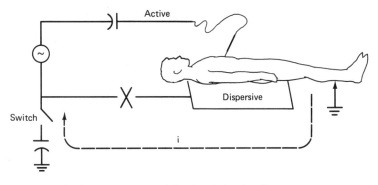

**FIGURE 10.14.** Consequences of a break in the dispersive electrode cable in a ground-referenced output (switch closed) and in an isolated output (switch open).

Power distribution systems in operating rooms are frequently ungrounded systems monitored by a line-isolation monitor to indicate the degree of isolation. Electrosurgical units have been responsible for causing these monitors to alarm due to electromagnetic interference.

At present, the conducted and radiated emissions of electrosurgical units are exempt from controls promulgated by the Federal Communications Commission, though this is under review and may be changed in the future.

## 10.9 DESIGN FOR SAFETY

The risk of inadvertent burns can be reduced simply by taking care to activate the unit only when the active electrode is in place at the site of intended electrosurgical effect. However, a failure may occur in the dispersive cable, hidden as it may be under the drapes and out of sight. A failure such as this could easily lead to electrosurgical currents in unintended ground pathways that might cause patient burns unless intentional design features have been incorporated to minimize the risk. Several design approaches specifically intended to enhance the safety of the electrosurgical unit and its accessories are discussed in this section.

### *Output Configuration*

Figure 10.14 shows that a point of contact of the patient with a grounded object forms a closure of the patient circuit in the event of a failure in the cable connecting the dispersive cable with its associated output terminal on the generator when it is of the grounded configuration (switch closed). If the area of the patient contact is small, the risk of burn at that point is great. Moreover, it may not even be apparent to the operator that anything is wrong, because the impedance of the alternate pathway may not alter the total circuit impedance sufficiently so that electrosurgical action at the active electrode would be affected.

In contrast, inadvertent contact to grounded objects does not close the patient circuit when an electrosurgical unit with well-isolated output (Fig. 10.14, switch open) is used. Consequently, when a break in the dispersive electrode cable occurs, there is no significant current in the incidental ground contact. Also, electrosurgical effect at the active electrode is markedly diminished as a result of the reduction of current in the active cable.

These factors, seemingly, would pose a convincing argument for the use of isolated-output units in preference to grounded devices were it not that other factors tend to reduce the safety differences, as we point out later.

## Alarms and Indicators

Alarms and indicators, both visual and audible, are usually provided to identify conditions that could result in injury.

Every electrosurgical unit should have a means of alerting the operator that the output of the unit has been switched on. The potential for injury is great whenever the active electrode is energized, particularly if unknowingly activated. Activation can—and has—occurred when someone has inadvertently stepped on the foot-operated switch, a component has failed within the generator, or moisture has entered an unprotected hand-controlled switch. An audible indication of activation is preferred because the attending personnel may not see a visual indicator. Sound level can be adjustable to adapt for differing ambient noise levels, but it should not be silenced. Convincing arguments might be made that, in some applications in which the patient is conscious during the electrosurgical procedure, the well-being of the patient would be compromised if an audible indicator were used. When such situations prevail, a visual indicator is a necessary alternative. However, the surgeon who has experienced a burn incident without the benefit of an audible indicator of activation is difficult to convince that there are valid situations in which the audible indicator can be omitted.

Continuity of the active-electrode cable is generally self-diagnosing. A break results in a noticeable failure to achieve therapeutic effect. The same is not necessarily true for the dispersive electrode cable, particularly those used with grounded-output units, as we have just discussed. Moreover, to operate with a broken dispersive electrode cable is to unduly risk patient burns. Therefore, visual indicators and audible alarms are incorporated. These are activated when an interrogation current, normally coursing out to the dispersive electrode and back to the generator through the two-conductor cable (see Fig. 10.15), is interrupted because of a break. Additionally, activation of most units is inhibited by continuity failure that results in an alarm.

Failure of the interrogation circuit in this continuity monitor to reach beyond the dispersive electrode connector and include the electrode itself should be considered a design deficiency. Because isolated-output units have an inherent ability to limit currents to ground under the condition of an interrupted dispersive electrode cable and to reflect the situation with reduced activity at the active electrode, some manufacturers of isolated units, somewhat justifiably, opt not to include a dispersive electrode cable continuity monitor.

The dispersive cable continuity monitor does not confirm that the dispersive

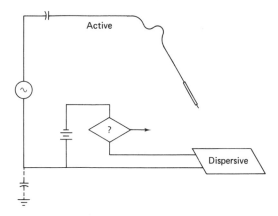

**FIGURE 10.15.** Dispersive cable continuity monitor.

electrode is in contact with the patient, though an occasional user makes the presumption. Contact of the dispersive electrode with the patient, together with integrity of the patient circuitry, can be monitored if the interrogation current includes the entire patient circuit (Fig. 10.16). In this case, an audible alarm is not provided because it is usual to inhibit activation of the unit until continuity is established, thereby avoiding the risks of an open patient circuit. Units having this type of continuity monitor usually retain foot- or hand-switched control over activation (providing continuity is established), though there have been systems that have capitalized on this monitor scheme to control activation. In this case, the surgeon does not have to actuate a footswitch but simply touches the active electrode to the surgical site—seemingly a convenience. However, the convenience is offset by a significant disadvantage and risk. If the active electrode is inadvertently laid on the patient, either directly or through a moist drape, continuity could be established and the unit activated, thus causing a burn or fire.

In designing this type of continuity monitor, precautions must be taken to assure that continuity is verified only when the interrogation current traverses the intended patient circuit, rather than possible alternative paths. Interrogation current that might return to the generator through a grounded pathway that bypasses the dispersive electrode cable must not satisfy the monitor.

This continuity monitor, with interrogation circuit encompassing the patient, also has a significant operational disadvantage. It does not easily permit fulguration (sparking to the tissue without direct electrode contact) because contact with the patient is necessary to activate the electrosurgical unit.

Another type of protective circuit alerts the surgeon to the existence of electrosurgical currents in other than the intended pathways. Though this type may be implemented in different ways, the net effect is that the monitoring circuit establishes the extent to which electrosurgical currents do or do not return to the generator by other than the intended pathway. In one form, it makes comparison between active electrode cable and dispersive electrode cable currents. To the extent that the ratio of these currents differs from unity, alternate pathways are involved and, when a threshold is exceeded, it disables output from the unit. Another method monitors the RF current in the impedance that provides the ground-

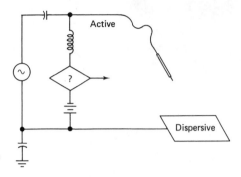

FIGURE 10.16. Patient circuit continuity monitor.

reference for the output circuit. Any current in that link can be attributed to currents returning through paths that bypass the dispersive electrode cable and, hence, reflect currents that could have passed from the patient through alternate ground pathways. When these currents exceed a predetermined limit, this deactivates the unit and protects the patient from burns at points of contact with alternate ground paths.

## Interlocks

We have already encountered one form of interlock—the locking out of activation of the generator on the failure to confirm continuity in the patient circuit. Interlocks can also effectively control another type of hazard.

As we have previously seen, it is usual to use a common electrode for cutting and coagulation, with the selection of the mode accomplished by pushing the appropriate pedal on a foot switch or button on a hand-switched active electrode handle. The control circuits of some units are implemented with interlocks that, in the event that both foot pedals or hand-controlled switches are inadvertently depressed simultaneously, either disable the generator or, more commonly, result only in energization of the coagulation mode. The coagulation mode, usually operating at a lower power level than the cut mode, is inherently less destructive to tissue than is the cut mode.

Increasingly, more complex surgery is being performed during which it is necessary to have two surgical sites under development at the same time. Consequently, there is a need for multiple electrosurgical sources and these are sometimes provided from the same generator unit. Although newer units offer the capability of two independent outputs, it is not uncommon that a single generator be implemented with, for example, one hand-switched active electrode handle and another one under foot-switch control. In those units that provide multiple output terminals, prudence suggests that suitable interlocks should be provided within the equipment so that one electrode will not be energized on a command intended for the other.

## Shielded Leads

Although shielding of the active and dispersive electrode cables would undoubtedly reduce the possibility of burns due to insulation failure and the risk, if any, of exposure of personnel to the high electromagnetic fields that surround these leads, shielding has not been widely used in electrosurgical applications. One notable exception is its use in dental electrosurgery. Practical reasons probably make this so. In general purpose electrosurgery, especially those in which higher voltages and powers are used, shielded cables would have been cumbersome and performance less well controlled than has been the case with unshielded leads. The broadband currents from spark-gap sources together with widely ranging patient load impedances lead to problems of excessive variation of standing wave ratio on shielded cables so that output is variable. Time and technical improvments are changing this and it is likely that the future will see increased use of shielded leads in all types of electrosurgery.

## 10.10 RECOMMENDED PRACTICES AND STANDARDS

There have been virtually no regulations or standards specifically applied to electrosurgical devices. The document that comes closest is the National Fire Protection Association's (NFPA) Publication 76C "Safe Use of High Frequency Electricity in Health Care Facilities (1980)." As a Recommended Practice, it is intended to be advisory in nature and is frequently, but wrongly, assumed to carry binding or legal authority. It carries information both for the designer and for the user. Though it is devoted to the broad class of high-frequency devices, it, nevertheless, has substantial information pertaining specifically to electrosurgery. NFPA 76C outlines the common hazards associated with electrosurgery and makes recommendations related to circuit design intended to reduce the risks. It calls for means to isolate the output circuit from low-frequency currents that might arise from the power supply or be produced by rectification phenomena in the patient circuit and means for monitoring continuity of the dispersive cable.

Marketing pressures have resulted in ever-increasing numbers of electrosurgical generator manufacturers submitting their product to Underwriters Laboratories (UL) for listing in conformity with the requirements of their standard, UL544, Medical and Dental Equipment. Typical of UL standards, this standard does not make requirements of the device that assure therapeutic benefit or necessarily otherwise affect performance. The standard ensures that construction and performance characteristics do not lead to the risk of shock to the patient or operating personnel or injury that would likely be due to overheating, fire, smoke, and so on. The standard, furthermore, does not impose requirements that are specific for electrosurgical devices but, rather, are applicable to medical devices in general.

The Council on Dental Materials and Devices of the American Dental Association has, for several years, had an acceptance program wherein manufacturers could submit their dental electrosurgical units for approval. For acceptance, the unit must conform to a set of criteria. Certain safety features and performance capabilities must be present.

The Medical Device Amendments of 1976 amended the Food, Drug, and Cosmetic Act and empowered the federal government with the regulation of the manufacture of medical devices. Several Food and Drug Administration (FDA) Device Classification Panels identified electrosurgical devices as high-priority items for which safety and performance standards are to be developed. Work has proceeded on the development of such standards and the Bureau of Medical Devices, FDA, has a draft version that is undergoing further refinement. AAMI has a draft standard for electrosurgery units and will develop a standard for dispersive electrodes. At the international level, Working Group 2 of the International Electrotechnical Commission Sub-Committee 62D has been drafting a set of standards for high-frequency surgical equipment. In order not to inhibit foreign trade any more than is necessary, efforts are underway to achieve as complete harmonization as is possible between requirements satisfying the FDA and those of the IEC. Citing significant differences between dental and general purpose electrosurgical units, the dental community is seeking FDA recognition of a separate standard for dental electrosurgical devices.

These matters are likely to be resolved in the early 1980s, though whether the FDA offering will be in the form of required standards or, rather, guidelines is not established at this point. It is likely that their direct impact will be upon the manufacturer rather than the user. Of course, the user will be indirectly affected by them as they affect resulting performance, safety, and cost.

## 10.11 INSPECTION AND PREVENTIVE MAINTENANCE

We have shown that electrosurgical units have both the potential for harm to patient and attending personnel and a past history of inflicting injury. Regular inspection of these devices is an important keystone in a preventive maintenance program. Each electrosurgical unit should be examined during incoming inspection prior to introduction into service and inspected periodically thereafter. Incoming inspection verifies that the electrosurgical unit meets the manufacturer's and user's specifications for performance and safety. Periodic inspection helps to detect any deterioration that might otherwise go unnoticed. Correction of a minor deficiency can prevent catastrophic failure, downtime, and the possible need for emergency repairs. The frequency of periodic inspections depends on a number of factors, including the frequency of use of the equipment and the rate at which problems occur with the equipment. A thorough inspection should be performed annually with a less comprehensive examination—items identified with an asterisk (*) in the procedure given below—carried out at three-month intervals in the intervening time.

The following outlines the important elements of an inspection procedure for electrosurgical devices. More detailed procedures are given in such publications as Health Devices (ECRI, 1973) and "Medical Equipment Management in Hospitals," available from the American Hospital Association (1978). Material supplied by the manufacturer should also be consulted.

### Features Shared with Other Electrically Operated Devices*

A number of basic visual checks and measurements commonly performed on general electrically operated patient-care medical devices should be carried out. The general condition of the equipment case and chassis, line cord, plug, strain reliefs, and control knobs should be examined for evidence of abuse or damage. This should include signs of liquid spillage and entry. Fuses (including spares) and/or circuit breakers should be checked. Resistance between a grounded point on the chassis and the grounding pin on the power plug should be made to confirm continuity of grounding. Conductivity through casters that may be required of equipment of this sort in certain operating room environments should be measured where necessary. Grounding of the foot switch case to the chassis should be confirmed. Fans, and associated filters, should be examined for dust accumulation and cleaned, if necessary (outside the operating room area, please!). Lamps and audible indicators should function properly.

### Leakage Current

Leakage current of power-line frequency from the chassis as well as from active and dispersive electrodes should be measured. Worst-case values should be noted and confirmed to be below accepted or specified limits. Typically, they should be below 100 $\mu$A from chassis to ground and below 50 $\mu$A from patient-contacting electrodes (active and dispersive) to ground. Measurements should be made when the unit is powered from a grounded distribution system. Many electrosurgical units are used in operating rooms supplied from an isolated power distribution system and worst-case leakage current measurements made on such systems may be unrealistically low. Leakage current meters may be susceptible to the radiated energy of the electrosurgical unit as evidenced by leakage current readings during activation of the electrosurgical unit but when the meter is not connected to the equipment under test. A capacitor across the input terminals of the leakage current meter (of the order of 0.1 $\mu$F) will often remedy this problem. Leakage current measurements should not be made from the active electrode while the unit is activated unless the test instrument is specifically provided with protective circuitry and filters to permit such a measurement. In general, it is satisfactory to make all leakage current measurements with the output controls set to minimum.

### Electrodes and Cables*

The condition of all reusable electrodes and cables should be checked for evidence of abuse. Examine cables for cracking following repeated sterilization. Make sure that any reusable dispersive electrode is smooth, free of cracks, and without dried electrode gel. Check to make sure that the gel associated with the instrument is of a conductive type, suitable for use in electrosurgery. Occasionally, nonconductive lubricating jelly is improperly stored with the electrosurgical accessories.

### Degree of Grounding of Dispersive Electrode Terminal

By connection either to the dispersive electrode terminal on the unit or directly to a dispersive electrode connected to the unit with an appropriate cable, confirm with an ohmmeter that the resistance from this point to ground is appropriate. Isolated-output units and units with the output referenced to ground by a capacitor should reflect a high resistance (several megohms or higher). In units whose output is directly grounded, this measurement should be of the order of a fraction of an ohm. This measurement may reflect the current necessary to charge the ground-referencing capacitor, in which case the resistance should settle to a high value within several seconds.

## Patient-Circuit Safety Devices*

Verify the function of alarm features associated with the safety devices monitoring the patient circuit. The most common type of monitor is that which confirms continuity of the dispersive electrode cable and connection of an electrode. Either by disconnecting the dispersive electrode from its cable or (where the dispersive electrode is permanently attached to its cable) by using an open-circuited mating plug in the outlet, check to see that appropriate visual and audible alarms are given. In most units, the alarm also prevents activation of the output and this should be checked to be sure that it occurs. Check units that monitor the complete output circuit for continuity by attempting to operate the unit while open-circuited. Establish by panel indicators or other means that the unit is not being activated.

Test electrosurgical units that compare active and dispersive cable currents using an appropriate load or a tester for measuring output. Set the unit to a typical working level and confirm that power is delivered to the load. Leaving the active lead to the load (tester) hooked up, connect the other lead from the load to a grounded point on the electrosurgical generator instead of to the dispersive electrode terminal on the unit. Confirm that an appropriate alarm is given and/or no output results when attempts to activate the unit are made.

Electrosurgical units having other forms of patient-circuit safety devices may need to be tested by special means detailed in the manufacturer's literature.

## Spark-Gap Performance

With the electrosurgical unit unplugged, remove the appropriate cover to gain visual access to the spark-gap assembly. Using caution, override any interlocks and energize the electrosurgical unit. Activate the unit in all modes that make use of the spark-gap assembly and observe that all gaps have approximately the same amount of spark activity. Confirm that spark-gap operation is consistent over the range of output control settings. Marked differences in spark uniformity suggest that maintenance may be necessary. Look for sparking across other capacitors and insulators. Electrosurgical analyzers are described (Miodownik, 1978) and commercially available that can measure crest factor of the output waveform and these may provide an effective way of assessing spark-gap performance.

## Output Current/Power*

Measure the output power or current using a test instrument intended for the purpose or a load consisting of noninductive resistors and a current meter satisfactory for the frequencies and waveform measured. The load resistance should be appropriate, preferably that specified by the manufacturer. Select a range of control settings on the electrosurgical unit that encompasses the entire output range. Use all the operating modes available on the electrosurgical unit. The output should increase smoothly from zero, or nearly zero, to maximum. Do not operate the unit at high output for prolonged periods of time because this places an unrealistic and unnecessary strain on both the electrosurgical unit and the test equipment.

### Output Isolation*

Make measurements to determine whether isolation has been degraded in those electrosurgical units in which output is not intentionally referenced to ground. Make measurements of power (or current) both from active electrode to ground and from dispersive electrode to ground. Unless the manufacturer specifies load resistances for these tests, use a typical load impedance of a few hundred ohms. When measuring the power from the active electrode to ground, make sure that the dispersive electrode, if it must be connected, is not in direct contact with ground and, preferably, is suspended to minimize capacitance to ground, as this degrades the degree of isolation. When the power from dispersive electrode to ground is measured, connect a hand-controlled active electrode to the electrosurgical unit, because capacitance in the control wiring sometimes adversely affects isolation. Make measurements in each of the operating modes. The extent of output reduction, when compared with comparable measurements made of output power when the load is connected across the output of the generator, gives direct evidence of the degree of isolation of the unit.

### Waveform

If there is a discrepancy between measured output power (current) and published specifications, make waveform measurements from an output jack on the electrosurgical analyzer with an oscilloscope of adequate bandwidth. It is sometimes difficult to make waveform measurements accurately, particularly with coagulation waveforms, and this can frequently be considered an optional measurement.

## 10.12 EDUCATION FOR USE

The safe and effective use of electrosurgical units is substantially dependent upon the degree of knowledge the user has of the equipment. Moreover, it is often the user's perception that the radio-frequency currents of these devices do not behave as predictably as the lower frequency currents or dc, with which they are more familiar. The biomedical and clinical engineer is, therefore, frequently called upon to participate in the development and presentation of educational programs for users.

The engineer has the responsibility to convey to the user the basics of electrosurgical devices to the extent that he or she feels that it is important for the user to know them in order to more effectively use the device. The engineer must correctly perceive the level on which the communication and teaching can take place, for there is frequently considerable distance between the technical levels of comprehension of the user and the engineer.

The engineer should also seek to understand the perceptions held by the user as to the operation of electrosurgical instruments. There are mistakenly held impressions about the role of the conductive floor in electrosurgery (e.g., that it is believed it plays a significant role in the return pathway or contributes importantly to the shock the physician might have received). Users may fail to conceive of alternate pathways for electrosurgical currents or have an imprecise view of the nature of capacitively coupled pathways. They may ascribe to the applied voltage the ability to leap vastly greater distances than the physics of gap breakdown predict. Occasionally, the user may fail to appreciate a difference between conductive gels intended for use with dispersive electrodes and nonconductive lubricating gels, which have no place in electrosurgery.

Both surgeon and nurse frequently find themselves in positions in which they may, in different operating rooms, necessarily have to use different generators and accessories. The problem for the physician may be compounded by the fact that he or she may operate in two or more hospitals, where there may be different equipment. The physician's response is frequently to relegate the setting up of the electrosurgical unit, and even the adjustment of output levels, to the nursing staff or operating room technicians without ever feeling a need to confront and understand the individual devices.

Clinical and biomedical engineers can build their own effective collection of teaching aids, such as slides, for teaching programs—and this is to be encouraged if the resources are available. Increasingly more and better interpretive material is being made available by the manufacturers of electrosurgical devices. This is because a substantial portion of the misadventures that occur during the use of electrosurgery happens due to operator error, not equipment failure.

Actual demonstrations of electrosurgical effects that can frequently be carried out on acceptable substitutes for the human body are particularly effective. Often a piece of meat, such as flank steak or liver, lying on a plate-type dispersive electrode can be used to demonstrate cutting characteristics or, alternatively, the extent of lack of cutting characteristics associated with coagulation or desiccation waveforms. Also, this is an effective preparation to show how, with the connection of a small-area contact to the meat, alternate paths can contribute to patient burns. Coagulation is somewhat more difficult to demonstrate. The white of an egg will sometimes convey the principles to be put forth. On special occasions, when the training needs justify it, demonstrations carried out in an animal laboratory can prove very effective.

Place posters, such as that prepared by ECRI (1975) (Fig. 10.17), in an appropriate prominent place to provide a constant reminder of the many factors that can reduce the incidence of injury.

Many patient burns have been wrongly attributed to electrosurgical devices. Quite often, the presenting lesion is so reminiscent of an electrical burn that the conclusion is immediately drawn that the electrosurgical device must have been to

# ELECTROSURGERY IS DANGEROUS

## Before the procedure

*Examine the equipment and accessories. DON'T USE:*
1. *Cables and accessories with damaged (cracked, burned, or taped) insulation or connectors*
2. *Cracked, dirty, or bent return plates\**
3. *Endoscopes with inadequately insulated eyepieces*

*Don't reuse disposable accessories*

*Check operation of a return cable sentry (buzzer or light)*

*Place the return electrode\* close to the surgical site and assure good patient contact*

*Keep ECG electrodes far from the surgical site and the return electrode\**

*Keep electrosurgical cables clipped away from the patient and from monitoring cables*

*Avoid pools of prepping agents and other fluids around any patient electrodes*

*Don't spark the blade[†] to ground or the return plate\**

## During the procedure

*Observe appropriate precautions when using oxygen of flammable anesthetics*

*Activate the unit only when touching the blade[†] to tissue*

*Avoid unnecessary or prolonged activation*

*Don't continue to increase power settings if you aren't getting results—look for other problems. They could injure you or the patient*

*Check contact with the return electrode\* after repositioning the patient*

## After the procedure

*Look for possible patient burns, especially near the return electrode\* and ECG electrode sites*

*Clean, inspect, sterilize, and store reusable cables and accessories carefully*

*\*Also called ground plate, patient plate, butt plate, grounding pad*
*†Also called pencil, knife, loop, ball, active handle*

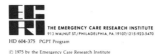

**THE EMERGENCY CARE RESEARCH INSTITUTE**
913 WALNUT ST/PHILADELPHIA, PA.19107/(215)923-5470

HD 604-375  PGPT Program

© 1975 by the Emergency Care Research Institute

Your hospital is a member of the *Health Devices Program*, a nonprofit information service. Additional information on electrosurgery was published in *HEALTH DEVICES*, Vol. 2, Nos. 8, 9, 11, and 12. To read these issues and learn more about the membership benefits of the program, contact

_____ , Extension _____ .

**FIGURE 10.17.** Electrosurgical safety poster. (Courtesy of *Health devices*, ECRI, Plymouth Meeting, PA.)

blame. Further investigation might even have shown that no alternate pathway could have existed, nor were there other explanations that could have made it plausible for the injury to have arisen from the electrosurgical unit. Often other devices were in use, such as a hypo/hyperthermia unit, which may have been subject to failure. Prepping agents can produce chemical injuries of the skin that mimic electrical burns. Pressure necroses may occur that are sometimes mistaken as having their origin with the electrosurgical unit. Various mechanisms of skin injury have been addressed in the literature (ECRI, 1980; Gendron, 1980). It is important for the biomedical or clinical engineer to appreciate these possibilities as they are called upon to investigate electrosurgical incidents and to convey to users, in educational programs, these alternate possibilities in order that they, the users of electrosurgical devices, can provide the best care with the least possible risk of injury.

# REFERENCES

## *Cited References*

AMERICAN SOCIETY FOR HOSPITAL ENGINEERING (1978). *Medical equipment management in hospitals.* Chicago: American Hospital Association.

BECKER, C. M., I. V. MALHOTRA, and J. HEDLEY-WHYTE (1973). The distribution of radio frequency current and burns. *Anesthesiology,* 38: 106–22.

BOND, J. H., M. LEVY, and M. D. LEVITT (1976). Explosion of hydrogen gas in the colon during proctosigmoidoscopy. *Gastrointest. Endosc.,* 23: 41–42.

CUSHING, W. T., and W. T. BOVIE (1928). Electrosurgery as an aid to the removal of intracranial tumors. *Surg. Gynecol. Obstet.,* 47: 751–84.

ECRI (1972). IVAC infusion pumps: Hazard. *Health Devices,* 1: 291–92.

ECRI (1973). Inspection of electrosurgical units. *Health Devices,* 2: 284–91.

ECRI (1975). Electrosurgery is dangerous. Available as a poster from ECRI, 5200 Butler Pike, Plymouth Meeting, PA 19462.

ECRI (1977). Electrosurgical units: Evaluation. *Health Devices,* 6: 59–86.

ECRI (1979). Disposable electrosurgical dispersive electrodes: Evaluation. *Health Devices,* 8: 43–65.

ECRI (1980). Skin injury in the OR and elsewhere: Hazard. *Health Devices,* 9: 312–18.

ELLIOTT, J. A. (1966). Electrosurgery. *Arch. Derm.,* 94: 340–50.

FINLAY, B., D. COUCHIE, L. BOYCE, and E. SPENCER (1974). Electrosurgery burns resulting from use of miniature ECG electrodes. *Anesthesiology,* 41: 263–69.

GEDDES, L. A., W. A. TACKER, and P. CABLER (1975). A new electrical hazard associated with the electrocautery. *Med. Instrum.,* 9: 112–13.

GENDRON, F. (1980). "Burns" occurring during lengthy surgical procedures. *J. Clin. Eng.,* 5: 19–26.

HARRIS, F. W. (1978). Desiccation as a key to understanding electrosurgery. *Proc. AAMI Ann. Meeting,* 121.

HUNGERBUHLER, R. F., J. P. SWOPE, and J. G. REVES (1974). Ventricular fibrillation associated with use of electrocautery. *JAMA,* 230: 432–35.

LEEMING, M. N., C. RAY, and W. S. HOWLAND (1970). Low-voltage, direct-current burns. *JAMA,* 214: 1681–84.

MIODOWNIK S. (1978). Electrosurgical output measurement: A review of methods and a new approach. *J. Clin. Eng.,* 3: 229–36.

NATIONAL FIRE PROTECTION ASSOCIATION (NFPA) (1980). *High frequency electrical equipment in hospitals.* Available as No. 76C from NFPA, 470 Atlantic Ave., Boston, MA 02210.

O'DONOGHUE, J. K. (1973). Inhibition of a demand pacemaker by electrosurgery. *Chest,* 64: 664–66.

PLUMLEE, J. E. (1973). Operating-room flash fire from use of cautery after aerosol spray: A case report. *Anesth. Analg.,* 52: 202–3.

SPIERDIJK, J., A. NANDORFF, and A. VAN BIJNEN (1968). Burns caused by monitoring in anesthesia. *Acta. Anesthesiol. Belg.,* 29: 305–11.

### Additional Readings

CURTISS, L. E. (1973). High frequency currents in endoscopy: A review of principles and precautions. *Gastrointest. Endosc.,* 20: 9–12.

DOBBIE, A. K. (1969). The electrical aspects of surgical diathermy. *Bio-Med. Eng.,* 4: 206–216.

ENGEL, T., and F. W. HARRIS (1975). The electrical dynamics of laparoscopic sterilization. *J. Reproductive Med.,* 15: 33–42.

GONSER, D. I., and O. F. KRAFT (1976). Design hazards of electrosurgical devices. *Med. Instrum.,* 10: 130–37.

HONIG, W. M. (1975). The mechanism of cutting in electrosurgery. *IEEE Trans. Biomed. Eng.,* BME-22: 58–62.

ORINGER, M. J. (1975). *Electrosurgery in dentistry,* 2nd ed. Philadelphia: W. B. Saunders.

OVERMYER, K. M., J. A. PEARCE, and D. P. DEWITT (1979). Measurements of temperature distributions at electrosurgical dispersive electrode sites. *J. Biomech. Eng.,* 101: 66–72.

TAYLOR, K. W., and J. DESMOND (1970). Electrical hazards in the operating room, with special reference to electrosurgery. *Can. J. Surg.,* 13: 362–74.

## STUDY QUESTIONS

**10.1** Explain the essential differences between electrosurgery and electrocautery.

**10.2** Discuss and compare factors in the use of ground-referenced and isolated-output electrosurgical units that affect the safety of these devices. What design features can be incorporated to minimize differences in the risks of each of these two types of units?

**10.3** A surgeon says that it seems that the performance of an electrosurgical unit she has been using is changing adversely. Particularly, she feels she is having more difficulty controlling bleeding. What needs to be checked if she is using a spark-gap type generator? A solid-state generator? What errors in surgical technique may also be responsible for the change?

**10.4** Discuss the recommendation that, contrary to initial impressions, it may be desirable and safer to use a "cutting" current rather than a "coagulation" waveform for desiccation of tissue masses such as the fallopian tubes. Review the recommendation in the light of the waveforms the generator delivers. Consider electrode geometry as a factor in the selection of waveform.

**10.5** A nurse tells you, after a report of occurrence of a skin lesion during a surgical procedure, that he is sure the dispersive electrode was properly placed because the dispersive cable alarm did not come on at all during the procedure. What further information must you have to determine whether or not deficiencies in the implementation of the electrosurgical patient circuit occurred?

**10.6** A patient, undergoing a minor electrosurgical procedure, reports that she feels a "shock" when the electrosurgical unit is applied. The physician also reports concurrent muscle stimulation. What things should the clinical engineer look for to determine whether this is likely to have happened? What equipment failures may have occurred? Are there any errors of technique that could aggravate the situation?

# Energy Transfer

# 11 Instruments in Surgery

*David C. Auth*

## 11.1 LEARNING OBJECTIVES

Upon completing this chapter you should be able to:

- State the principal methods for imparting or extracting energy to accomplish a surgical function.
- Describe the physical attributes of commonly available energy generators and make judgments concerning their overall effectiveness in anticipated surgical procedures.
- Describe the tradeoffs between cutting and coagulation efficiency.
- Describe the possibilities of conveying and delivering energy to remote areas of the body to accomplish a surgical function.
- Describe the technical literature discussing these new and evolving methods.
- Advise others on the feasibility of various energy devices for surgical procedures.

## 11.2 INTRODUCTION

Energy and one of its common forms, heat, are found everywhere in nature. We use energy, in one of its many forms, in nearly everything we do. Physicists use "conservation of energy" more than any other conservation property of nature to solve equations that deal with changes in matter. The ancients placed fire, one form of energy, into an elite category as one of the four elements. This chapter, and Chapter 10, concentrate on two of the most common forms of energy used for medical therapy: electrical and thermal.

Chapter 10 points out that the primary consequence of the use of radio-frequency electrical current in surgery is the generation of heat, which in turn results in a desired therapeutic effect. However, the subject of electrosurgery is sufficiently complex as to require a separate chapter. Thermal cautery for control of bleeding dates to the ancient Egyptians. With the widespread use of hot tools in early civilization, the reduction of bleeding in accidental transcutaneous injuries, compared to accidents occurring with cold sharp instruments, must have been noticed. In more recent times, the use of a hot iron for cautery is well known to the student of American Civil War history. When heat is applied to tissue, two important chemical changes occur:

1. The vapor pressure of the entrained tissue water increases, resulting in the release of water vapor, which in turn dries out the tissue (desiccates). This desiccation process causes a shrinkage of the tissue and a contraction of blood vessels.

2. The protein of the tissue and blood undergoes a change of physical state (denaturation) generally accompanied by a change of physical consistency from fluid to solid.

Both of these changes serve to reduce the loss of blood when thermal cautery is applied. It is precisely because of this heat-induced hemostasis that energy transfer devices have become important in surgery and repair of damaged tissue.

### Definition of Terms

**Surgery.** This is not an easily defined field of therapy. To some practitioners, surgery is the cutting of tissue. Others prefer to include the manipulation of tissue in some aggressive modality. Recently, many practitioners are referring to pure control of bleeding, when it is performed by energy transfer, as surgery. This reference is especially apparent in the recent development to stop bleeding of the gastrointestinal tract via peroral tubes that convey cautery energy to the bleeding lesion.

**Hemostasis.** From the Greek roots for "blood" and "stop," this word refers to the cessation of bleeding. The surgeon frequently secures hemostasis by suturing or ligating a bleeding vessel and, classically, surgeons pride themselves on suturing vessels with great dexterity and speed.

**Heat.** The physical form of contained energy in a substance is heat. Energy transfer devices either add to or take away heat from a substance. The hotter a substance becomes, the greater the contained energy and the greater the agitation of the molecules comprising the substance. Many chemical and biological transformations of a substance are directly associated with heat content or its commonly used measure, temperature.

**Coagulation.** This term has two very distinct meanings. A definition cherished by hematologists refers to the elaborate biochemical process in animals that allows the precipitation of platelets, which assemble in a plug, or clot, to inhibit the flow of blood. Another definition is indiscriminately used to refer to the disruption or denaturing of biological material usually associated with a stiffening of protein material. When we cook an egg on the stove, for example, the egg white, which contains a high percentage of the protein, albumin, becomes "denatured" protein. A chemical transformation dramatically results in a clearly visible stiffening of the material. This second definition of coagulation is the one associated with thermal hemostasis or cautery; because the blood plasma contains a high percentage of protein, it can be readily "coagulated" when heated.

**Cryosurgery.** This term refers to the utilization of "cold" for some surgical function. The placement of a cold substance adjacent to tissue results in the transfer of heat or energy away from tissue.

**Laser.** This term is an acronym for "light amplification by stimulated emission of radiation." This device has been a very important part of energetic surgery during the past 15 years, as it enables unique transport and deposition of thermal energy for surgical therapy.

**Endoscopy.** This word refers to the medical utilization of special optical instruments that permit the physician to visualize various regions of the body through a distal viewing port. The optical image is transported via a series of lenses, mirrors, or optical fibers to the outside of the body. Recently, the treatment of disease through such instruments has become quite practical and extensively used.

**Necrosis.** Refers to the death of tissue and it is frequently used in discussing thermal coagulation, as it normally accompanies coagulation. Necrosis may not cause undue consequences, because viable tissue can sometimes replace it without complication.

## Surgical Goals

**Cutting.** The severing of tissue is a primary function of many surgical procedures and various techniques may be utilized. Several techniques provide a cutting action by simultaneously employing more than one physical mechanism. Most cutting operations result in bleeding unless some specific action is taken to prevent it.

**Coagulation.** Prevention of the loss of blood is of paramount importance. Transfusions always contain an element of risk to the patient, one of the most common being infection. Acquiring blood suitable for transfusion is an expensive procedure even when the blood is donated. An important consideration for the cost-conscious engineer is the tradeoff between the cost of the transfusion and the cost of the instrumentation that eliminates the need for transfusion. Thermal knives in surgery always have a measure of coagulation associated with their cutting action. We discuss the level of coagulation efficiency and performance in the next section.

**Destruction.** There are many occasions when removal of tissue by a cutting or resecting maneuver is overly cumbersome. In recent years, the utilization of thermal devices to evaporate or freeze tissue for the express purpose of destruction has become increasingly popular. One of the best examples is use of supercooled liquids (liquid nitrogen) for the removal of warts. Another application gaining acceptance is the use of color pigmentation selective lasers for the preferential obliteration of tattoos and naturally occurring vascular birthmarks. These techniques permit selective removal of unwanted areas of tissue with only slight damage to adjacent tissue. Obviously, many of these procedures would involve microscopic precision if conventional resection using a steel scalpel were used. Furthermore, additional scarring would probably result.

### Remote Delivery

In addition to providing simultaneous cutting and coagulation, energy transfer devices frequently enable the delivery of surgical technique to otherwise inaccessible regions of the body. Perhaps the best example is the use of visible laser light to coagulate bleeding in the eye. Because the eye is transparent to light, we can direct a laser beam through the eye to the retina where its coherent optical energy is converted to thermal energy by absorption in hemoglobin molecules. This device permits direct, real-time coagulation of retinal tears under constant surveillance of the ophthalmologist. Not only is the action transmitted through the vitreous of the eye, but the vessel repair takes place in a space totally surrounded by tissue. An extensive armamentation of instruments is now developed for delivering therapeutic energy into remote areas of the human body.

## 11.3 HEMOSTASIS, COAGULATION, AND CAUTERY

### Adjuncts to Successful Cutting

As discussed in Chapter 10, thermal energy that is used for the evaporative cutting of tissue also provides some measure of coagulation. Depending on the temperature and tissue interaction of the thermal knife, the coagulation necrosis may extend several millimeters into tissue. With monopolar electrosurgery, electrical conduction to a distal patient plate results in tissue heating that is very intense in the region adjacent to the cutting scalpel. When the carbon dioxide, $CO_2$, laser scalpel is used, a small amount of heat is transferred to the tissue adjacent to the incision. The heat is able to coagulate protein molecules in the blood plasma adjacent to the incision, thereby "shrinking and plugging" the capillaries supplying that segment of tissue. We discuss other thermal knives in Section 11.4. Each thermal knife functions on a variation of this "shrinking and plugging" principle for hemostatic cutting.

### Physical Transformations

**Optical to Thermal.** Electromagnetic radiation in the visible or near infrared region of the spectrum is frequently referred to as optical radiation. Because short wavelength electromagnetic waves are easily confined to ducts or pipes and directed with high precision at biological structures, these waves acquire special importance in energetic coagulation. As optical waves are absorbed by matter, they excite the constituent atoms or molecules to a different quantum energy state. When the excited atom decays, it gives off either the same energy photon as that of the excitation process or a lower energy photon. The atom may also give up its energy to the environment in the form of vibrational quanta or mechanical quanta commonly referred to as *heat*. Solar heating is an example of this latter transformation.

**Thermal to Thermal.** Thermal energy may be exhibited in different ways. A hot gas is represented as a collection of rapidly moving molecules. If this collection of hot gaseous molecules impinges on a solid structure, that solid is heated by virtue of energy transfer at the impact interface. There may be a phase transition at the interface that provides even greater energy transfer. As an ice cube melts in a water bath, the heat of fusion is supplied by the water environment. If a hot substance touches the skin, a burn results because thermal energy is transferred to the skin with a resultant denaturation and dehydration of the affected tissue and, in severe cases, an evaporation of the tissue. Electrocautery probes and wires sometimes refer to heated objects made hot by the dissipation of heat in resistive electrical wires. Unfortunately, electrocautery also refers, in some authors' vocabularies, to direct RF electrosurgery as discussed in Chapter 10.

**Protein Denaturation.** As mentioned previously, protein molecules can be transformed or denatured by heat. Transformation typically takes place when the temperature of the protein reaches a temperature of 50–100°C. The extent of denaturation depends, to a small degree, on the time duration of the temperature evaluation. Normally, the process of denaturation results in necrosis.

**Vessel Shrinkage.** The process of protein stiffening secondary to denaturation results in obstruction of a bleeding vessel. The vessel itself also naturally tends to shrink when heated. We can explain some of this shrinkage by dehydration. The combination of vessel shrinkage and protein stiffening makes thermal coagulation effective in accomplishing hemostasis.

**Tissue Freezing.** Contrary to other methods of thermal denaturation discussed in this chapter, cryosurgery extracts energy from the tissue and forces a physical change. The transfer of the energy is accomplished by thermal conduction from the tissue to a cold probe that is placed against the tissue. The change in physical state associated with this cooling varies from temperature reduction to below normal physiological levels to actual freezing or solidification. When the tissue is frozen in this manner, the cell may be destroyed because of electrolytic changes within the cell or mechanical rupture due to the volume increase of the ice crystals. At the very least, temporary hemostasis can be accomplished using cryosurgery.

## Energy Transfer

**Radiation.** If light of a wavelength that is not highly absorbed by tissue is present, it penetrates into the tissue depth, gives up a portion of its energy, and provides for deep coagulation (Kiefhaber et al., 1975). We can argue that this deep and essentially instantaneous coagulation is of value in stopping bleeding in the presence of massive flow rates or in some circumstances in which intervening tissue is otherwise in the way; however, deep tissue damage also occurs.

**Conduction.** Heat conduction is a familiar process. Conduction is governed by a linear equation wherein the quantity of energy transfer is proportional to the area of interaction, the temperature difference, and the thermal conduction coefficient of the substance involved. In biological structures that are highly complex and inhomogeneous, simple thermal conduction modeling is normally impossible. However, the use of approximate models can sometimes yield useful results. Thus, for example, the use of the water as a medium similar to actual tissue can provide some insight into the ability to transport energy within tissue. When we use laser light to coagulate tissue, the radiative heating propagates quickly by optical absorption. As time progresses, some of the surface energy is transferred into the depth by radiation or thermal conduction.

**Convection.** The movement of matter that contains thermal energy is referred to as convection. In surgery, convection normally hampers the surgical procedure by draining away energy. The circulation of blood in tissue beneath a deliberately coagulated zone can remove heat energy that might otherwise build up, causing further tissue destruction or denaturation in the depth. In some applications of massive hemorrhage, it is necessary to first stagnate the flow of blood before attempting to provide hemostasis (Kimura et al., 1978).

## Energy Generators

**Electrical Resistance Heating.** These devices depend upon the generation of heat within themselves as electrical current flows through a conductor. Although electrocautery is sometimes confused with electrosurgery, electrocautery refers to the actual formation of heat in a probe or wire, which is then transferred (normally by thermal conduction) to the tissue to be coagulated or cut. Figure 11.1a shows a simple electrocautery or thermal probe. A voltage generator forces current to flow in a resistive coil of wire embedded in the probe. The flow of current causes heat formation as the electrons collide with the crystalline boundary layers in the metal wire. Nichrome wire is a popular material for this purpose because it has high electrical resistance and is stable at moderately high temperatures. In particular, it does not undergo severe oxidation at elevated temperatures. The heat generated by the hot coil of wire is transferred by thermal conduction through a ceramic matrix filling the space between the wire coil and the surrounding metal cup. If the metal cup, measuring approximately 2 mm in diameter, is touched to tissue, coagulation results. It is important to control the temperature of the probe in order to control hemostasis. If the probe tip temperature is too low, the coagulation will not start or will take a protracted length of time to occur, or it may cause deep tissue injury because of extensive thermal conduction into the depth.

Figure 11.1b shows a modified probe. This probe has a thermocouple imbedded in the ceramic matrix, which is used to monitor and control the tip temperature. Protell et al., (1978) have used such a device for endoscopic coagulation of GI bleeding. The electrical voltage produced by the imbedded thermocouple controls

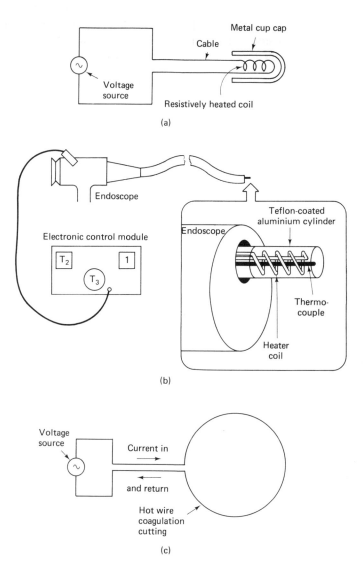

(a)

(b)

(c)

**FIGURE 11.1.** Three forms of electrocautery (thermal coagulation). (a) Simple electrical resistance probe. (b) Endoscopically passable electrocautery probe with thermocouple servo control of temperature. (Reprinted from *Auth, Gastroenterology,* 74(2), Part I, 258, 1978, with permission.) (c) Hot wire electrocautery for coagulation or cutting.

the supplied electrical resistance heating and thus ensures a preset temperature. Controlled studies show that contact temperatures for rapid coagulation should be 70–100°C for bare metal probes and 100–170°C for probes with dielectric coatings used for easy tissue release. This property of tissue release is especially important. Protell et al., (1978) report that the aluminum metal cup surrounding the ceramic matrix is coated with Teflon for easy detachment after coagulation. If this release property is not incorporated in the construction of the probe, the denatured clot of blood is frequently pulled off when the probe is removed, causing additional bleeding. Small probes are now available so that they can be delivered through operating channels of approximately 3 mm.

Figure 11.1c shows another type of electrocautery. The electrical resistance heating takes place in a metal wire that is the very element directly applied to the tissue. The heated wire may be made of nichrome or stainless steel. The hot wire exhibits a cutting action when touched to tissue but also can provide a considerable level of local hemostasis, depending upon the temperature and pressure of application. The instrument's use is dependent upon the skill of the operator; the wire can stick in the tissue if the speed is not carefully controlled. Excessive charring and mechanical adhesion can result.

**Optical Generators.** As mentioned previously, the energy contained in an optical electromagnetic wave or light beam can be converted to useful heat for coagulation purposes when it impinges on tissue or blood. Much of the interest in recent years in optical generators has focused on the use of lasers. The reason is twofold: (1) the laser provides light of pure spectral color and thus can be tuned to a specific absorption band for a particular chemical/molecular interaction; and (2) the laser light has a property referred to as *spatial coherence,* which implies high directionality or the ability to be focused into very small areas.

Figure 11.2 shows the difference between incoherent and coherent optical sources. Figure 11.2a shows a typical incandescent filament light source. If its light is collected and refocused by a lens, an image of the hot filament is obtained. With proper focusing, the resultant image may be smaller than the original filament. When this happens, the radiance of the image can be no greater than the original filament itself. It is an important property of light that the intrinsic radiance of an optical source can never be increased by a passive collection of optical elements, such as lenses, mirrors, and so on. Radiance is defined as the power per unit solid angle per unit projected area. In mathematical terms,

$$N_\theta = \frac{P_\theta}{(d\Omega_\theta) \, ([\cos \, \theta] \, dA_\theta)}$$

Thus, the radiance $(N_\theta)$ in direction $\theta$ degrees from the source axis is given as the power $(P_\theta)$ per unit solid angle $(d\Omega_\theta)$ per unit projected source area $[(\cos \, \theta) \, dA_\theta]$. In most practical applications, the radiance of an actual instrument is much less than the original radiance of the generating source. The laser, by virtue of its spatial coherence, possesses high radiance; that is, a laser's power density per unit of projected source area per unit of solid angle of illumination is high. A surgical laser can have a radiance greater than $10^{12}$ W/m$^2 \cdot$sr, whereas the radiance of a tungsten filament light bulb is approximately $10^6$ W/m$^2 \cdot$sr.

It is well known that we can generate and propagate a pencil-thin beam of laser light over a long distance. This property is referred to as *collimation.* A well-collimated beam of light may be obtained from an incandescent source if nearly all the optical intensity or power per unit area is sacrificed. When we perform such a

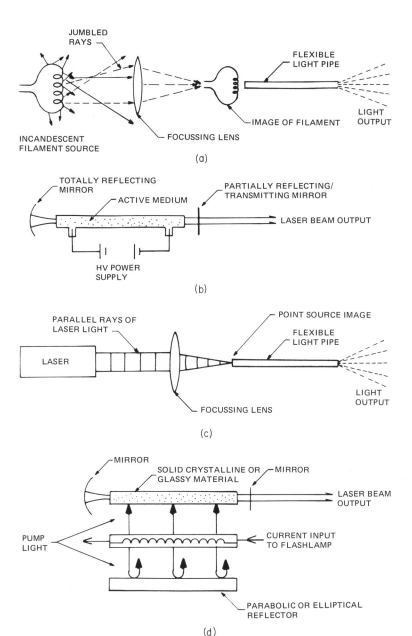

JUMBLED
RAYS

FLEXIBLE
LIGHT PIPE

IMAGE OF FILAMENT

LIGHT
OUTPUT

INCANDESCENT
FILAMENT SOURCE

FOCUSSING LENS

(a)

TOTALLY REFLECTING
MIRROR

ACTIVE MEDIUM

PARTIALLY REFLECTING/
TRANSMITTING MIRROR

LASER BEAM OUTPUT

HV POWER
SUPPLY

(b)

PARALLEL RAYS OF
LASER LIGHT

POINT SOURCE IMAGE

FLEXIBLE
LIGHT PIPE

LASER

LIGHT
OUTPUT

FOCUSSING LENS

(c)

MIRROR

SOLID CRYSTALLINE OR
GLASSY MATERIAL

MIRROR

LASER BEAM
OUTPUT

PUMP
LIGHT

CURRENT INPUT
TO FLASHLAMP

PARABOLIC OR ELLIPTICAL
REFLECTOR

(d)

**FIGURE 11.2.** Characteristics of surgical lasers contrasted to incandescent light. (a) Because of its low radiance, the incandescent source couples poorly to an optical fiber. (b) Elementary schematic of an electrical discharge gas laser of the argon or $CO_2$ type. (c) Efficient coupling of a high radiance laser source to an optical fiber. (d) Optically pumped solid state laser of the Nd:YAG type. (Reprinted from *Progress in hemostasis and thrombosis*, Vol. 4, New York: Grune and Stratton with permission.)

collimation experiment using incandescent light, we select a very small portion of the incandescent source and locate it at the focal point of a lens or mirror. The lens converts this point source of light into a set of parallel rays. The amount of energy from the point area of the incandescent source is indeed very small.

The laser, by contrast, operates by supplying atomic energy to an oscillating collimated beam of light set in motion between two parallel mirrors. The mirrors form a resonant electromagnetic structure that permits sustained reflection of light that is very well defined in its collimation. It is the property of stimulated emission of light that the wavelength and direction of light given off by the stimulated atoms are the same as the light causing the stimulation. Thus, as the light oscillates between parallel mirrors, it stimulates atoms between the mirrors to do likewise. Soon a large collection of electromagnetic radiation is circulating between the mirrors, which then can be "tapped" for a useful application.

The normal method of tapping this radiation is utilizing a partially transmitting mirror on one side of the optical resonator. Figure 11.2b depicts this structure with radiation emerging from the right side. In Fig. 11.2b, the atoms that supply the optical power are in a gaseous form in which they become excited by the discharge of electrical current. Thus, the atoms are energized by the flow of electricity, but they then give up their energy in a more organized way by supporting the highly directional oscillation between the mirrors. The partially transmitting mirror leaks some of the light out of the cavity and, in so doing, is sampling and preserving the directional character of light within the cavity. This sampling function is much the same as the capacitive extraction of electrical power from an oscillating electrical circuit. The limited bandwidth of circulating electrical energy in an electronic oscillator is replicated when extracted for work in the external world.

An important feature of a modern dielectric optical mirror is low total loss. Low total loss means that nearly all the energy not reflected by a dielectric mirror is transmitted. In contrast, for a metallic mirror (e.g., silver or aluminum) that would typically provide a reflection coefficient of 94% with 1% transmission, approximately 5% of the energy is lost. Energy loss is critical in laser systems because the trapped power in the resonant cavity can be quite high and a 5% loss factor would be, in some cases, much more energy than is coupled out for work. Figure 11.2c shows the laser light focused into a small light pipe by a conventional optical lens. Because many laser light applications require transport of coagulating radiation into remote areas of the body, the conveyance via microminiature waveguides is important. Furthermore, glass optical fibers used as the waveguides for low-loss purposes must be relatively slender to provide mechanical flexibility when needed.

Figure 11.2a shows incandescent light focused by a lens. If the focused light is directed at a slender optical waveguide, only a tiny percentage will actually be trapped in the guide; the rest will be wasted or, worse, may cause thermal damage to adjacent assemblies. Other familiar sources of spatially incoherent or diffuse light (low radiance) are gaseous discharges such as a neon sign, or the high-pressure xenon arc lamp. High-pressure discharges can emit high levels of radiant intensity compared to conventional incoherent sources but are, nonetheless, much lower in optical radiance than even a modest laser source.

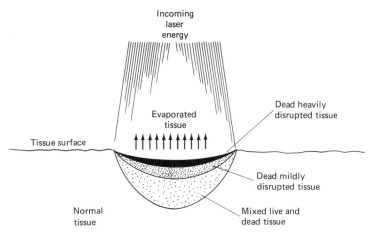

Incoming
laser
energy

Evaporated
tissue

Dead heavily
disrupted tissue

Tissue surface

Dead mildly
disrupted tissue

Normal
tissue

Mixed live and
dead tissue

**FIGURE 11.3.** Interaction of laser light with tissue. In this picture, the light is spread out causing a smooth coagulation rather than surgical cutting.

Laser sources utilizing gaseous atomic media or solid crystalline media are the most common for medical therapy. Figure 11.2d shows a typical crystalline laser. To obtain an electrical discharge within a solid or crystalline medium is impractical and, thus, an external light source is used to optically "pump" the laser medium. The optical pumping takes the place of the electrical discharge depicted in Fig. 11.2b. A therapeutic laser using this configuration is the Nd:YAG, the symbolic name referring to a neodymium-doped yttrium aluminum garnet crystal that serves as the agent for atomic amplification of the electromagnetic wave of the optical cavity resonator.

When the laser is used for coagulation, a beam of light is directed at the bleeding tissue either directly from the laser generator, via a system of lenses and mirrors, or via a fiberoptic cable. Figure 11.3 shows the interaction of a diverging beam of light (laser) when it impacts a tissue surface. The optical energy causes a rapid elevation in temperature of the tissue. At the surface, the tissue may evaporate if the energy density is high. At lower energy densities, coagulation may proceed with only a small release of water vapor. The amount of coagulation and the extent of desiccation is a function of the temperature of the tissue and, to a lesser extent, the length of time at which the temperature is elevated. Predicting the actual temperature rise following a known energy exposure of laser radiation is not an easy calculation because several undetermined variables are present, including scattering from the tissue matrix, inhomogeneous distribution of pigmentation (blood), convection cooling by moving blood in the local vascular structure, reflection from the tissue surface, formation of char at the surface, change of conductivity of the tissue following desiccation, and so on. In general, deep damage is associated with deep penetrating radiation (which is weakly absorbed by the tissue) and thermal applications, which are intense and protracted. As Fig. 11.3 shows, the profile of coagulation and tissue disruption graduates to normalcy into the depth of

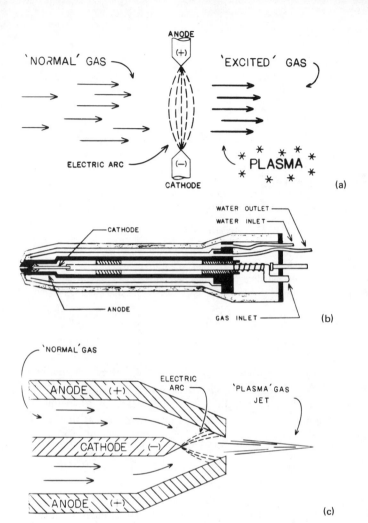

FIGURE 11.4. Schematic of the plasma scalpel. (a) Physical process. (b) Electrical schematic. (c) Overall system. (Reproduced with permission from Glover, J. L., Bendick, P. J., and Link, W. J., The Use of Thermal Knives in Surgery: Electrosurgery, Lasers, Plasma Scalpel, in Ravitch, M. M., et al. (eds.), *Current problems in surgery*. © Copyright 1978 by Year Book Medical Publishers, Inc., Chicago, IL.)

the tissue where the laser energy density and the subsequent temperature rise diminish.

**Plasma Sources.** The plasma scalpel (Glover et al., 1978) is a relatively new device available to surgeons for hemostatic incisions and local cutting. Figure 11.4 shows the typical instrument design; the plasma or electrically charged particles of gas are formed as they exit a metallic nozzle. A strong electric field causes the particles issuing from the nozzle to become charged, and therefore energetic. Their kinetic energy arises partially from motion and partially from the thermal excitation within the inert gas atoms. When the gaseous atoms impinge on tissue, the atoms give up energy to the tissue, and the result is local heating and hemostasis. Use of an inert gas avoids chemically deleterious effects.

**Other Sources.** We can propose a large array of other devices that will impart thermal energy to tissue. Thus far, most of these other techniques, such as

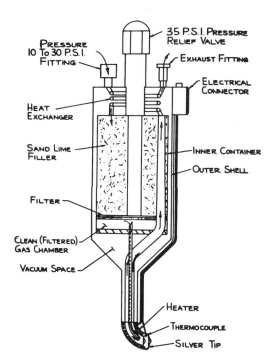

PRESSURE
10 TO 30 P.S.I.
FITTING

35 P.S.I. PRESSURE
RELIEF VALVE

EXHAUST FITTING

ELECTRICAL
CONNECTOR

HEAT
EXCHANGER

SAND LIME
FILLER

INNER CONTAINER

OUTER SHELL

FILTER

CLEAN (FILTERED)
GAS CHAMBER

VACUUM SPACE

HEATER

THERMOCOUPLE

SILVER TIP

**FIGURE 11.5.** Cryoprobe with liquid nitrogen as the working fluid. (From Rand, Cryosurgery, 1968. Courtesy of Charles C Thomas, Publisher, Springfield, IL.)

hot oil sprays and so on, are not practical in most applications, and we do not discuss them in detail.

**Cryoprobes.** Figure 11.5 shows a conventional cryosurgical probe. Liquid nitrogen is circulated adjacent to a metallic endpiece that makes actual contact with the tissue. Liquid nitrogen boils at 77°K or −196°C. Because a great amount of energy must be supplied to provide the boiling process, liquid nitrogen provides a well-calibrated source of refrigeration; in effect, the liquid nitrogen clamps its own temperature at 77°K until all the liquid converts to gas. This reference temperature applies to a standard atmospheric pressure "head" above the nitrogen. If the probe is inserted into a body cavity, the sides of the probe must be thermally insulated from adjacent organs.

The process of hemostasis with cryosurgery differs from that of heat denaturation of protein. The near term effect is to freeze the tissue and blood into a solid or congealed mass, which does not permit fluid transport. Another benefit of cryotherapy is to slow vascular circulation and thus transport of fluid, hence to slow bleeding. At present, the hemostatic benefits of cryotherapy for long-term management of bleeding problems are not well documented.

Other cryogenic surgery devices utilizing the Joule-Thompson expansion of gas (i.e., similar to normal Freon refrigeration systems) and the Peltier effect have been devised and may serve a particular purpose better than a liquid nitrogen probe. Maintenance of the liquid nitrogen gas requires a special "dewar" or "thermos bottle." This contains the gas without excessive loss of material due to boiling caused by energy leakage into the containment vessel.

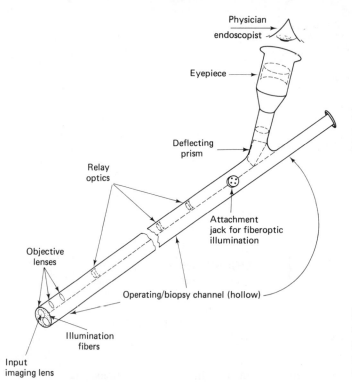

Physician
endoscopist

Eyepiece

Deflecting
prism

Relay
optics

Objective
lenses

Attachment
jack for fiberoptic
illumination

Operating/biopsy channel (hollow)

Illumination
fibers

Input
imaging lens

**FIGURE 11.6.** Rigid endoscope for visualization of internal body cavities. The operating channel permits insufflation, biopsy, or therapeutic operations.

## *Special Delivery Systems*

**Endoscopy.** A vast array of optical imaging systems now exists to aid the physician in the diagnosis of disease. These devices are also becoming increasingly important for therapy. Unlike the x-ray machine, the endoscope permits direct visualization of the diseased area in the body and affords the opportunity, via an operating channel, to administer therapy under direct surveillance. There are two basic types of endoscopes: rigid and flexible. Figure 11.6 shows a rigid endoscope, which uses a series of lenses to convey to the physician an image of a remote organ. Many applications of such an instrument in the management of diseases of the ear, throat, urinary tract, bone joints, and abdominal cavity have become routine. In applications in which a naturally occurring opening is not available, a small incision is made to enable passage of the endoscope. Thus, for example, a short (approximately 1 cm) incision is made in the abdominal wall to facilitate passage of the laparoscope to provide visualization of the Fallopian tubes during tubal ligation. These scope incisions are generally atraumatic and heal in a few days.

The sigmoidscope is an older instrument that consists of a hollow cylinder permitting direct viewing of the rectum and sigmoid colon. A much more sophisticated instrument that makes use of large self-focusing optical fibers permits visualization through an aperture of about 1.5 mm. A special optical fiber or cylinder

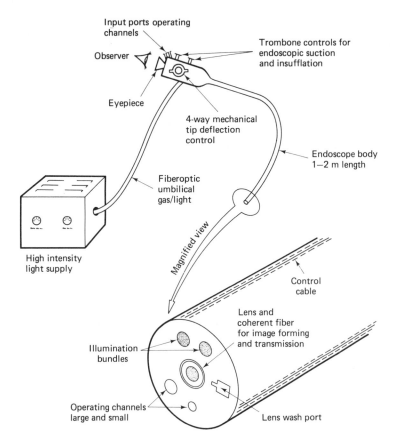

**FIGURE 11.7.** Flexible fiberendoscope with dual operating channels.

with a graded index of refraction from the center to the periphery produces, in effect, a continuum of closely packed low-power lenses. As such, it accomplishes the same mission as the rigid endoscope of Fig. 11.6 with a very small instrument diameter.

Figure 11.7 shows a conventional fiberoptic endoscope for flexible intubation and observation of remote anatomy. The image is first focused onto the distal array of optical fibers by a remote lens and is then broken up into an array of picture elements or "pixels." Each component of the picture is transported back to the proximal eyepiece by an individual optical fiber. If the picture is to have a field resolution of 200 × 200 elements, 40,000 fibers are required. This requirement is well within the realm of current technology.

Figure 11.7 shows that the endoscope is provided with longitudinal metal cables for distal guiding of the scope. A proximal control handle allows four-way vectoring of the distal tip. Some endoscopes can be deflected greater than 180°, allowing the scope to "look" at itself. Endoscopes have been specifically developed for visualization of the entire human colon, the stomach and duodenum, and

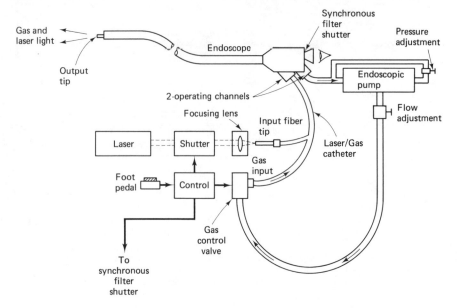

**FIGURE 11.8.** Laser photocoagulator for gastrointestinal endoscopy. A two channel operating endoscope allows for gas evacuation from one channel and simultaneous gas-jet assisted laser through the other.

bronchus. Their outer diameters range from approximately 6–15 mm, depending upon the application. The smaller scopes sacrifice some level of resolution but permit bronchoscopic or pediatric applications. Originally, the full-length hollow channel extending from the physician to the remote organ was used primarily for biopsy of suspicious lesions.

Much effort is currently devoted to exploration of diverse therapeutic methodology that can be transmitted through the endoscope. One therapeutic technique is the use of laser light for coagulation of gastrointestinal bleeding (Auth et al., 1976). This procedure utilizes laser light conducted along a single low-loss optical fiber of the type developed for optical communications. The fiber must have low loss so it will not be destroyed by the high optical power density, which may exceed 100 $kW/cm^2$. Furthermore, the use of an array of fibers is precluded because the laser light would destroy the optical fibers if it were focused into the interstices of the optical array.

New endoscopy systems have been developed (Kimura et al., 1978) in which the adjunctive use of pressurizing gas allows temporary stagnation of bleeding to assist the laser in denaturing and clotting bleeding vessels. This adjunctive gas pressurization scheme is especially important in episodes of severe bleeding in which an actual jet of blood is present. Figure 11.8 shows an example of such an endoscopic system. Overinsufflation of the patient's stomach must be avoided when the instrument is used for controlling massive gastric ulcer bleeding; one of the best methods to avoid overinflation is a closed-loop gas recycling system, wherein gas is

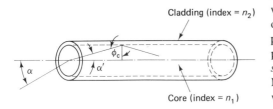

Cladding (index = $n_2$)

Core (index = $n_1$)

**FIGURE 11.9.** Cladded optical waveguide. Note the trapping of optical radiation by the transparent cylindrical core. (Reprinted from *Progress in hemostasis and thrombosis,* Vol. 4, New York: Grune and Stratton with permission.)

pumped out of the stomach before being reinjected as a gas jet assist (Auth et al., 1978). To further enhance clinical utility, the use of a servo control of flow rate preserves the volume of the hollow organ being examined. Thus, the physician performing the endoscopic therapy retains good apposition to the particular lesion being treated without volume change and the associated lesion motion during the procedure.

Instruments that allow distal and relatively noninvasive control of bleeding are particularly important to reduce mortality and morbidity in very ill patients who are poor surgical risks. In addition, these instruments reduce the cost of transfusions and surgery.

**Optical Fibers.** Figure 11.9 shows a typical fiberoptic waveguide used in laser photocoagulation or image transport. For low loss, the fiber is constructed of glass. Glass is somewhat flexible in fibers up to 1 mm in diameter. Fibers of 600-$\mu$m outer diameter permit bends down to about 2-cm radius of curvature. The larger the diameter, the greater is the elastic stress that is built up in the outer regions of the glass cylinder when the fiber is bent. Plastic fibers for optical wave conduction have been widely used but are not available with low loss. In Fig. 11.9, the outer cylinder consists of a lower index of refraction glass ($\eta_2$) or, in some cases, a plastic or silicone compound. The optical rays are reflected when they impinge on the interface, provided they have an angle of incidence (measured from the normal to the interface) that is larger than the critical angle of internal reflection. Reflection from such dielectric interfaces can be made to have almost no loss; for this reason, optical fibers with core (inner cylinder) diameters of the order of 100 $\mu$m can have attenuation coefficients of less than 5 dB/km.

In order to package endoscopes with a sufficiently large number of fibers to permit good optical resolution and yet retain small dimensions for insertion into body cavities, the individual fibers must be small. Typical sizes used by the endoscope makers are 10 $\mu$m outside diameter. Of course, for endoscopic imaging applications, the arrangement of the fibers with respect to each other must be preserved from input to output in order to preserve the image. Light rays that fall below the critical angle for internal reflection will be lost from the fiber. For this reason, the numerical aperture (NA) is frequently specified to formally state the maximum angle at which light can be trapped within the fiber and hence be allowed to exit. The numerical aperture is analogous in definition and application to that commonly used to describe microscope objective lenses. It is the sine of the maximum half-angle of the radiation that will be trapped and propagated by the fiber. For a structure such as Fig. 11.9, the value of numerical aperture is given as:

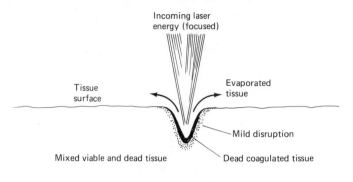

Incoming laser
energy (focused)

Tissue
surface

Evaporated
tissue

Mild disruption

Mixed viable and dead tissue

Dead coagulated tissue

Normal tissue

**FIGURE 11.10.** Use of focused laser radiation for evaporative cutting of tissue with associated coagulation and hemostasis.

$$NA = \frac{(\eta_2{}^2 - \eta_1{}^2)^{\frac{1}{2}}}{\eta_1} = \sin \alpha$$

With values of $\eta_2$ only slightly larger than $\eta_1$, it is possible to have values of NA that arc about 0.2 and, thus, the corresponding full acceptance angle ($2\alpha$) is equal to 23°.

## 11.4 CUTTING INSTRUMENTS

### General

As discussed previously, the energy associated with heat transfer may lend itself to a cutting function in addition to pure coagulation. Chapter 10 discusses ways of configuring electrosurgery to enhance the cutting effectiveness. Two principal characteristics are involved in thermal knife cutting: (1) evaporation of tissue in a serial fashion leaving a linear crater; or (2) increase in temperature, making possible blunt scalpel dissection or enhancing sharp scalpel dissection. In the first instance, we desire a thermal knife that favors rapid evaporation. Tissue may simply be transformed into a vapor state with resultant cratering, or steam vesicles can be formed that provide microexplosions, thereby rupturing the tissue. The latter method is typical of the cut mode of operation in electrosurgery.

### Laser Cutting

**Specific Laser Types.** The carbon dioxide laser has been widely utilized (Kaplan, 1976) for evaporative cutting of tissue. Because the 10.6-$\mu$m wavelength of this laser is in the middle-infrared region of the spectrum, it is rapidly absorbed by the water molecule. Because water is a major constituent of tissue, steam is formed when radiation strikes the tissue surface. Figure 11.10 shows the interaction of a focused laser beam on the surface of tissue. The laser cuts when the beam is

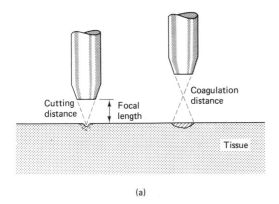

(a)

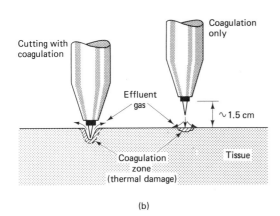

(b)

**FIGURE 11.11.** Cut mode versus coagulation mode for the laser and plasma scalpel. (a) A focused laser beam provides cutting action with some coagulation at the margin of the incision. A defocused beam provides coagulation with cutting. (b) The plasma scalpel cuts and coagulates simultaneously when in direct contact with the tissue surface. Coagulating without cutting can be performed readily by holding the tip of the handpiece approximately 1-2 cm from the tissue surface. (Reproduced with permission from Glover, J. L., Bendick, P. J., and Link, W. J., The Use of Thermal Knives in Surgery: Electrosurgery, Lasers, Plasma Scalpel, in Ravitch, M. M., et al. (eds.), *Current problems in surgery.* © Copyright 1978 by Year Book Medical Publishers, Inc., Chicago, IL.)

focused or coagulates when it is defocused, as shown in Fig. 11.11a. Ablation of tissue can be accomplished if a focused beam is rapidly swept over a surface. The hemostasis that accompanies a cutting instrument is inversely proportional to its cutting efficiency. Tissue is evaporated, thereby forming a crater or incision. A firm layer of carbonized tissue may be present at the surface. Directly beneath this zone a solid layer of coagulated tissue and blood is present, thereby sealing off further bleeding. Further into the depth, the tissue is in the normal condition. The depth of the coagulation zone (necessarily necrotic) is a function of the penetration depth of the laser used (see Fig. 11.12). Thus, if the wavelength of the radiation used for cutting is quickly absorbed by the tissue, it produces a less hemostatic incision than if the radiation penetrates more deeply into the bulk. The physical basis for this phenomenon is quite simple; as the radiation penetrates more deeply, more power is needed to bring the temperature of the entrained water to the boiling point. At the same time, adjacent tissue, not being boiled, is being coagulated to depths proportional to the penetration depth. Thus, when the incision is accomplished, a residue of unboiled and unfractured but denatured and coagulated tissue is left.

Figure 11.12 lists the tissue penetration depths of the $CO_2$, argon, and Nd:YAG lasers. Due to the shallow penetration depth of the $CO_2$ laser, we expect less coagulation with an incision. At the same time, we expect less necrosis to

|  | $CO_2$ | Argon | Nd:YAG |
|---|---|---|---|
| Wavelength (nm) | 10600 | 488–515 | 1050 |
| Red tissue | 0.05 mm | 0.5–0.8 mm | 3–5 mm |
| Whole blood | 0.05 mm | 0.1 mm | 0.6 mm |

**FIGURE 11.12.** Penetration depth for three surgical lasers in vascular tissue and whole blood (approximate values, depending upon hemoglobin concentration).

adjacent tissue. With the deeper penetration of the argon (wavelength: 488–515 nm) laser, we anticipate more coagulation in the wake of the incision. However, with a limited amount of power for evaporation and with the greater volume exposed (by virtue of the greater penetration depth), cutting efficiency is substantially reduced. Due to this inefficiency, the argon laser has not been extensively used by itself as a cutting scalpel. The Nd:YAG (wavelength: 1060 nm) laser penetrates quite deeply into tissue and is widely recognized as a very effective coagulating laser. The ND:YAG laser, however, is even less efficient as an evaporating-cutting laser than the argon laser.

**Plasma Scalpel.** Section 11.3 describes this device as a coagulation device. Without making any changes in configuration, the plasma scalpel is useful as a scalpel. Figure 11.11b shows the change in position necessary to convert the surgical result of hemostatic cutting to simple hemostasis. Although early work suggested a hazard of gas embolism by the use of the plasma scalpel in liver surgery, more recent work has diminished this fear (Glover et al., 1978). The plasma scalpel has an advantage over the $CO_2$ laser by its ability to cut effectively in the presence of blood, because the blood is automatically cleared from the field by the plentiful flow of gas. A gas assist, of course, can also be incorporated with a $CO_2$ laser to clear the field of obscuring water-laden blood, thereby allowing the infrared laser radiation to incise the tissue.

**Laser Blade Scalpel.** Figure 11.13 shows a hybrid scalpel that uses argon or Nd:YAG laser radiation trapped within a transparent mechanical scalpel blade (Kaplan, 1978). The scalpel's advantage is rapid cutting performance when utilized with wavelengths that alone are inefficient cutting modalities. Using fiberoptics, the laser radiation is flexibly coupled from the laser generator to the transparent blade. The laser radiation is injected into the transparent blade and then propagates to the sharp edge, as shown in Fig. 11.13. As the radiation propagates in the tapered waveguide zone proximate to the sharp edge, it begins to change its angle with respect to the plane of the blade. The radiation is confined to the plane of the blade because the angle of the optical rays is beyond the critical angle for internal reflection. Radiation leakage begins to occur as propagation in the tapered zone causes the component rays to fall below the critical angle. Thus, radiation is coupled out along the facets of the blade near the sharp cutting edge. The tissue is mechanically incised and subsequently coagulated by the proximate laser radiation. The facets of the blade press the immediately incised vessels shut, and the radiation is absorbed and simultaneously welds and cauterizes the bleeding vessels. If moderate hemostasis is desired, the argon laser provides selective damage to the bleeding vessels. For more extensive hemostasis (e.g., liver surgery), the Nd:YAG laser is preferable.

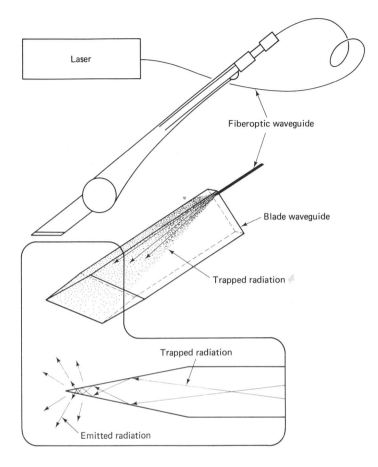

Laser

Fiberoptic waveguide

Blade waveguide

Trapped radiation

Trapped radiation

Emitted radiation

**FIGURE 11.13.** The laser blade scalpel combines mechanical parting of tissue with the coagulation efficiency of argon and ND:YAG laser radiation.

**Performance Tradeoffs.** The evaporative cutting characteristic of the $CO_2$ laser is very useful for surgical procedures in which a direct viewing telescope or large rigid endoscope may be employed. It conveys the radiation to the remote zone where hemostatic removal of the tissue is desired. The $CO_2$ laser scalpel uses the "articulating arm" shown in Fig. 11.14 to transport radiation from the laser generator to the operating field. This articulating arm is a series of mirrors that allows for rotation around an axis of 45° to a mirror plane. As the rotation proceeds, the radiation follows a path along the cylindrical structure containing the beam. This complicated device is required to provide some measure of flexibility to the surgeon during the operating procedure. If a flexible fiberoptic waveguide were available to carry high-power radiation at this wavelength, it would be of great help in surgery.

The plasma scalpel and the laser-blade scalpel both offer flexible conduits to convey the power to the operating field. One criticism that surgeons frequently make of the articulated arm $CO_2$ laser scalpel is the absence of tactile feedback during the cutting procedure. The radiation is focused at some predetermined point in space where the intense radiation facilitates rapid cutting. The surgeon, with the

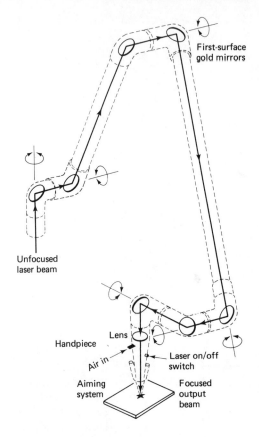

First-surface gold mirrors

Unfocused laser beam

Handpiece

Lens

Air in

Laser on/off switch

Aiming system

Focused output beam

**FIGURE 11.14.** Articulating arm for quasiflexible conveyance of carbon dioxide middle infrared laser light. (Reprinted with permission from Goldman, *Applications of the laser*. © Copyright by the Chemical Rubber Co., CRC Press, Inc.)

aid of a low-power visible light laser, is able to project the cutting action at some distance beyond the hand-held distal delivery system. All of these thermal knives, with the exception of the electrocautery wire, are intrinsically quite expensive and their use is not warranted unless we can identify specific benefits to the patient. When excessive blood loss may accompany a cold steel knife incision, one of the thermal knives could be safer and less expensive considering the cost of multiple blood transfusions.

## 11.5 TISSUE DESTRUCTION AND REMOVAL

The cutting efficiency of various thermal knives is used to remove lesions. In many instances, it is impractical to excise a malignant growth of tissue and, in some cases, the ability to ablate tissue in a controlled manner is preferable. The $CO_2$ laser is especially adept for controlled tissue ablation because material is boiled off the surface without excessive tissue necrosis. To accomplish this superficial evaporation of tissue, it is necessary to provide high-peak power densities to the tissue so that substantial evaporation can occur before heat is conducted into the depth of the tissue. This can be accomplished in two ways: (1) use of a focused spot of light that is rapidly scanned over the tissue; (2) use of a repetitively pulsed laser having a low-duty cycle.

The cryoprobe is useful to freeze undesirable cell masses, resulting in cell death. The speed with which freezing occurs is of importance in determining the extent of tissue destruction. Also, extensive freeze/thaw cycles may be necessary to secure cell destruction. Using a solid-tube endoscope, polyps or hemorrhoids inside various anatomical cavities may be conveniently removed. If unwanted tissue can be destroyed without affecting desirable tissue nearby, selective removal of the lesion can proceed.

Some surgeons use the cryoprobe to secure frozen mechanical contact of a tissue mass to the probe tip, which can then be used for mechanical extraction. This method has been used for removal of brain tumors. Controlled partial destruction or irritation of tissue can provoke a beneficial tissue response. Cryosurgery has been used to irritate the choroid of the eye, whereupon a locally formed exudate acts as a physiological binder to reattach the retina. Ophthalmologists have used cryoadhesion to extract cataracts and the advantages of this technique have been documented.

Cryosurgical methods in the management of cancer are primarily directed at the destruction of all cells in the diseased target area. Cryosurgery offers the special advantage of preventing dissemination of malignant cells because they are retained in a frozen zone.

## 11.6 EXAMPLES

### Ophthalmic Laser Photocoagulator

This device permits coagulation of bleeding vessels in the human eye. It is normally a part of an ophthalmologic slit-lamp biomicroscope. The ophthalmologist is able to visualize the process of vessel coagulation. The xenon arc lamp (Meyer-Schwickerath, 1960) has been successfully used for coagulation of bleeding ophthalmic disorders. The lamp's rather diffuse source characteristic (low radiance) frequently resulted in lesion production of a scale larger than desired. With the advent of laser technology in the 1960s, various investigators (Koester et al., 1962) began successfully to use the more easily controlled light from the laser for retinal coagulation. The ruby laser was replaced by the argon laser, which permitted a continuous beam of blue-green light to be directed with high precision and control at the retina to weld and coagulate bleeding vessels (L'Esperance, 1968).

Figure 11.15 shows the schematic diagram for an argon laser retinal photocoagulator. An orange filter separates and protects the physician's eye and enables continuous surveillance with full safety and comfort. The laser supplies power of approximately 1 W that is directed at the cornea; the eye itself focuses the incoming collimated radiation onto the retina. The laser radiation can be heavily attenuated, which enables the ophthalmologist to precisely target his lesion before firing the surgical pulse at high power. A pulse less than 1 s produces a well-defined and delimited lesion on the retinal surface. Lesions as small as 10 $\mu$m can be produced

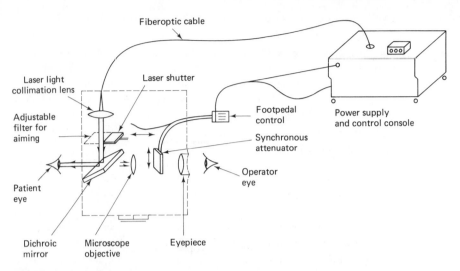

FIGURE 11.15. Schematic diagram of a laser photocoagulator for ophthalmology.

on the retina. Using the argon laser, the power densities calculated at the retina are quite remarkable. If a 1-W laser is used at full power to produce a 100-$\mu$m coagulated lesion, the approximate power density is 12 kW/cm$^2$. The fact that the actual laser spot size on the retina is so small allows for very efficient and rapid diffusion of the thermal energy away from the impact zone.

### Carbon Dioxide Laser Surgery

Figure 11.16 shows the three fundamental variations in delivery of $CO_2$ laser radiation for surgical therapy. Figure 11.16a shows the system attached to an articulating arm of the type shown in Fig. 11.14. A handpiece grasped by the surgeon permits flexible control of the delivered laser energy. The light is pre-focused at some distance (of the order of centimeters from the end of the hand-piece) to a small spot where the cutting action is maximized. The focal length of the output lens is selected to provide a useful working distance while retaining good control over the operation. If the surgeon wishes to diminish the cutting action but retain the ability to thermally coagulate, the beam may be applied to the tissue in an out-of-focus zone away from the focal spot. With larger working distances, the focused beam is more difficult to hold steady and the laser spot increases in size. As the spot size increases, the cutting efficiency diminishes. A special lens mounted in the handpiece focuses the radiation. Because the wavelength of 10.6 $\mu$m is approximately 20 times that of visible light, normal glass lenses do not transmit the radiation. Visibly opaque materials, such as germanium, are used for $CO_2$ laser lenses.

Figure 11.16b shows another method of delivering the $CO_2$ laser radiation to the operating field. The laser electrical power supply is attached, via an electrical umbilical cord, to the laser tube head; the tube head is either mounted on a

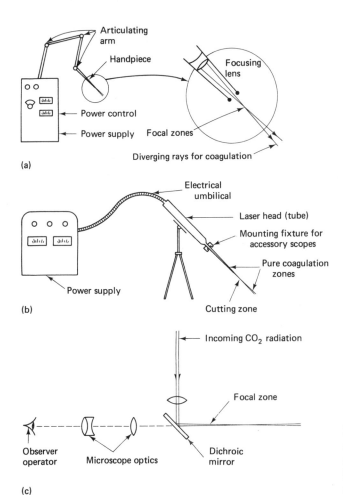

**FIGURE 11.16.** Three basic delivery systems for $CO_2$ laser surgical radiation. (a) Articulating arm. (b) Laser head. (c) Operating microscope.

pedestal, as shown, or hand held. By utilizing a movable laser tube, the articulated arm of Fig. 11.16a is eliminated. Articulating arms are expensive to manufacture due to the severe mechanical tolerances on the series of conveyer mirrors. With the movable laser head tube design, an endoscope and microscope may be affixed directly to the tube housing.

Figure 11.16c shows the use of an operating microscope in conjunction with the $CO_2$ laser beam. Laser light is brought into the microscope assembly from above and reflected to the right by a mirror. The microscope optics are arranged to the left of the deflecting mirror and have an axis that is the same as the axis of the focused laser beam. To see through the deflecting mirror, a special dichroic coating is necessary to provide reflection of 10.6 $\mu$m radiation, while transmitting visible light. Alternatively, the deflecting mirror can be made very small and the microscope optical field arranged so that a small deadband in the transfer system is not bothersome. With a microscope attachment, the $CO_2$ laser scalpel can be conveniently maneuvered with a joy-stick control and applied successfully for removal of tissue in the brain (Ascher, 1977) or throat (Strong and Jako, 1972) The beam focus is projected to a point in space for comfortable entry into various anatomical organs. The microscope telescope provides the surgeon with precise vision of the operating field. The glass optics of the microscope automatically block the scattered 10.6 $\mu$m radiation, thereby protecting the surgeon's eyes.

## REFERENCES

ASCHER, P. W. (1977). *Der CO$_2$-laser in der neurochirurgie*. Wien-München-Zürich-Innsbruck: Verlag Fritz Molden.

AUTH, D. C., V. T. Y. LAM, R. W. MOHR, F. E. SILVERSTEIN, and C. E. RUBIN (1976). A high-power gastric photocoagulator for fiberoptic endoscopy. *IEEE Trans. Biomed. Eng.*, BME-23: 129–35.

AUTH, D. C., C. GULACSIK, F. E. SILVERSTEIN, C. E. RUBIN, R. L. PROTELL, and D. A. GILBERT (1978). A clinically useful endoscopic laser coagulator with recirculating gas-jet assist. *Dig. Conf. Laser Electro-Opt. Syst.*: 46.

GLOVER, J. L., P. J. BENDICK, and W. J. LINK (1978). The use of thermal knives in surgery: Electrosurgery, lasers, plasma scalpel. *Cur. Prob. Surg.*, XV: 7–72.

KAPLAN, I. (1976). *Laser surgery*. Jerusalem: Jerusalem Academic Press.

KAPLAN, I. (1978). *Laser surgery II*. Jerusalem: Jerusalem Academic Press.

KIEFHABER, P., G. NATH, and K. MORITZ (1975). Eigenschafter und Eignung verschiedener Lasertransmissions-systeme fur die endoskopische Blutstillung. *Proc. 7. Kong. Gastroenterol. Endoskopic*, Wien: 1–13.

KIMURA, W. D., C. GULACSIK, D. C. AUTH, F. E. SILVERSTEIN, and R. L. PROTELL (1978). Use of gas jet appositional pressurization in endoscopic laser photocoagulation. *IEEE Trans. Biomed. Eng.*, BME-25: 218–24.

KOESTER, C. J., E. SNITZER, C. J. CAMPBELL, and M. C. RITTLER (1962). Experimental laser retina coagulator. *J. Opt. Soc. Amer.*, 52: 607.

L'ESPERANCE, F. A. (1968). An ophthalmic argon laser photocoagulation system: Design, construction, and laboratory investigations. *Trans. Am. Ophthalmol. Soc.*, 66: 827.

MEYER-SCHWICKERATH, G. (1960). *Light coagulation*. St. Louis: C. V. Mosby.

PROTELL, R. L., C. E. RUBIN, D. C. AUTH, F. E. SILVERSTEIN, F. TEROU, M. DENNIS, and J. R. A. PIERCEY (1978). The heater probe: A new endoscopic method for stopping massive gastrointestinal bleeding. *Gastroenterology*, 74: 257–62.

STRONG, M. S., and G. J. JAKO (1972). Laser surgery in the larynx—Early clinical experience with continuous CO$_2$ laser. *Ann. Otol. Rhinol. Laryngol.*, 81: 791–98.

## STUDY QUESTIONS

**11.1** An electrocautery loop of the type illustrated in Fig. 11.1c is required to cut and cauterize small tissue pedicles. The loop diameter is 1 cm (round).

    (a) If a 150 $\mu$m diameter steel wire is required to provide the proper cutting and coagulation properties, what voltage is required on the input to the loop to provide a power dissipation of 30 W? Assume that the electrical resistance of the connecting wires is negligible and electrical resistivity of steel $\rho =$ 11.8$\mu\Omega$•cm. Is this hazardous? See Chapter 10.

(b)  If nichrome wire of the same dimensions is used, what is the necessary voltage? $\rho$ of nichrome $= 100\ \mu\Omega$•cm.

**11.2**  A laser is operating with an output power level of 10 W. All of the power is injected into an optical fiber having a numerical aperture (N.A.) of 0.15 and a core diameter of 400 $\mu$m. Only 50% of the available N.A. is used on the input and output coupling.

(a)  What is the output beam divergence?

(b)  What is the output radiance at $\theta = 0$, assuming that the radiation intensity is uniform over the output beam angle and the full core area is equally illuminated?

**11.3**  If an incandescent filament light source is coupled to a bundle of closely packed cylindrical, cladded fibers, what would be the maximum radiance of the fiber bundle as a percentage of the input radiance? Given: fiber core diameter $= 9\ \mu$m and cladding thickness $= 0.5\ \mu$m. Assume that the packing is such that each fiber occupies a square space of area $= $ (o.d.)$^2$ where o.d. is outside diameter of fiber.

**11.4**  Given a 60-W $CO_2$ surgical laser that is focused by the output lens to a beam spot of 1-mm diameter:

(a)  What is the peak power density in the focal plane?

(b)  If all of the 60 W of power is converted to steam at 100°C, how many g/s of steam is formed? Assume starting temperature of 38°C.

(c)  Given the circumstances of (b), explain why a $CO_2$ laser of this power is considered to be a rapid cutting instrument. Discuss.

**11.5**  Compare and discuss the relative optical resolution of a fiberoptic endoscope (50,000 fibers and a square field of view) with a standard high-quality commercial broadcast TV with a 525-line raster scan.

**11.6**  Given the following table of representative values for delivered energy for a variety of thermal devices for coagulation of a single 1-mm artery:

- Argon laser (2.5 mm spot): 14 J
- YAG laser (2.5 mm spot): 40 J
- Electrofulguration (point electrode, see Chapter 10) (4-mm spot of tissue impact): 30 J
- Electrocautery (see Fig. 11.1b) (3-mm contact area): 6 J

Estimate depth of partial tissue necrosis. Assume tissue temperatures below 50°C cause no permanent damage. This table of values is typical of the real case; however, the calculation that is called for is very difficult for reasons already mentioned in Section 11.3 (optical generators). Compare your calculated values with the empirical values given below:

- Argon laser: 1 mm
- YAG laser: 5 mm
- Electrofulguration: 4 mm
- Electrocautery: 2 mm

Make any necessary approximations that you feel are justified and state the reasons.

**11.7**  Calculate the conversion efficiency of a high-power argon laser that delivers 25 W of radiation in the range of 454–514 nm when the input electrical power is 480 V, 3Φ, 60 A/phase, and unity power factor.

**11.8** In endoscopy, it is frequently necessary to insufflate the hollow body cavity with air or $CO_2$ gas in order to provide distension for more complete visualization. Compute the maximum pressure of insufflation in $Pa$ if a relatively flat zone of the stomach of area equal to 100 cm² is to have less than $13.3 \mu N$ of total force exerted by the insufflation.

**11.9** (a) Given a probe of the type depicted in Fig. 11.1a with an end cap of aluminum and Teflon, compute the necessary temperature of the inner surface of the aluminum if 3 W/mm² of heat flux density is to be transported across the surface into tissue. Take the thickness of the aluminum as 300 $\mu$m and the thickness of the Teflon as 2 $\mu$m.

Thermal conductivity data:

- Aluminum: 210 W/(m·k)
- Teflon: 0.10 W/(m·k)

Assume that the tissue temperature directly adjacent to the probe surface is 100°C.

(b) The thermal conductivity of copper is 390 W/(m·k) and for brass, 120 W/(m·k). What would be the relative advantages and disadvantages of these materials for the construction of the thermal probe described?

**11.10** (a) Given a tissue surface temperature of 100°C, calculate the energy transport rate through tissue (per cm²) into the interior to a depth of 2 mm. Assume for simplicity that the tissue temperature at the 2 mm depth is 38°C and that the heat capacity of the intervening tissue can be ignored. Take the thermal conductivity of tissue to be the same as water: 0.60 W/(m·k).

(b) If the intervening heat capacity were considered, how would it affect the energy transport rate? Give only a qualitative answer.

**11.11** In order to get superficial ablation of tissue with a $CO_2$ laser, it is judged necessary to provide a power density at the tissue surface of 20 W/mm² with a duty cycle of 10%. Using a continuous wave $CO_2$ laser with a power output of 15 W and a focal spot size (round) of 500 $\mu$m, calculate the rate of linear displacement (scan rate) to accomplish the above goal. Discuss.

# Anesthesia Delivery Apparatus

**12**

*Ronald S. Newbower*
*Jeffrey B. Cooper*
*James H. Philip*

## 12.1 CHAPTER OBJECTIVES

Upon completing this chapter you will be able to:

- Define the goals of anesthesia and various methods for achieving them.
- Describe the role of the anesthetist.
- Describe the environment in which anesthesia is used.
- Explain the operation of typical anesthesia delivery apparatus.
- Describe the general nature of monitoring procedures and devices used in anesthesiology.
- Discuss the areas of anesthesia practice needing further technological innovation.

## 12.2 INTRODUCTION TO ANESTHESIA

Anesthesia is a state of insensibility. The techniques for achieving it are not, in themselves, therapeutic tools. However, little surgical therapy would be possible without them. Before the discovery and application of methods for achieving general anesthesia, surgeons were judged primarily by speed. The best could amputate a leg in less than 45 seconds, assisted by several strong men to restrain the patient. In 1846, William T. G. Morton, a Boston dentist, performed the first successful public demonstration of general anesthesia, using ether, in the surgical amphitheater of the Massachusetts General Hospital in Boston. An earlier attempt by Horace Wells with nitrous oxide was a dismal failure and set back the acceptance of that very useful anesthetic by more than ten years. An earlier success by Crawford Long in Georgia went unpublished and hence mostly unnoticed [see Collins, (1976) for historical background]. Today, nitrous oxide is still widely used, but ether has been largely abandoned because of its explosive nature.

With the advent of anesthesia, surgeons were able to concentrate on matters other than speed. Long procedures requiring delicate skill became possible. Surgeons eventually accepted the use of sterile procedures around the turn of the century and, by the 1920s, the surgical scene had taken on the general features we see today. Monitoring has since increased in sophistication, new anesthetics and drugs have appeared, and the training of personnel has advanced. However, the basic features of the surgical arrangment—the sterile field, the anesthetist at the head of the bed, the anesthesia machine, the anesthetic record, and the human factors of the operating room—have remained almost unchanged since then. They now comprise a familiar tradition.

The general protocol and implementation of anesthesia is nearly the same for a tonsillectomy or hernia repair as for major abdominal surgery to repair an organ injured by trauma. Yet, the risk that might be acceptable for the life-saving procedure becomes unacceptable for the tonsillectomy. The pressure for error-free technique is great. Anesthesiologists have always responded by being carefully critical of their own craft. They have searchingly examined any anesthesia-related morbidity and mortality, both in the general literature and within the smaller scope of their own departmental conferences and seminars. And the safety record in anesthesia is good. Fewer than 1 in 3,000 surgical patients die from an anesthesia-related cause (Epstein, 1978), yet it appears possible and desirable to improve that figure. "Vigilance" is the motto of the American Society of Anesthesiologists and the often-repeated byword of most anesthetists. Anesthesiologists tend to be interested in technology and recognize their dependence on it, but rely primarily, perhaps excessively, on human vigilance to ensure safety in anesthesia. Healthy skepticism for complex technology is common.

Many factors tend to inhibit change in the nature of anesthesia technology. The (approximately) 20,000,000 general anesthetics administered each year in this country require the assistance of only about 30,000 anesthesia machines, and the turnover of these devices is very slow. Thus, the market for anesthesia equipment, which is shared by many manufacturers, is small. There is little incentive for investment in research and development. It is, therefore, not surprising that most current anesthesia equipment has been unaffected by the tremendous advances in technology of the last 20 years.

## 12.3 CURRENT ANESTHESIA PRACTICES

There are two major categories of anesthetic technique—general and regional. In general anesthesia, the patient's entire body, including the brain, is anesthetized. In regional anesthesia, only a portion of the body is anesthetized. This is a lesser physiological intervention and is therefore thought to be a safer technique. Cullen and Larson (1974) give a compact introduction to the speciality of anesthesia; we will present an overview here.

## *Regional Anesthesia*

Achieving regional anesthesia involves inhibiting the action of particular nerves that innervate a specific area of the body. Knowledge of neuroanatomy allows the anesthetist to place a needle tip adjacent to a given nerve or group of nerves and to inject a volume of drug that anesthetizes those nerves and causes the appropriate portion of the body to lose sensory as well as motor function. Minor regional blocks anesthetize areas of the body such as portions of the mouth, individual fingers, toes, hands, or feet. Major blocks are those of entire extremities such as a brachial plexus block of an arm.

Spinal anesthesia can anesthetize the lower portion of the body. It requires passage of an extremely thin needle (22–26 gage) between the lumbar vertebrae into the subarachnoid space (containing cerebrospinal fluid—CSF) and injection of a quantity of local anesthetic, which anesthetizes all nerves passing through that and possibly higher areas of the spinal cord. An occasional (5–15%) complication of this technique is headache, caused by leakage of CSF during several subsequent days.

Epidural anesthesia requires passage of a needle to the space just outside of the spinal canal and injection of anesthetic that bathes the nerves as they emerge. In intravenous regional anesthesia, the anesthetist exsanguinates an arm with a tight elastic wrapping and injects a large volume of liquid anesthetic to fill the venous system of the extremity. A tourniquet prevents loss of the anesthetic from that region.

We do not completely understand the mechanism of action of local anesthetics. We know that they increase the threshold for electrical excitation, reduce the rate of rise of the nerve action potential, and slow impulse propagation. There are various theories postulated for a mechanism, but they are beyond the scope of this text. Some common local anesthetics are cocaine, procaine (Novocaine), and lidocaine (Xylocaine). These and others have their own individual advantages and disadvantages.

## *General Anesthesia*

Anesthetists employ general anesthesia for most operations involving areas other than the arms or lower half of the body. There are, however, many specific indications and contraindications for both regional and general anesthetic techniques.

General anesthesia usually implies obliteration of consciousness, elimination of recall, abolition of pain, and paralysis of musculature. Loss of consciousness and amnesia benefit the patient psychologically. Insensibility to pain protects the body from its own normal physiological pain responses. Paralysis (referred to commonly as muscle relaxation) allows a quiet surgical field to simplify the surgeon's task.

There are two broad classes of general anesthetics. *Inhalational anesthesia* employs inhaled gases, usually administered with the aid of an anesthesia machine. These gases are complete anesthetic drugs in that they provide all four of the constituents of general anesthesia just described. *Balanced anesthesia* refers to techniques in which individual drugs are needed to perform one or more of the needed functions.

The major inhalation anesthetics are nitrous oxide; the fluorocarbons—halothane, enflurane, methoxyflurane; and the flammable agents—cyclopropane and ether. Most anesthesia today uses only nonflammable anesthetics and consists of the administration of nitrous oxide combined with one of the other more potent (fluorocarbon) anesthetics or one or more of the various intravenous drugs. Nitrous oxide by itself does not have the potency to provide surgical anesthesia. Although anesthetists can induce (begin) anesthesia with inhalation anesthetics, this process is often slow and therefore they frequently administer ultrashort-acting barbiturates, such as thiopental (Pentothal), intravenously to accelerate the process. We still do not understand the mechanism of general anesthesia, but it seems to be related to the solubility of the drugs in the lipid bilayer of nerve-cell membranes.

Balanced anesthesia usually consists of administering nitrous oxide for consciousness obliteration and amnesia, an intravenous narcotic for pain relief, and an intravenous muscle relaxant (neuromuscular blocking agent) for decreasing muscle tone and response to surgical stimulus. Commonly used narcotics are morphine and meperidine (Demerol). One can accomplish muscle relaxation (paralysis) in one of two ways. A nondepolarizing neuromuscular blocking agent provides prolonged action. These drugs (curare, pancuronium, gallamine) occupy receptors on the motor endplate of the neuromuscular junction and prevent the receptors from being occupied and excited by locally released acetylcholine. Because there is no depolarization and no initial muscle concentration, these drugs are termed *nondepolarizing agents*. At the termination of the anesthesia, the anesthetist can reverse blockade due to these agents by intravenously administering drugs that prevent acetylcholinesterase from metabolizing released acetylcholine. This allows acetylcholine to competitively reoccupy the receptor sites to regain normal neuromuscular junction function. The principal reversal agent is neostigmine (Prostigmine). Because there are other effects of acetylcholine inhibitors on the parasympathetic nervous system, the anesthetist also administers atropine to prevent bradycardia, bronchospasm, salivation, and gastrointestinal constriction.

The patient often requires intubation of the trachea with a cuffed endotracheal tube to guarantee a patent airway, prevent aspiration of gastric contents, oral secretions, or blood, or allow positive-pressure ventilation during surgery (see Fig. 12.1). This requires a short-lived muscle relaxant to facilitate intubation. As yet, there is no short-acting nondepolarizing muscle relaxant and only succinylcholine, a depolarizing muscle relaxant, is available. This agent acts by occupying the receptor site for acetylcholine but excites the neuromuscular junction that causes muscle fasciculation (spasmodic contractions) at the onset of muscle relaxation. Circulating plasma cholinesterase in the blood stream and at the neuromuscular junction quickly metabolizes the succinylcholine in normal individuals.

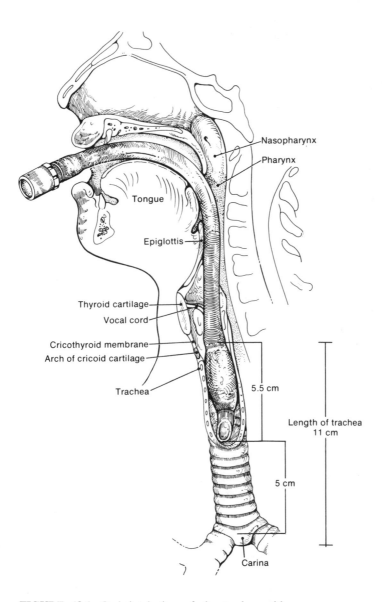

**FIGURE 12.1.** Oral intubation of the trachea with a cuffed endotracheal tube. The device is inserted with the aid of a conventional or fiberoptic laryngoscope to visualize the vocal cords and facilitate passage of tube through them. The cuff is inflated to a modest pressure to seal the tube in the trachea and permit positive pressure ventilation. Intubation may also be performed through the nose. (Reprinted from Wilkins (ed), *Textbook of emergency medicine*. © (1978), The Williams and Wilkins Co, Baltimore, MD.)

## Monitoring Drug Effects

Various techniques are useful in evaluating the depth of general anesthesia. The inhalation anesthetics cause depression of most of the body's systems. The effect of these agents on the pupils of the eyes combined with the effect on respiration, circulation, and musculature allows astute clinicians easy qualitative assessment of anesthetic depth. In addition, there are relatively consistent EEG changes that occur with most anesthetics, but these are not of clinical use in most situations because of difficulties in monitoring and interpreting the EEG during surgery. Computerized signal-processing and display techniques are attracting attention as aids in this process.

Anesthetists can assess muscle relaxation by observing the response to electrical nerve stimulation. Clinically used stimulators produce specific waveforms that make evaluation relatively simple. Response to tetanic stimulation (at 50–100 Hz) fades rapidly with nondepolarizing muscle relaxants. In contrast, depolarizing relaxants depress the response in a constant manner for all forms of stimuli, without fade. We can also evalute the effects of nondepolarizing muscle relaxants by observing the responses to a train-of-four stimuli at a 2-Hz rate. The ratio of the fourth response to the first response is a quantitative measure of muscle relaxation that the anesthetist can evaluate at any time without need for a baseline response prior to drug administration (Savarese and Ali, 1979). Quantitative measures of muscle force or action potential would allow automated assessment of neuromuscular blockade, although products based on that concept are not yet available.

## Uptake, Distribution, and Elimination of Anesthetics

Intravenous anesthetics such as thiopental are usually injected as a bolus and achieve high blood concentrations rapidly. They are very useful for a smooth induction of anesthesia. However, redistribution of the drugs from active sites to inactive sites, such as fat and muscle tissue, limit the length of action. Prolonged administration of an intravenous drug, in an attempt to sustain anesthesia, can lead to substantial accumulation in the inactive areas, ultimately achieving some sort of general equilibrium. Emergence from anesthesia then depends on metabolism and/or renal excretion of a large pool of drug and may be unacceptably slow. This is one of several factors encouraging the anesthetist to switch to inhalation agents for the prolonged maintenance of general anesthesia. These drugs leave the body as efficiently as they enter—through the lungs.

The partial pressure of anesthetic in the brain determines the depth of anesthesia. Thus, in using the volatile anesthetics, the anesthetist needs to control a variable that is not directly accessible. To infer the probable behavior of that variable during induction and maintenance of anesthesia requires an appreciation for the issues of uptake of anesthetic by blood from the alveoli and subsequent distribution of that anesthetic to various regions of the body. A proper theoretical analysis requires a multicompartmental model whose parameters include blood flow, anesthetic solubility, and tissue volume for every tissue type in every organ (Eger,

| Anesthetic | Formula | Vapor Pressure @ 20°C | | Solubility in Blood (Ostwald Coefficient) @ 37°C | MAC Vol% |
|---|---|---|---|---|---|
| | | mm Hg | Pa | | |
| Cyclopropane | $C_3H_6$ | $3.88 \times 10^3$ | $5.17 \times 10^5$ * | 0.55 | 9.2 |
| Ether | $(C_2H_5)_2O$ | 440 | $5.86 \times 10^4$ | 12 | 1.9 |
| Enflurane | $CF_2HOCF_2CFHCl$ | 175 | $2.33 \times 10^4$ | 1.9 | 1.7 |
| Halothane | $C_2F_3HBrCl$ | 243 | $3.24 \times 10^4$ | 2.4 | 0.75 |
| Methoxyflurane | $CHCl_2CF_2OCH_3$ | 23 | $3.07 \times 10^3$ | 11 | 0.16 |
| Nitrous oxide | $N_2O$ | $3.85 \times 10^4$ * | $5.14 \times 10^6$ * | 0.47 | 101 |

*gas, at room temperature and pressure

**FIGURE 12.2.** Characteristics of common inhalational anesthetics. (Values from Steward et al., 1973.)

1974). Our inability to measure or estimate all of these parameters limits practical clinical calculations to simple empirical relationships (Aldrete et al., 1979). In general, alveolar partial pressure tends to be in equilibrium with arterial partial pressure (blood leaving the alveoli). The brain partial pressure tends to follow the arterial partial pressure closely, because the ratio of cerebral blood flow to brain tissue capacity for anesthetic (the product of solubility and volume) is large. Thus, the concept has arisen of describing anesthetic potency in terms of a more accessible variable—the minimum alveolar concentration (MAC, expressed in volume percent) necessary (at equilibrium) to achieve the state of anesthesia (insensitivity to a surgical stimulus). Because it is the partial pressure in the brain that is important, the MAC has physiologic meaning only if the barometric pressure is specified and equilibrium has been achieved. Thus, its use can be confusing. Figure 12.2 gives some of the relevant parameters of common inhalational anesthetics.

During induction, the assumption of equilibrium is clearly not valid. Anesthetic enters from the anesthesia machine into the gas volume formed by the breathing circuit and the lungs (approximately 10 l). An amount of anesthetic is carried into the alveoli with each inspiration. An equilibrium is then achieved between blood flowing through the capillaries (which may already contain anesthetic from previous uptake) and alveolar gas. If the solubility of the particular anesthetic in blood is high, the partial pressure achieved after each breath's equilibration with accessible blood will be low during the uptake process. Thus, the rate of rise of partial pressure in the brain will be proportional to the concentration delivered to the lungs and to the rate of ventilation and inversely proportional to blood solubility and (surprisingly) cardiac output. As uptake continues, other tissue compartments (in parallel with the brain) absorb anesthetic as well. Some (heart and kidneys) reach significant levels faster than the brain. Eventually a general state of near equilibrium is reached.

In the equilibrium situation with inhalation anesthetics, a great simplicity emerges because metabolism is near zero. The partial pressure delivered from the anesthesia machine will be nearly matched by the partial pressure in the brain. Thus, the anesthetist can bring the partial pressure in the patient's brain to the desired level simply by administering a safe and steady concentration to the lungs and waiting for equilibration. More commonly, the anesthetist will accelerate the process of induction by administering a concentration of several times MAC and then tapering off to the desired equilibrium level (perhaps 1.3 MAC) at the appropriate time. As indicated earlier, this timing involves estimation and judgment.

The rate of emergence from anesthesia after termination of delivery of anesthetic gas is a complicated function of past history, continued ventilation, cardiac output, regional distribution of blood flow, and other variables. Some tissues accumulate large quantities of anesthetic, which are slowly released into the blood pool and washed out through the alveoli. It is part of the anesthetist's responsibility to control the depth as well as the time of emergence from anesthesia to match the surgical requirements. Unnecessarily deep or prolonged anesthesia can increase the probability of complications. Given the limitation of available data and of practical models of uptake and distribution, the anesthetist's best guide, frequently, is observation of the clinical signs of anesthetic depth.

## Physiological Stability

Because anesthesia depresses some or all of the body's own natural defenses, it is the anesthetist's duty to protect the patient from all unnecessary insults. Any insult that would arouse a protective response from an awake or naturally sleeping patient produces no such response from an anesthetized patient. As a result, even careless patient positioning can result in musculoskeletal, neurological, or corneal injuries. In effect, the anesthetist has contracted with the awake patient to protect and maintain him or her during this period of deliberate helplessness, and this responsibility overrides all others during the course of anesthesia and surgery.

Prior to the administration of any anesthetic, the anesthetist requires certain preliminaries to assist in the later maintenance of the patient. These include placement of a blood-pressure cuff (and associated stethoscope) and other appropriate cardiac monitors (e.g., precordial stethoscope and/or ECG). In addition, establishment of intravenous access is crucial. Intravenous drugs may be required as major components of a general anesthetic or as minor components to supplement a regional anesthetic. An intravenous infusion site also allows rapid treatment of any untoward complications or side effects of anesthesia.

Anesthetics depress the cardiovascular system. Therefore, pulse and blood pressure are of critical importance throughout the course of anesthesia and surgery. The anesthetist often monitors the ECG as well, watching for heart rate, occurrence of arrhythmias, and signs of coronary ischemia (ST segment changes). Anesthesia tends to stabilize the heart rate but predisposes to certain arrhythmias that are somewhat different from those seen elsewhere in medical practice. Most anesthetics depress blood pressure unless some specific mechanism releases catecholamines.

Because anesthetics often depress the contractile performance of the heart and because surgery is frequently performed on patients with cardiovascular or pulmonary disease, assessment of myocardial function is occasionally useful. Right heart catheterization, using a balloon-tipped flow-directed catheter, can provide pulmonary capillary wedge pressure as an estimate of left ventricular end-diastolic pressure. The same catheter can serve for performance of thermal-dilution measurements of cardiac output. Although some workers have occasionally used pulse-contour analysis to estimate cardiac output on a beat-to-beat basis, there is as yet no generally accepted continuous monitor of cardiac output. A finger plethysmograph can allow qualitative assessment of finger perfusion, although this information is of uncertain usefulness.

Most of the inhalation anesthetics, as well as barbiturates, narcotics, and muscle relaxants, depress respiration. In addition, these drugs dull the pharyngeal reflexes, which normally help the patient protect his own airway. As a result, obstruction by soft tissues is common during general anesthesia. Placement of a nasal or oral pharyngeal airway device provides relief in most instances. The patient may require endotracheal intubation if the airway devices are not adequate.

The anesthetist's hand on the breathing bag routinely monitors respiration during spontaneous, assisted, or controlled ventilation. Alternatively, a mechanical ventilator can provide sustained ventilation in a more controlled manner. The anesthetist can evaluate adequacy of gas exchange by sampling arterial blood for measurement of blood-gas partial pressures. Convenient intravascular sensors for blood parameters may become available in the forseeable future. End-expired respiratory and anesthetic gas concentrations can be useful in evaluating adequacy of ventilation as well as appropriateness of anesthetic tension.

Surgery frequently causes fluid and electrolyte imbalance. Intraoperative bleeding can cause a decreased intravascular volume, which, in turn, causes observable patterns of change in heart rate, blood pressure, urinary output, and central venous pressure. Blood volume per se is not easy to measure, but the anesthetist estimates losses from used sponges, and so on. Plasma volume losses to the interstitium occur in addition to blood loss. Electrolyte abnormalities occasionally occur due to absorption of fluids (e.g., distilled water used during transurethral resection of the prostate). This causes decreased serum osmolarity as well as hyponatremia, which can produce loss of consciousness or seizures.

All of these complications require prompt intravenous therapy. Typical intravenous (IV) apparatus includes a small catheter (20–14 gage) that is introduced percutaneously, with the aid of a needle, into a hand or arm vein under sterile conditions. The catheter is secured with tape and connected to a convenient length of plastic tubing. Conventional IV apparatus utilizes a manually controlled restrictive device for flow control and a drip chamber for flow measurement. Gravity provides the usual pressure source for infusion of fluids. In recent years, automated infusion devices using pumps and flow sensors of various kinds have allowed more consistent fluid administration.

Intravenous fluids are usually isotonic with plasma and include such solutions as 5% dextrose, 0.9% saline (normal saline), and lactated Ringer's solution (balanced salt solution). The anesthetist can add other fluids and drugs to the IV bags or bottles or inject them directly into the running IV line. Complications of intravenous therapy can include local inflammation or infection at the site of skin or vessel entry, inadvertent excessive fluid or blood administration, fluid extravasation, or occlusion due to blood clot formation in or near the catheter tip.

### Anesthesia Personnel

An anesthetist is anyone who administers anesthesia. Graduate registered nurses can take two years of specialized training followed by examination to become certified registered nurse anesthetists (CRNAs) and function under the supervision of a physician (an anesthesiologist or, occasionally, a surgeon). General practitioners occasionally administer anesthesia, although this practice is diminishing as anesthesiology evolves as a recognized specialty. Physicians desiring to specialize in anesthesiology continue their training following medical school with one year of general clinical training (internship) followed by two years of anesthesia training (residency) with an optional additional year of subspecialty training or research. They are then eligible for examination to become Fellows of the American Board of Anesthesiology (board-certified anesthesiologists). The special equipment required for anesthesia delivery often requires the assistance of technical support personnel. In addition, sophisticated monitoring needs often require engineering assistance or collaboration.

## 12.4 THE ANESTHESIA MAN–MACHINE SYSTEM

The anesthetist and his equipment constitute an almost classic man–machine system, expected to achieve a level of performance and safety approaching that of the pilot–airplane system in commercial aviation. In both systems, the personnel work for long stretches at fairly repetitive tasks that involve careful planning, manual skills, and vigilance, with occasional, and sometimes abrupt, requirements for bursts of intense activity. In aviation, a great deal of thought has gone into designing the equipment and procedures to optimize human performance and minimize error. However, in anesthesia, little effort has gone into design of the "cockpit" (Fig. 12.3), even though people are asked to work longer hours with less assistance and fewer technological aids to vigilance (Cooper and Newbower, 1975).

Figure 12.4 is a block diagram of the man–machine system in anesthesia. The patient is the focus. Measurements and observations produce information for the anesthetist. Some of the measurements (ECG, blood pressure, etc.) utilize technological assistance and some (skin tone, eye signs, chest movements, etc.) utilize the anesthetist's own senses. The anesthetist—the controller in a feedback loop—processes these data, makes decisions, and then carries them out with the aid of additional technological devices (intravenous apparatus, anesthesia machine, ventilator), with the aid of drugs (anesthetics, neuromuscular blocking agents, narcotics, etc.), and with his or her own hands. These actions cause changes in the patient's status—deepening or lightening the anesthesia, increasing or decreasing oxygenation, increasing or decreasing blood pressure, and so on. The anesthetist, repeating the observations, judges the adequacy of the changes and the process continues. Stability of the feedback loop is desirable, but achieving and maintaining stability requires experience on the part of the controller, adequate information from the sensors, and adequate control through the effectors. Even then, stability may not

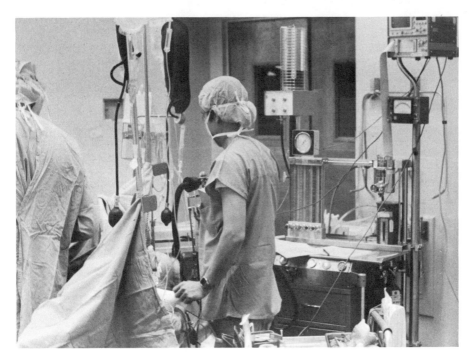

**FIGURE 12.3.** Typical operating-room setting showing the anesthetist at the head of the bed with a standard anesthesia machine and basic monitoring apparatus.

always be possible because of intrinsic or extrinsic influences on the patient (e.g., myocardial infarction, or an extreme maneuver by the surgeon). But the anesthetist's goals are to maintain physiologic stability while controlling anesthetic depth, muscle relaxation, fluid and electrolyte balance, and ventilation.

Fairly standard equipment and procedures are involved in the anesthesia delivery process. The anesthesia machine has two basic functions. It generates the desired mixture of oxygen, inhalation anesthetics, and other gases, and it provides a means for assisting or controlling the patient's ventilation. Its detailed structure and function are presented in Section 12.5. Most anesthesia machines are similar in concept. Indeed, some universal performance and design standards have evolved. For example, the Z-79 committee of the American National Standards Institute has a national standard for anesthetic gas machines (American National Standards Institute, 1979a). It constrains the design of most of the controls and displays to reduce the probability of human error. It also sets minimum standards for performance and accuracy.

The anesthesia machine forms the framework for the anesthetist's tools (see Figs. 12.3 and 12.5). The countertop may hold the drug tray and anesthetic record, and the drawers may contain supplies of disposables. Monitors and alarm devices are frequently bolted to the anesthesia machine.

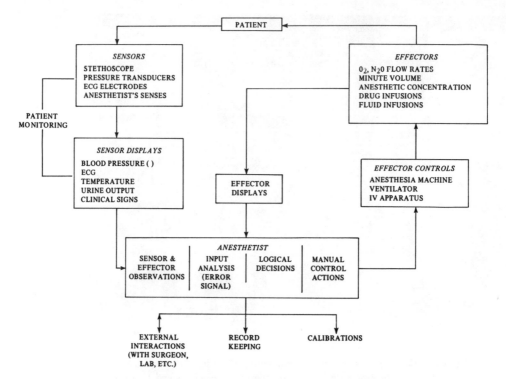

**FIGURE 12.4.** Schematic representation of the man-machine system in anesthesia. The anesthetist formulates decisions based on information about the performance of anesthesia apparatus and patient response. Effector apparatus carries out the desired actions. (From Gravenstein, *Monitoring surgical patients in the operating room*, 1979. Courtesy of Charles C Thomas, Publisher, Springfield, IL.)

## Monitoring Apparatus

The repertoire of monitoring devices is fairly simple for most surgical procedures. Saidman and Smith (1978), Gravenstein et al. (1979), and Leonard (1974) provide detailed discussions of current anesthesia monitoring practices. ECG monitors are similar to those in coronary care units but are usually much less sophisticated, with little or no alarm capability. Blood-pressure measurements may be intermittent and indirect (with a cuff and stethoscope for Korotkoff sounds) or continuous and direct (with an arterial catheter, transducer, and electronic monitor). Automated noninvasive blood-pressure instruments can supplant the invasive techniques in many cases. Right-heart catheters may provide supplementary pressure and flow information, with the use of multichannel pressure monitors and a thermodilution cardiac-output computer.

The anesthetist may assess pulmonary function by visual observation of skin tone and chest movements, by manually assisted ventilation to sense compliance

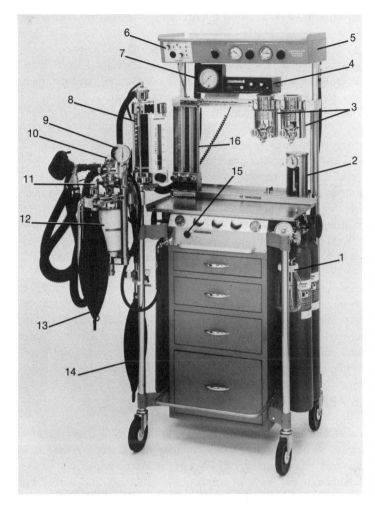

**FIGURE 12.5.** Typical anesthesia machine configuration with attached breathing circuit and monitoring devices. (1) Tracheal suction reservoir, (2) measured flow vaporizer, (3) direct reading vaporizers, (4) oxygen analyzer, (5) anesthesia ventilator, (6) ventilator disconnect alarm, (7) aneroid blood pressure manometer, (8) ventilator bellows, (9) airway pressure gage, (10) unidirectional valve, (11) breathing-circuit relief valve, (12) carbon-dioxide absorbent canister, (13) breathing-circuit reservoir bag, (14) waste-gas disposal reservoir bag, (15) oxygen flush, (16) rotameter flowmeters. (Courtesy of Foregger Medical Division, Puritan-Bennett Corporation.)

and flow, by continuous or intermittent spirometry, and by occasional measurement of arterial blood-gas partial pressures.

One of the anesthetist's most effective, general-purpose monitoring devices is the stethoscope. A conventional or modified stethoscope head can be applied to the chest of an awake patient. After anesthesia induction and tracheal intubation, an esophageal stethoscope (a balloon-tipped tube inserted into the esophagus via the mouth) may be very useful. The sounds picked up by either of these devices travel to the anesthetist's ear via a thin plastic tube and fitted monaural earpiece. Such a monitor conveys clear heart and lung sounds without intervening electronic devices. It is thus unaffected by interference from the electrosurgical unit (Chapter 10) or by power failure. It has its limitations, but its simplicity is desirable. The esophageal stethoscope can also serve as a substrate for other sensors such as thermistors for core-temperature measurements and electrodes for ECG sensing.

Neuromuscular function may be assessed intermittently with the aid of a nerve stimulator.

Temperature is an important variable to monitor in anesthesia, because anesthesia interferes with some of the normal mechanisms of thermal homeostasis, allowing progressive cooling. Anesthesia can even trigger a thermal runaway phenomenon known as malignant hyperthermia, which requires immediate attention for successful reversal. This, fortunately, occurs only rarely (perhaps once in 15,000 patients).

It is good practice to monitor some aspects of machine performance in anesthesia to alert the anesthetist to equipment or system failures that may occur. Desired variables include delivered oxygen concentration (which can be measured with an oxygen analyzer to assure proper life support) and airway pressure (which is generally measured by an aneroid gage on the machine). It may also be appropriate to monitor airway pressure with a "disconnect alarm" to assure that the mechanical ventilator is properly performing positive pressure ventilation. Because these monitoring devices are really part of the delivery apparatus, Section 12.5 describes them in more detail.

The anesthesiologist or clinical engineer must integrate all of this technology into a functioning system. Such a system may be coherent or haphazard, efficient or cumbersome, effective or not, depending on the thought, study, and design that go into the process of integration. Most of the systems in use today represent a loose collection of mechanical and electronic apparatus, in which the incompatibility of the electronic and mechanical components has limited the integration process.

## 12.5 ANESTHESIA DELIVERY APPARATUS

The basic anesthesia machine is a relatively simple and, in almost every case, a purely mechanical device. With few exceptions, manufacturers employ the same basic design principles and component configurations in their various competing models of machines. Although the basic principles have changed little during the past 30 years, there have been some significant changes in machine design that have improved reliability, accuracy, and safety. In this section, we describe the architecture that is found in most modern anesthesia machines. However, anesthesia machines may be used in routine service for as long as 15 years. Thus, many that are still in use do not represent the best of current design. Dorsch and Dorsch (1975) provide detailed descriptions of the various brands of anesthesia machines and their individualized components.

### A Typical Anesthesia Machine

Figure 12.6 shows a generalized schematic diagram of a prototypical basic anesthesia machine. It delivers controlled flows and concentrations of oxygen and anesthetic gases and vapors to a patient breathing circuit, which is most often directly attached to the machine itself. We will discuss the machine first and then consider various configurations of breathing circuits.

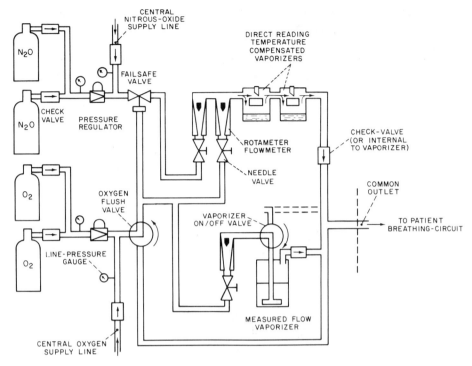

**FIGURE 12.6.** Schematic diagram of a hypothetical generalized anesthesia machine. Actual machines represent variations on this basic theme.

Oxygen, nitrous oxide, and any other compressed gases (e.g., carbon dioxide, helium, compressed air) used in anesthetic management are contained in cylinders that are mounted on yokes attached directly to the machine (see Fig. 12.5). In most applications, the nitrous oxide and oxygen compressed gas cylinders serve as emergency or temporary supplies while the primary source of gases is a central storage facility, with plumbing going directly to individual operating rooms. Most anesthesia machines can accommodate one or two cylinders each of nitrous oxide and oxygen while other gases are optional accessories for specific applications. The yokes of virtually all anesthesia machines now in service have indexing pins that mate into corresponding holes in the compressed gas cylinder valve. The purpose of this "Pin-Index Safety System" is to prevent the accidental mounting of a gas cylinder into the incorrect yoke (see Section 13.6). The yoke also contains a unidirectional (check) valve to prevent loss of gas from the hospital piping system or from a second cylinder when an empty cylinder is replaced. This valve also prevents transfer of gas from one cylinder to another (transfilling). A pressure gage (usually a Bourdon-type) mounted downstream of the check valve, indicates the cylinder contents. Because nitrous oxide is stored as a liquid [at its vapor pressure of 745 psi (5.14 MPa) at room temperature], its cylinder pressure remains constant until approximately ¾ of the contents are depleted and then begins to drop toward zero with further use. Oxygen is compressed to a pressure of 2250 psi (15.5 MPa) in a "full" cylinder, and that pressure drops steadily and nearly linearly as the gas is consumed.

A regulator (pressure-reducing valve), the design of which varies among manufacturers, reduces each compressed gas pressure to a working level of approximately 45 psi (310 kPa). When a central supply provides the gases, they enter the gas stream downstream of the regulator and at a pressure slightly higher than the regulator pressure so that gas flows preferentially from the piped source rather than the cylinder source. The gas at its regulated pressure flows to a variable-orifice, flow-control valve (usually a needle valve). The control knob of each valve is color-coded according to an industry standard mandated by ANSI requirements (American National Standards Institute, 1979a). Interestingly, the international and U.S. color codes for oxygen (white and green, respectively) are still not the same.

All machines manufactured after the early 1970s have some form of pressure-actuated, oxygen-supply-failure safety device. Usually a safety value is installed between the regulator and control valve of each anesthetic gas. The safety valve reverts to its normally closed state when the oxygen supply pressure drops below a preset value [usually about 30 psi (207 kPa)]. This safety valve thus prevents the delivery of *other* gases when the oxygen supply pressure has been lost or significantly reduced from any of a number of causes. Thus, the loss of oxygen pressure should become obvious to the anesthetist. Of course, this does not prevent the anesthetist from accidentally delivering an unsafe gas mixture by inadvertently shutting off the oxygen flow-control valve, misreading flowmeters, and so on. Some models of anesthesia machines manufactured after the late 1970s employ other protective systems that require either a minimum oxygen flow rate or a minimum oxygen concentration in order to deliver gases.

A rotameter flowmeter, which consists of a tapered tube containing a float, measures the flow rate of each gas resulting from the flow-control valve setting. Each rotameter is calibrated for a specific gas and is typically accurate to within ±3% of the full-scale flowmeter reading. On anesthesia machines manufactured after the mid 1970s, the manifold of flowmeters (see Fig. 12.5) has the oxygen flow control on the far right (on the downstream end) for standardization so that a leak in any one flowmeter is more likely to produce a loss of anesthetic gases than of oxygen. This reduces the danger of inadvertent delivery of an hypoxic mixture.

Figure 12.6 shows that the combined oxygen and anesthetic gas mixture is directed to the inlet of one or more devices that vaporize potent anesthetic liquids (e.g., halothane, enflurane). Figure 12.7 shows the schematic of a typical anesthetic vaporizer. A portion of the oxygen/anesthetic gas mixture flows into the vaporizing chamber that contains the liquid anesthetic. This portion of the gas becomes completely saturated with anesthetic vapor, either by flowing over wicks or by bubbling directly through the liquid. Thus, upon exiting this chamber, the gas mixture contains volatile anesthetic at the vapor pressure of the liquid. This mixture of oxygen, anesthetic gas and anesthetic vapor then rejoins the main stream to form the total fresh gas flow that eventually goes to the breathing circuit. The vaporizer control valve, calibrated in volume-percent of the liquid anesthetic, controls the

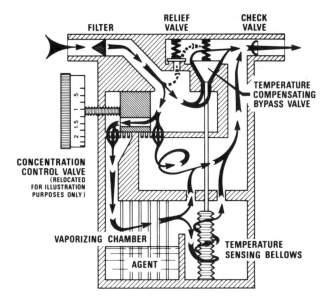

FILTER    RELIEF    CHECK
          VALVE     VALVE

TEMPERATURE
COMPENSATING
BYPASS VALVE

CONCENTRATION
CONTROL VALVE
(RELOCATED
FOR ILLUSTRATION
PURPOSES ONLY)

VAPORIZING CHAMBER

AGENT

TEMPERATURE
SENSING BELLOWS

**FIGURE 12.7.** Schematic diagram of a typical anesthesia vaporizer. The concentration control varies the mixture of fresh gas and gas saturated with anesthetic vapor, while the temperature compensation device makes additional adjustments in the mixing ratio to counteract the effects of variations of vapor pressure with temperature. (Courtesy of Ohio Medical Products.)

fraction of gas that flows into the vaporizing chamber. Most vaporizers of this type have a second variable-orifice valve, which has a flow resistance determined by a temperature-sensitive element, such as a bimetallic strip. This compensates for changes in liquid temperature (and hence vapor pressure), that occur due to changes in ambient temperature or to the consumption of heat of vaporization by the evaporation process. Thus, the goal is to deliver the dialed concentration of vapor under varying conditions. Each anesthetic vaporizer is specific for one anesthetic, because the vapor pressures of the various liquid anesthetics are all different. To prevent inadvertent filling of a vaporizer with the wrong anesthetic, there are various forms of indexing systems available for the liquid containers, but these are not universally employed. There are also certain design restrictions in the ANSI standard to assure isolation of vaporizers from each other and to preclude simultaneous operation of more than one. Old machines are not likely to offer these protections.

There is a more basic type of vaporizer that operates on the "measured flow" principle and that is frequently employed even on modern anesthesia machines. A separate control valve and rotameter supply an accurately metered flow of oxygen to the vaporizer. This oxygen bubbles through the liquid and is entirely saturated with anesthetic vapor. This vapor-laden gas mixture then flows into the main gas stream. The anesthetist must compute the oxygen flow required through the vaporizer to attain the desired concentration based on the total gas flow. He uses the temperature and the vapor pressure/temperature characteristics of the anesthetic liquid. He either uses a slide-rule-type calculator or simply memorizes the most frequently used total and vaporizer flow rates and sets accordingly for the desired anesthetic level. The advantage of this type of vaporizer is that it can be used with any anesthetic. Of course, confusion is possible concerning which anesthetic liquid the vaporizer contains.

The different types and brands of anesthetic vaporizers have a variety of idiosyncrasies that affect the concentration delivered. For instance, sudden increases in back pressure caused by flushing of oxygen into the fresh gas mixture or by a restriction in the fresh gas outflow can cause retrograde flow of *liquid* back to the rotameter of a measured-flow vaporizer. Either special internal design features of the vaporizer or a check valve in the vaporizer outflow can prevent this. In addition, some models of vaporizers can deliver variable concentrations with low total flow rates because of the fluctuations in back pressure during positive-pressure ventilation. Here again, the placement of check valves somewhere in the piping downstream of the vaporizer can diminish this problem. Figure 12.6 shows possible locations of such check valves.

All anesthesia machines are equipped with a valve that permits the addition of high flows of oxygen for flushing the system of anesthetic gases and vapors. The flush valve may divert oxygen pressure from the fail-safe device, thus causing the flow of anesthetic gases to cease during an oxygen flush. When a machine is equipped with a measured flow vaporizer, the oxygen flush valve is sometimes incorporated into the valve that switches the vaporizer in and out of the anesthetic circuit. (That incorporation of dissimilar functions has tended to encourage error in operation.)

Some anesthesia machines employ a pressure relief valve to prevent high pressures from being inadvertently generated with the piping system. Also, pressure relief valves are sometimes employed to prevent retrograde flow of anesthetic liquid in some types of measured flow vaporizers.

## Breathing Circuits

The anesthesia machine generates a continuous supply of the desired mixture of life support and anesthetic gases. The patient requires an intermittent flow of such gases during the course of respiration. The patient may also benefit from rebreathing some of the expired gases to conserve body heat and moisture. If rebreathing is to be used, some means is necessary for removing carbon dioxide from the expired gases. The collection of apparatus attached to the anesthesia machine to meet all these needs is known as the breathing circuit.

Probably the most commonly employed breathing circuit for adult anesthesia in the U.S. is the "circle system." Figure 12.8 shows a typical arrangement of components. One manufacturer's model can be seen in Fig. 12.5. Two unidirectional valves cause the gas to flow in a circle, which includes a chemical means for absorption of carbon dioxide. In this system, fresh gas from the anesthesia machine enters the breathing circuit at a point downstream of the carbon-dioxide-absorbent canister and upstream of the inspiratory unidirectional valve. This gas mixes with that already in the system, flows through the inspiratory unidirectional valve, and through either reusable or disposable corrugated tubing to the Y-piece. Expired gas from the patient flows through the other (expiratory) limb of the circle, through the

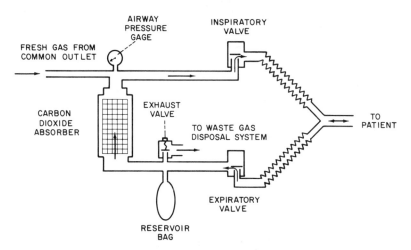

**FIGURE 12.8.** Schematic diagram of a typical "circle" type patient breathing circuit for use with an anesthesia machine.

expiratory unidirectional valve, and then into a reservoir bag. When positive pressure is generated in the reservoir bag by a squeeze, the collected gas is driven through the carbon-dioxide absorbent to the patient.

Because the fresh gas inflow to the system is much greater than that consumed by the patient and the absorbent, a positive pressure relief valve (located between the expiratory unidirectional valve and the carbon-dioxide-absorbent canister) allows for the escape of excess gas when a set threshold pressure is exceeded.

The absorbent canister forms the bulk of the circle system and the other components are joined to it. It contains either soda lime (a mixture of sodium, potassium, and calcium hydroxides) or barium hydroxide lime (a mixture of barium hydroxide octahydrate and calcium hydroxide). These absorb carbon dioxide chemically and liberate heat and water in the process. (The water may contribute humidification to gas in the circle). An indicator in the absorbent changes color as the capacity is exhausted. The canister is designed to allow easy replacement of the absorbent.

The unidirectional valves, attached at both inspiratory and expiratory connections to the carbon-dioxide-absorbent canister, are typically of simple design, with a caged disk resting atop the inflow tube. Relief valves for exhausting excess gas have many more design variations. Often, they are simply spring-loaded valves that provide for adjustment of the spring tension, which controls the circuit pressure at which the valve will open. This allows controlled exhaust of excess gases. The minimum exhaust pressure is usually about 1–2 cm $H_2O$ (100–200 Pa). At maximum, the valve is fully closed. When the anesthetist assists the patient's ventilation (by squeezing the reservoir bag), he sets the relief valve pressure at approximately 20 cm $H_2O$ (1,960 Pa). Most such valves (popoffs) do not have calibration markings, so the anesthetist adjusts the valve empirically.

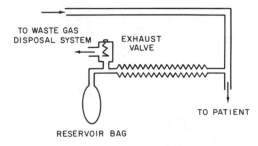

FRESH GAS FROM
COMMON OUTLET

TO WASTE GAS
DISPOSAL SYSTEM

EXHAUST
VALVE

TO PATIENT

RESERVOIR BAG

**FIGURE 12.9.** Schematic diagram of a Mapleson D breathing circuit frequently used in pediatrics. Some rebreathing of exhaled gas (including carbon dioxide) is an intentional feature of the design. The fraction rebreathed can be adjusted by changing the fresh-gas flow.

The circle system is common because it is the most flexible for adult anesthesia. If the patient breathes spontaneously, the relief valve is left in the open position and breathing proceeds with minimal resistance to inspiratory or expiratory flow. If the patient is deeply anesthetized and/or paralyzed, the anesthetist can assist or control ventilation by partially or fully closing the relief valve and squeezing the reservoir bag to fill the lungs.

There are many variations of the circle system, involving differing placements of the fresh gas inlet, reservoir bag, relief valves, and unidirectional valves. Each particular configuration has certain advantages and disadvantages (Dorsch and Dorsch, 1975). The system shown in Fig. 12.8 meets most of the objectives of conserving fresh gas and absorbent, maximizing humidification, and minimizing dead space and resistance to respiration. Circle systems also usually include a pressure gage for monitoring the circuit pressure. Because some components of the breathing circuit are difficult to sterilize, the circle system may include a disposable bacterial filter to combat the alleged problem of patient cross-infection (DuMoulin and Saubermann, 1977). Also, certain types of anesthetic vaporizers may be used within the circle system, although this has become an infrequent practice.

Other types of breathing systems, of a simpler design than the circle system, are often employed, particularly in pediatric anesthesia in which one desires minimal resistance to breathing and minimal rebreathing of expired gas. A basic system can be built around a straight metal tube with a side arm (Ayre's T-piece). The fresh gas flow is usually directed into the sidearm and the patient is connected to one end of the straight tube, the remaining end going to the expiratory limb of the system. There have been many variations to this concept in attempts to optimize one or another variable without losing the simplicity. Figure 12.9 shows one of the more common breathing circuits of this type: the Mapleson D System. It consists of a length of corrugated tubing connecting the expiratory end of the T-piece to a relief valve and reservoir bag. Other configurations of these components exist that differ, for instance, in the position of the fresh gas inlet or relief valve (Dorsch and Dorsch, 1975).

Until the mid 1970s, nitrous oxide and the potent volatile anesthetics were routinely exhausted into operating rooms from anesthesia circuits. Research has indicated that these trace gas levels in the ambient air were a health hazard to operating-room personnel (Spence et al., 1977) and, in addition, may have had a slight but significant anesthetizing effect on the anesthetist. For this reason, most operating rooms now provide some means of capturing and exhausting waste anesthetic gases. Various schemes accomplish this. In the simplest system, the waste gases travel through a hose from the escape part of the relief valve to the return duct of the operating room's single-pass ventilation system. If the operating-room ventilation recirculates, a separate exhaust duct may be used to draw waste gases to the outside. Alternatively, in more complicated techniques, the hospital vacuum system can serve by continuously flushing a reservoir that accepts the intermittent flows of waste gases. Some such scavenging systems may present new hazards by allowing extreme positive or negative pressures to reach the patient's lungs in certain failure modes, and the ANSI has promulgated a standard for their performance and design (American National Standards Institute, 1979b).

## Anesthesia Ventilators

When the surgical procedure requires the patient to be paralyzed, the anesthetist frequently utilizes an automatic ventilator rather than manually ventilating by squeezing the reservoir bag. This not only relieves tedium, but also provides more freedom to perform other necessary tasks.

Anesthesia ventilators use the same basic principles as the more complicated intensive care ventilators (Chapter 13). The anesthesia version includes some type of isolating bellows that is intermittently compressed and expanded and replaces the manual breathing bag in the circuit. It forces the anesthetic gas mixture into and out of the patient breathing circuit and lungs. Traditionally, anesthesia ventilators have been pneumatically powered becasuse of the explosion hazard of flammable anesthetics. However, with the decline in use of flammable agents, electronically powered and controlled ventilators are becoming more common.

Anesthesia ventilators usually have few controls. The anesthetist can vary tidal volume (the volume of a single breath) and ventilation rate. However, with most designs, he does not set these variables directly but rather controls them by setting other variables, such as the duration of inspiration, the flow rate during inspiration, and the time between the end of one inspiration and the beginning of the next. Thus, he has flexibility to adjust the ventilatory pattern to the varying needs of the patient and of the surgeon. Minute ventilation (the total volume of ventilation during 1 min) is an important variable, and it must be monitored carefully. The movement of the bellows along a calibrated scale indicates tidal volume; control markings or manual timing indicate rate. Minute ventilation can be estimated as the product of tidal volume and ventilation rate assuming there are no leaks in the breathing circuit. However, an accurate estimate requires correction for fresh gas flow during the inspiratory portion of the cycle (a slight addition to tidal volume) and allowance for compressibility of the gas and compliance of the breathing circuit components (a subtraction from the tidal volume). The actual tidal volume or minute ventilation can be measured with a ventilation meter, such as the Wright respirometer (see Section 13.8), or an electronic spirometer.

Many models of anesthesia ventilators also include provisions for limiting the peak inspiratory pressure, slowing the rate of exhalation, assisting ventilation only when the patient is not making inspiratory efforts, and maintaining a positive airway pressure during the exhalation phase (PEEP—Positive End Expiratory Pressure). Also, it is becoming increasingly common to find ventilators with integral disconnect alarms or other types of ventilation monitoring functions (see Section 13.8).

## 12.6 PERFORMANCE OF EQUIPMENT AND OPERATORS

Anesthesia apparatus is fundamentally simple in its design and function. However, there are many subtle and overt ways in which equipment can fail and operators can err, producing life-threatening situations that require rapid detection and correction. Though the risk of mortality or morbidity from modern anesthesia is relatively low, a major portion of that residual appears to be attributable to either mechanical failures or human errors. There have been many accounts of preventable mishaps (Cooper et al., 1978a), creating an increased recognition of the need for improved human-factors design and organization of equipment and of the need for the use of devices that monitor machine and operator performance.

Machine or operator failures can result in the delivery of gas mixtures to the patient that are either hypoxic (low in oxygen content), hypercapnic (high in carbon dioxide concentration), or lethally high in anesthetic concentration. Many possibilities also exist for hyperventilation, high airway pressure leading to compromised cardiac output or pneumothorax, or outright asphyxiation due to disconnection of the patient from the breathing circuit when the patient is paralyzed and mechanically ventilated. When such failures occur, the anesthetist can almost always recognize and deal with them promptly and effectively. However, unusual distractions or stresses may be present that diminish the anesthetist's ability to react quickly. These include surgical or physiological complications, anesthetist fatigue, or emotional stress. Fortunately, devices that aid the anesthetist's vigilance in such situations are available and are finding increasing acceptance. For example, anesthesia machines are now often equipped with instrumentation for monitoring the delivery of oxygen and the adequacy of ventilation.

Modern instrumentation for monitoring the oxygen concentration in anesthesia or intensive care breathing apparatus most often uses the polarographic sensor principle (Cobbold, 1974). Oxygen diffuses through an oxygen-permeable membrane and is reduced at a noble-metal cathode. By maintaining the cathode potential at approximately $-0.7$ V, oxygen reduction occurs exclusively and the current is linearly proportional to oxygen partial pressure. The sensors can be either reusable, rechargeable, or disposable. Most such monitoring devices directly display oxygen concentration in volume percent and are equipped with alarms to warn of inappropriately low or high oxygen concentrations. Oxygen monitors may be adversely affected by the presence of water condensing on the sensor, the use of electrosurgical units, or, under some conditions, nitrous oxide in the anesthetic gas mixture. As with other anesthesia apparatus, ANSI has promulgated a national standard to improve the safety and reliability of these devices (American National Standards Institute, 1979c) (see Section 13.8 for additional discussion).

Alarms for warning of significant leaks or disconnections in breathing apparatus connected to the patient have found extensive use in intensive care applications.

These alarms have only recently found acceptance in anesthesia. Such alarm devices usually employ an inexpensive pressure transducer. They alarm when the rate of ventilation, as indicated by positive excursions of airway pressure, appears to decrease below a limit. Thus, these devices do not actually measure flow and can give false indications under some circumstances. Flow-sensitive ventilation monitors are also available but are more complicated in design and operation, more expensive, and have not been widely accepted in anesthesia (see Section 13.8).

## 12.7 FUTURE DIRECTIONS

There are trends toward increasing length and increasing complexity in surgical procedures and towards operating on patients who are so ill that they would have been rejected as candidates for anesthesia only a few years ago. These trends reflect increasing physiological knowledge, improved pharmacologic tools, and new techniques (e.g., induced hypotension, blood reinfusion, and hemodilution, to reduce blood requirements; and induced hypothermia, to reduce oxygen requirements). Such trends create, however, increasing demands on the performance and sophistication of equipment. Coupled with demands for greater safety, these have triggered searching reappraisals of anesthesia technology (Ream, 1978) and there are several identified needs. New or improved drugs would be desirable. Intravenous drugs will eventually meet more and more of anesthesia's requirements, but changes in this area will come slowly. Many physiological variables that are of interest are not now available to the anesthetist or are not available on a continual basis. Assurance of adequate ventilation and cardiac output, with minimal cost and minimal invasion, would be very desirable. Greater capability in gas sensing is desirable, and progress is being made in this area.

Proper management of anesthesia depends on a proper flow of information. Adequate data about the patient, effectively presented to the anesthetist and properly stored for future reference, are essential. Modern technology, if carefully applied, can contribute much in this area. We require a truly integrated monitoring and delivery system that does not suffer from incompatible mechanical and electronic technologies. Were such a system available, it would facilitate more effective, more automated record-keeping. The handwritten anesthetic record is important, but it suffers in times of crises and heavy workload. Studies have convincingly demonstrated the weaknesses of the man-made record of blood pressure, in particular, during an anesthetic procedure (Zollinger et al., 1977). At busy times, such as anesthesia induction, the anesthetist cannot sample these variables rapidly and objectively. We need more work on resolving the issues of automated record-keeping—what to record, how to record and display data, how to enter data, and how to achieve adequate levels of confidence in such a system.

Some groups have begun to apply minicomputer or microcomputer technology to the processing and presentation of available data. In general, these record-keeping systems suffer from the fact that the anesthesia-machine's variables (flows, pressures, concentration, etc.) are not in electronic form. Attempts at attaching electronic transducers to a conventional mechanical machine have been clumsy and ineffective. A more fundamental approach requires redesign of the basic anesthesia

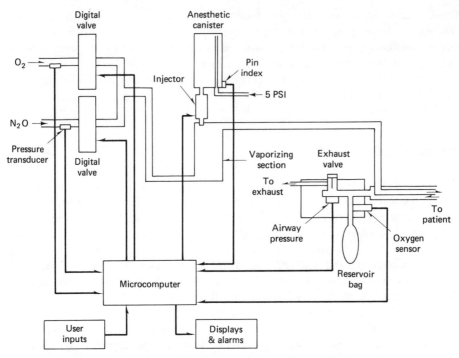

**FIGURE 12.10.** Diagram of the architecture of the Boston Anesthesia System, a microprocessor-based anesthesia machine. All the electronic and electromechanical devices are inherently digital and designed for extended reliability. (Reprinted from *Anesthesiology,* 49: 310–318, 1978, J. B. Lippincott with permission.)

machine, using technologies that are more compatible with electronic data processing, monitoring, and recording.

## New Anesthesia Delivery Systems

New technology is entering into the design of anesthesia machines. However, the level of integration of electronics with mechanical hardware is still fairly superficial. In commercially available machines, we see a larger amount of electronic alarm capability and more attention to human-factors engineering but, as yet, no fundamentally new approaches. At the prototype level, we see greater innovation, which may begin to have direct impact during the next decade. Figure 12.10 shows one particular prototype—the Boston Anesthesia System (Cooper et al., 1978b), which may serve as a focal point for discussion of potential technological changes.

That system is microprocessor-based and uses solenoid devices to control gas flows and anesthetic concentrations. Specifically, flows of the compressed gases are controlled by digital valves—banks of calibrated orifices that deliver predictable flows based on measured upstream pressures. The values of flow for the eight nozzles represent a binary sequence, so that the entire bank can generate any flow

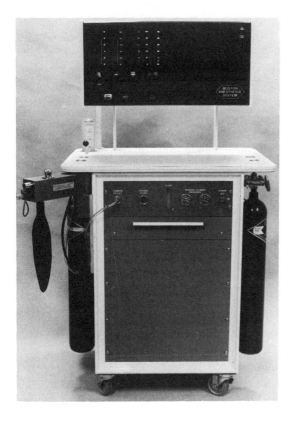

**FIGURE 12.11.** Photograph of the Boston Anesthesia System prototype, illustrating an electronic approach to improved human factors. Displays are grouped together in a logical array, with formats recognizable by anyone familiar with traditional machines.

between 0 and 10 l/min, with a resolution of $\pm$ ½ of the least significant bit ($\pm$ 20 ml/min), by opening and closing the correct controlling valves. The design of the nozzles is such that sonic velocities occur in their throats, virtually eliminating flow variation due to back pressure.

The volatile anesthetics, stored in sealed plug-in canisters, enter the gas stream in liquid form through a metering injection device and evaporate completely in a passive thermal-exchange chamber.

The system was designed with the constraints of the environment in mind (Fig. 12.11). A console contains all controls and displays, an alphanumeric message panel for alarm and status information, and a flat x–y dot-matrix display screen for plotting trends of physiologic variables sensed by conventional electronic monitors. The anesthetist can move the entire console around or even detach it from the base of the machine and place it in the optimal location.

With the increasing interest in reevaluating anesthesia technology, with the continuing pressures for absolute safety in the midst of complicated surgeries, and with the availabity of powerful new electronic technologies, it is clear that we are entering a period of change in the design and technology of anesthesia systems. Some of the potential clinical implications of these changes are significant. We have already indicated the interaction between available technology and record-keeping practices. We can further imagine that, given more quantitative control of anesthetic delivery, there will be a greater appreciation for and application of the concepts of uptake and distribution. Some feel that "closing the loop," that is, using feedback to regulate anesthetic depth, is a desirable goal. Although the new systems discussed might be necessary for such control, they are not sufficient. Better sensors and greater understanding of the physiologic issues are needed for any serious clinical application of these concepts. The anesthetist's place as the controller in the feedback loop is not likely to change significantly in the near future. The various discussions in this chapter of the anesthetist's functions in patient management should indicate that management of the anesthetic drugs is a component of a larger and more complex role. Gradually, the better understood and more routine of the anesthetist's tasks may be separated out and assigned to technological control, but the process will clearly be a cautious one.

## REFERENCES

ALDRETE, J. A., H. J. LOWE, and R. W. VIRTUE (eds) (1979). *Low flow and closed system anesthesia.* New York: Grune and Stratton.

AMERICAN NATIONAL STANDARDS INSTITUTE (1979a). Minimum performance and safety requirements for components and systems of continuous-flow anesthesia machines for human use. New York: ANSI, Z79.8-1979.

——— (1979b). Requirements for anesthesia gas pollution control. New York: ANSI, Z79.11 (Draft).

——— (1979c). Requirements for oxygen analyzers for monitoring patient breathing-mixtures. New York. ANSI, Z79.10.

COBBOLD, R. S. (1974). *Transducers for biomedical measurements: Principles and applications.* New York: Wiley.

COLLINS, N. J. (1976). *Principles of anesthesiology,* 2nd ed. Philadelphia: Lea and Febiger.

COOPER, J. B., and R. S. NEWBOWER (1975). The anesthesia machine: An accident waiting to happen, in R. M. Pickett and T. J. Triggs (eds), *Human factors in health care.* Lexington, MA: Lexington Books.

COOPER, J. B., R. S. NEWBOWER, C. D. LONG, and B. McPEEK (1978a). Preventable anesthesia mishaps: A study of human factors. *Anesthesiol.,* 49: 399–406.

COOPER, J. B., R. S. NEWBOWER, J. W. MOORE, and E. D. TRAUTMAN (1978b). A new anesthesia delivery system. *Anesthesiol.,* 49: 310–18.

CULLEN, S. C., and C. P. LARSON (1974). *Essentials of anesthetic practice.* Chicago: Year Book Medical Publishers.

DORSCH, J. A., and S. E. DORSCH (1975). *Understanding anesthesia equipment: Construction, care and complications.* Baltimore: Williams and Wilkins.

DUMOULIN, G. C., and A. J. SAUBERMANN (1977). The anesthesia machine and circle system are not likely to be sources of bacterial contamination. *Anesthesiol.,* 47: 353–58.

EGER, E. I. (1974). *Anesthetic uptake and action.* Baltimore: Williams and Wilkins.

EPSTEIN, R. M. (1978). Morbidity and mortality from anesthesia: A continuing problem. *Anesthesiol.,* 49: 388–89.

GRAVENSTEIN, J. S., R. S. NEWBOWER, A. K. REAM, and N. T. SMITH (eds) (1979). *Monitoring surgical patients in the operating room.* Springfield, IL: Thomas.

LEONARD, P. F. (1974). Medical engineering in anesthesiology, in C. D. Ray (ed), *Medical engineering*. Chicago: Year Book Medical Publishers.

REAM, A. K. (1978). New directions: The anesthesia machine and the practice of anesthesia. *Anesthesiol.,* 49: 307–8.

SAIDMAN, L. J., and N. T. SMITH (eds) (1978). *Monitoring in anesthesia*. New York: Wiley.

SAVARESE, J. H., and H. H. ALI (1979). Monitoring in the operating room: The neuromuscular junction, in J. S. Gravenstein, R. S. Newbower, A. K. Ream, and N. T. Smith (eds), *Monitoring surgical patients in the operating room*. Springfield, IL: Thomas.

SPENCE, A. A., E. N. COHEN, B. W. BROWN, P. P. KNILL-JONES, and D. U. HIMMELBERGER (1977). Occupational hazards for operating room-based physicians. *J.A.M.A.,* 239: 955–59.

STEWARD, A., P. R. ALLOTT, A. L. COWLES, and W. W. MAPLESON (1973). Solubility coefficients for inhaled anesthetics for water, oil and biological media. *Brit. J. Anaesth.,* 45: 282–91.

ZOLLINGER, R. M., J. F. KREUL, and A. J. L. SCHNEIDER (1977). Manmade versus computer-generated anesthesiology records. *J. Surg. Res.,* 22: 419–24.

## STUDY QUESTIONS

**12.1** What physiological information should be monitored from the anesthetized patient?

**12.2** How does the anesthetist determine the depth of anesthesia?

**12.3** What design feature is commonly used in anesthesia machines to protect against the hazard created by the loss of the oxygen supply? Explain its operation.

**12.4** List five equipment failures or human errors that could result in inadequate delivery of oxygen to the patient.

**12.5** Given that the internal volume of an oxygen compressed gas cylinder on an anesthesia machine is 5 l and that the pressure in the cylinder is 2250 psi (15.5 MPa), how long could you supply oxygen to a patient from one cylinder at a flow rate of 5 l/min? (Assume that oxygen is an ideal gas at these pressures.)

**12.6** What are the advantages of the circle breathing system? What are its disadvantages if used in pediatric anesthesia?

**12.7** Using a measured-flow vaporizer with halothane, what flow of oxygen into the kettle is required to achieve a 1% concentration of anesthetic if the total fresh gas flow to the patient is 5 l/min? (Use the anesthetic data in Fig. 12.2.)

**12.8** A direct-reading vaporizer intended for use with methoxyflurane has inadvertently been filled with halothane. What will be the concentration of halothane delivered if the vaporizer is set to deliver 2% methoxyflurane? What are the implications for the patient? (Use the anesthetic data in Fig. 12.2.)

**12.9** Design a device that would allow the delivery of no less than 25% oxygen from the anesthesia machine.

**12.10** Considering their blood solubilities, which anesthetic would be expected to induce anesthesia more rapidly, halothane or ether?

**12.11** What are the constituents of general anesthesia?

**12.12** Why will a greater cardiac output cause a slower induction with an anesthetic such as methoxyflurane?

**12.13** Many patients receiving general anesthesia believe that the total anesthetic consisted of Pentothal. Discuss the reason for this common misconception.

**12.14** Why doesn't the anesthetist use Pentothal for the whole duration of anesthesia?

**12.15** List three reasons for intubation of the trachea during general anesthesia.

**12.16** What are the two classes of muscle relaxants? How do they differ with respect to mechanism, duration of action, reversibility (natural or pharmacologic), and monitoring techniques used?

**12.17** What is the major factor determining duration of action of most intravenous anesthetic drugs?

**12.18** If the MAC of nitrous oxide is 101% at sea level, what is the MAC for a diver at a depth of 10 m in water?

**12.19** List the possible complications of intravenous therapy.

# Ventilators and Respiratory Therapy Equipment

## 13

*Warren D. Smith*

## 13.1 LEARNING OBJECTIVES

Upon completing this chapter you will be able to:

- Categorize the diseases requiring respiratory therapy and the equipment available for treatment.

- Describe normal and abnormal respiratory system function in a manner useful in the design of therapeutic equipment, in assessing therapeutic effects, and in characterizing patient–equipment interaction.

- Explain the physical principles of operation of basic respiratory therapy devices.

- Solve problems involving the effects of therapeutic equipment on the state of the patient and the effects of the patient on the operation of the equipment.

- Convert patient needs and therapeutic goals into equipment design specifications.

- Delineate the safety hazards involved in the use of respiratory therapy equipment and ways to minimize the hazards.

## 13.2 INTRODUCTION

The field of respiratory therapy is rapidly advancing in sophistication as it assumes a more prominent role in health-care delivery. This chapter introduces the therapeutic devices used in this and related fields for treating respiratory system problems. We present concepts of device function and patient interaction to aid in understanding equipment design and application.

Sections 13.3 and 13.4 review normal and abnormal respiratory system function. Section 13.5 then surveys the spectrum of respiratory therapy equipment, and the remaining three sections provide additional information on selected devices. Ventilators or breathing machines receive the most attention. They are the most complex devices covered, and their discussion provides a synthesis of the topics of gas delivery, humidification, and monitoring. Their use overlaps with the areas of emergency equipment, IPPB therapy, neonatal care, and anesthesia delivery.

Throughout the chapter, we give partial pressures of gases in the body in millimeters of mercury (mm Hg or torr) at saturation ($P_{H_2O}$ = 47 mm Hg at 37°C), and the hydrostatic pressures of ventilation in centimeters of water (cm $H_2O$). The interrelationship is: 1 mm Hg (= 1 torr) = 1.36 cm $H_2O$. The conversions to the metric unit of pressure, the $N/m^2$ or pascal (Pa), are: 1 mm Hg = 133.3 Pa, and 1 cm $H_2O$ = 98.1 Pa. We express quantities of gas as equivalent volumes in liters (l) under the conditions of body temperature (37°C) and sea level barometric pressure (1 atm or 760 mm Hg). We denote this set of standard conditions in the body BTPS (body temperature and pressure saturated).

We give the pressure of a gas source such as a gas cylinder in pounds per square inch, gage (psig), which means pounds per square inch (psi) above atmospheric pressure. The conversions to other units are: 1 psi = 6895 Pa = 70.3 cm $H_2O$ = 51.7 mm Hg. For a gas source, we express the quantity of gas as the equivalent gas volume in liters at the STP standard conditions of 0°C and 760 mm Hg. We can use the gas laws found in physics texts and reviewed in virtually any treatment of the respiratory system to convert from one set of conditions to another.

The symbols we use in this chapter are a compromise between the conventions of engineering systems analysis on one hand and pulmonary physiology on the other. Our general rule is to use the engineering convention of lower case symbols for time variables and upper case symbols for system parameters. Thus, we use lower case $p$ for hydrostatic pressure, $g$ for gas flow, $v$ for volume, and $c$ for concentration. We make exception to this rule for the commonly encountered pulmonary symbols for particular volumes ($V_T$ for tidal volume, $V_A$ for alveolar volume, $V_D$ for dead space) and flows ($\dot{V}_A$ for alveolar ventilation rate, $\dot{Q}$ for volume flow of blood) and for gas partial pressure or tension $P$ and gas fractional concentration $F$. We prefer $V_{FRC}$ to the physiologist's FRC for functional residual capacity. We generally follow the physiologist's conventions for the secondary (subscript) symbols used to modify the partial pressures, gas fractional concentrations, and blood-gas concentrations (A for alveoli, I for inspired gas, E for expired gas, a for arterial blood, mv instead of v for mixed venous blood).

## 13.3 NORMAL RESPIRATORY FUNCTION

The respiratory system contributes in several ways to homeostasis, that is, the body's tendency to maintain a suitable internal state. Primarily, it functions with the cardiovascular system to transport oxygen to the tissues and carbon dioxide away from the tissues. Its specific task is to regulate lung ventilation to control the (systemic) arterial partial pressures (tensions) of oxygen and carbon dioxide. The respiratory system also works with the kidneys to regulate pH and participates in thermoregulation and fluid balance. Other functions of the respiratory system include conditioning the inspired air (heating, humidifying), guarding against invasion by airborne particles, chemicals, and organisms (ciliary action, secretions, coughing, sneezing), and communication (vocal, nonvocal) (Selkurt, 1976).

The "state" or condition of the "controlled system" or "plant" is regulated by a complex closed-loop control system (Grodins and Yamashiro, 1978). Oxygen sensors are located at chemoreceptor sites in the arteries of the neck (the carotid bodies) and the upper thorax. Sensors for carbon dioxide and pH are located in the brain and at the arterial chemoreceptor sites. Based on input from these sensors, as well as a variety of other inputs, the brain adjusts ventilation rate and also cardiac output to maintain the controlled system in a suitable state. The control system also includes feedback loops to optimize the mechanical process of ventilation and the distribution of ventilation and pulmonary perfusion (Comroe, 1974).

The processes that make up the controlled system include *ventilation* of gases between the lungs and the outside air, *pulmonary gas exchange* by diffusion between the lungs and the blood, *bulk transport* of gases by the circulation, and *systemic gas exchange* by diffusion between the blood and the tissues. In reviewing these processes, we first consider the mechanics of ventilation separately and then incorporate them into the overall gas transport system.

### *Mechanics of Ventilation*

**Mechanical Structure.** Figure 13.1 shows that the lungs are suspended within the thoracic cavity and communicate with the outside through the airways. At rest, subatmospheric intrapleural pressure $p_{pl}$ holds the lungs against the inner lining of the thorax, thus keeping the lungs inflated and pulling in on the thoracic wall. We call the total volume in the lungs and airways at rest the functional residual capacity $V_{FRC}$.

Each inspiration, driven by the contraction of muscles in the chest wall, the diaphragm, and the neck, adds tidal volume $V_T$ of fresh air to $V_{FRC}$. The muscle force does two kinds of work: Potential energy is stored in the expansion of the compliant (elastic) components of the lungs and thoracic wall, and energy is dissipated in overcoming both the resistance to gas flow in the airways and the resistance to motion in the tissues of the lungs and chest wall. Expiration is normally passive; as the inspiratory muscles relax, the stored compliance energy forces air back out of the lungs.

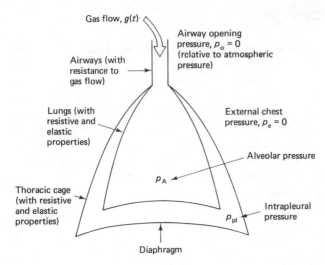

**FIGURE 13.1.** The mechanical structure involved in ventilation.

We can model the breathing mechanism in terms of compliance and resistance elements, as inertial effects are generally negligible (Grodins and Yamashiro, 1978). The compliance $C$ of an enclosure is a measure of the ease with which it can be expanded and is defined as the ratio of the incremental increase in its volume to the related incremental increase in the pressure inside relative to outside. The compliance components of the breathing structure are generally nonlinear, with compliance decreasing as volume and pressure increase. In the tidal volume range of normal breathing, compliance is approximately constant; that is, changes in volume are linearly related to changes in pressure. The energy stored in compliance $C$ by pressurizing it to value $p_C$ is $_0\int^{p_C} Cp\,dp$, which, if $C$ is a linear element, is $\frac{1}{2}Cp_C^2$. Figure 13.2a shows the properties of a typical compliance element. For convenience, we represent mechanical compliance by the symbol for its electrical analog, capacitance.

A pressure gradient along a passageway is required to move gas through it. Airflow resistance $R$ is a measure of how difficult it is to force the gas to flow and is defined as the ratio of the incremental increase in pressure to the related incremental increase in flow. Airflow resistance encountered in ventilation is also nonlinear, increasing with increasing flow, but linearization is acceptable for the moderate flows of normal breathing. The rate of energy dissipation, or power loss, in resistance $R$ due to gas flow $g$ and pressure difference $p_R$ is $gp_R$, which becomes $g^2R$ for a linear resistance. Figure 13.2b summarizes the properties of airflow resistance. We can model the energy dissipation caused by tissue motion in a similar fashion. For convenience, we represent mechanical resistance by the symbol for its analog, electrical resistance.

Figure 13.3 shows two models of the normal breathing mechanism. Each is driven by a pressure source $p_{mus}(t)$ developed by the inspiratory muscles. The first-order model in Fig. 13.3a lumps all the energy storage effects into single compliance $C$ and the dissipative effects into gas-flow component $R_g$ and tissue component $R_t$. This model is useful for relating resistance and compliance effects to the

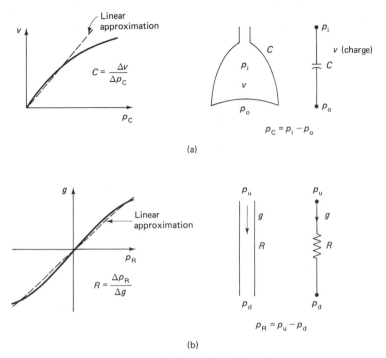

**FIGURE 13.2.** Elements used in lumped models of ventilatory mechanics. (a) Compliance element and its electrical analog, the capacitor. (b) Resistance element and its electrical analog, the resistor.

applied pressure and to the resultant flow $g(t)$, volume $v(t)$, and alveolar pressure $p_A(t)$. The top four graphs of Fig. 13.4 show these variables for a normal breath. Note that the inspiratory muscles are active during both inspiration and expiration. During inspiration, the source pressure is the sum of a compliance and a resistance component. During expiration, the source pressure acts against the compliance pressure to retard deflation.

In order to include the behavior of intrapleural pressure $p_{pl}(t)$ shown in Fig. 13.4e, we must use the more complex model of Fig. 13.3b. This second-order model separates tissue resistance and compliance into lung (subscript l) and thoracic wall (subscript w) components. Note that intrapleural pressure reflects the resistance and compliance components of the lungs alone in a manner analogous to the way $p_{mus}(t)$ reflects the combined properties of the lungs and thoracic wall.

If the respiratory muscles were 100% efficient, then the normal work of breathing would consume only about 0.5% of the resting metabolic oxygen influx (Grodins and Yamashiro, 1978). Instead, the muscles may be only 5% efficient (Comroe, 1974); if so, normal ventilation would consume 10% of the oxygen influx.

**Ventilatory Gas Flows.** Most of the gas within the resting lungs resides in small air sacs called alveoli. Figure 13.5 represents this gas, which is continuously exchanging with the blood, as alveolar volume $V_A$. The remaining amount of gas lies in the so-called dead space volume $V_D$ in the airways and does not participate

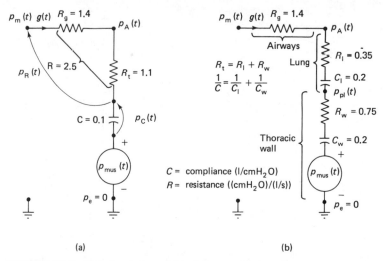

FIGURE 13.3. Two lumped models of the mechanics of ventilation. Numerical values are representative of a normal 70-kg adult. (a) Lumped compliance but separate airway and tissue resistances. (b) Separate models for airways, lungs, and thoracic wall.

in gas exchange. The functional residual capacity is the sum of the alveolar and dead space volumes at the end of a passive exhalation; that is, $V_{FRC} = V_A + V_D$. When we inspire tidal volume $V_T$ of fresh air, amount $V_D$ lies inert in the dead space, and the remainder $V_T - V_D$ mixes with the alveolar contents. During expiration, volume $V_T$ of mixed gas leaves the alveoli. Volume $V_D$ of this gas remains in the airways, and we expel the net amount $V_T - V_D$ from the body. Thus, with each breath, there is a ventilatory replacement of $V_T - V_D$ l of mixed alveolar gas by the same volume of fresh air. If the respiratory frequency is $f$ breaths per minute (bpm), then the rate at which the alveolar space is ventilated is

$$\dot{V}_A = f(V_T - V_D) \text{ l/min} \qquad (13.1)$$

Assume an individual at sea level is breathing dry air that has an oxygen partial pressure of $P_{IO_2} = 159$ mm Hg and negligible carbon dioxide ($P_{ICO_2} = 0.3$ mm Hg $\simeq 0$ mm Hg). As the air flows into the body, it is warmed to body temperature (37°C) and humidified to saturation ($P_{H_2O} = 47$ mm Hg). Hence, in the airways, $P_{IO_2}$ drops to

$$P'_{IO_2} = \left( \frac{760 - 47}{760} \right) P_{IO_2} = 149 \text{ mm Hg} \qquad (13.2)$$

The partial pressure of carbon dioxide in the inspired air $P'_{CO_2}$ remains negligible. Denote the average alveolar partial pressure of oxygen by $P_{AO_2}$ and that of carbon

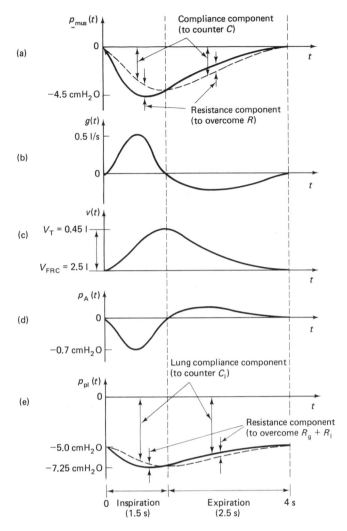

FIGURE 13.4. Pressure, flow, and volume waveforms developed during a breath cycle. Numerical values are representative of a normal 70-kg adult. (a) Pressure developed by inspiratory muscles. (b) Gas flow into the lungs. (c) Lung volume. (d) Alveolar pressure. (e) Intrapleural pressure.

dioxide by $P_{ACO_2}$. Then the average net flow of oxygen into the lungs by ventilation is

$$\left(\begin{array}{l}\text{Net rate of } O_2 \\ \text{ventilation}\end{array}\right) = \frac{1}{760}(P'_{IO_2} - P_{AO_2})\dot{V}_A \text{ l/min} \qquad (13.3)$$

Similarly, the average net flow of carbon dioxide out of the lungs by ventilation is

$$\left(\begin{array}{l}\text{Net rate of } CO_2 \\ \text{ventilation}\end{array}\right) = \frac{1}{760}(P_{ACO_2} - P'_{ICO_2})\dot{V}_A$$

$$= \frac{1}{760}P_{ACO_2}\dot{V}_A \text{ l/min} \qquad (13.4)$$

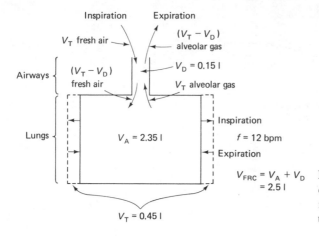

Inspiration    Expiration

$V_T$ fresh air →    $(V_T - V_D)$ alveolar gas

Airways {
$(V_T - V_D)$ fresh air    $V_D = 0.15$ l
                           $V_T$ alveolar gas

Lungs {
$V_A = 2.35$ l             Inspiration
                           $f = 12$ bpm
                           Expiration

                           $V_{FRC} = V_A + V_D$
                           $= 2.5$ l

$V_T = 0.45$ l

**FIGURE 13.5.** Ventilatory gas exchange in a breath cycle. Numerical values are representative of a normal 70-kg adult.

## Overall Gas Transport

Figure 13.6 models the overall process of oxygen transport from the outside air to the tissues. Figure 13.7 shows the corresponding model of carbon dioxide transport from the tissues to the outside air. The models assume that the tissues consume oxygen at the rate of $M_{O_2}^-$ l/min and give off carbon dioxide at the rate of $M_{CO_2}^+$ l/min. These two rates are generally close but not equal, and their ratio depends on the particular type of metabolic processes taking place in the tissues (Comroe, 1974).

Though we use them here just to provide steady state relationships among the respiratory variables, we can also extend these models into simple kinetic descriptions of the respiratory system (Talbot and Gessner, 1973). The insight into the dynamics of the controlled respiratory system provided by these and more complex models (e.g., Dickinson, 1977) is essential to the development of sophisticated respiratory therapy equipment.

**Pulmonary Gas Exchange.** In the normal resting individual, the diffusion of oxygen and carbon dioxide between the alveoli and pulmonary capillary blood proceeds essentially to equilibrium (Comroe, 1974). Thus, the difference between $P_{AO_2}$ and arterial oxygen tension $P_{aO_2}$ is small, and, to a close approximation,

$$P_{aO_2} = P_{AO_2} \qquad (13.5)$$

Because carbon dioxide diffuses 20 times more readily than oxygen (Grodins and Yamashiro, 1978), the arterial carbon dioxide tension $P_{aCO_2}$ closely satisfies

$$P_{aCO_2} = P_{ACO_2} \qquad (13.6)$$

**Bulk Transport.** If we neglect dynamic transients and metabolic processes in the blood, the net circulatory transport of oxygen from the lungs to the tissues equals the rate oxygen is delivered to the tissues by the arterial blood minus the rate oxygen is returned to the lungs by the venous blood. In terms of cardiac output $\dot{Q}$

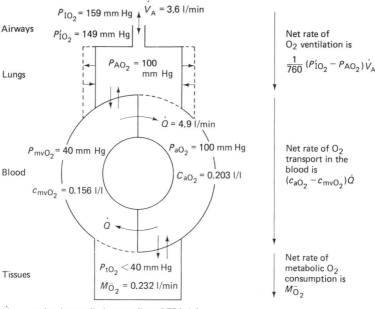

$P_{IO_2} = 159$ mm Hg   $\dot{V}_A = 3.6$ l/min

Airways   $P'_{IO_2} = 149$ mm Hg

Net rate of
$O_2$ ventilation is

$$\frac{1}{760}(P'_{IO_2} - P_{AO_2})\dot{V}_A$$

Lungs   $P_{AO_2} = 100$ mm Hg

$\dot{Q} = 4.9$ l/min

$P_{mvO_2} = 40$ mm Hg   $P_{aO_2} = 100$ mm Hg

Net rate of $O_2$
transport in the
blood is
$(c_{aO_2} - c_{mvO_2})\dot{Q}$

Blood   $C_{aO_2} = 0.203$ l/l

$c_{mvO_2} = 0.156$ l/l

$\dot{Q}$

Tissues   $P_{tO_2} < 40$ mm Hg

$M_{\bar{O}_2} = 0.232$ l/min

Net rate of
metabolic $O_2$
consumption is
$M_{\bar{O}_2}$

$\dot{V}_A$ = alveolar ventilation rate (l gas BTP/min)
$\dot{Q}$ = cardiac output (l blood/min)
$P_{IO_2}$ = partial pressure of $O_2$ in inspired air (mm Hg)
$P'_{IO_2}$ = partial pressure of $O_2$ is saturated inspired air at 37°C (mm Hg)
$P_{AO_2}$ = average alveolar partial pressure of $O_2$ (mm Hg)
$P_{aO_2}$ = systemic arterial partial pressure of $O_2$ (mm Hg)
$c_{aO_2}$ = systemic arterial $O_2$ concentration (l $O_2$ BTP/l blood)
$P_{mvO_2}$ = systemic mixed venous partial pressure of $O_2$ (mm Hg)
$c_{mvO_2}$ = systemic mixed venous $O_2$ concentration (l $O_2$ BTP/l blood)
$P_{tO_2}$ = effective partial pressure of $O_2$ in the tissues (mm Hg)
$M_{\bar{O}_2}$ = metabolic rate of $O_2$ consumption (l $O_2$ BTP/min)

**FIGURE 13.6.** A model of the oxygen transport plant. Numerical values are representative of a normal 70-kg adult.

(l-blood/min) and arterial and mixed venous oxygen concentrations $c_{aO_2}$ and $c_{mvO_2}$ (l-$O_2$/l-blood), this flux is

$$\left(\begin{array}{c}\text{Net rate of } O_2 \text{ transport}\\ \text{in the blood}\end{array}\right) = (c_{aO_2} - c_{mvO_2})\dot{Q} \text{ l-}O_2/\text{min} \qquad (13.7)$$

In an analogous way, the net circulatory transport of carbon dioxide from the tissues to the lungs is

$$\left(\begin{array}{c}\text{Net rate of } CO_2 \text{ transport}\\ \text{in the blood}\end{array}\right) = (c_{mvCO_2} - c_{aCO_2})\dot{Q} \text{ l-}CO_2/\text{min} \qquad (13.8)$$

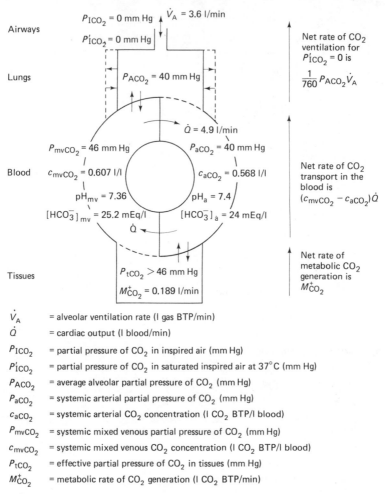

$\dot{V}_A$ = alveolar ventilation rate (l gas BTP/min)

$\dot{Q}$ = cardiac output (l blood/min)

$P_{ICO_2}$ = partial pressure of $CO_2$ in inspired air (mm Hg)

$P'_{ICO_2}$ = partial pressure of $CO_2$ in saturated inspired air at 37°C (mm Hg)

$P_{ACO_2}$ = average alveolar partial pressure of $CO_2$ (mm Hg)

$P_{aCO_2}$ = systemic arterial partial pressure of $CO_2$ (mm Hg)

$c_{aCO_2}$ = systemic arterial $CO_2$ concentration (l $CO_2$ BTP/l blood)

$P_{mvCO_2}$ = systemic mixed venous partial pressure of $CO_2$ (mm Hg)

$c_{mvCO_2}$ = systemic mixed venous $CO_2$ concentration (l $CO_2$ BTP/l blood)

$P_{tCO_2}$ = effective partial pressure of $CO_2$ in tissues (mm Hg)

$M^+_{CO_2}$ = metabolic rate of $CO_2$ generation (l $CO_2$ BTP/min)

**FIGURE 13.7.** A model of the carbon dioxide transport plant. Numerical values are representative of a normal 70-kg adult.

where $c_{mvCO_2}$ and $c_{aCO_2}$ are the respective mixed venous and arterial concentrations of carbon dioxide (1-$CO_2$/1-blood).

The relationship between a particular oxygen blood-gas tension and oxygen concentration is given by the blood dissociation curve for oxygen, adjusted for the specific conditions of temperature, pH, carbon dioxide tension, and hemoglobin concentration (Comroe, 1974). A similar relationship exists between the tension and concentration of carbon dioxide in the blood. These dissociation curves are non-linear but, under normal conditions, linearized relationships can be useful (Talbot and Gessner, 1973).

The amount of carbon dioxide in the blood is closely related to blood pH by the chemical reaction

$$H_2O + CO_2 \leftrightarrow H_2CO_3 \leftrightarrow H^+ + HCO_3^- \qquad (13.9)$$

The Henderson-Hasselbalch equation, derived from this reaction, is

$$pH = pK + \log_{10} \frac{[HCO_3^-]}{[H_2CO_3]}$$

which, using Henry's law, we may rewrite as (Grodins and Yamashiro, 1978)

$$pH = 6.10 + \log_{10} \frac{[HCO_3^-]}{0.0301 P_{CO_2}} \qquad (13.10)$$

Normally, the renal system regulates the arterial bicarbonate concentration to a value of about $[HCO_3^-]_a = 24$ mEq/l. For $P_{aCO_2} = 40$ mm Hg, equation 13.10 gives the arterial pH as $pH_a = 7.4$.

A change in pH affects bicarbonate concentration. Prior to renal compensation, which takes days or weeks (Comroe, 1974), the relation in normal blood $[\,[H_b] = 150$ g/l-blood$]$ between a deviation from the normal pH and the deviation in bicarbonate concentration is (Grodins and Yamashiro, 1978)

$$\frac{\triangle[HCO_3^-]}{\triangle pH} = -36.1 \text{ mEq/l per pH unit} \qquad (13.11)$$

Equations 13.10 and 13.11 together describe the effects of a change in $P_{aCO_2}$ on $pH_a$ and arterial $[HCO_3^-]$ due to passive chemical buffering. These expressions also describe the effects of a change in $P_{mvCO_2}$ on $pH_{mv}$ and mixed venous $[HCO_3^-]$, where the normal values are, say, $P_{mvCO_2} = 46$ mm Hg, $pH_{mv} = 7.36$, and $[HCO_3^-]_{mv} = 25.2$ mEq/l.

**Systemic Gas Exchange.**  The final step in each of the transport models is gas exchange between the blood and tissues. Just as in the lungs, this exchange across the systematic capillary walls takes place by diffusion driven by partial pressure gradients.

**Steady State Relations.**  In the steady state, the net ventilatory flow of oxygen into the lungs equals the net circulatory flow of oxygen to the tissues, and this equals the metabolic rate of oxygen consumption. That is, from equations 13.3 and 13.7,

$$\frac{1}{760}(P'_{IO_2} - P_{AO_2})\dot{V}_A = (c_{aO_2} - c_{mvO_2})\dot{Q} = M_{O_2}^- \text{ l-O}_2/\text{min} \qquad (13.12)$$

Similarly, for carbon dioxide, equations 13.4 and 13.8 are equal in the steady state, and both equal the metabolic rate of carbon dioxide generation; thus,

$$\frac{1}{760}P_{ACO_2}\dot{V}_A = (c_{mvCO_2} - c_{aCO_2})\dot{Q} = M_{CO_2}^+ \text{ l-CO}_2/\text{min} \qquad (13.13)$$

We can use steady state models, equations 13.12 and 13.13, to predict the asymptotic effects of a change in one respiratory variable on the other variables (see, e.g., problems 13.5 and 13.23).

## 13.4 PROBLEMS REQUIRING RESPIRATORY THERAPY

The mechanical and gas-transport models introduced in the previous section provide a convenient structure for classifying respiratory system problems. First, we can distinguish between abnormalities in the controller and those in the controlled system. The controller may be totally nonfunctional due to damage to the central nervous system, or it may control but at the wrong gas tensions or with inadequate sensitivity. Damage to the brain can also result in abnormal breathing patterns (Comroe, 1974). In the controlled system, there may be problems with ventilation, with pulmonary gas exchange, with circulatory transport, or with systemic gas exchange.

### Ventilatory Problems

Ventilation may be insufficient because the ventilatory mechanism lacks muscle drive, because there are abnormalities in resistance, compliance, or dead space, or because the lungs are nonuniform in structure. The driving force may be inadequate because of muscle weakness or paralysis, damage to the thoracic wall structure, or excessive pain with breathing effort.

**Resistance Problems.**   Diseases characterized by abnormally high resistance are termed *obstructive* diseases. Resistance can increase due to mechanical abnormalities such as tumor growth, muscle constriction of the airways (bronchial spasm), inflammation and swelling of the airway linings (mucosal edema), or excessive secretions into the airways. Allergic bronchial asthma can cause both muscle spasm and edema (Egan, 1977).

A high resistance increases the dissipative work of breathing and prolongs lung filling and emptying. The resultant larger tidal volume increases compliance-related work. Also, if the lungs do not empty, $V_{FRC}$ is elevated, resulting in less efficient action of the breathing muscles (Egan, 1977).

Pulmonary destructive diseases such as emphysema (also called COLD for chronic obstructive lung disease), bronchiectasis, and cystic disease destroy the cartilage supporting the airways, leading to bronchiolar collapse. In this condition, the airways are held open during inspiration, but they are squeezed down during expiration, making it difficult and sometimes impossible for the patient to exhale. These diseases also destroy the elasticity of the lungs, which contributes to the problem of excessively large $V_{FRC}$. Also, the resultant nonuniform lung structure interferes with ventilation distribution (Egan, 1977).

Tissue resistance may increase in a variety of diseases, such as pulmonary sarcoidosis and fibrosis, diffuse carcinomatosis, asthma, and kyphoscoliosis (abnormal curvature of the spine), but rarely is it the major problem in a disease (Comroe, 1974).

**Compliance Problems.**   Diseases characterized by abnormally reduced compliance are termed *restrictive* diseases. Restriction of the chest wall can occur in diseases leading to skeletal deformations, such as kyphoscoliosis, tuberculosis, and osteoporosis, or in diseases that reduce flexibility, such as arthritis, scleroderma, and fibromyositis. Traumatic damage, as in an automobile accident, can also lead to thoracic restriction.

Lung compliance can be reduced by pulmonary fibrosis and by excessive fluids in the vasculature (congestion) or tissues (edema) (Egan, 1977). Adequate surfactant at the alveolar surface is essential to maintaining normal lung compliance. A lack of surfactant causes restrictive problems in infants with respiratory distress syndrome (RDS) and in adults suffering the pulmonary ischemia of shock lung (also called adult respiratory distress syndrome or ARDS) (Comroe, 1974). Other restrictive problems include adhesions between the pleural surfaces of the lungs and thoracic wall and pressure against the diaphragm due to abdominal tension, excessive gas or fluid in the abdomen, or obesity.

## Gas-Exchange Problems

Pulmonary gas diffusion can be retarded by a thickening of the alveolar–pulmonary capillary membrane, as in pulmonary fibrosis, edema, granuloma, or connective tissue proliferation (Egan, 1977). Alternatively, the exchange between the lungs and blood can be diminished by inadequate ventilation $\dot{V}$ or pulmonary capillary perfusion $\dot{Q}$ or by a mismatch in the distribution of ventilation and perfusion. An abnormally high $\dot{V}{:}\dot{Q}$ ratio can occur because of some actual increase in dead space, as in the destructive diseases mentioned previously, or because of a virtual increase in dead space due to blocked perfusion, as with a pulmonary embolism. This condition lowers $P_{aO_2}$ and elevates $P_{aCO_2}$, but can usually be countered by increased ventilation. A low $\dot{V}{:}\dot{Q}$ ratio can occur because of actual shunting of blood past the pulmonary capillaries or because of virtual shunting due to inadequate alveolar gas mixing or diffusion. Because the hypoxia produced by this condition is the result of the venous admixture of shunted blood, it may not respond to increased ventilation (Comroe, 1974).

In a patient with gas exchange problems, the difference between alveolar and arterial oxygen tensions may be large, so that equation 13.5 is no longer a good approximation. Less frequently, equation 13.6 for carbon dioxide may be inappropriate.

## Bulk-Transport Problems

The bulk-transport mechanism may be deficient because of inadequate cardiac output or because the gas-carrying capacity of the blood, that is, the amount of gas carried per given gas tension, is too low. Cardiac output may be low due to shock, heart failure, or valve or other structural defects, or because of the increased blood viscosity of polycythemia (Egan, 1977).

Anemia, with the consequent reduction in hemoglobin concentration, lowers the blood's carrying capacity for both oxygen and carbon dioxide. The presence of abnormal hemoglobin or hemoglobin bound to carbon monoxide can also reduce oxygen-carrying capacity (Comroe, 1974).

### Tissue Problems

Oxygen uptake can be retarded locally by blood shunting or vasoconstriction and system-wide by histotoxin poisoning of the cytochrome oxidase system, as with cyanide (Comroe, 1974).

## 13.5 SURVEY OF RESPIRATORY THERAPY EQUIPMENT

### Emergency Equipment

A *resuscitator* is a compact, portable device for on-the-scene, short-term ventilatory support and delivery of oxygen. It is used with a face mask and perhaps an *oropharyngeal* airway to keep the tongue from blocking airflow. Also, an *esophageal obdurator* may be used to prevent the stomach from being inflated and to prevent regurgitation and aspiration of stomach contents. The *bag resuscitator* (Fig. 13.8a) delivers a breath of oxygen to the patient when the operator squeezes the bag. Upon release, the bag fills with oxygen again, while the patient exhales to the air through the inspiratory/expiratory (I/E) valve. The *demand valve* (Fig. 13.8b) is essentially a simple artificial ventilator. It consists of a "smart" (I/E) valve coupled to an oxygen source through a flow resistance. The I/E valve is designed to open following the pressure drop of an inspiratory effort, after a built-in expiratory interval has elapsed, or when manually triggered by the operator. It remains open until a preset pressure is delivered (McPherson, 1977).

### Gas-Delivery Equipment

Pressurized sources of gas are required for ventilatory support and for delivery of therapeutic gases and medicated aerosols to the patient. Gases encountered include air, oxygen, carbon dioxide, helium, and nitrogen. Prior to delivery to the patient, the gases must be of suitable composition, temperature, and humidity, and pressure and flow must be carefully regulated. Section 13.6 describes equipment for these purposes.

### Vacuum-Delivery Systems and Suction Devices

*Suction devices* are used to aspirate fluids from the patient's repiratory passages and, in the case of air (pneumothorax) or fluid (hydrothorax) in the intrapleural cavity, to maintain a steady subatmospheric pressure of, say, $-50$ mmHg in this cavity (Egan, 1977). Safety valves and vacuum regulators protect the patient against excessive vacuum gradients. Fluid-collection containers with overflow shutoff

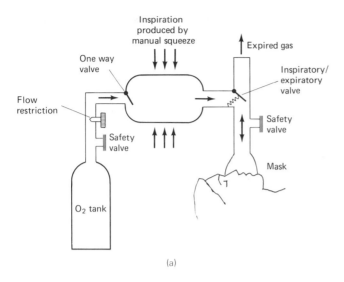

(a)

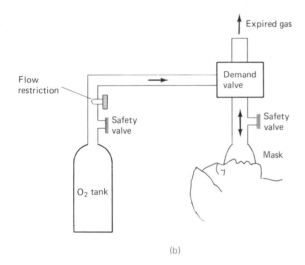

(b)

**FIGURE 13.8.** Two types of emergency resuscitators. (a) Manual bag resuscitator. (b) Demand valve.

valves prevent contamination of the vacuum system. Vacuum delivery systems operate below 460 mm Hg ($-300$ mm Hg relative to atmospheric) and are like gas-delivery systems in reverse in that the vacuum line is attached to the intake port of a rotary vane gas pump. The two systems include similar storage tanks, gages, regulators, and safety valves. The Compressed Gas Association (CGA, 500 Fifth Ave., New York, NY 10036) has developed specifications for both types of delivery systems.

### Humidifiers and Nebulizers

A *humidifier* increases the water-vapor content of gas delivered during gas or IPPB therapy or during artificial ventilation. A *nebulizer* generates a controlled aerosol of of water or medication for delivery into the patient's lungs. Section 13.7 treats these devices in more detail.

### Intermittent Therapy Equipment

*Intermittent positive pressure breathing* (IPPB) refers to the mechanical ventilation of a patient over a period of 15–30 min on a schedule of, say, from one to four times a day. IPPB therapy treats diseases such as acute and chronic bronchitis, pulmonary emphysema, bronchiectasis, lung abscess, acute bronchial spasm, and pulmonary edema. This therapy improves ventilation and gas exchange, delivers elevated oxygen levels, delivers medicated aerosols, and, in the case of pulmonary edema, reduces cardiac output by elevating intrathoracic pressures. The therapist administers the treatment with care, as it requires patient cooperation and is physically demanding on the patient.

Medications open up the airways, loosen mucous deposits, and kill infection organisms. *Bronchodilators* open the airways by relaxing bronchiolar muscles, while *decongestants* work by *vasoconstriction* of the pulmonary vessels or by *anti-inflammatory* action on the swollen tissues. Mucous secretions may be freed by the nebulized delivery of a variety of agents, including water or saline, ethyl alcohol, detergents, mucolytics capable of breaking down the mucous proteins, or proteolytics that act on the components of purulent sputum (Egan, 1977).

The compact "pressure" ventilators described in Section 13.8 can deliver IPPB, and special purpose devices are also available. These include small gas-powered devices, such as the Ohio Hand-E-Vent II (Ohio Medical Products, Madison, WI), which are similar to the demand valve mentioned previously. Manual nebulizers may also be used.

### Ventilators

A ventilator is a device that either controls or assists the mechanical ventilation of a patient's lungs. Such a machine is also called a *breathing machine* or a *respirator*. The latter term is losing favor, because it also refers to a breathing mask for filtering out dust and chemicals. Section 13.8 discusses ventilators more extensively.

### Extracorporeal Oxygenators

If ventilation is not feasible, as during thoracic surgery or with severe respiratory disease, then we must transfer gases directly into and out of the patient's blood via an *extracorporeal oxygenator* or *artificial lung*. Part or all of a patient's cardiac output circulates through the oxygenator, where a large surface area exposes it to the desired gas mixture. Section 4.6 discusses designs for achieving the required blood–gas interface for diffusive transport. Gille and Bagniewski (1976) and Peirce (1972) review the use of oxygenators for treating respiratory insufficiency.

## Monitoring Instrumentation

The use of therapeutic devices requires instrumentation for monitoring the patient. Sections 13.6 through 13.8 describe the monitoring required during gas and nebulizer therapy and artificial ventilation. See medical instrumentation texts such as Webster (1978) or Cromwell et al. (1973) for additional information on specific devices.

## Patient-Training Devices

To optimize ventilation distribution and gas exchange while minimizing the work of breathing, respiratory patients need to learn to breathe properly. In severe cases of bronchiolar collapse, for example, the emphysema patient must learn to exhale gradually against pursed lips, or air may become trapped and impossible to force out (Egan, 1977). Training devices using visual or aural biofeedback enable such patients to compare their airflow or volume patterns against desired patterns. Cutter Resiflex (Covina, CA), for example, offers respiratory exercisers that provide visual incentive to the patient via either flow (Model 970-20) or volume (Model 970-21) feedback.

## Environmental Control Equipment

To avoid intubation or a mask, a plastic tent or box over the patient's head can deliver oxygen. We must control the gas composition, temperature, and humidity of the tent and take precautions to avoid combustion in the oxygen-enriched atmosphere (Egan, 1977). An incubator completely encloses the infant and totally controls its environment, including the gas breathed (Section 15.5).

Hyperbaric therapy treats problems related to respiratory insufficiency due to inadequate ventilation or circulatory problems (Innes, 1970; Meijne, 1970). By totally enclosing the patient in a pressure chamber, we can raise oxygen tensions so high that anemic blood can carry useful amounts of oxygen. Also, oxygen can diffuse directly through the skin to tissues suffering from circulatory damage. We must guard against the hazards of decompression and oxygen-enriched atmospheres. Single person units are smaller and less costly, but larger units allow a therapist to be in the chamber with the patient in case of emergency.

## Neonatal Equipment

The problems of respiratory therapy are compounded with the neonatal patient (Epstein and Epstein, 1979; Rogers, 1972). A small infant may need a tidal volume of 10 ml and a respiratory frequency of 60 bpm versus, say, 500 ml and 12 bpm for the adult. Also, compliance may be low, requiring relatively high delivery pressures. Thus, the therapist uses specialized devices that minimize dead space, deliver small volumes precisely, and are sensitive enough to trigger off the neonate's delicate breathing efforts.

Available neonatal equipment includes the Bourns Infant Ventilator Model LS-104-150 (Bourns Life Systems, Inc., Riverside, CA), the Ohio Neonatal Respirator (Ohio Medical Products, Madison, WI), and the Babybird (Bird Corporation, Palm Springs, CA).

## 13.6 GAS-DELIVERY SYSTEMS

### Supply Systems

Gas may be provided by a source near the patient, or it may be piped from a central location. In either case, the pressurized cylinder is the most common source for gases such as oxygen, carbon dioxide, helium, and nitrogen. Air reconstituted from nitrogen and oxygen may also be provided in this manner, or filtered room air may be compressed as needed. In the latter case, a rotary pump or one of piston or diaphragm design typically cycles on and off to maintain a specified pressure in a storage tank, and a water condenser partially dries the air leaving the tank (McPherson, 1977).

Pressurized tanks range in size from the small Style A (about 8 cm $\times$ 28 cm) to the large Style H (about 23 cm $\times$ 127 cm). At a typical pressure at room temperature of 2200 psig, a Style H tank can hold about 10 kg or 7,000 l (STP) of oxygen. In contrast, the same size tank can hold about 31 kg or 16,000 l (STP) of carbon dioxide at a pressure of only 840 psig. More carbon dioxide can be stored at less pressure because, unlike oxygen, $CO_2$ liquefies under pressure at room temperature. For gases such as $O_2$, tank pressure is a good index of the amount of gas remaining. Because pressure remains essentially constant until the liquid phase is gone, we can only determine the amount of gas remaining in a $CO_2$ cylinder by weighing the tank. For a mixture of $O_2$ and $CO_2$, $CO_2$ partial pressure is kept low enough to avoid a liquid phase and hence to avoid a change in the composition of the gas delivered as the tank is emptied (Garrett and Donaldson, 1978).

Another common source of oxygen is the cryogenic container, which may be large enough to hold millions of liters (STP) of $O_2$ or small enough for the ambulatory patient to carry. Cryogenic storage requires special tanks that are like large thermos bottles to hold the very cold liquid oxygen ($O_2$ boils at $-182.96°C$ at 760 mm Hg), but offers more compact storage at less pressure (200 psig). The stored oxygen is kept cold by its own gradual evaporation as it flows into the delivery system or is vented to the atmosphere (McPherson, 1977).

Figure 13.9 shows a typical delivery system. Each cylinder on a manifold has its own shutoff valve and high-pressure safety relief valve and is isolated by a one-way check valve to protect the system. Other valves can isolate various legs of the system for safety and maintenance. Regulators downstream drop the pressure to a typical working value of 50 psig.

### Regulation of Pressure and Flow

Figure 13.10 shows a simple pressure regulator. The spring-loaded valve opens only when downstream pressure drops below the regulated value. Pressure is

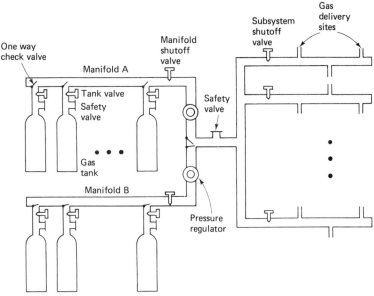

**FIGURE 13.9.** A representative gas delivery system. Manifold A is delivering gas, while manifold B is in reserve.

measured by a mechanical gage, either of the Bourdon design (pressures > 200 psig), or the diaphragm type (pressures < 200 psig), in which the distension with pressure of a metal chamber is linked to a dial pointer.

The measurement and regulation of flow are less straightforward. Sometimes a pressure gage upstream of a known orifice is calibrated in units of flow. We should only interpret the reading on such a gage to be the flow achievable if there were no downstream flow resistance; for constant upstream pressure, the reading on this "flow" regulator would not change, even if the true flow were zero. The Thorpe tube (rotameter) shown in Fig. 13.11 is a common gage in flow regulators. The position of the float is highly dependent on density as well as volume flow, and a tube is calibrated for a specific gas at a given temperature and pressure. To minimize changes in pressure at the float due to downstream resistance, the tube is often "compensated" by placing it on the regulated pressure (upstream) side of the flow control (Fig. 13.11b).

## Gas Mixing

Figure 13.12 shows several ways to mix gases such as oxygen and air before delivery. The delivered gas composition of the *gas adder* (Fig. 13.12a) is dependent on the airflow rate, and that of the *entrainment device* (Fig. 13.12b) (e.g., a Venturi tube) depends on $O_2$ flow and downstream backpressure. We know the gas mixture out of the *dual Thorpe tube* device (Fig. 13.12c) if the Thorpe tubes are operated at their calibrated pressures, but adjustments of total flow and mixture are

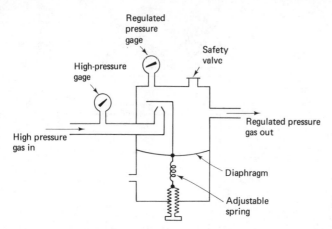

FIGURE 13.10. A single stage
pressure regulator.

highly interdependent. By incorporating the dual pressure regulator, the *controller*
or *blender* (Fig. 13.12d) can accurately deliver the gas mixture specified by the
calibrated needle valve adjustment over a broad range of flows.

## Safety Considerations

A Style H cylinder of, say, nitrogen pressurized to 2,200 psig, has a potential
energy of about 3 MJ (about 1 kW h), which, if suddenly converted to kinetic
energy, could accelerate the heavy tank (about 70 kg) to a velocity of roughly
Mach 1 and wreak considerable havoc. To guard against this hazard, the Department of Transportation regulates the construction, testing, and marking of gas
cylinders. Oxygen and flammable gases present additional hazards. The Compressed
Gas Association (CGA) has developed regulations for safety labeling, approved by
the American Standards Association (ASA). In addition, the CGA, the National
Fire Protection Agency (NFPA), and local authorities have developed recommenda-

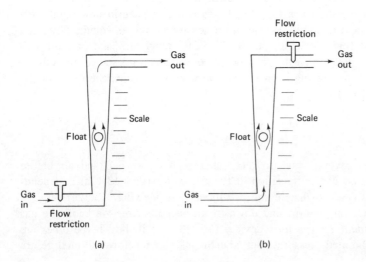

FIGURE 13.11. Two Thorpe
tube configurations for measuring gas flow. (a) Uncompensated. (b) Compensated.

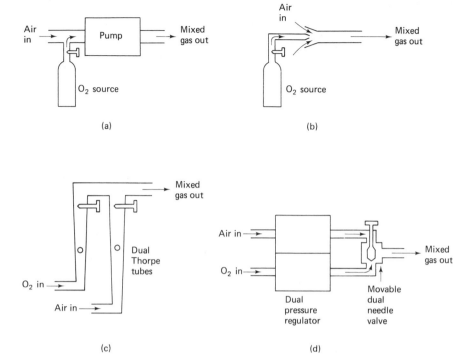

FIGURE 13.12. Four ways to mix gases for delivery to the patient.
(a) Gas adder. (b) Entrainment device. (c) Flowmeter mixer. (d)
Controller or blender.

tions and regulations regarding the storage, transport, and use of gas cylinders. The
NFPA has also developed safety specifications for cryogenic oxygen storage systems
(McPherson, 1977).

We must also take safety precautions to reduce the chance of delivering the
wrong gas to the patient. The contents of each pressurized cylinder must be shown
on the label and must meet purity standards of the Food and Drug Administration
(FDA) as listed in the United States Pharmacopia (USP). In addition, the Bureau of
Standards recommends the use of a color-coding system designed by the CGA
(e.g., green for $O_2$, gray for $CO_2$) (McPherson, 1977).

The valves and outlets for large cylinders are indexed to gas type by thread
size, type, and rotation direction and coupling design. The Pin Index Safety System
(PISS) of the ASA serves the same function for smaller tanks. In this system, the
cylinder yoke on the delivery system has a built-in combination of pins so that it
can only accept a gas cylinder having holes drilled in the proper locations on the
valve body (Garrett and Donaldson, 1978). A Diameter Index Safety System
(DISS), in which a unique combination of coupling diameter and thread design is
used for each gas, has been developed for low-pressure (less than 200 psig)
couplings in the delivery system. Station outlets may consist of a DISS connector
and a manual valve or be of the "quick-connect" type developed by various
manufacturers. NFPA regulations cover these connections as well as the structure of

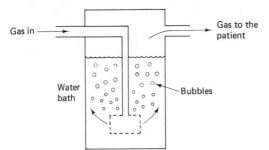

**FIGURE 13.13.** A bubble humidifier.

gas supply and piping systems (McPherson, 1977). For satisfactory operation, the components of a gas delivery system must be designed to work together. Anyone involved in the design of such a system needs to keep in mind the system-wide significance of the decision to use a particular connector type or manufacturer's product.

## 13.7 HUMIDIFIERS AND NEBULIZERS

### Humidifiers

As gas enters the airways, it is heated to body temperature and saturated with water vapor, reaching a water content of 43.8 mg/l at 100% relative humidity. The delivery of dry gas causes the patient discomfort and, especially if the upper breathing passages are bypassed, damages the airway tissues. Humidifiers of various designs add water vapor by providing a water–gas interface. The *bubble humidifier* in Fig. 13.13, for example, bubbles the gas through a reservoir of water on the way to the patient.

At an operating temperature of, say 20°C, saturated gas can only hold 18.4 mg/l of water, which, at body temperature, corresponds to a relative humidity of 42%. Hence, some humidifiers incorporate heaters to increase the amount of water vapor delivered to the patient. Others generate aerosols of water droplets that add to the water vapor content by evaporating in the warm airways (McPherson, 1977).

### Nebulizers

For maximum effectiveness with minimum side effects, we must control both the volume flow and the site of deposition of a water or medication aerosol delivered into a patient's lungs. The site of deposition is affected by the size of the water droplets, with larger droplets being deposited in the upper airways, and droplets on the order of 1 $\mu$m in diameter being maximally deposited in the small airways. The aerosol produced by a simple *atomizer* contains such a broad range of particle sizes that much of the water and medication is lost to the upper respiratory tract. To control the size range of delivered particles, nebulizers of various designs are available (Fig. 13.14). The simplest is a modified atomizer (Fig. 13.14a). A baffle

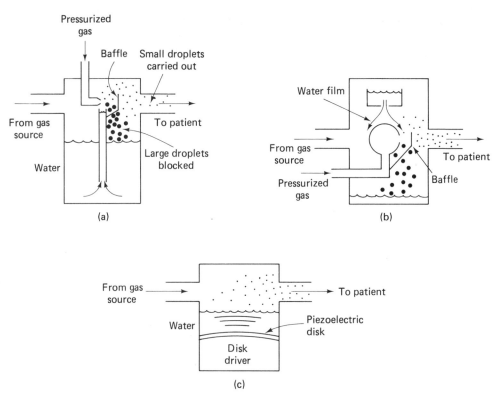

**FIGURE 13.14.** Three types of nebulizers. (a) Atomizer with baffle.
(b) Babbington nebulizer. (c) Ultrasonic nebulizer.

blocks and recovers excessively large particles, but at the expense of reducing the
output volume flow rate. To produce a higher flow of small droplets, the *Babbington nebulizer* (Fig. 13.14b) uses a high velocity gas jet to blast apart a thin film
of fluid flowing across the jet orifice. The piezoelectrically-driven *ultrasonic
nebulizer* (Fig. 13.14c) vibrates the water at a frequency (e.g., 1.35 MHz) selected
to produce droplets with the desired size range (e.g., from 1 $\mu$m to 10 $\mu$m). These
latter nebulizer types can deliver such high volumes of water that the airways can
be overloaded, and it is even possible to overhydrate the patient. These effects are
of particular concern with patients already suffering excessive airway obstruction,
those in critical water balance, and small neonates (Egan, 1977).

## 13.8 VENTILATORS

This section introduces concepts basic to understanding the design and operation of
ventilators. We emphasize positive pressure ventilation of the passive adult patient
and briefly discuss other therapeutic situations. Chapter 12 considers breathing
machines for surgery, and Chapter 15 reviews the special requirements of the
neonate.

## Patient Requirements and Safety Considerations

The therapeutic goals of ventilation are to maintain appropriate arterial levels of oxygen, carbon dioxide, and pH, while minimizing patient risk, discomfort, and time on the ventilator. Of the patient's physiological needs, an adequate level of oxygen tension is the most crucial, though abnormally low or high levels of oxygen, carbon dioxide, or pH are all harmful to the patient. As a rule of thumb, therapy is indicated if $P_{aO_2}$ is less than 50–60 mm Hg, $P_{aCO_2}$ is greater than 50–55 mm Hg, or arterial blood pH is less than 7.25 (Egan, 1977).

We regulate blood-gas levels and pH by adjusting the composition of the inspired gas and by selecting a breathing pattern to deliver the desired level of ventilation. The choice of breathing pattern includes a selection of tidal volume $V_T$ and respiratory frequency $f$, which together determine alveolar ventilation rate $\dot{V}_A$ by equation 13.1. A third factor in the breathing pattern is the ratio of the durations of inspiration and expiration (I:E ratio). We may also select different time courses of pressure or flow delivery, or "waveform shapes."

The therapist initially estimates the ventilatory needs of a patient from past experience and with the aid of a nomogram. The Radford nomogram, for example, relates a patient's body mass and sex to appropriate combinations of tidal volume and respiratory frequency (Mushin et al., 1969). This nomogram covers body masses from less than 3 kg to over 110 kg and includes adjustments for fever, altitude, and changes in dead space $V_D$. Specified combinations of tidal volume and respiratory frequency range from 12 ml at 50 bpm for a small infant to 900 ml at 8 bpm for a large adult male. Equation 13.1 shows that more than one combination of $V_T$ and $f$ delivers the same $\dot{V}_A$. In practice, the therapist selects the specific combination based on other needs of the patient. For example, we can use a combination of low $V_T$ and high $f$ to avoid the buildup of undesirably high transthoracic pressures. On the other hand, low $f$ coupled with high $V_T$ minimizes problems due to airway resistance and enhances ventilation distribution (Petty, 1974).

To ensure complete emptying of the lung, expiration should be at least as long as inspiration. Typically, we set the I:E ratio at 1:2, to allow twice the time for expiration as for inspiration. Other factors also affect the choice of I:E ratio. A relatively long inspiratory phase, for example, allows more time for ventilation distribution and may improve gas exchange but also increases average intrathoracic pressure and hence the potential for the pressure-induced side effects mentioned later (Mushin et al., 1969). Whatever breathing pattern we select, we usually interrupt it at regular intervals by larger, longer breaths (sometimes called *sighs*) to avoid atelectasis, that is, the gradual closing of alveoli in regions of the lung which occurs during steady ventilation (Egan, 1977).

Once the therapist initiates ventilation, he adjusts the breathing pattern and gas composition on the basis of gas tensions and pH measured in blood samples collected periodically. In patients with normal lungs and blood, we can maintain a suitable oxygen level by ventilating with room air at a rate that holds arterial carbon dioxide tension at the desired level of $P_{aCO_2} = 40$ mm Hg. This rate meets the patient's oxygen needs because the arterial blood is essentially saturated with oxygen. In patients with impaired gas exchange, ventilation sufficient to ensure adequate carbon dioxide removal may not provide enough oxygen to the blood, because oxygen diffuses less readily than carbon dioxide. In such patients, we may avoid hypoxia by hyperventilating their lungs or by increasing $F_{IO_2}$, the oxygen fraction of the inspired air. If the patient is hyperventilated, we can maintain the desired carbon dioxide level by increasing the dead space and, hence, the amount of expired gas the patient rebreathes, or by including carbon dioxide in the inspired gas mixture (Egan, 1977).

As with other therapeutic interventions, ventilating a patient carries with it the potential for undesirable side effects. A breathing machine must satisfy the general requirements for safety in a therapeutic device. The patient and therapist must be protected from electrical shock and thermal burns, and there must be no electromagnetic radiation that could interfere with other devices such as cardiac pacemakers. Also, the controls and indicators on the machine must be accurate, and the machine must be able to deliver ventilation according to the performance claimed. In addition, because the interruption of ventilation for only a few minutes can lead to irreversible damage or death, the breathing machine must be reliable and have appropriate alarms and safety features to protect against malfunction (ANSI, 1976).

In general, we provide ventilation to the patient in a manner as close as possible to the conditions of normal breathing. In this way, we minimize risk and usually shorten the process of weaning the patient from the ventilator (Petty, 1974). Exposure to elevated oxygen levels is toxic. Hence, we should keep $F_{IO_2}$ as close as possible to that of normal air (Heironimus and Bageant, 1977). To minimize the hazard of airway drying, the inspired gas should be at a temperature between 32 and 39°C and have a water content of at least 33 mg-$H_2O$/l, thus ensuring at least a 75% relative humidity at the nominal body temperature of 37°C. In no instance should the inspired gas temperature exceed 41°C (ANSI, 1976). In addition, the inspired gas should be filtered free of particles and should not pass through any regions contaminated by chemicals or microorganisms.

The pressures that result in the thorax and other parts of the body during ventilation may have undesirable effects. If the ventilation produces pressure at the airway (positive pressure ventilation), the resultant superatmospheric pressures in the thorax can reduce venous return and lower systemic blood pressure. These abnormal pressures can also act on the volume sensors in the thorax to alter fluid balance (Egan, 1977; Nordström, 1972). High intrapulmonary pressures can even burst a lung, causing a pneumothorax (Petty, 1974). Alternatively, if the ventilator reduces the pressure around the body (negative pressure ventilation), the resultant subatmospheric pressures in the tissues can induce blood pooling and thus also reduce venous return and alter fluid balance. To minimize these problems, we should keep the average pressure gradient over the breath cycle as small as possible and keep the peak intrapulmonary pressure low. As a safety precaution, applied airway pressure should not exceed 40 cm $H_2O$ (Egan, 1977).

Abnormalities in thoracic structures or in cardiovascular function can accentuate these undesirable side effects. A low lung and chest-wall compliance means we require higher pressure gradients to deliver the same tidal volume. If the compliance of the lungs is high relative to that of the chest wall, as in the destructive diseases such as emphysema, positive pressures applied at the airway have even more impact on the cardiovascular system (Petty, 1974). Alternatively, high airway resistance or a nonuniform distribution of resistance and compliance means more time is required for adequate inspiration and expiration. This increase in time accentuates the deleterious effects of the ventilatory pressures.

There is little problem in ventilating a patient with normal thoracic structure and cardiovascular function. Low pressure gradients of 10 cm $H_2O$ or less are sufficient, and we can attain adequate gas distribution and exchange for a broad range of breathing patterns. Also, the body easily compensates for the effects of any abnormal pressures. For such a patient, the performance of a breathing machine and the way it is used are not very critical. On the other hand, the delivery of optimal ventilation with minimum risk to patients with abnormal thoracic structure and cardiovascular function may require delicate tradeoffs involving the level of oxygenation and the choice of breathing pattern (Petty, 1974). Such cases require a flexible breathing machine, or a selection of machines, offering the therapist a broad choice of alternatives in gas composition and in the characteristics of the delivered pressures and flows.

## Methods of Delivering Pressure and Flow

Several schemes for classifying ventilators have been developed (Mushin et al., 1969; McPherson, 1977). In this chapter, we concentrate on those characteristics of breathing machines that most directly affect their therapeutic function. First, we present various ways of characterizing how ventilators move gas into and out of the patient's lungs and follow this by methods used to cycle between inspiration and expiration.

**Positive Pressure versus Negative Pressure.** The two most common ways of generating a pressure gradient to inflate the lungs are *positive pressure ventilation* (PPV), in which we apply pressure at the airway opening, and *negative pressure ventilation* (NPV), in which we reduce the pressure around the body, or at least the thorax. Figure 13.15 compares these methods. Note that the two methods can produce the same gas flow and volume waveforms but that the average pressure in the thorax is less with NPV than with PPV. Sometimes we use a combination of these methods. The most common means of emptying the lungs is to simply equalize the airway and extrathoracic pressures, and thus allow the compliance of the lungs and chest wall to passively push out the air.

During normal inspiration, the muscles generate subatmospheric (negative) intrapleural pressures. Hence, negative pressure ventilation is in a sense "natural." The "iron lung" or Drinker apparatus, used to ventilate numerous polio victims in earlier decades, is based on this principle. More recent devices of this type include the whole body Isolette Negative-Pressure Respirator (Air Shields, Inc., Hatboro, PA) for infants and the Emerson Curiass or thoracic shell (J. H. Emerson Co., Cambridge, MA). Units of this latter type apply negative pressures to the thorax alone rather than to the whole body.

Negative pressure machines are also "natural" in that special provisions for air delivery, such as intubation or tracheostomy, are usually not necessary, and

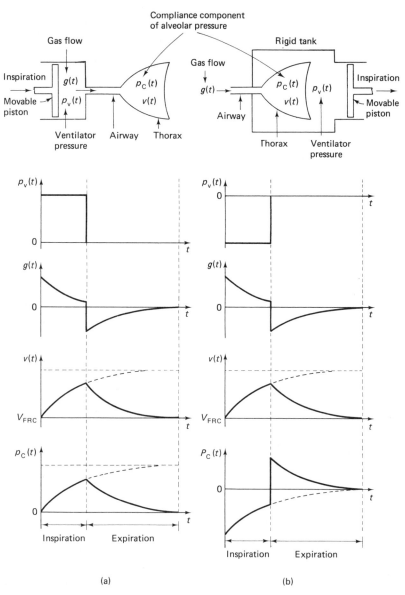

**FIGURE 13.15.** Comparison of (a) positive pressure and (b) negative pressure ventilation. For simplicity, we assume that the pressure generated by each machine is constant throughout inspiration. We assume that expiration is passive.

talking is possible. On the other hand, the whole body tank, and even the curiass, exert subatmospheric pressures not only on the chest but also on other parts of the body, which can cause the undesirable side effects discussed previously. Moreover, such devices severely reduce access to the patient, making patient care difficult, and

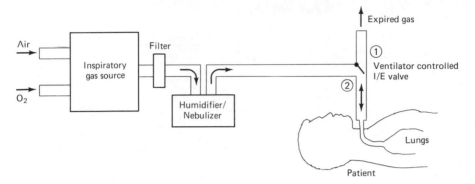

**FIGURE 13.16.** Patient circuit for intermittent positive pressure ventilation (IPPV).

create the problem of adequate air seals around the patient. Because of these problems, negative pressure ventilation is in limited use (Egan, 1977).

Most breathing machines in use today employ positive pressure ventilation, and we consider only this type of machine in the following discussions. This method of delivery provides free access to the patient but requires special care in interfacing the ventilator with the patient. In addition, the abnormally elevated pressures in the thorax may potentially cause the deleterious side effects discussed previously.

The application of positive pressure during inspiration, followed by passive expiration against atmospheric pressure, is called *intermittent* (or *inspiratory*) *positive pressure ventilation* (IPPV). We need to distinguish this continuous mode of ventilation from the periodic, short-duration therapeutic use of ventilators for IPPB and from a weaning mode called *intermittent mandatory ventilation* (IMV), in which breath cycles delivered by the ventilator alternate with the patient's own efforts (McPherson, 1977). In some patients, the ventilator assists the lungs during expiration by applying subatmospheric pressure at the airway, a mode called *negative end expiratory pressure* (NEEP). In other patients, it enhances ventilation distribution and gas exchange by increasing the average degree of lung inflation over a breath. The ventilator can hold the lungs open by *expiratory retard*, in which it inserts a high resistance in the expiratory pathway, or by *positive end expiratory pressure* (PEEP), in which it elevates the pressure against which passive expiration takes place. A similar technique, in which the patient is not artificially ventilated but is breathing from a source elevated in pressure, is called *continuous positive airway pressure* (CPAP) or *continuous positive pressure breathing* (CPPB). As discussed previously, the elevation in average intrathoracic pressure associated with increased lung inflation also increases the chance of undesirable side effects on circulatory performance (Petty, 1974).

**The Patient Circuit.** Figure 13.16 shows the patient circuit for a ventilator that delivers intermittent positive pressure ventilation. During inspiration, the ventilator moves the inspiratory/expiratory (I/E) valve to position 1, and this delivers to the patient the source gas of suitable composition, humidity, and temperature.

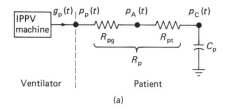

Ventilator | Patient

(a)

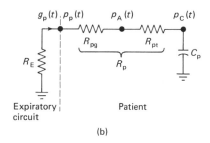

Expiratory circuit | Patient

(b)

**FIGURE 13.17.** Model of an IPPV ventilator-patient system. We model the patient as a resistance $R_p$ and compliance $C_p$. During inspiration (a) the ventilator delivers gas flow $g_p(t)$ and pressure $p_p(t)$, and during expiration (b) the lungs empty through expiratory resistance $R_E$. We denote the compliance component of alveolar pressure $p_A(t)$ by $p_C(t)$.

Expiration begins when the ventilator moves the I/E valve to position 2, which allows the air in the lungs to passively exhaust to the environment.

For long-term ventilation, the airway interface to the patient is of critical importance. A facemask can be used for short-term emergency ventilation, but a safe, effective seal to the face is difficult, and the airways may become obstructed by the tongue or by regurgitated gastric contents. For ventilation over a period of days or weeks, the patient must have an oral endotracheal or nasotracheal tube or a tube inserted through a tracheostomy. Tubes through the mouth or nose have the advantage of not requiring surgery, whereas the tracheostomy tube, being shorter, reduces dead space and improves access to the bronchi for the aspiration of secretions (Egan, 1977). These tubes have inflatable or spongy cuffs, which ensure a tight gas seal in the trachea and minimize the chance of blood or gastric contents entering the lungs. We must ensure that the localized pressure of the cuff on the airway wall does not damage the wall tissue (Petty, 1974). Because these tubes bypass the humidifying and warming upper airways, they accentuate the need to precondition the delivered gas.

In preparing a ventilator for use, we must ensure that there is no contamination from previous users. Thus, between patients, we must either sterilize or dispose of those parts of the patient circuit exposed to expired air.

**Pressure Sources versus Flow Sources.** The ventilator may be powered electrically or pneumatically from a central or local source of compressed gas. Inspiratory flow may come directly from a valved source of compressed gas or result directly from the push of a rotary or linearly driven piston. Alternatively, we may employ a "double circuit" system, in which we pressurize gas surrounding a bag or bellows, and this delivers the bellows contents to the patient (McPherson, 1977; Mushin et al., 1969). More fundamental than these specific mechanisms, however, is how the ventilator interacts with the patient system. Figure 13.17 shows a simple model of an IPPV ventilator–patient system during a breath cycle. The

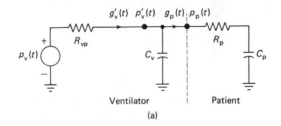

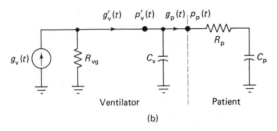

**FIGURE 13.18.** Equivalent source models of an IPPV machine during inspiration. (a) Model based on ideal pressure source $p_v(t)$. (b) Model based on ideal flow source $g_v(t)$.

patient model, with compliance $C_p$ and total resistance $R_p$, comes from Fig. 13.3a. In the passive patient, $p_{mus}(t) = 0$. Pressure $p_C(t)$ is the compliance component of alveolar pressure $p_A(t)$. During inspiration, the ventilator delivers to the patient gas flow $g_p(t)$ and pressure $p_p(t)$, which depend on the characteristics of both the ventilator and the patient. We assume expiration is passive, during which air flows out of the lungs and through some external expiratory resistance, $R_E$. The directional arrows for $g_p(t)$ in Fig. 13.17 are to show sign convention; that is, $g_p(t)$ goes negative during expiration.

We can model the dependence of ventilator performance on patient load in a manner exactly analogous to that used with electrical sources. That is, we can equivalently describe the output characteristics of the ventilator during inspiration in terms of either an ideal pressure source $p_v(t)$ (analogous to an ideal voltage source) or an ideal flow source $g_v(t)$ (analogous to an ideal current source) coupled with appropriate internal passive elements. This concept is illustrated by the simple equivalent source models shown in Fig. 13.18 in which the pressure source feeds a series airflow resistance $R_{vp}$ and the flow source feeds a parallel airflow resistance $R_{vg}$. Any ventilator that can be modeled by Fig. 13.18a can also be modeled by Fig. 13.18b. We have included an internal compliance element $C_v$ in each model to account for elasticity and gas compression effects in the ventilator and tubing.

We can consider the ventilator to behave like a *pressure source* during inspiration if the time course of $p_p(t)$ is not affected much by changes in the patient. Note that the lack of dependence on the *patient* is the deciding factor here, not whether $p_p(t)$ is constant with time. Though changes in the patient load may have little effect on $p_p(t)$ with a pressure-source ventilator, they strongly affect delivered flow. For example, an increase in the patient's resistance $R_p$ would proportionately reduce flow and, hence, the volume delivered during inspiration. The models of Fig. 13.18 more closely represent a pressure source as $R_{vp}$, $R_{vg}$, and $C_v$ decrease.

We consider the ventilator to be a *flow source* if the time course of inspiratory flow is not affected significantly by the patient load. In this case, though changes in the patient do not alter delivered flow, they may result in significant changes in pressures in the system. For example, a decrease in the patient's compliance $C_p$ would proportionately increase the pressure developed in the lungs during inspiration. The models of Fig. 13.18 move closer to flow sources as $R_{vp}$ and $R_{vg}$ increase and $C_v$ decreases.

Analogous to electrical sources, Fig. 13.18a shows that one way to make a flow source is to place a high-pressure source in series with a large resistance to flow. We can set some ventilators, such as the Bird respirators (Bird Corporation, Palm Springs, CA), to deliver flows to the patient that are driven by a pressure of 50 psig or about 3500 cm $H_2O$ (McPherson, 1977). For a typical flow on the order of 0.25 l/s, the internal series resistance of such a ventilator is 14,000 (cm $H_2O$)/(l/s). Because the ventilator source pressure and resistance are many orders of magnitude greater than the patient pressures and load, respectively, we can consider the machine to be a flow source. Also, for a constant driving pressure, flow is constant during inspiration. Another way to build a flow source, also analogous to techniques used in electrical power supplies, is to use feedback. This approach is taken in the Servo Ventilator 900B (Siemens Corporation, Union, NJ) and other recent machines (Engelman and Cook, 1977; Cox and Chapman, 1974). With this more flexible approach, we can make the ventilator behave like a flow source that is time-varying.

A ventilator must be "powerful" enough to ventilate the patient, and the models of Figs. 13.17 and 13.18 are useful for calculating ventilator power requirements. In addition to meeting the average power requirements to do the work of inspiration at the desired respiratory frequency, the ventilator must also be able to generate the desired pressures and have the instantaneous power capability to deliver the maximum flows required.

## Methods of Controlling the Breath Cycle

Automatic ventilators employ a variety of electronic, fluidic, and mechanical techniques for cycling back and forth between inspiration and expiration. The references provide details of these mechanisms. This section emphasizes the ways in which different control methods affect therapeutic performance. On a particular ventilator, the same method may trigger both inspiration and expiration, or a different method may be used for each. In addition to automatic cycling, ventilators usually provide some manual means of initiating an inspiration and expiration.

**Patient Demand.** If a patient has some residual ventilatory function, and his respiratory regulation mechanisms are intact, then the patient can control the ventilation delivered by means of an *assist* or *demand* mode. We can set the ventilator to initiate an inspiration when it senses a patient-induced drop in pressure at the airway. Similarly, the ventilator can sense a high airway pressure to end inspiration and begin the expiratory phase. We may permit the patient to trigger the onset of inspiration, expiration, or both. Once the patient initiates a phase, ventilator function may be predetermined, or, by incorporating feedback, the patient may

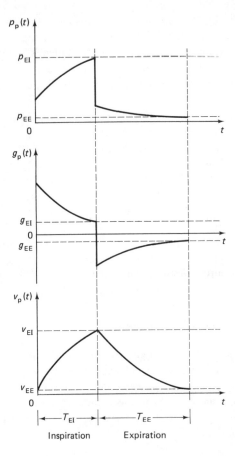

**FIGURE 13.19.** Threshold values of pressure, flow, volume, and time which can control the durations of inspiration and expiration. The subscripts EI and EE refer respectively to values which can be used to end inspiration and end expiration.

actually be able to control delivery throughout the entire phase. Also, we may set the ventilator to take over ventilation in the absence of adequate triggering by the patient. In this mode, the ventilator is an *assistor-controller* (McPherson, 1977).

**Time, Pressure, Volume, and Flow Cycling.** For the completely passive patient, the ventilator must control the duration of the inspiratory and expiratory phases of the breath cycle. The three most common control methods are to terminate a phase after a specified *time* has elapsed, after a specified airway *pressure* is attained, or after a predetermined *volume* of air has moved into or out of the lungs. It is also possible to end a phase by sensing when *flow* drops below some preset level.

Theoretically, we can use any combination of these methods to provide satisfactory ventilation to a stable patient. Figure 13.19 shows airway pressure $p_p(t)$, delivered gas flow $g_p(t)$, and volume $v_p(t)$ for a breath cycle. The subscripts EI and EE represent appropriate thresholds to trigger the end of inspiration and expiration. The waveforms correspond to either of the models in Fig. 13.18 with a constant pressure or flow source, $C_v = 0$, and $R_{vp}$ or $R_{vg}$ relatively small. The circuit in Fig. 13.17b models expiration.

The procedure involved in setting a ventilator to some desired $V_T$, $f$, and I:E ratio varies considerably with the type of gas source and method of cycle control.

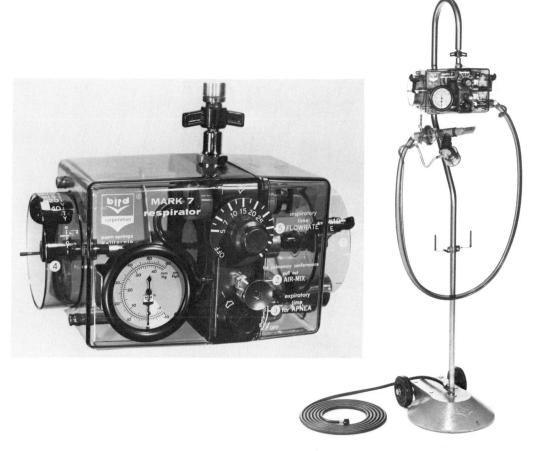

**FIGURE 13.20.** The Bird Mark 7 ventilator. (a) Main body. (b) With patient circuit. (*Courtesy* Bird Corp., 3M, 1980.)

The Bird Mark 7 ventilator (Fig. 13.20), for example, is driven by a 50-psig source and cycles according to complex interactions between pneumatic pressures and magnetic forces (McPherson, 1977). With the Air Mix knob pushed in and a passive patient, this machine is essentially a pressure-cycled constant-flow source during inspiration and has a time-cycled expiratory phase. To set $V_T$ and inspiratory duration $T_I$, we must achieve, by trial and error, the proper combination of Inspiratory Flow Rate (upper center in Fig. 13.20a) and Inspiratory Pressure Limit (on the right side). We then set the duration of expiration $T_E$ using the Expiratory Time control (lower center). The result is an I:E ratio of $T_I$:$T_E$ and a respiratory frequency of $f = 60/(T_I + T_E)$, with $f$ in bpm and $T_I$ and $T_E$ in seconds.

In contrast, Fig. 13.21 shows the Bennett MA-1 Ventilator (Puritan-Bennett Corp., Kansas City, MO). In this machine, an electrically powered compressor pushes gas out of a bellows and into the patient at a rate limited by the Peak Flow control. The Rate control sets an electronic timer, which determines respiratory

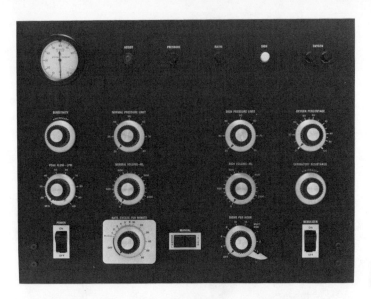

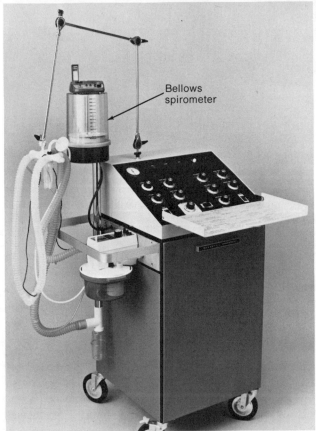

**FIGURE 13.21.** The Bennett MA-1 ventilator. (a) Control panel. (b) With patient circuit. (*Courtesy* Puritan-Bennett Corp.)

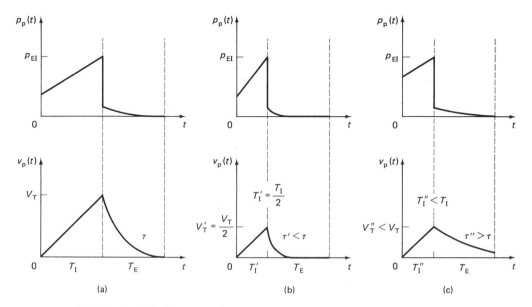

**FIGURE 13.22.** Response of a flow-source ventilator with pressure-cycled inspiration and time-cycled expiration to changes in the patient. We show volume $v_p(t)$ in excess of $V_{FRC}$ and represent the expiratory time constant by $\tau$. (a) Normal patient compliance $C_p$ and resistance $R_p$. (b) Compliance reduced to $C'_p = C_p/2$. (c) Resistance increased to $R''_p = 2R_p$.

frequency. Under conditions of moderate flows and pressures, the inspiratory flow is relatively patient-independent and constant. Flow continues until the volume specified by the Normal Volume control is delivered, as determined by the excursion of the bellows. The I:E ratio varies according to the flow rate and tidal volume selected, and the machine alarms if inspiration exceeds expiration in duration. If pressure in the patient circuit exceeds the threshold set by the Normal Pressure Limit control, then inspiration ends before the specified tidal volume is delivered. Other controls on the machine determine the delivery of "sighs," the delivered oxygen concentration, and the sensitivity to patient triggering in the assist mode.

Other ventilators have even different sets of controls, and there have been recent efforts to provide independent parameter controls (Engelman and Cook, 1977). Mushin et al. (1969) summarize all the possible combinations of parameters and their interrelationships by their "butterfly diagram."

The means by which a ventilator controls the breath cycle is important because, in addition to affecting the set-up procedure, it determines the way the ventilator responds to changes in the patient. For example, the Bird ventilator, when operated as described previously, behaves like a pressure-cycled source of constant flow during inspiration and has a passive, time-cycled expiratory phase. Figure 13.22a shows representative delivered pressure and volume curves for such a machine, where, for simplicity, we assume an I:E ratio of 1:1. When constant flow begins during inspiration, the lungs fill at a steady rate, and $p_p(t)$ shows an immediate resistance component to which is added a steadily increasing component due to the patient's compliance. During expiration, volume decreases exponentially (for a linear patient model) to zero, as does $p_P(t)$, now the result of flow through small expiratory resistance $R_E$ (see Fig. 13.17b).

Now assume that, with no change in ventilator settings, the patient's compliance drops to $C_p' = C_p/2$, due, say, to increased fluid in the lungs or to atelectasis. Figure 13.22b shows that inspiratory flow produces the same flow resistance component in $p_P(t)$, but pressure due to compliance builds up twice as fast as before. Hence, pressure limit $p_{EI}$ is reached in half the time, so that the patient receives a new tidal volume of $V_T' = V_T/2$. Also, the I:E ratio becomes 1:2, and the respiratory frequency changes to $f' = (^4/_3)f$. The reduced compliance also causes the lungs to empty faster during expiration.

With this type of ventilator, then, a change in the patient's compliance changes the tidal volume and respiratory frequency, which leads to a change in alveolar ventilation rate and ultimately to changes in the patient's blood gases and pH. To illustrate these changes, assume that the patient's dead space $V_D$ remains constant with a value equal to $^1/_5$ of the initial tidal volume (e.g., $V_T = 500$ ml and $V_D = 100$ ml). Then, the alveolar ventilation rate drops from the original value $\dot{V}_A$ to the new value,

$$\dot{V}_A' = f'(V_T' - V_D)$$

$$= \frac{\dot{V}_A}{2} \tag{13.14}$$

If we permit the consequences of the change in compliance to proceed to a new steady state, we can use equations 13.12 and 13.13 to predict the final gas tensions. Assuming the patient's metabolic level remains steady, the new steady state alveolar carbon dioxide tension $P_{ACO_2}'$ is related to the original value of, say, $P_{ACO_2} = 40$ mm Hg, by

$$\frac{P_{ACO_2}'}{760} \dot{V}_A' = \frac{P_{ACO_2}}{760} \dot{V}_A$$

or, using equation 13.14,

$$P_{ACO_2}' = 2P_{ACO_2}$$

$$= 80 \text{ mm Hg}$$

By equation 13.6, arterial carbon dioxide tension increases in the same manner as alveolar tension. This increase in carbon dioxide tension leads to a drop in pH. Specifically, for a normal hemoglobin concentration of 150 g/l, equations 13.10 and 13.11 show that the arterial blood pH drops from an assumed original value of 7.4 to a new value of 7.21 prior to compensation by the kidneys.

In a similar manner, the new steady state alveolar oxygen tension $P_{AO_2}'$ is given by

$$\left( F_{IO_2} - \frac{P'_{AO_2}}{760} \right)\dot{V}'_A = \left( F_{IO_2} - \frac{P_{AO_2}}{760} \right)\dot{V}_A$$

or, if $F_{IO_2} = 0.20$ (saturated room air) and $P_{AO_2} = 100$ mm Hg, then

$$P'_{AO_2} = 48 \text{ mm Hg}$$

If equation 13.5 is true, then arterial tension decreases in an identical fashion; if there is a significant alveolar–arterial difference in oxygen tension, then arterial tension decreases to maintain this difference.

We could also use equations 13.12 and 13.13, in conjunction with appropriate $O_2$ and $CO_2$ curves, to determine the resultant steady state venous blood–gas tensions. Without carrying out the detailed calculations, it is evident that $P_{mvCO_2}$ would increase, $pH_{mv}$ would drop, and $P_{mvO_2}$ would decrease.

In summary, if we do not take corrective action, the levels of oxygen, carbon dioxide, and pH all move to decidedly unacceptable values.

An increase in the patient's resistance, as with bronchoconstriction or a buildup of secretions in the airways, also changes the tidal volume and respiratory frequency delivered by this type of machine. Figure 13.22c illustrates the consequences of such a change. Changes in $V_T$ and $f$ with changes in the patient also occur in a pressure-source ventilator that is either pressure- or volume-cycled. Alternatively, if the phases of a pressure-source ventilator are time-cycled, then a change in the patient does not affect respiratory frequency or the I:E ratio but can still have a significant effect on ventilation by changing delivered tidal volume.

In contrast, a flow-source ventilator with either a volume- or a time-cycled inspiration and a time-cycled expiration continues to deliver the same breathing pattern during IPPV, in terms of $V_T$, $f$, I:E ratio, and inspiratory flow and volume waveforms, regardless of changes in the patient. In this sense, such a ventilator is "patient independent," though other aspects of ventilation do depend on the patient. The Bennett MA-1 ventilator, operated under the conditions described previously, is an example of this type of machine. Though an oversimplification, we often refer to machines of this type as "volume" ventilators to distinguish them from the so-called "pressure" ventilators, represented by the Bird Mark 7. Other differences between these types of machines are the high cost (thousands of dollars), larger size, and greater complexity of "volume" ventilators versus the less expensive (hundreds of dollars), smaller, simpler "pressure" ventilators. In practice, "volume" ventilators are used for long-term ventilation and "pressure" ventilators for shorter term ventilation, such as in IPPB therapy.

Figure 13.23 illustrates the performance of a time- or volume-cycled flow-source ventilator when the patient's compliance reduces by half (Fig. 13.23b) and when resistance doubles (Fig. 13.23c). For simplicity, we assume the flow source to be constant, so that volume builds up in the lungs at a steady rate during inspiration. Because inspiratory flow is independent of the patient, time-cycling and volume-cycling the inspiratory phase are equivalent. Note that, as predicted, a change in the patient's compliance or resistance has no effect on delivered tidal

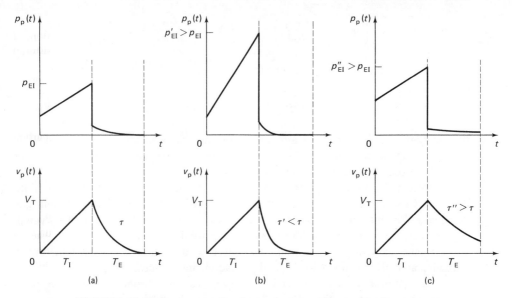

**FIGURE 13.23.** Response of a flow-source ventilator with time- or volume-cycled inspiration and time-cycled expiration to changes in the patient. We show volume $v_p(t)$ in excess of $V_{FRC}$ and represent the expiratory time constant by $\tau$. (a) Normal patient compliance $C_p$ and resistance $R_p$. (b) Compliance reduced to $C_p' = C_p/2$. (c) Resistance increased to $R_p'' = 2R_p$.

volume, respiratory frequency, or I:E ratio. The pressures developed at the airway and in the lungs, however, do change. To deliver the same volume into half the compliance requires twice the pressure, as reflected in the compliance component of $p_p(t)$ in Fig. 13.23b. We need to protect the patient against such potentially dangerous high pressures. An increase in the patient's resistance, shown in Fig. 13.23c, also increases the delivered pressure $p_p(t)$. Because the lungs empty more slowly in this case, the average alveolar pressure is elevated, though peak alveolar pressure remains unchanged.

**Flow or Volume Waveforms.** There has been recent interest in the therapeutic effects of the time course or waveform of flow, and hence volume, in IPPV (Chaney and Smith, 1977; Johansson, 1975; Jansson and Jonson, 1972). That is, for fixed values of $V_T$, $f$, and I:E ratio, it is possible that some patients would benefit from the delivery of an early inspiratory flow (EIF) waveform, shown in Fig. 13.24a. With this pattern, we deliver tidal volume early in inspiration, allowing time for ventilation distribution and gas exchange. Others might need a late inspiratory flow (LIF) waveform (Fig. 13.24b), in which the delivery of tidal volume late in inspiration would reduce average intrathoracic pressures. Still other patients might require some intermediate pattern of delivery, such as the constant inspiratory flow (CIF) pattern of Fig. 13.24c.

One way to deliver different patterns is to use different machines (Sullivan et al., 1977; McPherson, 1977), but this is cumbersome. We can change the inspiratory flow pattern on some ventilators by controls for inspiratory "hold," "pause,"

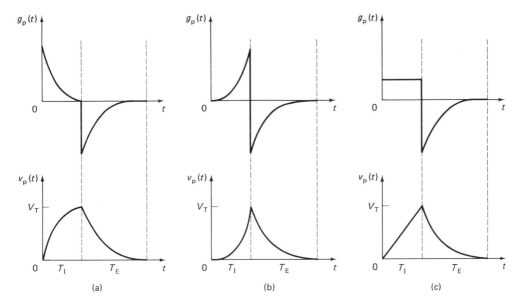

**FIGURE 13.24.** Three different inspiratory flow patterns and the corresponding volume waveforms. We show volume $v_p(t)$ in excess of $V_{FRC}$. (a) An EIF pattern. (b) An LIF pattern. (c) The CIF pattern.

or "plateau." Generally, however, the selection of different patterns is difficult or impossible because little or no choice of pattern is offered, because the adjustment controls involved are interdependent, or because the pattern delivered is strongly dependent on the patient.

Recently, efforts have been made to overcome these problems by developing time-cycled flow-source ventilators that offer patient-independent performance for a wide variety of inspiratory flow or volume waveforms (Engelman and Cook, 1977; Cox and Chapman, 1974; Nordström, 1972). For such machines, we can consider the breath cycle to be controlled not just in terms of the durations of inspiration and expiration but, at least during inspiration, in terms of the flow or volume delivered at each point in time.

Inspiratory flow waveforms are of therapeutic interest because they affect the degree and duration of lung inflation. As discussed previously, many other factors, such as the combination of $V_T$ and $f$, the I:E ratio, and the use of expiratory retard and PEEP, also affect the time course of lung inflation. Thus, the true value of different inspiratory patterns rests on the extent, *relative to these other factors,* to which they affect the degree and duration of lung inflation.

### Monitoring and Safety Features

The final test of whether a ventilator is functioning properly is the state of the patient, as determined by clinical observation and analysis of arterial blood gases and pH. Though we may closely watch the patient initially, with blood samples drawn as frequently as every 15 min, we watch the stable patient less closely and

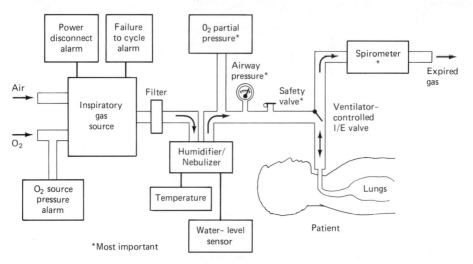

FIGURE 13.25. Composite of monitors and alarms used during artificial ventilation added to the patient circuit of Fig. 13.16.

may analyze blood gases and pH only a few times a day (Egan, 1977). Monitors and patient protection devices are essential, however, because only a few minutes of inadequate ventilation can kill the patient. The monitors should be independent of the ventilator controls and should monitor the parameters of interest in the most direct way possible. Figure 13.25 shows a composite of monitoring devices and safety features used during artificial ventilation added to the basic patient circuit of Fig. 13.16.

At its simplest, monitoring must include some means of assessing ventilation delivery rate and oxygen concentration or partial pressure. A spirometer in the expiratory flow pathway is the most common means of verifying the rate of ventilation delivered to the patient. Figure 13.21b shows the Bennett Monitoring Spirometer (Puritan-Bennett Corp., Kansas City, MO), which is one such device. The excursion of the bellows gives a visual indication of expired tidal volume. We can also check on the rate of ventilation delivery by accumulating expiratory flow for one minute. We call this measurement a *minute volume*. Figure 13.26 shows the Wright Respirometer (Fraser/Harlake, Cleveland, OH) to represent devices used for this purpose. This small device incorporates a rotating vane in the air stream coupled to a gear mechanism and readout dial. Recently, spirometers have been developed that are based on flow transducers utilizing thermistors, heated wires, ultrasound, or the development of pressure differentials (McPherson, 1977). A common device for monitoring delivered oxygen partial pressure is a small fuel cell powered by the oxygen itself, such as one of the BMI OA200 series (BioMarine Industries, Inc., Devon, PA). Oxygen monitors based on Clark-type electrodes (Webster, 1978) are also commonly used. The battery-operated Foregger 450 $O_2$ Monitor (Foregger Air Products, Allentown, PA) is an example of such a device.

Because of the dangers of overpressurization, we monitor the pressure in the patient circuit and incorporate a pressure relief valve or inspiration abort feature. The simplest such monitor is a mechanical gage, such as those visible on both the

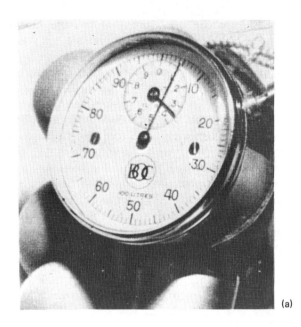

(a)

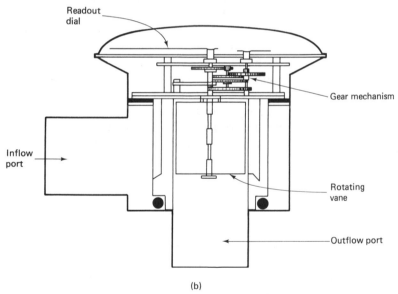

Readout
dial

Gear mechanism

Inflow
port

Rotating
vane

Outflow port

(b)

**FIGURE 13.26.** Wright respirometer. (a) Outside view (Reprinted from *Intensive care and rehabilitative respiratory care*, Lea and Febiger with permission). (b). Internal mechanism.

Bird respirator in Fig. 13.20 and the Bennett ventilator in Fig. 13.21. We monitor patient-circuit pressure because it is so accessible, but alveolar and intrapleural pressures are more appropriate indices of hazard to the patient. We cannot directly measure alveolar pressure, but we can estimate it from flow measurements using the patient models of Fig. 13.3. We can use esophageal pressure measured by a balloon-tipped catheter as an index of intrapleural pressure and, hence, as a measure of pressure hazard to the cardiovascular system.

More sophisticated monitors include audio or visual alarms to signal when certain ventilation parameters exceed range limits. Thresholds are often set, for example, for excessively high or low inspiratory pressures and sometimes for high end-expiratory pressure. Some ventilators alarm at a loss of electrical or pneumatic power and at a loss of oxygen source pressure. The ventilator may also alarm at the failure to complete a breath cycle or to cycle at an adequate rate.

Sometimes the monitors and alarms are built into the ventilator, and there are also stand-alone devices. The Monaghan 700 Ventilation Monitor (Monaghan, Division of Sandoz-Wander, Inc., Littleton, CO), for example, uses a flow transducer in the expiratory flow line to provide a digital readout of tidal volume, minute volume, and respiratory frequency. We can set thresholds on the monitor for high and low tidal volume and high and low rate, and an audio alarm sounds if a threshold is exceeded. Another self-contained unit, the Bourns Model LS-117-2 Ventilation Failure Alarm (Bourns, Inc., Life Systems Division, Riverside, CA), monitors patient airway pressure and alarms for conditions indicative of patient disconnect, excessive change in the patient, and ventilator malfunction.

The sophisticated PF-41 Pulmonary Monitoring and Display System (Research Development Corporation, San Francisco, CA), coupled to the same manufacturer's G-21 Respiratory Gas Monitor and VRP Respiratory Gas Monitor, can monitor both ventilator function and the condition of the patient. This system includes pressure and flow transducers and on-line analyzers for oxygen and carbon dioxide at the patient's airway. A built-in microcomputer generates displays of respiratory frequency, tidal and minute volumes, mean and maximum airway pressure, flow, volume, and $P_{CO_2}$ waveforms, pressure-volume plots, flow-volume plots, average airway $P_{O_2}$, and end-expiratory $P_{CO_2}$. The system can also estimate the patient's compliance and resistance, and, if blood-gas data are entered, can calculate dead space, acid-base balance, and shunt fractions.

### Closing the Loop

In the assist mode, the patient's own physiological mechanisms provide the necessary feedback to regulate the delivery of mechanical ventilation. Normally in this mode, the breathing machine responds to pressure signals generated as the patient attempts to initiate an inspiration or expiration, but other involuntary signals, such as efferent neural or EMG activity, or voluntary signals could also be used.

Mechanical ventilation of a passive patient requires some other means of regulation. At present, the feedback loop involves a human being making observations of the patient and measurements of arterial blood gases and pH and then making whatever changes are perceived as necessary in ventilator settings.

There is interest, however, in "closing the loop" around the patient–ventilator system by automating the measurement of the patient's respiratory state, the determination of the patient's ventilatory needs, and the setting of ventilation parameters.

Properly designed automatic systems excel in continuous, reliable monitoring of multiple variables and in coping with dynamic changes in complex systems. Recent technological advances have made closed-loop ventilation more practical. Ventilators are already using internal feedback loops to improve performance (Engelman and Cook, 1977; Cox and Chapman, 1974; Nordström, 1972). The incorporation of digital electronics, and especially microprocessors (Simes et al., 1976), is particularly promising, as conventional microprocessors are capable of serving as feedback controllers (Marsh and Smith, 1980).

It is a relatively straightforward matter to devise a closed-loop controller to maintain a stable respiratory state in the passive, but otherwise essentially normal, patient. It should be sufficient to have a linear PID (proportional, integral, derivative) controller acting on sensed end-expiratory $P_{CO_2}$ and controlling the respiratory frequency of an IPPV machine with other ventilation parameters fixed (Marsh and Smith, 1980). As discussed previously, end-expiratory $P_{CO_2}$ in such a patient is very close to $P_{aCO_2}$, and the control of $P_{aCO_2}$ to the proper level ensures that pH and $P_{aO_2}$ are also maintained at appropriate levels. Also, the pressure-induced side effects of IPPV are generally not a problem in such a patient.

The control problem becomes more difficult in patients with abnormalities of the lungs and chest, cardiovascular or blood deficiencies, or problems of fluid or acid-base balance. In these cases, the feedback system must incorporate a control policy involving not only the simultaneous regulation of the blood gases and pH but also the minimization of the deleterious effects of the delivered pressures. The design of the best controller requires the characterization of a very complex dynamic system (Dickinson, 1977; Bidani and Flumerfelt, 1976; Damokosh-Giordano et al., 1973) and, of at least as great importance, specification as to just what tradeoff of ventilation variables to meet competing goals is truly best for the patient. There have already been attempts to design controllers to optimize ventilation according to multiple performance criteria (Gupta et al., 1978; Mitamura et al., 1975; Woo and Rootenburg, 1975). Given the present debate among respiratory therapists regarding what constitutes the *best* therapy, however, the design of a comprehensive closed-loop ventilator lies some years in the future. Another problem is the need for simultaneous measurements of multiple indices of the patient's state. Though there has been progress in indwelling sensors and noninvasive monitoring techniques, a comprehensive closed-loop ventilator must still await the development of more suitable transducers.

# REFERENCES

ANSI (1976). *ANSI Standard Z79.7-1976*. New York: American National Standards Institute.

BIDANI, A., and R. W. FLUMERFELT (1976). Respiratory plant dynamics under open control loop conditions. *Proc. Annu. Conf. Eng. Med. Biol.*, 18: 91.

CHANEY, R. M., and W. D. SMITH (1977). The assessment of intrathoracic changes in pressure waveforms applied during artificial ventilation. *Proc. AAMI Annu. Meeting*, 297.

COMROE, J. H. (1974). *Physiology of respiration*. Chicago: Year Book.

Cox, L. A., and E. D. W. Chapman (1974). A comprehensive volume cycled lung ventilator embodying feedback control. *Med. Biol. Eng.*, 12: 160–69.

Cromwell, L., F. J. Weibell, E. A. Pfeiffer, and L. B. Usselman (1973). *Biomedical instrumentation and measurements*. Englewood Cliffs, NJ: Prentice-Hall.

Damokosh-Giordano, A., G. S. Longobardo, and N. S. Cherniack (1973). The effect of controlled system (plant) dynamics on ventilatory responses to disturbances in $CO_2$ balance, in A. S. Iberall and A. C. Guyton (eds), *Regulation and control in physiological systems*. Pittsburgh: Instrument Society of America.

Dickinson, C. J. (1977). *A digital computer model of respiration*. Baltimore: University Park Press.

Egan, D. F. (1977). *Fundamentals of respiratory therapy*. St. Louis: C. V. Mosby.

Engelman, F. A., and A. M. Cook (1977). Digital electronic control of automatic ventilators. *IEEE Trans. Biomed. Eng.*, BME-24: 188–90.

Epstein, M. A., and R. A. Epstein (1979). Airway flow patterns during mechanical ventilation of infants: A mathematical model. *IEEE Trans., Biomed. Eng.*, BME-26: 299–306.

Garrett, D. F., and W. P. Donaldson (1978). *Physical principles of respiratory therapy equipment*. Madison, WI: Ohio Medical Products.

Gille, J. P., and A. Bagniewski (1976). Ten years of use of extracorporeal membrane oxygenation (ECMO) in treatment of acute respiratory insufficiency (ARI). *Trans. Am. Soc. Artif. Int. Organs*, 22: 102–9.

Grodins, F. S., and S. M. Yamashiro (1978). *Respiratory function of the lung and its control*. New York: Macmillan.

Gupta, A. K., J. Sharma, and P. Mukhopadhyay (1978). Optimisation method applied to the design of ventilators. *Med. Biol. Eng. Comp.*, 16: 387–96.

Heironimus, T. W., and R. A. Bageant (1977). *Mechanical artificial ventilation*, 3rd ed. Springfield, IL: Charles C Thomas.

Innes, G. S. (ed) (1970). *The production and hazards of a hyperbaric oxygen environment: Proceedings*. Oxford: Pergamon.

Jansson, L., and B. Jonson (1972). A theoretical study on flow patterns of ventilation. *Scand. J. Resp., Dis.*, 53: 237–46.

Johansson, H. (1975). Effects on breathing mechanics and gas exchange of different inspiratory gas flow patterns in patients undergoing respirator treatment. *Acta Anaesthesiol. Scand.*, 19: 19–27.

Marsh, W. I., and W. D. Smith (1981). A flexible system for closed-loop ventilator development. *Proc. 14th Hawaii International Conference on System Sciences*, 457–62.

McPherson, S. P. (1977). *Respiratory therapy equipment*. St. Louis: C. V. Mosby.

Meijne, N. G. (1970). *Hyperbaric oxygen and its clinical value: With special emphasis on biochemical and cardiovascular aspects*. Springfield, IL: Charles C Thomas.

Mitamura, Y., T. Mikami, and K. Yamamoto (1975). A dual control system for assisting respiration. *Med. Biol. Eng.*, 13: 846–53.

Mushin, W. W., L. Rendell-Baker, P. W. Thompson, and V. W. Mapleson (1969). *Automatic ventilation of the lungs*, 2nd ed. Philadelphia: F. A. Davis.

Nordström, L. (1972). On automatic ventilators. *Acta Anaesthesiol. Scand., Suppl.* 47.

PEIRCE, E. C. (1972). The role of the artificial lung in the treatment of respiratory insufficiency: A perspective. *Chest,* 62: 1075–1175.

PETTY, T. L. (1974). *Intensive and rehabilitative respiratory care,* 2nd ed. Philadelphia: Lea and Febiger.

ROGERS, E. J. (1972). Physics vs. physiology in infant ventilation. *Respiratory Therapy.* 2: 45–49.

SELKURT, E. E. (ed) (1976). *Physiology,* 4th ed. Boston: Little, Brown.

SIMES, J., D. ASCHE, A. COOK, J. HATHAWAY, and R. ZUMSTEIN (1976). Microprocessors used in the monitoring and control of artificial ventilation of the human lung. *Proc. 1976 Joint Automatic Control Conf.,* 301–2.

SULLIVAN, M., M. SAKLAD, and R. R. DEMERS (1977). Relationships between ventilator waveform and tidal-volume distribution. *Respiratory Care.* 22: 386–93.

TALBOT, S. A., and U. GESSNER (1973). *Systems physiology.* New York: Wiley.

WEBSTER, J. G. (ed) (1978). *Medical instrumentation: Application and design.* Boston: Houghton Mifflin.

WOO, J. L., and J. ROOTENBERG (1975). Analysis and simulation of an adaptive system for forced ventilation of the lungs. *IEEE Trans. Biomed. Eng.,* BME-22: 400–411.

## STUDY QUESTIONS

**13.1** What parts of the respiratory system comprise the controlled system or plant? What parts make up the controller? What would you need to know in order to know the "state" of the plant?

**13.2** Define the volumes $V_{FRC}$, $V_T$, $V_A$, and $V_D$, and show their interrelationship. Justify equation 13.1.

**13.3** In terms of the simple model of Fig. 13.3a, write a mathematical expression for the total work of an inspiration $W_I$. Use the parameter values given in Fig. 13.3a to evaluate this expression. Assume for simplicity that inspiratory flow is given by $g(t) = 0.4/\sin \frac{\pi}{2} t$ l/s, $0 \leq t \leq 2$ s. For the same flow, find $W_I$ when $R$ is doubled. Repeat for $C$ halved.

**13.4** Under what conditions are equations 13.5 and 13.6 no longer true?

**13.5** Consider the respiratory system models for $O_2$ and $CO_2$ in Figs. 13.6 and 13.7, respectively, with the numerical values shown in the figures. Assume that $M_{O_2}^-$ and $M_{CO_2}^+$ both increase by 25% and that the respiratory controller increases $\dot{V}_A$ to maintain $P_{ACO_2}$ at its original value. Find the new steady state values for $\dot{V}_A$ and $P_{AO_2}$. If $\dot{Q}$ does not change, find the new values for $P_{mvCO_2}$ and $P_{mvO_2}$. Refer to the literature for the needed $CO_2$ and $O_2$ dissociation curves.

**13.6** State specifically how each of the following conditions would be reflected in the respiratory system models of Figs. 13.3 through 13.7:
(a) Asthmatic bronchial spasm.
(b) Pulmonary edema.
(c) Emphysema.
(d) Respiratory distress syndrome.
(e) Polio.
(f) Cyanide poisoning.

**13.7** Review the relative merits of all the ways to interface with the patient for repiratory therapy.

**13.8** Compare the use of aerosols for humidification and for nebulization.

**13.9** How do breathing machines for emergency use differ from those for long-term therapy?

**13.10** In what ways could $P_{aO_2}$ and $P_{aCO_2}$ be regulated during extracorporeal membrane oxygenation?

**13.11** In normal arterial blood with [Hb] = 150 g/l and $P_{aO_2}$ = 100 mm Hg, the $O_2$ concentration is $c_{aO_2}$ = 0.203 l-$O_2$/l-blood. What fraction of the $O_2$ is carried by the plasma? Now assume that in a hyperbaric chamber, $P_{aO_2}$ in this blood is elevated to 3 atm. What is the new $c_{aO_2}$, and what fraction of the $O_2$ is carried by the plasma? See the literature for the needed $O_2$ dissociation curve.

**13.12** Describe the systems that have been developed to guard against the inadvertent delivery of the wrong gas to the patient.

**13.13** Explain why, in the presence of back pressure, a Thorpe tube underestimates (grossly, if "uncompensated") the true volume flow, while a "flowmeter" based on a pressure gage upstream of a known orifice overestimates the true flow.

**13.14** Illustrate the need for monitoring delivered $F_{IO_2}$ in the context of the methods used for mixing gas flows.

**13.15** Assume IPPV is delivered with $f$ = 12 bpm and I:E = 2:3 and with a constant inspiratory flow of $g(t)$ = 0.25 l/s. For the patient model and parameter values shown in Fig. 13.3, make a sketch to scale of $v(t)$, the lung volume above $V_{FRC}$. To the same scale, sketch $v(t)$ for $g(t)$ twice as big. Repeat to show the effect on the original waveform of: doubling $f$; halving the I:E ratio to 1:3; using an early inspiratory flow pattern.

**13.16** Review the safety and monitoring features that should be incorporated in long-term artificial ventilation.

**13.17** Define
(a) Delivered pressure $p_p(t)$.
(b) Alveolar pressure $p_A(t)$.
(c) Compliance pressure $p_C(t)$.
(d) Intrapleural pressure $p_{pl}(t)$.
Which pressure is the best index of the hazard of a pneumothorax? Which is the best index of hazard to the cardiovascular system? Which is most readily monitored?

**13.18** Describe the ways by which we can increase the average degree of lung inflation during IPPV. What are the hazards of increasing the average lung inflation?

**13.19** To show how gas compression "looks like" elastic compliance, calculate the apparent compliance, due to gas compression, of a 50-l rigid glass jar.

**13.20** In a manner similar to Figs. 13.22 and 13.23, show graphically the effects of halving $C_p$ and doubling $R_p$ during IPPV with a ventilator modeled by a low-value constant pressure source and series resistance (see Fig. 13.18a)
(a) With pressure-cycled inspiration and time-cycled expiration.
(b) With volume-cycled inspiration and time-cycled expiration.

**13.21** Describe what is meant by the terms "pressure" ventilator and "volume" ventilator. In what ways is this classification of ventilators an oversimplification?

**13.22** Compare automatic closed-loop control with the present method of controlling ventilation. Sketch a noninvasive feedback system for controlling $P_{aCO_2}$ in a passive patient with normal pulmonary and cardiovascular structure. Sketch a feedback system for controlling the respiratory system in a passive patient with cardiopulmonary abnormalities. Indicate the performance required of such a system and the current limitations to its implementation.

**13.23** Assume that a passive patient with the respiratory plant modeled by Figs. 13.5 through 13.7 is attached to a ventilator modeled by Figs. 13.17 and 13.18a that has a pressure-cycled inspiration and a time-cycled expiration. Assume further that $p_v(t) =$ 4.7 cm $H_2O$, $R_{vp} = 2.5$ (cm $H_2O$)/(l/s), $C_v = 0$, $R_p = 2.5$ (cm $H_2O$)/(1/s), $C_p = 0.1$ 1/(cm $H_2O$), and $T_E = 3.5$ s, and that inspiration ends when $p_p(t)$ reaches 4.58 cm $H_2O$. Calculate the effects on $f$, $V_T$, I:E ratio, $\dot{V}_A$, $P_{aO_2}$, $P_{aCO_2}$, and $pH_a$ of an increase in patient resistance to $R_p = 5.0$ (cm $H_2O$)/(l/s). Determine qualitatively the effects on $P_{mvO_2}$, $P_{mvCO_2}$, and $pH_{mv}$. Repeat for a drop in patient compliance to $C_p = 0.05$ 1/(cm $H_2O$).

# 14 The Artificial Kidney

*Robert L. Stephen*
*Allen Zelman*

## 14.1 LEARNING OBJECTIVES

Upon completing this chapter you will be able to:

- Describe the most common causes of renal failure requiring artificial aids.
- Define the major terms related to artificial kidneys. Describe the procedures of hemodialysis, peritoneal dialysis, hemofiltration and hemoperfusion.
- Describe the structure and functions of the normal kidney.
- Define the limitations of current dialysis methods.
- Describe the major types of artificial kidneys and the principles by which they operate.

## 14.2 INTRODUCTION

This chapter describes the bioengineering substitution of a biological system necessary to maintain life: the kidney. It must be clearly understood at the outset that the native (natural) kidneys have large reserves and that at least 90% of their excretory capacity will be nonfunctional before artificial kidney support is applied.

There are four recognized treatment modalities available: hemodialysis, peritoneal dialysis, hemofiltration, and hemoperfusion. Each modality is described in detail. When comparing the efficacy of the artificial kidney with that of a well-functioning natural kidney, these renal substitutions are imperfect to an obvious degree when assessing two things: (1) the average patient's general well-being; (2) the freedom of movement, an ordinary holiday excursion for example, of patients so treated. A general appreciation of the many deficiencies in the bioengineering field is emphasized by the following comparison.

The fundamental advantages of all biologic systems are:

1. Self-repair and regeneration.
2. Control and decision processes.
3. Distributed energy conversion and storage.
4. Large number of components.
5. Small component size.
6. Dynamic self-adaptation.

The limitations of man-made systems are:

1. Energy conversion and storage.
2. Biocompatibility.
3. Computation and control.
4. Fixation and attachment.
5. Signal acquisition and return.
6. Chemical transfer.

The kidney has little regeneration capacity but otherwise possesses all of the mentioned biologic attributes. Section 14.6 clarifies these properties.


## 14.3 DESCRIPTIVE TERMINOLOGY

**Hemodialysis.** The extracorporeal passage of blood through a semipermeable membrane allows the diffusion and, hence, removal of water and metabolic waste products from the circulating blood (Fig. 14.1).

**Peritoneal Dialysis.** The peritoneum is a living semipermeable membrane that lines the abdominal cavity. Instillation of fluid and electrolytes into the peritoneal cavity permits diffusion (dialysis) of metabolic waste products from the peritoneal blood supply into the fluid within the peritoneal cavity. Water diffuses across the peritoneum into the peritoneal cavity, following an osmotic gradient artificially created by the addition of glucose to the peritoneal fluid (Fig. 14.2).

**Hemofiltration.** The extracorporeal circulation of blood along a high-flux (porous) semipermeable membrane and the application of hydrostatic pressure removes large quantities of fluid, electrolytes, and waste products from the circulating blood. Fluid loss, which is relatively very large (20–80 l), is replaced by intravenous infusion of a physiologic electrolyte solution (Fig. 14.3).

**Hemoperfusion.** Blood passes directly over a bed of absorbing material—usually activated charcoal or amberlites. Metabolic waste products and/or toxins

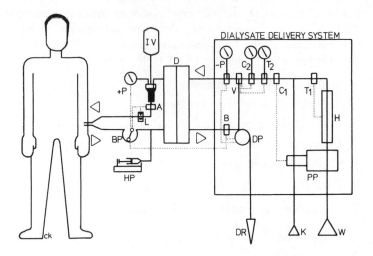

| | | |
|---|---|---|
| A | AIR DETECTOR | DR | DRAIN | P | PRESSURE |
| B | BLOOD DETECTOR | H | HEATER | PP | PROPORTIONING PUMP |
| BP | BLOOD PUMP | HP | HEPARIN PUMP | T | TEMPERATURE SENSOR |
| C | CONDUCTIVITY METER | IV | INTRAVENOUS FLUIDS | V | BYPASS VALVE |
| D | DIALYZER | K | CONCENTRATE | W | WATER |
| DP | DIALYSATE PUMP | L | LINE CLAMP | | |

**FIGURE 14.1.** Diagram of a typical hemodialysis arrangement using a proportioning system for dialysate delivery. Dotted lines indicate interaction between monitoring systems and major circuit components to ensure patient safety, e.g., diversion of dialysate through by-pass valve (V) should dialysate be found to have improper electrolyte concentration (C2) or temperature (T2).

(drugs, poisons) absorb onto the very large surface area of these microporous structures (Fig. 14.4).

**Uremia.** Patients suffering severe renal failure present a well-recognized, but vaguely defined, clinical picture. Invariably, there are elevated serum nitrogenous chemistries and usually there is: weakness, lethargy, anorexia, nausea, vomiting, an abnormal serum electrolyte ($Na^+$, $K^+$, $Cl^-$, $HCO_3^-$, $Ca^{++}$, $PO_4^-$) pattern, tissue wasting, and excess body water.

**Dialyzer (Hemodialyzer).** A semipermeable membrane is packaged in a supporting structure. Blood passes along one side of the membrane and a physiologic solution (dialysis solution, dialysate) along the other side (Fig. 14.5).

**Hemodialysis Machine.** This is popularly termed the *artificial kidney*. A system of pumps, clamps, timers, tubing circuitry, bubble traps, and heating coils passes blood and dialysate fluids through a dialyzer (Fig. 14.1).

**Dialysate Delivery System.** (1) This part of a hemodialysis machine pumps

## PERITONEAL DIALYSIS

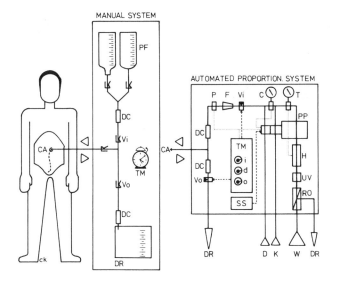

| C | CONDUCTIVITY METER | K | CONCENTRATE | TM | TIMER |
|---|---|---|---|---|---|
| CA | CATHETER | P | PRESSURE | i | inflow |
| D | DEXTROSE | PF | PERITONEAL FLUID | d | dwell |
| DC | DRIP CHAMBER | PP | PROPORTIONING PUMP | o | outflow |
| DR | DRAIN | RO | REVERSE OSMOSIS UNIT | UV | ULTRAVIOLET LIGHT UNIT |
| F | FILTER | SS | PUMP SPEED SELECTOR | V | VALVE (i inflow, o outflow) |
| H | HEATER | T | TEMPERATURE | W | TAP WATER |

**FIGURE 14.2.** Diagram of typical peritoneal dialysis arrangements using either manual or automated systems for dialysate delivery and cycle timing.

## HEMOFILTRATION
(POSTDILUTION)

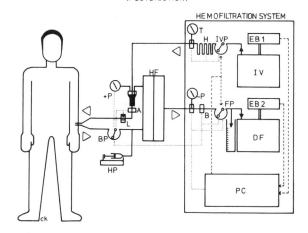

| A | AIR DETECTOR | FP | FILTRATE PUMP | IVP | IV FLUID PUMP |
|---|---|---|---|---|---|
| B | BLOOD DETECTOR | H | HEATER | L | LINE CLAMP |
| BP | BLOOD PUMP | HF | HEMOFILTER | P | PRESSURE |
| DF | FILTRATE | HP | HEPARIN PUMP | PC | PROCESS CALCULATOR |
| EB | ELECTRONIC BALANCE | IV | INTRAVENOUS FLUID | T | TEMPERATURE |

**FIGURE 14.3.** Diagram of a typical hemofiltration arrangement using the postdilution method for fluid replacement.

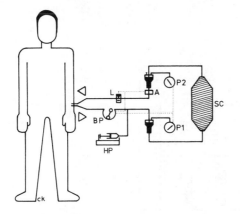

| | |
|---|---|
| A AIR DETECTOR | P1 PRE-CARTRIDGE PRESSURE |
| BP BLOOD PUMP | P2 POST-CARTRIDGE PRESSURE |
| HP HEPARIN PUMP | SC SORBENT CARTRIDGE |
| L LINE CLAMP | |

**FIGURE 14.4.** Diagram of a typical hemoperfusion arrangement.

blood and dialysate through a dialyzer. Different types of dialyzers may be used in conjunction with a single type of dialysis delivery system. (2) A delivery system that instills and removes peritoneal dialysis solution into and out of the peritoneal cavity.

**Blood Access.** Acute blood access that is equivalent to "one shot only" requires the insertion of a large-bore needle or cannula into a large blood vessel, usually the femoral vein, and it is withdrawn after a single treatment.

Long-term blood access consists of either an arteriovenous (A-V) shunt (Fig. 14.6) or an internal A-V fistula (Fig. 14.7).

**Peritoneal Access.** Acute peritoneal access is also equivalent to "one shot only" and requires the temporary insertion of a catheter through the abdominal wall into the peritoneal cavity by means of a sharp-pointed trocar (needle). (Fig. 14.8).

Long-term peritoneal access consists of the surgical implantation of a permanent catheter that, theoretically, is used indefinitely.

**Clearance.** The clearance is the volumetric rate (usually expressed in ml/min) at which a solute is removed from the blood; for example, if the clearance of urea for a specific dialyzer is given as $C_{urea} = 100$ ml/min, this means that the dialyzer has the capacity to clear all urea from 100 ml of blood every minute. Clearance is really a convenient mathematical expression. No dialyzer ever clears all of anything from a specific quantity of blood. However, a dialyzer with a $C_{urea}$ of 100 ml/min will clear approximately 200 ml of blood of half its quantity of urea in 1 min, which is mathematically equivalent to totally clearing 100 ml of blood every minute.

**Mass Transfer Rate.** The mass transfer of a substance is the amount of that substance transferred across a dialysis membrane over a specified period of time. There is an important difference between this concept and that of clearance that can be best illustrated by the following example. Hemodialysis performed only three

## COIL DIALYZER

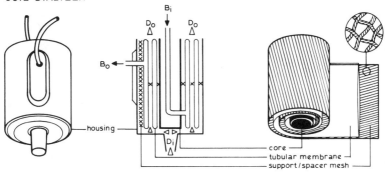

housing — core — tubular membrane — support/spacer mesh

## FLAT (PARALLEL) PLATE DIALYZER

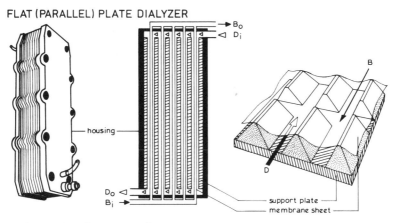

housing — support plate — membrane sheet

## HOLLOW FIBER (CAPILLARY) DIALYZER

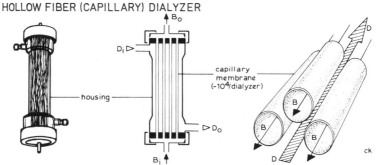

housing — capillary membrane ($\sim 10^4$/dialyzer)

**FIGURE 14.5.** Diagrams of main types of dialyzers currently in clinical use. D denotes dialysate, B blood, with subscripts i and o representing in- and outflow.

times weekly will remove (transfer) approximately the same amount of urea from the body (120–140 g) over the period of one week as will the native kidneys. Yet, the weekly urea clearance achieved by hemodialysis ($\sim$ 120 1) is far less than that achieved by the native kidneys ($\sim$ 1200 1). The reason for this apparent disparity is simple. Patients treated by long-term dialysis exist (the word is used advisedly) with far higher blood levels of urea (140–200 mg/100 ml) than do patients with

## ARTERIO-VENOUS SHUNT (EXTERNAL)

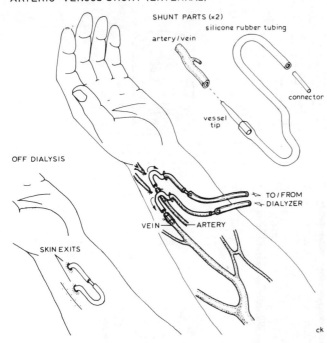

**FIGURE 14.6.** Diagram of arterio-venous shunt. Cannulae are implanted surgically into an artery and vein diverting blood flow through silicone rubber tubing which is partially externalized and can readily by connected to the dialyzer tubing or short-circuited when not in use.

## ARTERIO-VENOUS FISTULA (INTERNAL)

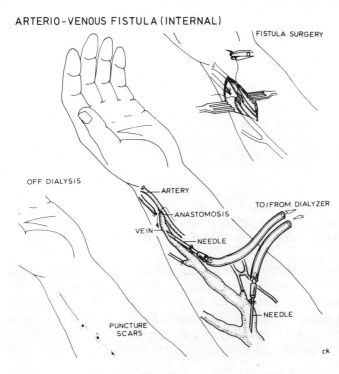

**FIGURE 14.7.** Diagram of arterio-venous fistula. An artery and a nearby vein of sufficient caliber are surgically connected. The diversion of arterial flow directly into the vein (by-passing the capillary system) leads to considerable enlargement of this vein, which then can easily be cannulated with large-bore needles for dialysis treatments.

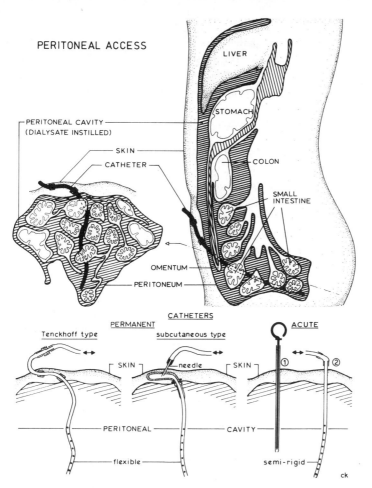

PERITONEAL ACCESS

LIVER

STOMACH

PERITONEAL CAVITY
(DIALYSATE INSTILLED)

SKIN

CATHETER

COLON

SMALL
INTESTINE

OMENTUM

PERITONEUM

CATHETERS

PERMANENT

Tenckhoff type

subcutaneous type

ACUTE

needle

SKIN

SKIN

① ②

PERITONEAL

CAVITY

flexible

semi-rigid

ck

**FIGURE 14.8.** Diagram of the peritoneal cavity and current access methods. For short-term (acute) access, a semi-rigid catheter is inserted repeatedly with the help of a steel mandrel (1,2). Long-term access requires the surgical implantation of a more flexible permanent catheter. Note the correct position of the catheter tip in the pouch of Douglas for maximum dialysate flow rates.

normally functioning kidneys (20–40 mg/100 ml). This is also true for almost all other metabolic waste products.

## 14.4 EVOLUTION OF ARTIFICIAL KIDNEY THERAPY

### Hemodialysis

Kolff and Berk (1944) achieved the first successful application of hemodialysis in the treatment of kidney failure, but, in that era, use of this therapy was restricted to patients suffering from acute, potentially reversible, renal failure. If 10% or more kidney function returned, patients usually recovered; if not, treatment was discontinued and the patients died. The reason for this approach was simply the decreasing availability, with time, of blood access routes. Prolonged hemodialysis requires recurrent access to vessels supplying relatively high blood flow ($> 150$ ml/min) through the extracorporeal circuitry. Repeated punctures or "cutting down" (surgically exposing) such sites meant their inevitable destruction and unavailability for further use.

Scribner et al. (1960) and Quinton et al. (1960) devised the first "permanent" blood-access route by suturing a plastic tube into an artery and a vein and short-circuiting the blood flow. A section of this tubing or shunt is sited external to the skin, rendering repeated blood access an easy technical procedure. Although clotting and infection caused multiple problems, this apparently simple innovation had far-reaching consequences. For the first time, the concept of long-term prolongation of life for a person suffering the lack of a vital organ could be attempted in a rational manner.

Unfortunately, the problems of blood clotting and infection with A-V shunts remained a major source of morbidity and mortality. Brescia et al. (1966) reported another major advance, the subcutaneous (under the skin) A-V fistula.

An artery is joined surgically to a vein through which blood then flows at a greatly increased rate. The sites chosen are usually the forearm, the upper arm, or the thigh, and the insertion of one or two large-bore (14-gage) needles into this vein usually supplies an adequate blood flow (200–300 ml/min) for hemodialysis or hemofiltration treatments. In more recent years, various synthetic substitutes for veins, bovine blood vessels and polytetraflurethylene for example, have been implanted and joined to an artery and a vein whose functional capacity is considered questionable.

Hemodialysis has not changed materially over the past 35 years. It still relies upon diffusion of chemical species down concentration gradients (conductive clearance) and a membrane, usually cellulosic, to remove metabolic waste products from uremic blood. The technique is inherently size-discriminatory, small molecular weight (MW) solutes clearing at a far more rapid rate than larger MW solutes.


## Peritoneal Dialysis (PD)

Ganter (1923) first clinically applied peritoneal dialysis in surgical patients, and his description of the problems associated with fluid preparation and measurements of even the simplest serum chemistries (not to mention the slow dissemination of information in that era) obviously discouraged even minimal use of this technique for more than 20 years.

In the late 1940s and in the 1950s, peritoneal dialysis was widely used for cases of acute renal failure. However, the trocar (Fig. 14.8) access methods used then allowed leakage of fluid around the catheter with consequent inevitable infection if the catheter were left in place for too long. The discomfort of repeated punctures led to the development of numerous access devices that allowed painless insertion of the peritoneal catheter (Merrill et al., 1962). Palmer et al. (1964) described the first permanent indwelling peritoneal access device. It was modified to a catheter shape called the Tenckhoff catheter (Tenckhoff and Schechter, 1968). Maxwell et al. (1959) introduced commercially prepared peritoneal dialysis solutions. Since that time, procedural simplicity has been an outstanding attraction of manual exchange peritoneal dialysis. With this technique, a bottle or plastic bag ($\sim$ 2000 ml) of peritoneal dialysis solution infuses by gravity into the abdominal cavity, where it remains for 15–45 min and then drains out by gravity into a disposable container. This procedure is repeated 6 to 12 times for each dialysis and literally can be performed almost anywhere, anytime by nearly anyone. Unfortunately, the multiple changing of tubes (6–12 times) from one bottle to the next breaks the sterile circuitry and there is an unacceptably high incidence of peritonitis (infection of the peritoneal cavity) accompanying the use of manual exchange peritoneal dialysis. A group at Seattle brought about a dramatic decline in the infection rate by automation of dialysate delivery systems that include only two breaks in circuitry: the catheter connect and disconnect maneuvers at the beginning and end of treatments (Tenckhoff, 1977).

There, the situation has rested for some years. Manual exchange with bottles or plastic bags runs a risk of peritonitis varying between 1–10% of all dialysis performed, whereas with automated delivery systems employed, the incidence is 0.1–1.5% (Golper et al., 1978). Manual exchange peritoneal dialysis is simple, convenient, guarantees mobility and easy travel, but has an unacceptably high incidence of peritonitis. Automated machines are bulky, travel means literally a travel van, and they require sterilization for each use; however, the incidence of peritonitis is low.

Continuous Ambulatory Peritoneal Dialysis (CAPD) is the most recent innovation in peritoneal dialysis technique (Popovich et al., 1978). CAPD uses the continuous presence of peritoneal dialysis shown in the peritoneal cavity, except for periods of drainage and instillation of fresh solution four or five times per day. There is no doubt that this technique represents a very real advance in dialytic therapy. Virtually all patients reported an increased sense of well-being, improved appetite, and absence of the "washed out" feeling that follows a standard dialysis. Dietary liberation is universal and blood pressure control improved in most cases; however, infection once again is proving to be the nemesis of this dialysis format. The technique is simple and the very antithesis of automation; patients are fully mobile in spite of an additional 2 l of fluid in the abdominal cavity, but the connect–disconnect procedures every 4–5 h have produced an alarming rate of infection, a problem that must be solved before the technique becomes widely accepted.

Like hemodialysis, peritoneal dialysis relies upon conductive clearance; however, there are certain differences that are important. Peritoneal dialysis exhibits much lower clearance values for small molecules, such as urea and creatinine, than does hemodialysis. For example, peritoneal urea clearance is 20–30 ml/min as compared to hemodialysis urea clearances of 100–180 ml/min. Thus, intermittent peritoneal dialysis treatments are of considerably longer duration (totalling 30–40 h per week) than are hemodialysis treatments, which total 12–18 h per week. Like hemodialysis, peritoneal dialysis is size-discriminatory, but the decrease in clearance with increase in molecular weight is not nearly so pronounced. There is no sharp "cut-off," and appreciable quantities of large molecules, including serum proteins, are removed during treatment. This difference is even more pronounced when CAPD is compared with standard thrice-weekly hemodialysis.

Because of the low small-molecule clearances achieved by peritoneal dialysis, a number of investigators have studied methods whereby these clearance values may be improved. Such methods include instillation of drugs into the peritoneal cavity (Nolph et al., 1977), the manipulation of dialysate volumes and flow rates (Lange et al., 1968; Kablitz et al., 1978), and the recirculation of dialysate through a sorbent system (Lai et al., 1975). As yet, reliable urea clearances $> 40$ ml/min have not been achieved and, furthermore, it would seem that the theoretical upper limit for $C_{urea} \sim 50$ ml/min (Popovich, 1978).

## Hemofiltration

Henderson et al. (1967) introduced hemofiltration, which utilizes convective transport of solutes. Blood circulates through a high-flux dialyzer (which contains more porous membranes) and a transmembrane pressure gradient $(\overline{\Delta P_m})$ ensures the removal of a large quantity (15–80 l) of ultrafiltrate, the volume of which is replaced intravenously with physiologic electrolyte solution. Hemofiltration, within a very wide range, is not size-discriminatory. In other words, the clearance of a solute such as inulin (MW $\sim$ 5,000 daltons) is comparable to the clearance of a solute such as urea (MW 60 daltons).

There are two techniques used, predilution and postdilution. The predilution technique requires the infusion of physiologic solutions into the blood before the blood passes through the dialyzer. Relatively enormous quantities of fluid (70–80 l) are used for each treatment. The result is that there is clearance of small molecular weight substances equivalent to that obtained by hemodialysis and far superior clearances for larger molecular weight species such as inulin. However, this technique is either extremely expensive or technically complicated and it also requires close monitoring. The postdilution technique involves infusion of physiologic solutions after blood has passed through the dialyzer, that is, simple volumetric replacement of the filtrate, some 18–30 l, which is much less expensive but clearances of small molecules suffer. These are often 50% or less than small molecule clearances obtained by standard hemodialysis. The situation is not static: Some recent investigations have demonstrated increased small molecule clearances with postdilutional hemofiltration (see Miller et al., 1979; Schaefer et al., 1978).

## Hemoperfusion

Yatzidis (1964) introduced hemoperfusion over activated charcoal for the purpose of removal of metabolic waste products or toxins from the blood. Early technical problems included denaturation of plasma proteins, destruction of formed blood elements, and charcoal particle emboli. Adequate preparation and pretreatment of charcoal, usually by cellulosic coating, overcame most of these problems and made safe clinical application possible. The very large surface area of this microporous structure adsorbs numerous substances from the blood including creatinine, uric acid, a wide variety of drugs, amino acids, vitamins, polypeptides, and some protein. Interestingly, one substance that is poorly adsorbed is urea. Present-day hemoperfusion technology does not permit major manipulation of electrolytes, acid-base balance, or water balance; therefore, the role of hemoperfusion in kidney disease is adjunctive only (Chang, 1978).

## 14.5 MOLECULAR WEIGHT AND SOLUTE CLEARANCE

The dialysance properties of numerous blood-borne substances is now an important area of research. The ease with which a certain solute crosses a dialysis membrane depends upon many factors: the size of the molecule, its charge, solubility, hydration shell, degree of protein or lipid binding, to name only a few.

The size of any molecule bears an approximate positive correlation to its molecular weight, and it is this area that is attracting most research effort. In brief, the ease with which any molecule crosses a dialysis membrane bears a rough inverse relationship to its molecular weight. Urea (MW 60 daltons), creatinine (MW 113 daltons), uric acid (MW 168 daltons), and electrolytes are low molecular weight species that freely traverse all membranes in clinical use. On the other hand, for all practical purposes, such membranes are impermeable to proteins whose molecular weights are measured in multiples of $10^4$, $10^5$, or even $10^6$ daltons.

To this point, the situation is relatively clear-cut; nevertheless, there is a gray region in which the molecular weights of many solutes vary from 500–20,000 daltons. Within this range, transfer of individual solutes across a membrane varies considerably with both the membrane material and the technique (hemodialysis, peritoneal dialysis, hemofiltration) utilized. Possibly this is irrelevant, but more likely it is very relevant because there is an increasing body of evidence that inadequate removal of certain substances in this molecular weight range ("middle molecules") is responsible for many symptoms of uremia (Kjellstrand et al., 1979).

At this point, a cautionary note is necessary. Some investigators state the middle molecule range is from 500–5,000 daltons, others state it is from 900–1,100 daltons (a precision that is probably unjustified), and yet others state that there are some middle molecules in the range of 10,000–20,000 daltons. Obviously, there is an element of tautology in all this. "Middle molecules" is a term that has become synonymous with "unidentified uremic toxins" in the molecular weight range of 500–20,000 daltons and various investigators quote middle-molecule ranges that correlate with their unidentified toxin of choice. Provided we are aware of these ambiguities, no misunderstandings should arise.

**Clearance Comparison of Different Formats.** Standard hemodialysis offers the most efficient clearance for small molecules, but the rate falls off sharply once the molecular weight exceeds 200 daltons. Postdilutional hemofiltration is less efficient in clearing small molecules but offers much more effective removal of middle molecules. CAPD, although less effective than hemodialysis in the removal of small molecules, promotes surprisingly good middle molecule clearance. Hemoperfusion absorbs solutes over an extremely wide range, making any form of prediction somewhat speculative.

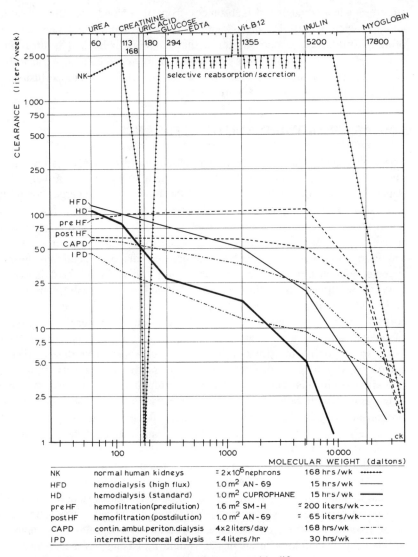

| | | | |
|---|---|---|---|
| NK | normal human kidneys | ≃ 2x10⁶ nephrons | 168 hrs/wk ••••••• |
| HFD | hemodialysis (high flux) | 1.0 m² AN-69 | 15 hrs/wk ———— |
| HD | hemodialysis (standard) | 1.0 m² CUPROPHANE | 15 hrs/wk ━━━━ |
| pre HF | hemofiltration (predilution) | 1.6 m² SM-H | ≃ 200 liters/wk ----- |
| post HF | hemofiltration (postdilution) | 1.0 m² AN-69 | ≃ 65 liters/wk ------ |
| CAPD | contin. ambul. periton. dialysis | 4x2 liters/day | 168 hrs/wk —·—·— |
| IPD | intermitt. peritoneal dialysis | ≃ 4 liters/hr | 30 hrs/wk —··—··— |

**FIGURE 14.9.** Comparative weekly clearances with different forms of treatment, including the normal kidneys (logarithmic scale). Note selectivity of kidneys which clear substances of essentially equal molecular weight at rates varying from 0 to ∼ 6000 l/week.

Hemodialysis with high-flux rather than standard hemodialyzers is receiving increasing attention. This treatment supplies good small molecule clearance and effective (equivalent to postdilutional hemofiltration) clearance of middle molecules up to a molecular weight of ∼ 1,500 daltons.

Figure 14.9 shows clearances versus a MW range from 0–17,800 daltons. Clearances are standardized to l/week to allow meaningful comparison of different modes of treatment. Average treatment times are also shown. Note: (1) Weekly treatment times for hemodialysis and hemofiltration (3 × 5 h) are considerably shorter than for intermittent peritoneal dialysis (3 × 10 h) and CAPD (168 h); (2) the wide range of excellent clearance values obtained with predilutional hemofiltration; (3) the marginal small molecule, but good middle molecule, clearance of postdilutional hemofiltration as compared to standard hemodialysis; (4) similar small molecule and improved middle molecule clearance of high-flux hemodialysis as compared to standard hemodialysis; (5) the slow decrease in clearance values in both forms of peritoneal dialyses as the molecular weight of solutes increases; (6) weekly clearance differences between all artificial kidney formats and that of the native kidneys; (7) the zero clearance (tubular reabsorption) of glucose by the native kidneys.

## 14.6 THE NORMAL KIDNEY AND ITS FUNCTIONS

The functional unit of the kidney is the nephron (Fig. 14.10), with each kidney containing approximately one million of these units.

The nephron is composed of: (1) the glomerulus, which is a membrane or filter; (2) the proximal convoluted tubule (PCT); (3) the loop of Henle; (4) the distal convoluted tubule (DCT). The hydrostatic pressure differential between the afferent (leading to the glomerulus) and efferent (leading from the glomerulus) arterioles (~ 70 mm Hg) causes a filtrate of the plasma fraction of blood to cross the glomerulus into the proximal convoluted tubule. This fluid (the glomerular filtrate) is not identical in constituents to plasma, there being a cut-off for solutes with molecular weight > 30,000 daltons. Collectively, all nephrons filter the plasma at approximately 120 ml/min, which is termed the *Glomerular Filtration Rate* (GFR). When standardized for 1.73 m$^2$ body surface area, a GFR ≤ 80 ml/min is pathological.

During the passage of the glomerular filtrate through the PCT, both active and passive processes account for the absorption of 65–75% of the water, the vast majority of the electrolytes and crystalloids, and also a great proportion of the amino acids, proteins, and polypeptides that have been filtered through the glomerulus. The remaining fluid and solutes continue along the loop of Henle, then the DCT, the collecting tubular ducts, into the renal pelvis and to the bladder via the ureters. During this passage, composition and concentration of the tubular fluid are altered by obligatory and selective reabsorption, secretion, diffusion, and osmosis in a constant exchange of solutes and water with the renal capillaries that originate from the efferent arteriole. The end result is the excretion of approximately 1.5 l of fluid (urine) per 24 h, which contains high concentrations of virtually all metabolic waste products that require elimination from the body. Also excreted are what may be termed "adjusted" concentrations of various electrolytes and other crystalloid substances. The exquisitely balanced modes of excretion by the kidney are the result of finely tuned control and decision processes, in which respect the artificial kidney is extremely limited.

An excellent example of these control and decision processes is the behavior of the sodium ion (Na$^+$). When crossing the glomerulus in the glomerular filtrate,

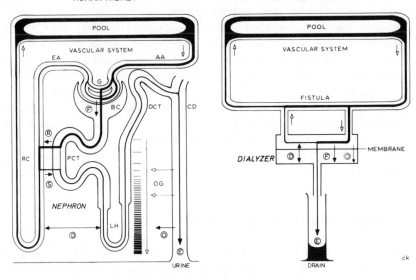

HUMAN KIDNEY     ARTIFICIAL KIDNEY

**FIGURE 14.10.** In the human kidney, water and solutes are removed by filtration (F) from the blood entering the glomerulus (G) through the afferent arteriole (AA). The filtrate is collected in Bowman's Capsule (BC) and then passes through the proximal convoluted tubule (PCT), the loop of Henle (LH), the distal convoluted tubule (DCT) and the collecting duct (CD). During this passage, composition and concentration of the tubular fluid are altered by obligatory and selective reabsorption (R), secretion (S), diffusion (D) and osmosis (O) in a constant exchange of solutes and water with the renal capillaries (RC) which originate from the efferent arteriole (EA). The overall solute concentration (osmolality) of the final product, urine, may be higher or lower than the plasma osmolality when finally excreted (E) as water is selectively re absorbed from the collecting duct following an osmotic gradient (OG) established by countercurrent multiplication involving active solute transport mechanisms in the hairpin-shaped loop of Henle. In the artificial kidney solutes are exchanged between blood and dialysate by diffusion (D) and/or removed by filtration (F), water is removed by filtration (F) or osmosis (O). Limited selectivity is achieved by manipulation of the dialysate composition and membrane selection.

the concentration of $Na^+$ is virtually the same as that in plasma $\sim$ 140 mmol/l. In the proximal tubule, energy-requiring metabolic processes actively reabsorb 65–75% of the $Na^+$ back into the bloodstream against a concentration gradient and water follows down the resulting osmolar gradient. A further fine adjustment to the amount of sodium reabsorbed takes place in the loop of Henle and the DCT under the action of certain steroid hormones produced by the adrenal gland.

The behavior of metabolic waste products is much simpler and is exemplified by the behavior of urea (a protein breakdown product), creatinine (a waste product of muscle metabolism), and uric acid (a nucleic acid breakdown product). Urea is predominantly removed from the body by glomerular filtration, some being reabsorbed in the loop of Henle. Creatinine is almost totally excreted by glomerular filtration. Uric acid is secreted into the DCT from the tubular cells and is then excreted in the urine.

## Acid-Base Balance

In addition to the excretion of metabolic waste products and the maintenance of normal body water and electrolyte composition, the kidney plays an important role in the maintenance of body acid-base balance. Each day, a total excess of 30–100 mmol of hydrogen ions are produced by metabolic processes and/or ingested in various foodstuffs, primarily protein. The kidney assists in correction of this potential $H^+$ loading problem by exchanging $H^+$ for $Na^+$ in the renal tubules and then buffering $H^+$ by three processes: (1) carbon dioxide/bicarbonate buffer; (2) hydrogen/dihydrogen phosphate buffer; (3) ammonia/ammonium buffer.

When cations, predominantly $Na^+$, are reabsorbed from the renal tubules, they exchange for $H^+$, which is secreted into the renal tubular fluid, and the reactions shown in Figure 14.10 take place. The end result is the urinary excretion of buffered $H^+$, certain radicals ($A^-$) such as $SO_4^{--}$, the production of $CO_2$, some of which is excreted via ventilation through the lungs, and the conservation of $Na^+$ (Fig. 14.11). The above description is a bare outline only; the production of $NH_3$ by tubular cells is itself a complex process.

## Synthetic and Regulatory Functions of the Kidney

The kidney is primarily responsible for the synthesis of the most active form of vitamin D, which is 1,25 dihydroxycholecalciferol (vitamin $D_3$). The parent compound cholecalciferol is ingested by mouth, hydroxylated at the carbon 25 position in the liver, and then the final hydroxylation at the carbon 1 position is undertaken in the kidney. Vitamin $D_3$ assists the absorption of calcium from the gut and plays a role in maintaining skeletal homeostasis.

The kidney also produces a precursor to the hormone responsible for the release of red cells from the bone marrow into the circulation: erythropoietin. A simple illustration best describes the effect of this hormone. In normal persons, the number of red blood cells circulating is approximately 5 million/mm³, the hemoglobin content is 15 g/dl, and the hematocrit is 40–45%. In a person suffering end-stage renal disease, there are classically 2–3 million circulating red cells/ml, the hemoglobin is 6 to 9 g/dl, and the hematocrit varies between 18 and 25%.

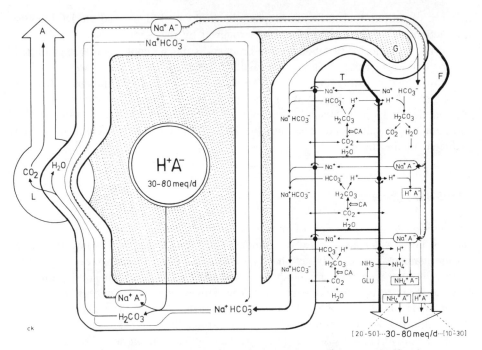

**FIGURE 14.11.** Acids produced in metabolism ($H^+A^-$) are buffered in the blood by sodium bicarbonate ($NaHCO_3$). While blood pH thus is kept constant, $NaHCO_3$ is constantly lost as $CO_2$ is exhaled through the lungs (L) and $Na^+A^-$ is removed from the blood by filtration (F) in the kidneys (glomerulus, G). Additional $NaHCO_3$ is lost directly to filtration. In the kidney tubules (T), the filtered $NaHCO_3$ is recovered by reabsorption of $Na^+$ in exchange for $H^+$ derived from the formation of carbonic acid from $CO_2$ and water under the influence of the enzyme carbonic anhydrase (CA). Additional $NaHCO_3$ is formed by the same reaction from the sodium filtered as $Na^+A^-$. Acids are thus excreted as either $H^+A^-$ or $NH_4^+A^-$ (combining with $NH_3$ produced in the tubular cells from glutamate (GLU)) without a net loss of sodium bicarbonate.

## 14.7 RENAL FAILURE

Renal failure is traditionally divided into acute renal failure and chronic renal failure. Although this is somewhat arbitrary, it has proven useful in prognosticating the outcome of the disease. When acute renal failure occurs and the patient survives, either complete or at least useful renal function usually returns. On the other hand, chronic renal failure denotes an inexorable deterioration of renal function over a time period that may vary from a few months to many years.

### *Acute Renal Failure*

In general terms, acute renal failure occurs when there has been some direct insult to the urinary system and a useful classification is as follows:

1. *Volume depletion.* This may occur as a result of: (1) direct blood loss, which can follow a wide variety of natural or artificial disasters such as severe injuries, surgical misadventure, and certain bleeding disorders; (2) dehydration, which may be caused by lack of available fluids, vomiting, and/or diarrhea over a prolonged interval; (3) burns and crush injuries to various bodily tissues. These situations may bring about acute renal failure simply because of the shunting blood flow away from the kidneys to other vital regions such as the heart and brain. Kidney cells, notably those lining the tubules, are deprived of their blood supply and undergo first swelling and if the situation is not rapidly corrected, necrosis. With the malfunction and blocking of the tubules, the excretory component of the kidneys is sharply reduced or virtually disappears. As a consequence, accumulation of meta-bolic waste products, acid-base imbalance, possible fluid overload, and electrolyte derangement occur. This is a serious clinical situation with an often quoted mor-tality of 50–60%. However, a prime factor in this rather high mortality rate is the severity of the original injury itself.

2. *Nephrotoxins.* A wide variety of drugs, certain organic compounds, some com-mon industrial substances, and heavy metals may directly damage the kidneys. Rapid withdrawal of the agent responsible usually leads to recovery.

3. *Obstruction/infection.* Major obstruction at any site along the urinary tract, with or without accompanying infection, causes acute renal failure. Relief of the obstruc-tion usually rectifies the situation.

### End-Stage Renal Disease

On a population basis, approximately 100 people/million/year will present with the condition known as End-Stage Renal Disease (ESRD). This simply means that the kidneys are no longer capable of sustaining any form of useful life and, unless some form of active intervention is undertaken, the person so afflicted usually will die within a short period of time. Although not invariably the case, ESRD is usually the final stage of progressive, chronic renal failure. The causes of chronic renal failure are many and the majority of them are still ill understood. They may be divided into hereditary conditions such as *hereditary nephritis* and polycystic kidneys; obstructive/infective causes such as ureteric reflux with pyelonephritis; drug-induced renal failure, predominantly caused by easily obtained "over-the-counter" proprietary analgesic drugs; kidney disease caused by certain common metabolic disorders such as diabetes mellitus; a heterogenous (by far the largest group) termed *glomerulonephritis*. In this latter disorder(s), the glomeruli are damaged by as yet ill-defined causes, the condition is progressive, variable (some months to many years), and stabilization of renal function rarely occurs.

### Therapy of Acute Renal Failure

Routine and preferably rapid measures for treatment of acute renal failure include volume replacement (blood, plasma, electrolyte solutions), withdrawal of any sus-pected drug or other agent that may be implicated in the etiology of the disorder, use of antibiotics and supportive therapy for severe infections, and the surgical relief of any obstruction. Meticulous attention to detail is required. It is all too easy to overload a patient with fluid, and if renal function does not return rapidly, the patient may literally drown as a result of this enthusiastic therapeutic maneuver. Careful monitoring of serum levels of nitrogenous waste products and electrolytes (particularly potassium, a high level of which is rapidly lethal) is mandatory. Worsening serum chemistries and/or obvious fluid overload, in the face of almost complete renal shutdown, is an absolute indication to undertake more active therapy (i.e., dialysis).

Under these circumstances, dialysis techniques are fundamentally sound. Patients are invariably hospitalized, they are in a precarious condition, and mobility is the least of their concerns. Although a few patients may progress to End-Stage Renal Disease, the usual outcomes are either recovery of both kidney function and the patient, or death. Therapy is intensive and expensive, but it is temporary. Therefore, the ungainliness of most dialysis systems is not an impediment to limited (days to weeks) effective treatment. Nor is relative isolation from the more sophisticated medical centers a contraindication to performing successful, if temporary, dialysis treatments. An acute peritoneal catheter, some bottles of peritoneal dialysis solution, a place to hang the bottles, and some tubing are the only requirements to carry out a lifesaving maneuver. In a nutshell, dialysis techniques are therapeutically satisfactory, often gratifying so, when used in the treatment of Acute Renal Failure.

## 14.8 THERAPY OF END-STAGE DISEASE

### Kidney Transplant: Artificial Kidney

A successful kidney transplant is by far the treatment of choice for End-Stage Renal Disease. However, this fortunate result is still beyond reach of more than 50% of patients in the U.S. A shortage of donor kidneys, rejection by the body of the transplanted kidney, and severe infections (often life-threatening because of the drugs used to prevent kidney rejection) are the main contributors to this unsatisfactory situation.

The alternatives to transplantation are hemodialysis, peritoneal dialysis, and hemofiltration. Hemoperfusion may be used as an adjunctive form of therapy. Unlike treatment of acute renal failure, these therapies are far from satisfactory, the prolonged time factor exposing the obvious deficiencies of this particular artificial organ. Perhaps the best description of patients so treated is that, although they are not near death, they do not feel well: Theirs is a twilight state of health.

Some treatment deficiencies are due to a failure of the synthetic functions of the kidney, for example, skeletal thinning that is due in part to lack of vitamin $D_3$ and anemia due to lack of erythropoietin. Probably the best approach to such problems is the use of oral or injectable substitution therapy rather than incorporation of specific corrective mechanisms into an artificial kidney. Allowing this, we can confine improvement of existing techniques to a more efficient substitution of the kidney's excretory role. There is ample room for improvement.

If we list the problems confronting patients, dialysis staffs, and investigators in order of ease of solution, they are: (1) optimizing existing equipment and techniques; (2) impaired freedom of movement of most patients; (3) problems with access routes; (4) inadequacy of dialysis.

**Optimizing Existing Equipment and Techniques.** For a complete study of problems amenable to corrective measures in the field of hemodialysis, the reader is urged to consult the excellent treatise by Keshaviah and Luehmann (1979). The authors discuss problems with water supplies, including the presence of heavy metals, aluminum (strongly suspected of causing first dementia and then death), organic compounds (e.g., pesticides), and the growth of bacteria in dialysate reservoirs. Considering that a vast number of potentially lethal substances are separated from direct blood contact by a single sheet of membrane whose thickness is only 11–20 $\mu$m, it is remarkable there are not many more disasters than have actually been reported. Nevertheless, the mortality from contamination of dialysate water is very real and morbidity is assumed to be widespread. More general use of reverse osmosis units, charcoal filters, and deionizers is reducing the extent of this problem.

The authors also discuss errors in dialysate electrolyte composition, which have a definite morbidity and mortality, imperfect pressure monitoring, which leads to unpredictable ultrafiltration rates, and even such apparently mundane occurrences as the kinking of blood and dialysate lines. These "occurrences" are not inconsequential; kinked blood lines have caused dialyzers to rupture, with consequent severe hemorrhage leading to some deaths.

The list is long and only a few examples are listed here. Suffice it to say that most defects are correctable either by redesign or improvement in dialysis techniques.

**Impaired Freedom of Movement.** Although there have been many changes in hemodialysis machines since their inception, the great majority of these changes have had a cosmetic rather than technological impact. This is not to say that innovation has been nonexistent. For example, in the 1960s a "batch" device in which the operator diluted a concentrated salt solution in a large (100–200 l) tank was the only system available. Such batch systems are simple, reliable, and inexpensive. The disadvantages include bulkiness, poor mobility, considerable operator time in preparing the dialysate, and the opportunity for major human error. Omission of concentrated salt solution to the dialysate means dialysis of blood against tap water, which results in massive hemolysis (shattering of red blood cells) and, often, death. The advent of proportioning ("single-pass") dialysate delivery systems has simplified dialysate preparation and continuous monitoring of the electrical conductivity of diluted dialysis concentrate affords a check on the accuracy of its ionic concentration. The single-pass dialysis delivery system is a convenient space-saver and large batches of dialysate are no longer an absolute requirement for any dialysis center.

Nevertheless, virtually all delivery systems simply grew as the years passed, responding to various requests from users. Periodic, fundamental redesign has rarely occurred. We may judge these devices by the following criteria: safety, chemical "processing," reliability, dialysis time required, patient acceptance, social acceptability, cost, convenience, mobility, space occupied, and energy requirements. Most systems rate poorly when judged on the last four criteria. The traditional artificial kidney utilizes a complex and cumbersome array of pumps, timers, clamps, accumulators, dialyzers, bubble traps, tubes, and large tanks or self-proportioning systems. For many years, the "Christmas tree" effect has been in evidence: Another device is integrated into an existing system to enhance performance, or safety, or both. Furthermore, virtually all dialysis delivery systems are powered from a 120- or 220-V source, a situation that has discouraged energy-efficient design.

Most patients must return to their hemodialysis or automated peritoneal dialysis machines either at home or in-center three times a week. There is no question that most of these unnecessarily large, overly complicated pieces of apparatus with their plumbing and electrical hookups cannot accompany the traveling patient. This in itself is a frustrating and embittering experience for many persons. Attempts have been made to tackle this problem with some modest success. Portable systems exist. They include: "hanging-bottle" peritoneal dialysis, in which increased risk of peritonitis and lower small molecule clearances are the only real deficiencies; CAPD, the Redy hemodialysis system (Gordon et al., 1971), which has also been adapted to peritoneal dialysis (Gordon et al., 1976); and the "suitcase kidney" designed by Friedman et al. (1977). In spite of carbon dioxide production and unstable calcium–magnesium balance in the Redy system, or the relatively large volume ($3 \times 21$ l) of dialysate needed for the suitcase kidney, these two artificial kidneys satisfy all the criteria for portability, provided a line power source is available.

At the University of Utah, a small, easily portable dialysis delivery system has been in clinical use for nearly five years. It consists of a fully wearable module powered by rechargeable batteries. The module has a "dry weight" of 4.5 kg when fully loaded and is connected to a 20-l bath, which may be changed once or twice during the course of dialysis (40–60 l total), depending upon patient chemistries. From a strictly chemical processing viewpoint, the system is almost conventional in that blood is withdrawn from and returned to the patient via a single-needle catheter and exchanges with dialysate fluids via a standard dialyzer. From a hydraulic and hardware standpoint, however, the machine is considerably different from its predecessors, and the design incorporates a pulsatile blood and dialysis pump, which operates in synchrony with two passive valves, the antirecirculation valve (which is in the blood line) and the ultrafiltration regulation valve (which is in the dialysate line) (Jacobsen et al., 1975). The patient cannot remain detached from the 20-l bath throughout the entire course of dialysis, but he may do so for a limited time (15–30 min), during which there continues a restricted form of dialysis. Neither urea nor potassium are removed, but adsorption of other nitrogenous waste products and ultrafiltration continue (Stephen et al., 1975).

All three of the above systems can be improved. More compact energy storage, more efficient pumping modes, and improved sorbents are within the capacity of present-day technology.

**Problems with Access Routes.** Blood access has been termed the Achilles' heel of hemodialysis/hemofiltration. The lack of truly blood-compatible synthetic materials means that any form of A-V shunt is predisposed to blood clotting, often causing infection and usually leading to a short (weeks or months) functional lifetime.

A natural vein used in an A-V fistula is blood-compatible but access supplying a reasonable blood flow (200–300 ml/min) means the insertion of one or two large-bore 14-gage needles or cannulae. Patients accept this as a necessary evil on a thrice-weekly basis, but many would not accept it on a daily basis. If the cannula is simply left strapped in place between dialyses, clotting and infection are inevitable. Furthermore, repeated venipunctures damage the wall of the fistula and a damaged vessel wall is more predisposed to the deposition of a clot or thrombus. Fortunately, this latter process is more retarded than in an A-V shunt, and an A-V fistula lasts months to years.

Innovations required are the implantation of a totally biocompatible material carrying a high blood flow and a "plug in" infection-proof device for attachment of the artificial kidney. These requirements bristle with difficulties, which will not be overcome easily.

## 14.9 INADEQUACY OF DIALYSIS

**Dialyzers and Membranes.** General standards for hemodialyzers have improved greatly: they are reliable (i.e., they perform closely to specifications), batch manufacture is reasonably consistent, they now have a good safety record (very few leaks or ruptures and no obvious toxic effects), and the "splicing" of ruptured cellophane tubing is very much in the past. More efficient solute extraction has been effected by improving membrane manufacturing technique, altering dialyzer configuration to provide even distribution of blood and dialysate over the total membrane area, and minimizing the thickness of the blood layer. Nevertheless, membrane material has varied little; most dialyzers contain cellulosic membrane, a material that has some definite drawbacks.

**Depletion Syndromes.** Figure 14.10 schematically shows a nephron and a dialyzer. The tubular apparatus profoundly affects the ultrafiltrate of plasma that passes through the glomerulus, both fluid and solutes are reabsorbed into the circulation, and certain substances are secreted into the luminar fluid. The dialyzer in Fig. 14.10 represents hemofiltration and hemodialysis, although circulating dialysate is not depicted. For the purpose of this discussion, this is immaterial; the following principles apply equally to hemodialysis, hemofiltration, or to peritoneal dialysis.

The crucial functional difference between the dialyzer and the nephrons of the native kidney is that all substances, be they water, vitamins, polypeptides, carbohydrates, or lipids, crossing the artificial membrane arc totally excreted. On the other hand many, if not most, substances passing through the glomerulus are at least partly reabsorbed in the renal tubules. Thus, treatments with dialyzers have the potential to cause depletion syndromes in patients. For example, glucose, amino acids, and vitamins filtered through the glomerulus of a normal kidney are almost totally reabsorbed back into the body by tubular processes and at the same time virtually all similar-sized molecules of metabolic waste products are excreted in the urine. Using a dialyzer, all the previously mentioned solutes, and many more, are filtered (or dialyzed) and therefore excreted indiscriminately.

Although it is a simple matter to add glucose to dialysate or intravenous fluids, it becomes increasingly expensive and impractical to do so with amino acids, vitamins, and probably a host of other ingredients, many of which are neither cataloged nor are their functions in the body fully understood. The construction of a physiologic artificial nephron is beyond the limits of present-day knowledge. To avoid this potential depletion problem, a diet containing a generous supply of first-class protein (essential amino acids), adequate calories, and vitamin supplementation is necessary. Nevertheless, many authorities regard depletion syndromes in dialysis patients as a major cause of their poor general health. The problem is compounded because intestinal absorption of most essential substances is impaired in uremic persons. An underdialyzed patient demonstrates decreased intestinal absorption as compared to a well-dialyzed patient. In turn, this well-dialyzed patient loses more essential solutes across the dialysis membrane than does the underdialyzed patient. The present consensus is to "eat well and dialyze well," a disturbing generalization.

**Uremic Toxins.** As well as a total deficiency in "conservation," standard hemodialyzers demonstrate an uneven excretory performance. The membranes in these dialyzers are size-discriminatory, and inadequate clearance of certain toxic middle molecules is suspected of causing nerve damage, red blood cell damage, suboptimal platelet function, and numerous other syndromes associated with long-term dialysis treatments. We may well ask: Why not routinely use hemofiltration with high-flux membranes? Preinfusion hemofiltration is either too expensive or too complicated to be used routinely and postinfusion hemofiltration demonstrates relatively poor small-molecule clearances. There is at present heavy emphasis on middle molecule toxicity; however, a balanced perspective must be maintained. As yet, the only middle molecule unequivocally designated as a toxin is parathyroid hormone. Excess levels of this hormone (almost invariable in uremia) participate in the pathogenesis of bone deformity, cerebral dysfunction, itching, soft tissue deposition of calcium salts, anemia, nerve damage, and tissue destruction. Apart from parathyroid hormone, a specific chemical description of even one toxic middle molecule has not appeared. It is no accident that middle molecule clearance characteristics of dialyzers are measured using innocuous "markers" such as cynanocobalamin (vitamin $B_{12}$) and inulin. Conversely, excessive amounts of many small molecules are undoubtedly toxic: sodium, water, calcium, potassium, magnesium, phosphate, hydrogen, urea, uric acid, guanidine, and polyamines to name only a few. With this background, hemodialysis with a high-flux dialyzer is a theoretically attractive measure. It is much less expensive than hemofiltration and supplies both good small molecule clearance and good middle molecule clearance.

However, ultrafiltration rate (removal of fluid from the patient) is difficult to control accurately and if too much fluid is removed too quickly, the result can be disastrous. Various hybrid formats are undergoing experimental evaluation. High-flux dialysis combined with limited hemofiltration reduces the expense and complexity of routine hemofiltration and supplies good small molecule and reasonable middle molecule clearances.

The innovations required are: (1) a reliable dialysis delivery system with volumetric ultrafiltration control regulated to within ± 100 ml/h (because the average dialysate flow rate is 500 ml/min, design constraints for such a system are rigorous); (2) a series of membranes with "cutoffs" at molecular weights approximating 500, 1,000, 1,500, 2,000, 3,000, 5,000, 10,000, and 20,000 daltons. Clinical trials with such membranes will assist materially in demonstrating the range of middle molecule toxicity or indeed if such toxins exist at all.

**Periodicity of Treatments.**  Normal kidneys function continuously 168 h/week and constantly adjust all excretory processes, whereas long-term dialysis is most often carried out $3 \times 3$–6 h/week for hemodialysis and $3 \times 9$–15 h/week for peritoneal dialysis. Thus, solute and water levels throughout the body oscillate, sometimes in a violent manner.

Only a small minority of patients state that standard hemodialysis improves their feeling of well-being at the time of procedure itself, that is, when fluid, electrolytes, and serum nitrogenous chemistries are at least partially corrected. The majority comment with varying degrees of emphasis upon the unpleasantness of the side effects, a general feeling of malaise, and finally the need to sleep it off. This "dialysis disequilibrium syndrome" is a frequent ($> 50\%$) complication of hemodialysis; the incidence in patients undergoing peritoneal dialysis and hemofiltration is far less. Major symptoms of the disequilibrium syndrome are headache, nausea, vomiting, asterixis, muscle cramps, hypotension, hypertension, convulsions, confusion, stupor, coma, and sometimes death. Minor symptoms include dizziness, restlessness, and anxiety (Kjellstrand et al., 1975). The syndrome is most pronounced during rapid, overefficient dialysis and occurs more frequently in severely uremic patients (Arieff and Massry, 1976).

One explanation is the "trade-off" hypothesis, in which marked oscillations in the concentration levels of ions and toxins in the blood of dialyzed patients may cause subclinical damage to the cells of the body, adding up to progressive damage with time. This is comparable to "fatigue damage" in a plastic material subjected to a cyclic stress pattern. Other explanations include a falling serum osmolality (primarily because of urea removal) causing vascular paralysis and slow metabolizing of acetate by some patients, also causing vascular paralysis.

Some more recent publications tend to define this complex issue a little more clearly (Koch and Baldamus, 1980; Shaldon et al., 1980). When changing osmolalities and the effects of acetate loading are factored out, hemofiltration treatments cause less symptomatology than do equivalent (time: rate of fluid removal) standard hemodialysis treatments. It appears that patients' vascular systems compensate well for simple ultrafiltration (fluid removal alone) and for hemofiltration (fluid removal + partial replacement). Vascular compensation during standard hemodialysis plus ultrafiltration (a routine hemodialysis treatment) simply does not occur; in fact, patients actually decompensate as dialysis time passes. The term *vascular compensation* should be clearly understood. When any person loses fluid, blood vessels reflexly constrict, thus maintaining blood pressure and adequate blood flow to vital regions such as the brain and heart. A good measurement of vascular compensation is vascular resistance, which increases with both ultrafiltration alone and with hemofiltration but usually decreases with hemodialysis plus ultrafiltration. The etiology of decompensation with routine hemodialysis treatments is obviously multifactorial; however, there is an attractive hypothesis to explain the difference between hemofiltration and standard hemodialysis. Hemofiltration effectively removes a toxic middle molecule, which causes vascular paralysis, and standard hemodialysis does not.

Whatever the reason(s), hemodialysis with high-flux membranes is one possible solution and more frequent or even continuous dialysis is another. Disequilibrium is treatment-time dependent and trials conducted with hemodialysis performed for 2–3 h on a daily basis have demonstrated a definite reduction in incidence of disequilibrium. Nevertheless, with the exception of continuous ambulatory peritoneal dialysis, there are valid objections to this procedure being used on a broad scale with present-day technology.

1. The cost of each in-center dialysis is approaching $150.
2. True blood compatible materials have yet to be synthesized. Some blood clotting occurs in the extracorporeal circuitry, especially in dialyzers, and when used 7 days/week, the blood loss in patients already anemic is significant.
3. There is a problem of blood access.

**Iatrogenic Illness.** The kidney plays a crucial role in the elimination of many drugs, prescribed or otherwise, from the body. Patients treated by the artificial kidney ingest more than their share of such drugs, a situation that often leads to much confusion when evaluating their state of health. Certain drugs such as aminoglycoside antibiotics (streptomycin, kannamycin, gentamycin, tobramycin) are excreted unchanged almost totally by the kidneys. This is a relatively simple circumscribed situation: Measurement of serum levels, measurement of the amount removed by dialysis, and adjustment of dosage usually permits satisfactory therapeutic results and an acceptably low incidence of side effects.

Unfortunately, the previous simple rules do not apply to the vast majority of drugs. Phenytoin sodium (Dilantin) is used widely in patients with chronic renal failure. This drug exists in both the free and bound (to albumin) forms in serum. In persons with normal kidney function, the total serum level is used to monitor the effective therapeutic dose. In patients with renal failure, the drug's binding sites on albumin are occupied by excess metabolic waste product(s). Thus, an effective therapeutic dose is reflected by a lower Dilantin serum level. Dialysis (three times weekly) removes some of the competitive waste products, making more binding sites on the albumin molecule available for the drug but also removes some of the free Dilantin from the serum. The end result is predictable confusion. Fortunately, satisfactory therapy is usually achieved by administering a standard dose for age and weight and avoiding measurement of serum levels. Attempts to attain orthodox therapeutic serum levels will almost certainly lead to Dilantin toxicity.

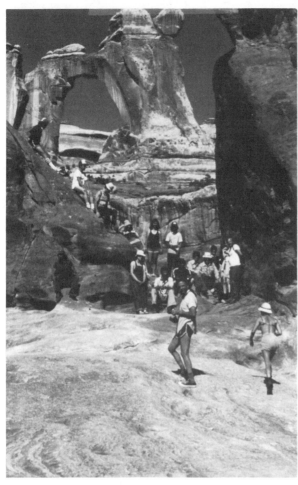

**FIGURE 14.12.** Dialysis patients and staff exploring Canyonlands National Park in southeastern Utah.

The most widespread problem is associated with the "sleeping drug-sedative compounds," of which there are a legion. Under normal circumstances, the majority of these drugs are first metabolized by the liver (hydroxylated, conjugated) to more inactive and usually water-soluble metabolites, which are then excreted by the kidneys. Many of these metabolically transformed drugs possess some of the activity of the parent compound and many are poorly dialyzed. The consequences of prescribing such drugs on a long-term basis are quite apparent. A population of dazed, irrational, and somnambulistic dialysis patients already exists. They request, and receive, such drugs to dissociate themselves from their plight.

**Attitudinal Illness.** If both dialysis personnel and the patients themselves regard persons treated by the artificial kidney as being ill, they are ill, or will become so very shortly. It has been shown quite conclusively that dialysis patients who undertake regular aerobic exercise (running, swimming, etc.) demonstrate improved blood pressure control, higher hematocrits, improved cardiac performance, less skeletel damage, and lower serum lipids than do their more sedentary

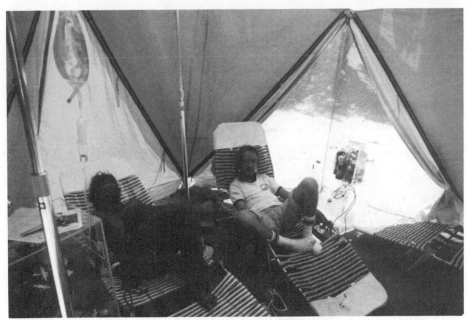

**FIGURE 14.13.** Dialysis patients being dialyzed on a national park campground within hours after completing a two-day backpacking hike. The equipment used is a battery-powered wearable artificial kidney (WAK) developed at the University of Utah.

brethren. If a patient arrives at a dialysis center in a wheelchair (as many do), there should be an excellent reason for this means of locomotion.

Figures 14.12 and 14.13 demonstrate a group of patients undertaking a 15-mile hike, complete with backpacks, and then dialyzing under canvas with the Utah WAK at the end of the day. Although one of patients folded temporarily, they, one and all, did not consider themselves capable of such an undertaking a scant 12 months prior to this expedition. Their sense of achievement was profound and justified.

### ESRD: Some Facts and Implications

In 1973, the Medicare program assumed responsibility for the major portion of funding for persons suffering ESRD. In the U.S. during 1979, there were over 40,000 patients maintained by the artificial kidney (the vast majority by hemodialysis) as a permanent life-support system. The cost has exceeded one billion dollars during this year and a simple projection indicates that in 1981 there will be over 60,000 patients so treated.

These expenditures are distributed as follows:

1. In-Center Dialysis: Patients with ESRD are dialyzed in a fully staffed and equipped dialysis center. Cost—~ $24,000 per patient per year.

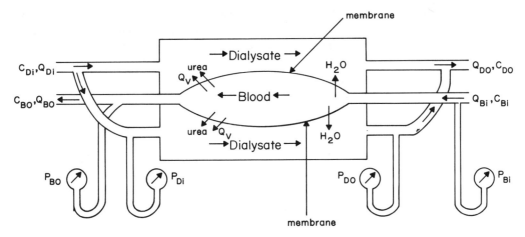

**FIGURE 14.14.** Schematic of a generalized artificial kidney.

2. Self-Care Dialysis Centers: Patients are dialyzed in fully equipped centers, but machine preparation, cleaning, and many of the maneuvers during dialysis are undertaken by the patients themselves. There is only a skeleton trained staff available. Cost—~ $17,000 per patient per year.

3. Home Dialysis: Patients have their machine installed at home and are dialyzed either by a relative or a paid technician.
Cost—~ $10,000 per patient per year with relative;
~ $14,000 per patient per year with a trained technician.

Arguments abound as to whether patients on home dialysis are preselected (less ill), whether they undergo more dialysis misadventures requiring more hospitalization, and so on. Nevertheless, the overall trend is quite plain: If patients are dialyzed at home or away from dialysis center settings, costs are markedly reduced and, if one thing is certain in the field of artificial kidneys, it is that the present rate of increase in expenditures cannot continue.

## 14.10 MASS TRANSPORT CHARACTERISTICS OF ARTIFICIAL KIDNEYS

The purpose of this section is to describe the functioning of the artificial kidney in terms of its contemporary manufacture, blood interactions, and mass transport characteristics.

Figure 14.14 is a schematic view of a typical blood path within all artificial kidneys now commercially available. The blood flows between two sheets of membrane material or inside a hollow fiber, with dialysate flowing on the outside of the membrane. When the dialysate and blood flow in the same direction within the dialyzer, the dialyzer is said to be operated in the "co-current" mode. When the blood and dialysate flow in opposite directions, the dialyzer is operated in the "counter-current mode," and when the blood and dialysate flow perpendicular to one another, the mode is "cross-current." The counter-current mode maximizes the average concentration difference across the membrane and is about 15% more efficient in solute removal than the co-current mode. The cross-current mode is somewhat less efficient than the counter-current mode but more efficient than co-current flows.

The artificial kidney serves two major functions: solute and water removal. Water removal can usually be predicted by

$$Q_v = A_m L_p \overline{(\triangle P_m} - \triangle \pi_p) \qquad (14.1)$$

where $Q_v$ (ml/h) is the water removed from the patient per hour (i.e., the ultrafiltration rate); $A_m$ (m²) is the area of the membrane, $L_p$ [ml/(h•m²•mm Hg)] is the ultrafiltration index of the membrane; $\overline{\triangle P_m}$ (mm Hg) is the mean hydrostatic pressure difference across the membrane; and $\triangle \pi$ (mm Hg) is the osmotic pressure of the proteins. The mean transmembrane pressure is often referred to as TMP, so TMP = $\overline{\triangle P_m}$. TMP can be calculated from

$$\text{TMP} = \overline{\triangle P_m} = \frac{P_{Bi} + P_{Bo}}{2} - \frac{P_{Di} + P_{Do}}{2} \qquad (14.2)$$

where $P_{Bi}$, $P_{Bo}$, $P_{Di}$, and $P_{Do}$ are the hydrostatic pressures at the blood inlet and output, and dialysate inlet and output, respectively. For Cuprophane PT-150, the most common hemodialysis membrane, $L_p \simeq 3$ ml/(h•m²•mm Hg). The osmotic pressure, $\triangle \pi_p$, is derived almost solely from the plasma protein and is essentially the same for all patients, 25 mm Hg. Thus, for a typical dialysis in which a patient needs to lose 3 lb (1.36 kg) in 4 h, the TMP will have to be set at 138 mm Hg. No commercial dialysate delivery machine has more than two hydrostatic pressure gages, and these usually read $P_{Do}$ and $P_{Bo}$. By accident, it happens that $(P_{Do} + P_{Bo})$ ~ $(\triangle P_m - \triangle \pi_p)$ within 5–25 mm Hg, depending on the dialyzer; thus, only two pressures are needed for clinical accuracy in predicting patient weight loss. There is an additional complication because as dialysis proceeds, proteins bind to the membrane and clots form in the blood channels, causing shunting within the dialyzer and decreased membrane area for mass transport. In addition, as ultrafiltration (patient water loss) occurs, proteins will be swept onto the membrane, forming a gelatinous layer through which water must also be transported. These factors taken together would indicate that the ultrafiltration index should decrease with time during dialysis and indeed it does. Figure 14.15 shows, for example, that $L_p$ decreases linearly with time at 7%/h for the RP-6 flat plate dialyzer.

The solute removal for artificial kidneys has traditionally been characterized by the equation for clearance, $C$ (ml/min), as

$$C = \left( \frac{C_{Bi} - C_{Bo}}{C_{Bi}} \right) Q_{Bo} + Q_v = \frac{C_{Do}}{C_{Bi}} Q_{Do} \qquad (14.3)$$

where $C_{Bi}$, $C_{Bo}$, and $C_{Do}$ (mol/cm³) are the blood input, blood output, and dialysate output concentrations, respectively; $Q_{Bo}$ and $Q_{Do}$ (ml/min) are the blood and dialysate output flow rates, respectively; and $Q_v$ (ml/min) is the ultrafiltration rate.

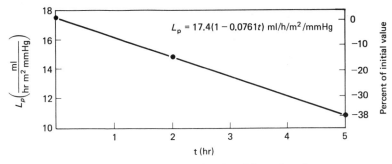

Ultrafiltration index as a function of time, $t$ (hours)
RP–6 Dialyzer, co-current operation
$Q_v = L_p(1 + \alpha t)(\overline{\Delta P}_m - 25 \text{ mmHg})$

**FIGURE 14.15.** The ultrafiltration index falls off linearly with time. (Courtesy of Allen Zelman, Edwin Bullock, Robert Stephen, Carl Kablitz, Douglas Duffey, and W.J. Kolff, "Controlled Ultrafiltration During Single Pass Dialysis with the RP-6 Dialyzer and Evaluation of Its Time Dependent Ultrafiltration Index," to be published in the *Journal of Artificial Organs*, 1980.)

Clearance is generally depicted by a clearance versus blood flow diagram given in Fig. 14.16. This format is a poor choice because clearance is a function of ultrafiltration and the $C$ versus $Q_B$ graph usually gives no information concerning ultrafiltration. Unfortunately, as yet there is no model accurately depicting clearance as a function of ultrafiltration and blood flow. For this reason, a format has been introduced by Zelman et al., (1979) with the in vitro clearance determined from equation 14.3 for a range of clearance values at different blood flows and ultrafiltration rates. These values are fitted to the equation

$$C = \alpha_0 + \alpha_1 Q_v + \alpha_2 \frac{1}{Q_B} \qquad (14.4)$$

This equation separates $Q_v$ and $Q_B$ into independent variables, which allows an unambiguous graph to be shown as depicted for the RP-6 dialyzer in Fig. 14.17. Equation 14.4 is an intuitive approach and the coefficients $\alpha_0$, $\alpha_1$, and $\alpha_2$ are not derived from a particular model. A considerable amount of description and experimental detail on hemodialysis is given by Klein (1977) and Zelman and Gisser (1979).

## 14.11 CONSTRAINTS ON DIALYZER SIZE AND TIME OF DIALYSIS

One would be tempted to believe that the larger the surface area of the dialyzer and the longer the patient is on the dialyzer, the better would be the dialysis. This is only true within limits. When the area of the dialyzer becomes large ($>2$ m²), the extra blood volume, necessary to prime the dialyzer, can become hazardous to the

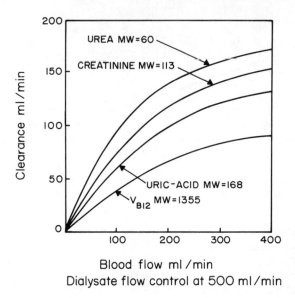

FIGURE 14.16. Clearance as a function of blood flow Asahi HF K-1 disposable, hollow fiber kidney. Effective surface area, 1.1 m².

cardiovascular status of the patient. A larger dialyzer will retain more blood after each dialysis; this is very hazardous to dialysis patients because they already have abnormally low red blood cell counts due to renal failure. Also, the larger the membrane area, the faster is dialysis, but the solute removal cannot be so rapid as to cause the plasma to decrease in osmolality while the osmolality of the cerebral-spinal fluid remains high. If this occurs, water from the plasma will be osmotically driven into the brain, increasing intracranial pressure and causing severe seizures, brain damage, and even death. During dialysis, the decrease in plasma osmolality is primarily due to urea removal. A urea clearance value between 130–150 ml/min appears to be safe, but large-area dialyzers or high-flux dialyzers may have urea clearances of 180 ml/min. This value is often too high for safe dialysis of patients with small mass ($< 70$ kg) unless blood flow is kept low to maintain clearance at a tolerable level.

During the first 30 years of clinical dialysis, a great many dialysis protocols have been tried. The most common dialysis schedule is for the average patient to be dialyzed with $Q_B = 200$ ml/min, $Q_D = 500$ ml/min with single pass dialysate delivery, a dialyzer with 1-m² membrane, and dialysis to be 4–5 h per dialysis three times a week. This regimen is varied somewhat for special patient needs. A clinical approach to the kinetics of hemodialysis has been given by Hampers et al. (1973).

## 14.12 TYPES OF DIALYZERS AND DIALYSIS

Dialyzers are labeled coil, flat plate, or hollow fiber based upon the manner in which the membrane is packaged.

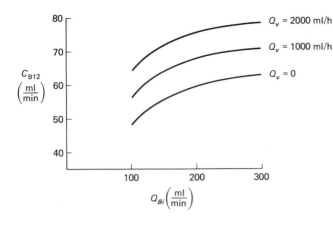

FIGURE 14.17. Counter-current vitamin $B_{12}$ clearance as a function of ultrafiltration. (Courtesy of A. Zelman and D. Gisser, "In Vitro Characterization of the RP-6 Dialyzer: Co-current and Counter-Current Clearance as a Function of Ultrafiltration," published in the *Journal of Dialysis*, Vol. 3, pp. 237-250, 1979.)

## Coil Dialyzer

Figure 14.5a shows a schematic of the membrane coil. The blood flows through a flattened tubing, which is wound around a cylindrical core. A plastic mesh is wound with the tubing to provide a separation through which the dialysate can flow. The mesh induces mixing of the dialysate as it passes through the dialyzer; this increases the transport of solute and solvent through the membrane. Because the blood is under pressure, the membrane is forced into the mesh, forming a more tortuous path for the blood; thus, the blood is also mixed by the dialysate side mesh. The coil dialyzer has cross-current flow paths. The dialysate delivery system for the coil is called "single pass recirculation" because dialysate is fed into and removed from a small volume chamber at 500 ml/min. Another pump draws dialysate from this chamber and recirculates it through the coil at 1,000–2,000 ml/min.

## Flat Plate Dialyzers

Figure 14.5b shows a schematic of the flat plate dialyzer. The blood flows between sheets of membrane, which are sandwiched between dialysate channels. The dialysate flows between sheets of membrane and a plastic plate, which usually has tortuous grooves to increase dialysate and blood mixing in a fashion similar to the coil. The flat plate dialyzer is usually run in the counter-current mode to obtain maximum efficiency with single pass flow at 500 ml/min.

## Hollow Fiber Dialyzer

Figure 14.5c shows a schematic of the hollow fiber dialyzer. In this dialyzer, the blood flows through a tube some 250 $\mu$m in diameter and perhaps 30 cm long. To gain the necessary 1 m² of area, the dialyzer must contain at least 4,244 tubules.

Because of tubule failure due to clotting, typical hollow fiber dialyzers contain up to 20,000 fibers. The bundle is held together by a plastic potting compound and the ends of each bundle are cut perfectly flat with a microtome. The dialysate inlet and outlet are positioned to minimize streaming. A uniform dialysate flow through the bundle is essential for efficient operation. The dialysate is usually run single pass at 500 ml/min in the counter-current mode.

## Solute Removal

Presently, there are no theories that relate membrane transport coefficients to the "clearance" of a dialyzer. However, understanding of dialysis can be improved by a rudimentary understanding of how membranes are characterized.

It should be realized that classical concepts such as diffusivity and viscosity are difficult to apply, if not totally inapplicable, to a membrane–solute–solvent transport situation. The close proximity of the membrane to the solute and solvent alter the character of viscous and diffusive processes inside the membrane. Thus, membranologists turn to an intuitive formula developed by Staverman (see Katchalsky and Curran, 1965) for characterizing membrane transport phenomena. The transport equations are cast into experimentally accessible parameters, namely solute flux, $J_s$ (mol/h·m$^2$), volume flux, $J_v$(m/h), transmembrane hydrostatic pressure and osmotic pressure, $\Delta P$ (mm Hg), $\Delta\pi$ (mmHg), and $\Delta C_s$ (mol/m$^3$), the transmembrane concentration difference. The transport equations can be written

$$J_v = - L_p(\Delta P - \sigma\Delta\pi) \qquad (14.5)$$

$$J_s = \bar{C}_s (1 - \sigma)J_v - P_m\Delta C_s \qquad (14.6)$$

where $L_p$ [ml/(h·m$^2$·mm Hg)] has been introduced before as the ultrafiltration index, $P_m$(m/h) is the solute permeability coefficient, $\sigma$ (dimensionless) is the Staverman reflection coefficient, and $C_s$ (mol/m$^3$) is the average concentration across the membrane. Each of these transport coefficients ($L_p$, $\sigma$, and $P_m$) has an analog that offers instructional interpretation. In particular, it can be shown that

$$L_p \propto \frac{r^2}{\eta l} \qquad (14.7)$$

$$P_m \propto \frac{K_m D}{l} \qquad (14.8)$$

$$\sigma \propto \frac{1}{r^2}(1 - K_m) \qquad (14.9)$$

where $r$ (m) is an effective pore radius through the membrane, $\eta$ (poise) is the "apparent viscosity" of the fluid permeating the membrane, $l$ (m) is the membrane thickness, $D$ (m$^2$/h) is the diffusivity of the solute through the membrane, and $K_m$ (dimensionless) is the solubility of the solute in the membrane relative to the external solution.

|  | $L_p$ (ml/h·m²·mm Hg) |
|---|---|
| Cuprophane PT-150 | 1.54 |
| Polyacrylonitrite RP-AN-69 | 30.4 |
| Polycarbonate N1SR-440.8 | 3.76 |
| Cordis-Dow | 1.22 |
| Amicon PMD | 21.5 |

**FIGURE 14.18.** Ultrafiltration index for various membrane materials.

Figure 14.18 gives a few values of $L_p$ for commercially available hemodialysis membranes. Figure 14.19 gives $\sigma$, $P_m$, and $R_m$ for the most common hemodialysis membrane, Cuprophane PT-150. Figure 14.20 is a plot of $1/P_m = R_m$ versus molecular weight, where $R_m$ is called the "membrane resistance."

In choosing a membrane for a particular dialysis process (hemodialysis, hemofiltration, etc.), one can select the type of membrane by specifying $L_p$, $\sigma$, and $P_m$.

### Hemoperfusion and Dialysate Regeneration

Hemoperfusion can best be described in conjunction with dialysate regeneration: The principles are identical in that both techniques rely upon the absorption of solutes onto a large surface area microporous structure. Nevertheless, it must always be remembered that dialysate regeneration allows greater latitude in clinical trials. It is one thing to run a nonsterile cell-free solution through a sorbent material. It is quite another to perfuse the sorbent directly with blood and its delicately structured cellular elements.

The most common practice in dialysate delivery is to provide dialysate at 500 ml/min to the dialyzer and allow the used dialysate to flow down the drain. Thus, for a typical dialysis period of 5 h, some 150 l of dialysate are used and the water wasted. Water and salt solutions are not expensive, so this is a very practical solution for most dialysis systems. However, for portability and convenience, it

| Solute | Molecular Weight Dalton | $P_m \times 10^2$ m/h | $\sigma$ Dimensionless | $R_m$ min/cm |
|---|---|---|---|---|
| urea | 60 | 3.18 | 0.0 | 18.9 |
| creatinine | 113 | 1.30 | 0.0 | 35.8 |
| uric acid | 168 | 1.14 | — | 52.6 |
| phosphate | 95 | 0.932 | — | 64.4 |
| sucrose | 342 | 0.526 | 0.157 | 114.0 |
| raffinose | 504 | 0.367 | 0.241 | 164.0 |
| vitamin $B_{12}$ | 1355 | 0.166 | 0.387 | 362.0 |

**FIGURE 14.19.** Values of constants for Cuprophane PT-150, the most common dialysis membrane.

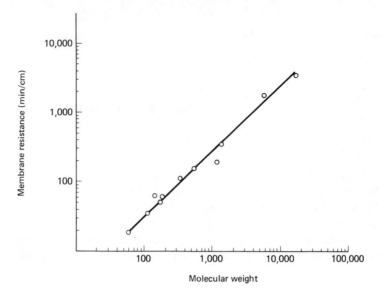

**FIGURE 14.20.** Plot of membrane resistance as a function of molecular weight for Cuprophane PT-150. (Courtesy of Elias Klein, James K. Smith, F.F. Holland, Jr., and Roy E. Flagg, "Membrane and Materials Evaluation," National Technical Information Service, U.S. Dept. of Commerce, EB-225 070.)

would be advantageous if the dialysate solution could be minimized in volume, recirculated through absorbents to remove the metabolic waste products, and returned to the dialyzer. Controlling the complex ion exchange processes that occur between the dialysate and sorbent material is extremely difficult, as are the engineering problems associated with minimizing the volume of the absorbent system. Therefore, it is not surprising that there is only one dialysate regeneration system commercially available (Redy Systems, Organon Teknika Corporation, Oklahoma City, OK) that will meet the daily needs of hemodialysis patients.

The complexity of the dialysate regeneration is exemplified by describing an ideal system designed with the following characteristics.

1. The system should provide a range of dialysate flows from 50 ml/min to 500 ml/min so that the regeneration system can be used interchangeably for peritoneal dialysis, hemodialysis, or hemofiltration.

2. The volume of fluid in the dialysate regeneration system should only include fluid that is necessary to fill the dialyzer, lines, and to submerse the absorbents in fluid.

3. Ultrafiltration should be avoided by a metering pump that can be regulated to withdraw set amounts of fluid from the recirculating dialysate.

4. The dialysate regeneration system must maintain rigorous control over certain

recirculating ions (calcium, magnesium, sodium, potassium, chloride, and bicarbonate) and should regulate pH.

5. With a single pass through the regeneration system, the following solutes must be reduced essentially to zero concentration: ammonium, sulfate, phosphate, urea, creatinine, and uric acid, as well as guanidines, indoles, organic acids, phenolic compounds, chloramines, and chlorine.

6. The system should be compatible with any water source.

7. The system must be able to remove some 60–70 g of urea for each dialysis.

8. The materials used for the absorption of the metabolic waste products must not be toxic; in the case of a membrane rupture during hemodialysis, if these materials should come in contact with the patient, the patient's safety must not be jeopardized.

9. It should be obvious that dialysate regeneration systems are tending towards the wearable artificial kidney and that significant organic and inorganic chemistry as well as engineering effort will be necessary to bring the size of the regeneration system to that of a truly convenient portable unit. Removal of urea remains one of the fundamental impediments.

## Hemoperfusion with Activated Charcoal

Activated charcoal is a highly porous material capable of removing a great variety of nonpolar solutes from aqueous solutions. However, its use in hemoperfusion must be accompanied by very careful removal of all particulates that may break off from the activated charcoal. In order to prevent charcoal microparticles from depositing in tissues or causing embolism in the capillaries, chronic use of charcoal necessitates its separation from the blood by an absolute barrier. Only in acute emergency cases should the charcoal be used directly in contact with the blood. To improve patient safety, techniques have been devised for encapsulation and/or thorough rinsing of the charcoal before use. Encapsulation includes coating whole charcoal particles as well as embedding within membranes and enclosing in polymer hollow fibers. However, encapsulation severely deters absorption on the activated charcoal by forming an additional barrier through which diffusion must occur. However, both coated and uncoated charcoal readily absorbs for substances such as creatinine, glutethimide, pentobarbital, chloramines, amino acids, polypeptides, and protein.

The kinetics of absorption onto activated charcoal is a tremendously complex problem for which no general solution has been developed. The problems associated with absorption involve the transfer of the solute from the bulk solution through the boundary layer next to the particulate materials, through the membrane surrounding the activated charcoal (if there is one), then through the fluid inside the porous structure of the charcoal, then absorption directly onto the charcoal. Obviously, every new granular form of activated charcoal will behave differently; thus, an analytical solution to the problem of absorption is very difficult to achieve and most data are depicted graphically as functions of the various variables of the system. On the other hand, the equilibrium properties of absorption are much more

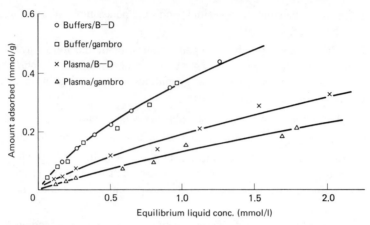

FIGURE 14.21. Absorption of creatinine from plasma and buffer solution. (Courtesy of M. Skulsky and P.C. Farrell, "Uptake Characteristics of Selected Biochemicals and Coded and Uncoded Activated Charcoal," 71st Annual Meeting of A.I.Ch.E., 1978.)

easily characterized analytically and experiments can be performed to show the capacity of the absorber in picking up any particular solute. The equations that are more frequently used to characterize the absorption of materials are the Freundlich equation and the Langmuir isotherm equation.

An example of absorption from plasma and saline is given in Fig. 14.21 (Skulsky and Farrel, 1978). The Gambro-Adsorba is a hemoperfusion cartridge filled with coated charcoal derived from peat moss and consists of cylindrically shaped particles (1 mm diameter, 1–8 mm length, surface area about 970 m²/g) encapsulated with a cellulose membrane 3–5 μm thick. The B-D charcoal (Pittsburgh ACT. Carbon Company, Pittsburgh, PA) hemoperfusion cartridge uses noncoated charcoal and consists of coconut shell material granules (0.3–0.84 mm diameter, surface area about 900 m²/g). From the graph it is seen that the Gambro absorption is somewhat lower then the B-D system. Conceivably, the membrane coating could alter absorption capacity, but the lower absorption could also be due to the altered pore structure of the Gambro charcoal as a result of the carbon extrusion into cylinders.

## 14.13 ACKNOWLEDGEMENT

The authors gratefully acknowledge the assistance of Carl Kablitz, M.D., who supplied Figs. 14.1 to 14.11.

## REFERENCES

Arieff, A. I., and S. G. Massry (1976). Dialysis disequilibrium syndrome, in *Clinical aspects of uremia and dialysis,* S. G. Massry and A. L. Sellers (eds). Springfield, IL: Charles C Thomas.

BRESCIA, M. J., J. E. CIMINO, K. APPEL, and B. J. HURWICH (1966). Chronic hemodialysis using venipuncture and a surgically created arteriovenous fistula. *N. Eng. J. Med.*, 275(20): 1089–92.

CHANG, T. M. S. (1978). Perspective of hemoperfusion. *Art. Organs*, 2(4): 359–62.

FRIEDMAN, E. A., J. T. HUTCHISSON, and G. R. BRIEFEL (1977). Complete clinical evaluation of compact travel hemodialyzer. *19th Ann. Contractors Conf. NIAMDD:* 67.

GANTER, G. (1923). Uber die Beseitigung giftiger Stoffe aus dem Blut durch Dialyse. Munch Med Wochenschr, 50: 1478–1480.

GOLPER, T. A., W. M. BENNETT, and S. R. JONES (1978). Peritonitis associated with chronic peritoneal dialysis: A diagnostic and therapeutic approach. *Dialy. & Transpl.*, 7(#11): 1173–78.

GORDON, A., O. S. BETTER, M. A. GREENBAUM, L. B. MARANTZ, T. GRAL, and M. H. MAXWELL (1971). Clinical maintenance hemodialysis with a sorbent-based, low volume dialysate regeneration system. *Trans. Am. Soc. Art. Int. Organs*, 17: 253–58.

GORDON, A., A. J. LEWIN, M. H. MAXWELL, and N. D. MOREALES (1976). Augmentation of efficiency by continuous flow sorbent regenera-peritoneal dialysis. *Trans. Am. Soc. Art. Int. Organs*, 22: 599–604.

HANAPERS, C. L., E. SCHUPAK, E. G. LOWRIE, and J. M. LAZARUS (1973). *Long-term hemodialysis*. New York: Grune and Stratton.

HENDERSON, L. W., A. BESARAB, A. MICHAELS, L. W. BLUEMLE, JR. (1967). Blood purification by ultrafiltration and fluid replacement (diafiltration). *Trans. Am. Soc. Art. Int. Organs*, 13: 216–22.

JACOBSEN, S. C., R. L. STEPHEN, E. C. BULLOCH, R. D. LUNTZ, and W. J. KOLFF (1975). A wearable artificial kidney: Functional description of hardware and clinical results. *Clin. Dial. Transplant Forum*, 5: 65–71.

KABLITZ, C., R. L. STEPHEN, S. C. JACOBSEN, R. KIRKHAM, and W. J. KOLFF (1978). Reciprocating peritoneal dialysis. *Dialy. & Transpl.*, 7: 3.

KATCHALSKY, A., and P. CURRAN (1965). *Nonequilibrium thermodynamics in biophysics*. Cambridge, MA: Harvard University Press.

KESHAVIAH, P., and D. LUEHMANN (1979). *Critical review of documentation of artificial kidney systems: Hemodialysis*. FDA, HEW Contract #223-78-5046.

KJELLSTRAND, C. M., A. ARIEFF, and S. MASSRY (1979). Inadequacy of dialysis: Why patients are not well. *Trans. Am. Soc. Artif. Int. Organs*, 25: 518–20.

KJELLSTRAND, C. M., R. L. EVANS, R. J. PETERSEN, J. R. SHIDEMAN, B. VON HARTITZSCH, and T. BUSELMEIER (1975). The "unphysiology" of dialysis: A major cause of dialysis side effects? *Kidney Int.*, 7(1): S-#2.

KLEIN, E. (ed) (1977) Evaluation hemodialyzers and dialysis membranes. *DHEW Publication No. (NIH) 77:* 1294.

KOCH, K. M., and C. A. BALDAMUS (1980). Sympathetic response and hemodynamic stability during volume removal in ESRD patients: A study comparing ultrafiltration (UF), hemodialysis (HD), and postdilution hemofiltration (HF). *Prog. Chronic Renal Disease Conf., NIAMDD:* 37–38.

KOLFF, W. J., and H. T. J. BERK (1944). The artificial kidney: A dialyzer with great area. *Acta. Med. Scand.*, 117: 121–27.

LAI, F., R. TANKERSLEY, M. SCOTT, H. WAYT, and A. ZELMAN (1975). Third generation artificial kidney. *Trans. Am. Soc. Art. Int. Organs*, 21: 346.

LANGE, K., G. TRESER, and J. MANGALAT (1968). Automatic continuous high flow rate peritoneal dialysis. *Archiv. für Klin Medizin.*, 214: 201.

MAXWELL, M. H., R. E. ROCKNEY, C. R. KLEEMAN, and M. R. TWISS (1959). Peritoneal dialysis: Technique and applications. *J.A.M.A.*, 170: 8, 917.

MERRILL, J. P., E. SABBAGE, L. HENDERSON, W. WELZANT, and C. CRANE (1962). The use of an inlying plastic conduit for chronic peritoneal irrigation. *Trans. Am. Soc. Art. Int. Organs*, 8: 252.

MILLER, J. H., J. H. SHINABERGER, J. A. KRAUT, and P. W. GARDNER (1979). A volume controlled apparatus for ultrafiltration and hemofiltration with acetate or bicarbonate solutions. *Trans. Am. Soc. Art. Int. Organs*, 25: 404.

NOLPH, K. D., A. J. GHODS, P. BROWN, J. VANSTONE, F. N. MILLER, D. L. WIEGMANN, and P. D. HARRIS (1977). Factors influencing peritoneal dialysis efficiency, *Dialy. & Transpl.*, 6: 2.

PALMER, R. A., W. E. QUINTON, and J. E. GRAY (1964). Prolonged peritoneal dialysis for chronic renal failure. *Lancet*, 1: 700–702.

POPOVICH, R. (1978). Physiological transport parameters in patients. *Dialy. & Transpl.*, 7:8.

POPOVICH, R. P., J. W. MONCRIEF, K. D. NOLPH, A. J. GHODS, Z. J. TWARDOWSKI, and W. K. PYLE (1978). Continuous ambulatory peritoneal dialysis. *Ann. Intern. Med.*, 88 (#4): 449–56.

QUINTON, W., D. DILLARD, and B. H. SCRIBNER (1960). Cannulation of blood vessels for prolonged hemodialysis. *Trans. Am. Soc. Art. Int. Organs*, 6: 104–113.

SCHAEFER, K. V., D. HERRATH, C. A. GULLBERG, G. ASMUS, M. HUFLER, G. OFFERMANN, H. CREMER, C. C. HEUCK, and E. RITZ (1978). Chronic hemofiltration—A critical evaluation of a new method for the treatment of blood. *Artificial Organs*, 2(4): 386–94.

SCRIBNER, B. H., J. E. Z. CANER, R. BURI, and W. QUINTON (1960). The technique of continuous hemodialysis. *Trans. Am. Soc. Art. Int. Organs*, 6: 88–103.

SCRIBNER, B. H., R. BURI, J. E. Z. CANER, R. HEGSTROM, and J. M. BURNELL (1960). The treatment of chronic uremia by means of intermittent hemodialysis: A preliminary report. *Trans. Am. Soc. Art. Int. Organs*, 6: 114–122.

SHALDON, S., M. C. BEAU, G. DESCHODT, P. RAMPEREZ, and C. MION (1980). Vascular stability during postdilutional high flux haemofiltration with acetate (HFA) or bicarbonate (HFB) compared to single pass haemodialysis with acetate (HDA) or bicarbonate (HDB). *Prog. Chronic Renal Disease Conf., NIAMDD*: 46–47.

SKULSKY, M., and P. C. FARREL (1978). Uptake characteristics of selected biochemicals and coated and uncoated activated charcoal. *71st Annual Meeting of A.I.Ch.E.*

STEPHEN, R. L., S. C. JACOBSEN, E. ATKIN-THOR, and W. J. KOLFF (1975). Portable/wearable artificial kidney (WAK): Initial evaluation. *Proc. E.D.T.A.*, 12: 511–18.

TENCKHOFF, H. (1977). Solutions and equipment. *Dialy. & Transpl.*, 6 (#2): 24–27.

TENCKHOFF, H., and H. SCHECHTER (1968). A bacteriologically safe peritoneal access device. *Trans. Am. Soc. Art. Int. Organs*, 14: 181–86.

YATZIDIS, H. (1964). A convenient haemoperfusion micro-apparatus over charcoal for the treatment of endogenous and exogenous intoxications: Its use as an effective artificial kidney. *Proc. E.D.T.A.*, 1: 83.

ZELMAN, A., and D. GISSER (1979). In vitro characterization of RP-6 dialyzer: Co-current and counter-current clearance as a function of ultrafiltration. *J. Dialysis*, 3: 237.

Zelman, A., P. Whittam, W. Edleman, J. Angell, M. White, and D. Gisser (1979). Standards for accurate in vitro characterization of dialyzers: Test case the vivacell. *J. Dialysis*, 3: 11–25.

## STUDY QUESTIONS

**14.1**  A patient was using a 1 m² dialyzer and lost 4 lbs in 5 h. What $\overline{\Delta P}_m$ must have been used if the ultrafiltration index of the dialyzer was 3 ml/(h•m²•mm Hg)?

**14.2**  For a patient with a BUN at 80 mg% and using a dialyzer with an urea clearance of 125 ml/min, what is the initial rate of urea removal in mol/h and g/h?

**14.3**  If the dialysate flow is increased, what happens to clearance?

**14.4**  If the blood flow and dialysate flow are increased, what happens to clearance?

**14.5**  If the $\Delta P_m$ is increased, what happens to clearance?

**14.6**  If the dialysate-out pressure is changed from zero to $-100$ mm Hg, what happens to clearance and ultrafiltration rate?

**14.7**  For Fig. P14.1, consider the following conditions.

- $P_{Bi} = 100$ torr; $P_{Bo} = 40$ torr; $P_{Do} = 150$ torr; $P_{Di} = -200$ torr
- $Q_{Bi} = 200$ ml/min; $Q_{Di} = 500$ ml/min; $L_p = 10$ ml/(h•m²•mm Hg); $\pi_p = 25$ mm Hg
- $C_{Bi} = 200$ mg% glucose; $C_{Bo} = 100$ mg% glucose; $A_m = 1$ m²

(a)  Neglecting ultrafiltration, calculate the clearance of glucose and the concentration of glucose in the dialysate output. Would these calculations differ for counter-current flows as opposed to co-current flow?

(b)  Calculate the mean transmembrane hydrostatic pressure, the ultrafiltration rate, the concentration of glucose in the dialysate-out, the dialysate-out flow rate, the blood-out flow rate and the clearance.

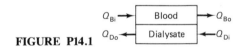

**FIGURE P14.1**

**14.8**  For Fig. P14.2, consider the following conditions.

- $C_u = 180$ ml/min; $A_m = 2$ m²; no ultrafiltration
- Urea store volume is roughly 60% of body mass and to be considered well stirred.
- Initial patient BUN = 100 mg%; patient weight is 70 kg.

(a)  Without a mathematical derivation, what is the clearance at $t = 0$ h, at $t = 100$ h, at $t = \infty$ ?

(b)  What is the urea concentration of the patient as a function of time?

(c)  What is the concentration of blood-out as a function of time?

(d)  What is the concentration of the dialysate-out as a function of time?

(e)  How long would it take for the patient's BUN to decrease to 30 mg%?

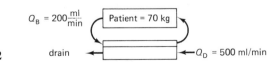

**FIGURE P14.2**

**14.9** For the hemodialyzer shown in Fig. P14.3, the dialysance, $D$, is 100 ml/min and constant, where dialysance is related to clearance by $C_{Bi}C = (C_{Bi} - C_{Di})D$. Note that when the dialysate-in flow concentration is not zero, clearance is not a constant, but dialysance is "nearly" constant.

- $C_{Bi}$ = (100 mg% BUN)$_{initial}$
- $C_{Di}$ = (0 mg% BUN)$_{initial}$
- $T = 37°C$
- $Q_D$ = 500 ml/min
- $Q_B$ = 200 ml/min
- Patient weight 70 kg

(a)  If no ultrafiltration occurred, how much urea would be removed in 6 h?
(b)  If ultrafiltration occurred primarily as a result of $\overline{\Delta P}_m$ (neglect $\pi_p$) and conditions were set so that

- $P_{B_{in}}$ = 250 torr; $P_{B_{out}}$ = 50 torr    Constant
- $P_{D_{in}}$ = 40 torr; $P_{D_{out}}$ = 0 torr    Initial
- $L_p$ = 2 ml/(h·m²·mm Hg); $A_m$ = 1 m²

what is the time-dependent rate of ultrafiltration and what volume would be transported in 5 h from start of dialysis?
(c)  What is the solute flow (g/min) initially and at 5 h?

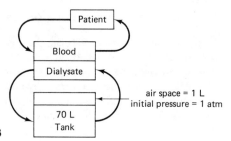

**FIGURE P14.3**

**14.10** For Fig. P14.4, consider the following conditions.

- Patient initial glucose = 100 mg%
- Dialysate initial glucose = 0 mg%
- Dialysance is constant at 100 ml/min.
- T = 37°C

(a)  Consider the case of no ultrafiltration.
(1)  Calculate initial $C_{Do}$ and $C_{Bo}$ (in mg%).
(2)  Calculate initial solute transfer in mol/(s·cm²). Molecular weight of glucose = 180.
(3)  Compute $C_{Bo}(t)$, $C_{Bi}(t)$, $C_{Do}(t)$, and $C_{Di}(t)$.
(4)  How long would it take for the bath to reach 90% of its equilibrium value?
(b)  Consider the case in which ultrafiltration occurs. Let $\overline{\Delta P}_m$ = 100 torr and $L_p$ = 10 ml/(h · mm Hg).
(1)  Calculate initial $C_{Bo}$ and $C_{Do}$ (in mg%).
(2)  How long would it take for the patient to lose 1 kg of weight (in h)?

(3) If one desired to decrease the body stores of urea by 50% in 3 h, what value of $\overline{\Delta P}_m$ would have to be set?

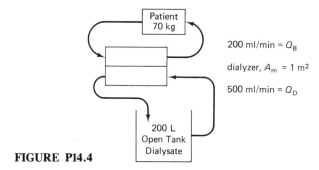

**FIGURE P14.4**

**14.11** The following data were collected on glucose for a 1 m² high-flux dialyzer with dialysate of 500 ml/min and counter-current flow.

| $C$ (ml/min) | $Q_{Bi}$ (ml/min) | $Q_v$ (ml/min) |
|---|---|---|
| 78 | 100 | 6.4 |
| 81 | 100 | 13.9 |
| 83 | 100 | 29.8 |
| 107 | 200 | 7.2 |
| 111 | 200 | 14.9 |
| 117 | 200 | 30.0 |
| 126 | 300 | 9.1 |
| 129 | 300 | 23.6 |
| 135 | 300 | 31.2 |

(a) Using multiple regression, fit these data to equation 14.4
(b) Find the "estimate of mean error" by calculating the standard deviation between the curve fit and the data.
(c) Make a plot of clearance at zero and at 2 l/h ultrafiltration rate as a function of blood flow. What would the error in the estimate of clearance be if ultrafiltration was not taken into account? Sketch in the estimate of mean error that brackets the curve.
(d) The clearance is equal to $A_m P_m$ at infinite $Q_B$ and $Q_D$ and zero ultrafiltration rate. Estimate $P_m$ from these data.

# Neonatology, Obstetrics, and Gynecology

## 15

*Michael R. Neuman*

## 15.1 LEARNING OBJECTIVES

Upon completing this chapter you will be able to:

- Describe the methods of thermal therapy in neonates.
- Describe the function of the neonatal intensive care unit.
- Describe neonatal respiratory assist devices.
- Describe methods of obtaining water and electrolyte balance.
- Describe bilirubin therapy methods and equipment.
- Describe devices used in obstetrics and gynecology.

In this chapter, we examine therapeutic devices used in neonatology, obstetrics, and gynecology. We look at the neonatal intensive care unit and see how it helps premature and other high-risk infants in the early days of their lives. We examine the devices that aid the neonatologist in giving intensive care and also describe that care. We also examine therapeutic devices used in obstetrics and gynecology for fertility control and induction of labor.

## 15.2 INTRODUCTION

Neonatology is the field of medicine concerned with the care of newborn infants. It is a subspecialty in pediatrics, and today it is also related to obstetrics and gynecology because many physicians now consider the care of mother, fetus, and newborn continuously. No longer is the obstetrician concerned only with the mother and fetus, and the pediatrician concerned only with the newborn. Instead, obstetricians and neonatologists work closely together in caring for their patients. This is especially true when there is some known risk. Often, obstetricians and pediatricians who are concerned with pregnancy, labor and delivery, and the neonate, are known as perinatologists and are especially interested in the perinatal period, that period of time including the final third of pregnancy and the first week of newborn life.

The perinatologist, and especially the neonatologist, are concerned in particular with special problems that are encountered by the premature infant and full-term infants who are at high risk. They must worry about providing life-support systems in situations in which these are needed for survival, as well as diagnosing and correcting any abnormalities present. In recent years, there has been great interest in the diagnosis and surgical repair of neonatal congenital abnormalities, which a few years ago would have meant certain death for the infant. Life-threatening abnormalities in the cardiovascular system of newborn infants can now be either temporarily or permanently repaired using modern surgical techniques.

## 15.3 THE NEONATAL INTENSIVE CARE UNIT

A major change in the method of care of neonates has occurred with the advent of the neonatal intensive care unit. The development of specialized centers for the care of ill neonates and transport systems for bringing these neonates to the centers has significantly reduced the neonatal death rate. These centers supply intensive and aggressive clinical care through highly trained staff assisted by various diagnostic and therapeutic devices.

### The High-Risk Neonatal Patient

Fortunately, the majority of pregnancies result in healthy infants who do not require any form of specialized care. However, in about 10% of deliveries, the infants are at risk and require intensive care for survival. These infants are often the result of so-called high-risk pregnancies in which the obstetrician has identified problems before birth, but this is not always the case. As a matter of fact, one of the major problems confronting modern obstetrics is the identification of those patients who are at risk during or, for that matter, even before pregnancy, so that they can receive specialized care as soon as possible.

Infants delivered before the pregnancy has run its full course are known as premature neonates and usually require intensive care, especially if they are under 2,500 g. Some of these infants are quite small and are unable to survive in the normal hospital environment. Diabetes is a significant risk factor in pregnancy and can produce neonates who require intensive care. Sometimes diabetic pregnancies are interrupted before the fetus has reached full-term maturity, thereby resulting in a premature neonate. Full-term infants of diabetic mothers have other problems that often require intensive care. Infants with life-threatening congenital abnormalities can benefit from intensive care. This is especially true for those infants suffering from abnormalities of the cardiovascular system and of the ventricular drainage system in the brain. Sometimes these infants require surgery, and the surgical patient should receive intensive care during recovery. There are other situations in which neonates require intensive care, and these frequently are related to problems during pregnancy and especially in labor and delivery.

## Function of Intensive Care

The neonatal intensive care unit permits physicians and nurses to continuously observe patients so that they can readily detect conditions requiring immediate intervention. Both the clinical staff and electronic instrumentation provide this continuous observation. The intensive care unit also maintains an optimal environment in which the neonate can grow and develop. Intensive care can also assist the patient with certain bodily functions such as breathing, temperature control, and detoxification. Finally, intensive care can provide optimal nutrition and fluid and electrolyte balance for the neonatal patient.

## Special Features of Neonatal Intensive Care Units

The most important component of a neonatal intensive care unit is the staff. It is followed in importance by the various therapeutic, diagnostic, and monitoring devices that assist the clinical staff in providing care. In addition to these, the structure of the intensive care unit itself is important. Because observation of the patient is one of the most important aspects of medical diagnosis, it is important that the intensive care unit be designed not to impede observation in any way. For example, skin color is useful in detecting neonatal jaundice, and so lighting in the intensive care unit must be neutral so that it does not interfere with determining skin color. Furthermore, the color of the walls of the unit must also be neutral because reflected light from them could affect the apparent skin hue. Radiant heat gain or loss by the neonate is an important factor in its temperature regulation, and so the intensive care unit should be designed with this in mind. Outside windows can frequently be a significant source of radiant heat during the day and a sink at night, especially during cold weather. For this reason, there should be few outside windows in a neonatal intensive care unit.

Ambient temperature and humidity in the intensive care unit can affect neonatal thermal balance. Ideally, the intensive care unit should be a walk-in incubator at a temperature of approximately 33°C, but this would be uncomfortable for the clinical personnel and could possibly reduce their efficiency to the point where advantages gained from the elevated ambient temperature would be lost. Specialized intensive care units have been constructed where these temperatures are maintained and where the walls of the room are also heated to minimize radiant loss from the infant. While these rooms have proven useful for research purposes, the general trend today is to avoid their use in the care of high-risk infants.

Additional features of the neonatal intensive care unit that are similar to those of an adult intensive care unit include adequate services available at each patient location, easy access to equipment required for resuscitation, ability to observe all patients from a central location, and easy and quick access to appropriate laboratory support.

## *Regionalization*

Neonatal intensive care is expensive and it is not necessary for every hospital to have a neonatal intensive care service. Instead, one hospital in a region should be set up to care for the high-risk neonate and a transport service established to bring neonates who require intensive care from other hospitals in the region. The intensive care unit should be set up in hospitals that handle the high-risk pregnancies for the region, because it is far better to have the neonatal intensive care facilities available at delivery rather than to require transport. Furthermore, it is well known that the best transport is achieved before delivery of the fetus and, so, by referring the mother to the high-risk center for delivery, she can obtain the best care from the entire high-risk perinatal service.

When infant transport is necessary, it requires specialized equipment and personnel. Transport teams of a neonatologist and neonatal intensive care nurse should go on all transport calls so that therapy can be begun at the neonate's originating hospital. Furthermore, special transport equipment to provide appropriate neonatal environment and monitoring should be available to the transport personnel. In many regions, transport is carried out by means of an ambulance, but in some regions that cover a large area, such as in predominately rural parts of the country, helicopters are used for transport.

An unfortunate side effect of neonatal transport is the separation of mother and child. Some pediatricians (Klaus et al., 1972) feel that this can significantly reduce maternal-infant bonding, and so they take great efforts to bring the family together in the neonatal intensive care unit as soon as possible. Often, the fathers are encouraged to come to the intensive care unit and to participate in the care of their child in whatever ways seem appropriate.

## 15.4 NEONATAL THERMAL BALANCE

The mechanisms of heat production and heat loss in the neonate are different from those of the adult. An important aspect of the care of the premature infant is to achieve a stable thermal environment to minimize excessive heat gain or heat loss. We must understand the basic concepts of heat production and loss in the neonate before we design appropriate environmental chambers to minimize thermal excesses. Neonatal thermal balance can be summarized by

$$Q_m = Q_c + Q_r + Q_\sigma + Q_e \qquad (15.1)$$

where $Q_m$ is the metabolic heat production and $Q_c$, $Q_r$, $Q_\sigma$, and $Q_e$ the convective, radiative, conductive, and evaporative heat losses, respectively. $Q_m$ must always be positive, but the terms on the right-hand side of the equation may be negative.

When this occurs, this represents heat gain rather than loss. For example, if the air surrounding the infant is warmer than the child, he will gain heat convectively. Thus, $Q_c$ in equation 15.1 will be negative.

## Heat Production

Heat is produced in the neonate by the oxidation of biochemical fuels. A particular aspect of heat production in the neonate that is not seen in the adult is nonshivering thermogenesis. The neonate can increase heat production in a cold environment without increased muscular activity or shivering as we usually see in adults. The neonate can also vasoconstrict skin vasculature to minimize heat loss from the skin. Nonshivering thermogenesis requires oxygen, and when oxygen supply to the tissues is limited, as in the case in some lung diseases, thermogenesis is reduced.

A source of neonatal heat that is not supplied by metabolism is radiant warming of the infant. When the neonate is in an environment in which large portions of skin are exposed to radiant energy, such as from an outside window on a warm day, from artificial light, or from radiant warmers, the result is a power input into the neonate. The infant must make an additional effort to dissipate the heat to avoid an increase in body temperature. Although we can use this principle to advantage in establishing adequate thermal balance for the neonate, it is important that the clinician understand the sources and effects of radiant power to fully evaluate thermal conditions surrounding the patient.

## Heat Loss

The physical mechanisms of heat loss from an object that is warmer than its environment apply to the neonate. These include radiation, convection, conduction, and, when water or other volatile materials are present, evaporation. The primary mechanisms of heat loss from the neonate are radiation and convection. At an environmental temperature of 30°C, these account for as much as 80% of the total heat loss. Because the surface-area-to-volume ratio is greater in the neonate than in an adult, the heat loss from radiation and convection is significantly larger. Also, the thermal conductance from deep body tissues to the skin is greater in the neonate than it is in the adult due to a smaller amount of subcutaneous fat. Conductive losses from the neonate are determined by his immediate environment and can be kept insignificantly small through the use of appropriate insulating materials. Evaporative heat loss comes from the lungs and the skin surface. It is affected to some extent by relative humidity, but the reduced evaporative heat losses at high relative humidity are generally outweighed by the inconvenience caused by such an environment. Heat loss can be controlled effectively by choosing appropriate environments for the neonate. Although convection is easily understood and controlled by determination of environmental air temperature and velocity, radiation is a bit more difficult. Not only must we understand the radiative losses from the infant, but also consider this with respect to radiative gain from the environment. An outside window can result in a greater radiation loss on cold nights than on warm days. Similarly, the wall temperature and emissivity of the immediate environment of the neonate play a strong role in the net radiative loss.

Sometimes thermal equilibrium is not maintained and equation 15.1 becomes an inequality. When this occurs, balance can once again be achieved by modifying the values of the terms of the equation. This can be accomplished by a change in physical properties or by a change in body temperature. In the former case, such physiologic changes as a variation of cutaneous perfusion can effect $Q_c$, $Q_r$, and $Q_\sigma$. All of the variables in equation 15.1 are affected by neonatal temperature, but each in a different way. For example, $Q_r$ is proportional to $T^4$ where $T$ is absolute temperature, while $Q_\sigma$ is proportional to $(T - T_0)$ where $T_0$ is the surrounding air temperature. Thus, the neonate cannot only change his heat production by changing his temperature, but he can also change the relative proportion of his different modes of heat loss.

### The Neutral Thermal Environment

Because oxygen is required for the production of energy in the neonate, and energy is necessary for heat production or cooling, there must be some optimal situation where neither thermogenesis nor cooling is necessary and so minimum oxygen is required by the neonate. These conditions are known as the neutral thermal environment and they include air temperature and flow, relative humidity, and radiating surface temperature. We must consider these factors to produce minimum oxygen consumption while maintaining neonatal core temperature at $37 \pm 0.5°C$. The specific conditions change with the age of the infant and its size. In actual practice, only the factor of environmental air temperature is usually considered. A newborn infant weighing less than 1,500 g should be in an environment in which the air temperature is 34.3°C, while a newborn full-term infant weighing more than 2,500 g only requires an air temperature of 33.0°C for neutral thermal conditions (American Academy of Pediatrics, 1971). These temperatures diminish as the infant ages and grows.

## 15.5 INCUBATORS

One of the most important factors in the care of the newborn infant is keeping him warm. Thus, the development of devices to warm and maintain the infant in a neutral thermal environment is important in the therapy of premature infants. It is interesting that the early incubators were not always used for therapeutic medical purposes. In the early part of this century, premature infants were displayed as a curiosity at expositions and fairs, and they were kept in glass incubators so that they could easily be seen by the spectators.

### Structure and Operation

Although there are several different manufacturers of neonatal incubators, Fig. 15.1 shows their basic structure and mode of operation. The neonate lies on a flat, covered foam mattress in the infant chamber. This part of the incubator is enclosed

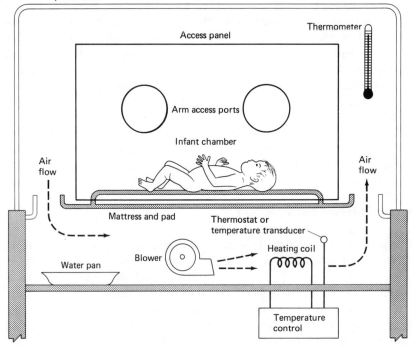

Clear plastic cover

Access panel

Thermometer

Arm access ports

Infant chamber

Air flow

Air flow

Mattress and pad

Thermostat or temperature transducer

Heating coil

Blower

Water pan

Temperature control

**FIGURE 15.1.** A neonatal incubator.

by a clear plastic hood. The two long sides of this cover have circular ports that can be opened so that the clinical staff can place their hands and arms in the incubator to manipulate the baby without introducing a lot of cool room air. One of these sides often has a panel slightly larger than the infant that can be opened for more unrestrained access to the patient. The plastic hood itself can be raised for further access if necessary but, of course, when this is done all temperature control is lost.

Under the base of the infant chamber, we find the heating and humidification plant. Air leaves the infant chamber through an opening in its base that is located at the end closest to the infant's feet. It passes over a pan of water that serves to humidify the air, when this is desired, and a blower then forces the air through the electrical heating coil. There can also be a water pan for humidification downstream from this heating coil. Finally the air passes over a temperature sensor for controlling the temperature in the infant chamber before reentering the chamber near the patient's head. In the switching type of incubator (two heating states, on and off), this is usually a simple thermostat. Incubators that use proportional electronic control employ a thermistor as a temperature transducer. It is connected to an electronic control circuit that provides electrical power to the heating coil that is proportional to the difference between the desired temperature and the actual temperature. In some incubators, the thermistor temperature sensor can be placed in the infant chamber just above the infant to provide more accurate temperature control of the infant's immediate environment. There are some incubators in which the temperature control does not fix the air temperature to a set point but, rather, it senses the skin temperature of the neonate by means of a thermistor placed on the abdomen, usually over the liver, and adjusts the air temperature to maintain a set infant skin temperature. This type of control is often referred to as infant servotemperature control.

Incubators often also have a thermometer, usually the mercury-in-glass type, installed in the infant chamber so that clinical staff can check the air temperature.

## Transport Incubators

Special incubators are needed to transport infants from the referring hospital to the intensive care center. These devices, although somewhat smaller, have the same basic design as the incubator of Fig. 15.1. They must operate from a variety of electrical sources. A secondary battery on the incubator itself is used when no power is available. So that they can easily be moved from one point to another, transport incubators must be light, have large wheels, and be capable of being securely fastened in the transport vehicle.

## Incubator Thermal Balance

We saw from equation 15.1 that the infant is in thermal equilibrium when the heat generated and received by the infant just equals his heat losses. We can write a similar equation for the incubator.

$$Q_h + Q_m = Q_\sigma + Q_r + Q_e + Q_\ell \qquad (15.2)$$

where $Q_h$ is the heat generated by the electrical heating element and $Q_\ell$ represents heat losses from warm air leaking from the infant chamber through ports and other openings. The left-hand side of the equation represents heat production, while the right-hand side represents heat losses, although $Q_r$ can sometimes be negative and represent a radiant heat gain. In most incubators, it is found that an electrical heating element capable of 100–150-W maximum power is sufficient to maintain a neutral thermal environment.

## Problems with Present Incubator Design

Figure 15.1 shows that, from the standpoint of temperature control engineering, this incubator design leaves much to be desired. But before we are too critical, let us remember that not only must an incubator design provide an adequate thermal environment, but it must allow easy access to the infant, both visually and through direct contact, so that appropriate clinical care can be given. Note that the infant chamber temperature does not necessarily have to be at the desired value because the temperature sensor for controlling the heating coil is usually not located in the chamber itself. The clear plastic hood over the infant chamber is not a good thermal insulator, and so there is heat loss through it. More accurate temperature control could be achieved with the temperature sensor located in the infant chamber, but even when this is done, the temperature in the infant chamber does not necessarily have to be uniform. Because warm air enters the chamber in the vicinity of the infant's head and air is withdrawn from the opposite end of the chamber, the air around the infant's feet is cooler than that around his head. Furthermore, turbulent flow patterns through the chamber also tend to produce nonuniform temperature distributions. This, of course, is further disrupted when access ports are open. Because air constantly flows over the infant, and this air is often a few degrees cooler than he is, the infant can be cooled by convection. New designs employing laminar flow of the air through the infant chamber and double-wall plastic covers for better insulation can overcome these problems, but access to the infant is not always as convenient, and these systems are much more expensive to produce commercially. Thus, the design of Fig. 15.1 remains the standard for infant incubators.

Although the newer incubators use proportional electronic control with the temperature sensor in the infant chamber, enough of the old thermostatically controlled on–off heaters are still used to warrant some comment. The heating coils generally have a rather high mass and, hence, a large thermal inertia, and this is true for the thermostatic element itself. Thus, this control system frequently over-shoots and oscillates. Incubator manufacturers use fairly high-mass mercury-in-glass thermometers with the bulb in a metal well in the infant chamber. This design produces a thermal low-pass filter so these do not show the oscillation. Amplitude of oscillation can be 1 or 2°C and vary throughout the infant chamber for reasons previously described. Perlstein et al. (1970) have found that in this type of incubator, infant apnea (cessation of breathing) occurred more frequently when the heater was on than when it was off. They, therefore, conclude that the use of proportional electronic control not only provides a more uniform temperature but is also safer for the infant with respiratory problems.

Proportional control can produce problems when it is used in infant servotemperature control systems. When we desire to control the incubator air temperature to yield a particular infant body temperature, it is crucial that the thermistor temperature sensor remain in good contact with the infant and that it detect a temperature indicative of his core temperature. Should this thermistor become loosened from the infant's skin, the control system will not know that this has happened and will servo the incubator air temperature to give the desired temperature at the thermistor. Thus, the air temperature will be regulated at the desired neonatal body temperature, and this might be outside of the patient's neutral thermal environment.

Radiation heat losses through the clear plastic hood of the incubator generally are not accounted for in present designs. We must worry about net radiant energy loss from the neonate and this includes considering not only heat radiated from exposed neonatal skin, but also heat reabsorbed from external radiant sources. The basic incubator design of Fig. 15.1 has little control over this radiation. There are, however, ways to circumvent this problem. One simple way is to provide a second clear plastic cover to go around the neonate so that the incubator, in effect, has a double wall. The inner cover is at the internal temperature of the incubator and serves as a radiant source to replace some of the radiant energy lost by the neonate. This double box type of construction is somewhat inconvenient and makes access to the neonate more difficult. Some new incubator designs incorporate electrical heaters in the walls of the hood of the incubator that are similar to the window defoggers on automobiles. In this way, the walls of the incubator can be heated to a temperature at which not only will they provide radiant energy to make up for radiant heat losses from the neonate, but they will also minimize the effects of conducted heat loss through the hood. In this case, $Q_r$ in equation 15.1 can be very small or even zero.

A third problem with present incubator designs is the high ambient noise level in the infant chamber. This noise comes from the blower mechanism located directly beneath the infant and the air rushing through the chamber. The noise level of typical incubators in use in neonatal intensive care units can be as high as 80 dB, and the effect of this continuous noise on infants is not fully understood. Closing the door of the storage cabinet under the incubator can produce a sound amplitude of 114 dB in the infant chamber. These high sound levels might cause future problems when we consider that healthy infants thrive best in a quiet home environment.

## Radiant Warmers

Although the incubator can be effective in maintaining the neonate at the neutral thermal environment, it is not very convenient to use when extensive clinical procedures must be carried out. Although walk-in incubator rooms in which the clinicians join the infant inside a large incubator remove the inconvenience of access to the neonate, they have other problems as stated earlier.

A way to avoid these problems is to use a radiant warmer. Figure 15.2 shows the basic structure of the device. It consists of a large radiant heater placed above the infant. The heater is located high enough so that clinicians working with the neonate do not accidentally bump their heads on it. It has a relatively low thermal mass so that it responds quickly to changes in its electrical power supply. The infant lies on a pad on the working surface of the radiant warmer. The sides are high enough to prevent the infant from falling off and to minimize drafts that could cool the infant by convection. The basic idea behind the radiant warmer is that, because the infant loses a lot of energy by radiation, this should be an effective means to replace it. The thermal balance equation in this case becomes

$$Q_{rs} + Q_m = Q_c + Q_\sigma + Q_{r\ell} + Q_e \qquad (15.3)$$

where $Q_{rs}$ is the radiant power that the infant receives from the radiant heater and $Q_{r\ell}$ represents radiant losses from the neonate.

For $Q_{rs}$ to replace radiant and other losses requires that there be careful

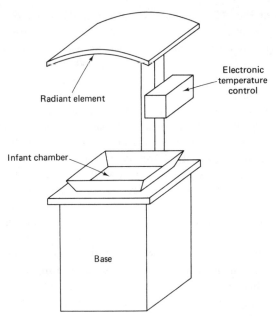

**FIGURE 15.2.** A neonatal radiant warmer.

control of this variable so that the infant does not become either too warm or too cold. Thus, this system must operate in a servo mode similar to that of the infant servo-controlled incubator. A thermistor is placed on the neonatal skin in such a way that it is protected from direct radiation from the radiant warmer and only responds to the neonatal skin temperature. This temperature, in turn, controls the electrical power to the radiant element so that the proportional control system tries to maintain the neonatal skin temperature at the desired value.

This device has problems similar to those of the infant servo-controlled incubator. In effect, what it tries to do is to control the thermistor temperature so that it will be at the set point. The question is whether the thermistor temperature is the same as the infant's temperature. If a thermistor becomes loosened from the neonatal skin or completely falls off, the radiant warmer can overheat the patient. On the other hand, if the thermistor becomes repositioned so that it is warmed by the radiant heater, there can be circumstances in which it will heat faster than the neonate, resulting in not enough radiant energy being supplied. For these reasons, radiant warmers are seldom used today for the long-term care of high-risk infants but, rather, find application in treatment areas in which the infant must undergo procedures such as placement of umbilical catheters, peripheral I-V lines, extensive physical examination, and so on and there is constant supervision from the clinical staff.

## 15.6 RESPIRATORY ASSISTS

One of the most significant changes that occurs in the newborn during birth is the transition from exchange of respiratory gases through the placenta to exchange through the lungs. This not only involves inflation of the lungs and exchange of air but also changes in the blood-flow circuit of the cardiovascular system. Thus, anomalies can be present before birth but not appear until after delivery.

### Neonatal Respiratory Distress Syndrome

Neonatal respiratory distress syndrome or Hyaline membrane disease is the most commonly seen pulmonary disorder in neonates and is the principal cause of neonatal death (Behrman, 1977). Premature infants are most susceptible and the incidence increases as the gestational age of the neonate decreases. The disease is usually seen in the first day of life, and it can first be detected by noting signs of respiratory distress in the infant such as rapid breathing, grunting on expiration, and intercostal and subcostal retractions. Histologically, the lungs appear to have a membrane of hyalin, an amorphous material, over the alveoli and alveolar ducts. This lining reduces the compliance of the lungs, making breathing more difficult, and also limits the transport of oxygen to the alveolar capillaries. Upon x-ray examination, a pulmonary infiltrate appears and the infant is often cyanotic and has low arterial oxygen tension.

The treatment of neonatal respiratory distress syndrome in intensive care units has dramatically improved the survival rate. In addition to supportive care, respiratory therapy is essential. This involves providing continuous positive airway pressure, continuous negative pressure, or ventilatory assist. Sections 13.3 and 13.7 and the following paragraphs describe some of the devices used. In addition, it is important to provide blood-gas monitoring either by indwelling sensors, frequent blood sampling, or transcutaneous oxygen tension measurement.

### Nasal Continuous Positive Airway Pressure

The administration of continuous positive airway pressure (CPAP) via the nasal route has been an important aspect of the treatment of neonatal respiratory distress syndrome. Special devices for the administration of nasal CPAP are available for the neonate. Figure 15.3 shows a neonatal nasal cannulae assembly. This device, molded of soft silicone rubber, allows the placement of a cannula in each side of the nose with a flange against the base of the nose to provide an effective seal. By using soft silicone rubber for both the cannulae and the flange, there is minimum of nasal irritation. In normal operation, the cannula is connected to a source of air and oxygen at a regulated elevated pressure.

In the early application of this type of nasal cannula, makeshift assemblies for providing the air and holding the cannula had to be used. These occupied a large portion of the area above the neonate in the incubator and tended to be quite inconvenient, especially when it was necessary to change the position of the infant. For this reason, a complete nasal CPAP administration system was developed to avoid these problems. Figure 15.4 shows that this system consists not only of the plumbing to connect the nasal cannula to the air–oxygen supply but also an assembly to permit convenient adjustment of the position, to regulate the pressure, to provide a safety valve for overpressure, and a means of positioning the infant's head. The head cradle is arranged so that the nasal cannula moves along with it,

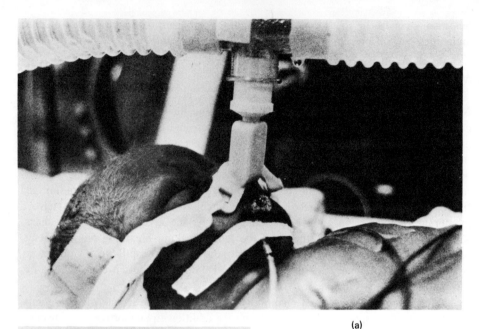

(a)

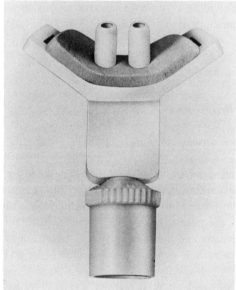

(b)

**FIGURE 15.3.** A nasal cannula for administration of neonatal continuous positive airway pressure. (a) Infant with nasal cannula in place. (b) The nasal cannula itself. (Courtesy Argyle Division, Sherwood Medical Products, St. Louis, Missouri.)

thereby allowing the neonate to be repositioned without the necessity of changing the position of the nasal cannula. This system makes it possible to administer CPAP without seriously interfering with other aspects of neonatal intensive care.

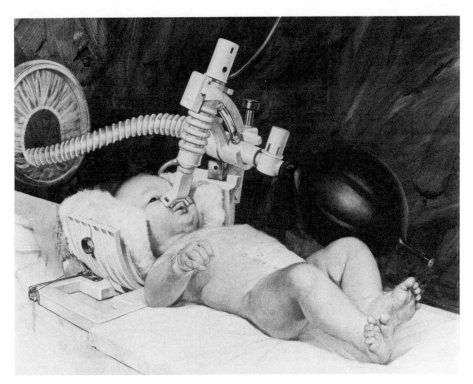

**FIGURE 15.4.** An administration system for continuous positive airway pressure through the nasal cannula. (Courtesy Citadel Division, Sherwood Medical Products, St. Louis, Missouri.)

## Oxygen Hood

Oxygen therapy can also be given in mild cases of respiratory distress syndrome using an oxygen hood. This is a small plastic box open on one side that can be placed over the neonatal head. This box is connected to a supply of heated, humidified oxygen–air mixture that flows into the incubator at a fairly high rate; thus, the neonatal head is exposed to gas containing a high oxygen content. It is easier to provide breathing air with a high percentage of oxygen in this way than it would be to fill the entire infant chamber of the incubator with air of increased oxygen concentration. The effects of mixing with outside air are minimized in this way in the critical area around the neonatal nose and, thus, smaller amounts of oxygen are required. Nevertheless, the maximum practical oxygen fraction that can be used with this system is about 45%. Higher oxygen concentrations require using a mask, nasal cannula, or trachial intubation.

A critical factor in providing special oxygen–air mixtures to the neonate either in a hood or through a more direct connection to the pulmonary system is the temperature and humidity control of the breathing air mixture. Generally, these factors are controlled outside of the incubator by means of regulating the temperature of the water in the humidifier or nebulizer (a device for providing a mist of

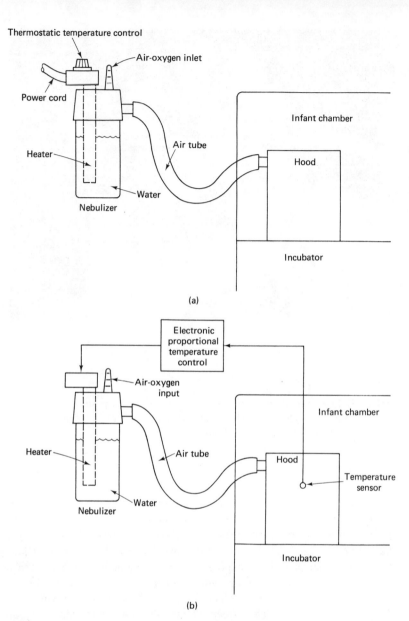

**FIGURE 15.5.** Administration of air-oxygen mixtures through a neonatal hood. (a) Conventional system with temperature control at the nebulizer. (b) Electronic proportional temperature control with the temperature sensor located in the neonatal hood.

small water particles) at the oxygen–air source near the incubator (see Section 13.7 and Fig. 15.5a). Note that this method of temperature control does not necessarily ensure adequate temperature regulation at the neonate because the humidified air must pass through a relatively long tube exposed to the nursery ambient temperature before entering the incubator and being available to the infant. Figure 15.5b shows a better system. Here, the heating still takes place at the humidifier or nebulizer outside of the incubator, but the heating element now is controlled by a sensor, usually a thermistor, located near the infant. The temperature sensor can be located above the infant's nose and used to signal a proportional controller that controls the heater. In this way, the temperature can be maintained at a much more constant level than would be possible with an on–off type of control.

### Retrolental Fibroplasia

This disease of the neonatal eye can be caused by oxygen therapy (Stern, 1973). An increase in its incidence was noted after the application of elevated oxygen in the treatment of neonatal respiratory distress syndrome. It is, therefore, extremely important to monitor neonatal arterial oxygen tensions when the infant breathes elevated oxygen fractions. It is generally accepted that the arterial partial pressure of oxygen should not exceed 60 mm Hg.

This disease involves fibrosis and detachment of the neonatal retina. In advanced cases, the fibrotic retina is pulled immediately behind the lens, resulting in a white appearance to the pupil. The disease results in impaired vision and often blindness. It is a preventable disease, and that is why it is so important to have careful management of oxygen therapy in the neonate. Arterial oxygen tensions can rise rapidly during the recovery phase of neonatal respiratory distress syndrome, and frequent or continuous blood-gas monitoring is essential to avoid this disease.

### Apnea

Cessation of breathing, known as apnea, is frequently encountered in premature infants and larger infants who suffer from neonatal respiratory distress syndrome. Apneic episodes are usually terminated by stimulation of the infant, such as touching a foot, stroking it, or gentle shaking. Thus, it is important in those neonates susceptible to apnea that they be constantly monitored either by human personnel or electronic devices. Apnea monitors determine if respiratory movements are taking place either by measuring transthoracic electrical impedance, measuring displacement of the chest wall, or detecting motion resulting from breathing activity. Several different types of monitors employing these principles are available in neonatal intensive care units (Neuman, 1979) and, although each type of monitor has some limitations, these devices are important in the care of infants susceptible to apnea.

## 15.7 FLUID AND ELECTROLYTE BALANCE AND NUTRITION

Water makes up a large percentage of the neonate. Because the premature infant is so small and there are various sources and losses of water, it is important that we pay special attention to water, electrolytes, and nutrients in caring for this patient.

## Water and Electrolyte Balance

If we consider a neonate who is not growing, we desire to have this infant in a situation in which the amount of water and the amount of electrolytes he takes in are equal to the amounts of each that he loses. Under these circumstances, he is said to be in water and electrolyte balance. In caring for infants in intensive care units, frequently intravenous fluids are administered and, thus, it is important to be able to administer just enough fluid to maintain the infant's needs. Excessive fluids can cause overhydration and its accompanying severe problems, while inadequte fluid therapy can result in dehydration. The small mass of premature infants means that slight variations in the amount of fluid administered can result in severe deviations from maintaining water balance. The same is true for electrolytes. Because water distribution is strongly related to electrolyte concentration, improper administration of electrolytes can cause osmotic water shifts.

In considering water and electrolyte therapy for neonates, we should be concerned with the intake of water and electrolytes and their losses. Water intake in the neonate results from the water content of milk and other fluids taken orally, $M_o$, and from carbohydrate metabolism, $M_m$. Losses of water occur in the urine, $M_u$, feces, $M_f$, insensible loss, $M_i$, and sweat, $M_p$. Another factor that we can consider a "loss" is the water needed for growth, $M_g$, that water incorporated into growing tissue. Thus, water balance occurs when

$$M_o + M_m = M_u + M_f + M_i + M_p + M_g \qquad (15.4)$$

We seldom see losses from sweating, $M_p$, in infants in intensive care units because of adequate temperature control, and young infants have not adequately developed sweating as a means of cooling. Insensible losses, $M_i$, include evaporation of water from the skin and from the lungs. Normally, approximately one third of the insensible loss comes from the lungs, but this can increase significantly in premature infants or for infants in low relative humidity environments. Insensible water loss can be a significant factor in neonatal water balance.

We can make similar arguments in considering electrolyte balance. $Na^+$, $K^+$, $Mg^{++}$, $Ca^{++}$, $Cl^-$ and other electrolyte intake is through the feeding of the infant, and output is by means of the urine and feces. In addition, some of these ions are incorporated into growing tissue. As with water, we must maintain a balance between intake and output.

## Intravenous Fluid Therapy

Neonates receiving intensive care frequently require the administration of intravenous solutions. This creates another input for water and electrolyte balance considerations. It is important in administering intravenous solutions containing electrolytes that we consider how both the water and electrolyte load and input correlate with the output. Small errors in the administration of intravenous solutions can result in significant imbalance in the neonate due to his small mass. It is, therefore, important to carefully monitor the infant in terms of the amount of fluids administered and the amount of fluid loss. Metering pumps to carefully control the administration of intravenous solutions should be used. Devices for use with neonates are essentially the same as those used with adults. These consist of peristaltic-type pumps, drop counting and clamping devices, or driven syringes.

The peristaltic-type pump design is frequently used. It is basically either the roller pump, as described for pump-oxygenators in Section 4.6, or the finger-type pump. Either the roller or a row of fingers compress a tube in series with the I-V line, thus creating a peristaltic wave. In either pump design, the rate of propagation in the peristaltic wave and the diameter of the tube determine the flow. Both types of pump can be controlled to give very low flows. The tubes used in these pumps can create problems for the patient. Because they are compressed and relaxed many times, small holes can occasionally develop. Generally, these holes are too small to let fluid leak out, but air can leak in. A bolus of air can thus leak into the intravenous line and advance into the patient. Although a small amount of air such as this introduced into an adult vein produces no serious problem, this is not the case in the neonate, and especially in the premature neonate. An air bubble as small as 5 ml can fill the neonatal left ventricle and stop the effective pumping of blood due to its high compliance. Under these circumstances, the cardiac output drops to zero and death ensues. It is, therefore, important to monitor the output of such pumping systems to detect air bubbles before they enter the neonatal circulation. Figure 15.6 shows such a system (Neuman, 1973). The I-V line serves as the dielectric of a capacitor, which is formed by placing a clamp containing electrodes

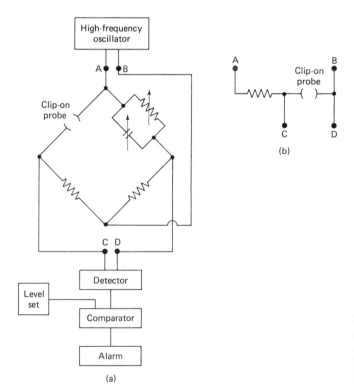

**FIGURE 15.6.** Block diagram of an air-bubble detector for use on neonatal intravenous infusion lines. (a) Bridge circuit. (b) Simple resonant circuit.

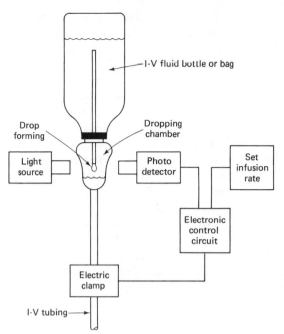

I-V fluid bottle or bag

Drop forming

Dropping chamber

Light source

Photo detector

Set infusion rate

Electronic control circuit

Electric clamp

I-V tubing

**FIGURE 15.7.** Drop counter type of neonatal intravenous infusion control.

over the line between the pump and the patient. The dielectric constant of water is considerably higher than that of air, and as long as water remains in the tube between the electrodes, there is a relatively large capacitance. If, on the other hand, air enters the segment of tube between the electrodes, the net dielectric constant is diminished and the capacitance reduced. This change in capacitance can be detected with an ac bridge circuit, or a simple RC voltage divider can feed a detector amplifier operating class C. The voltage increase due to a capacitance reduction activates the alarm and stops the pump.

Figure 15.7 shows the drop-counting intravenous fluid administration control. A standard intravenous administration tube connects to the fluid container and a light source shines through the drop chamber. A fluid drop falling into the chamber momentarily interrupts the light beam, which is detected as a pulse at the photodetector. Because the drop volume is relatively constant, the pulse rate corresponds to the drop rate and, hence, the amount of fluid administered. An electronic control circuit adjusts an electric clamp valve attached to the administration tube below the dropping chamber to administer a preset number of drops per unit time. Although the drop method does not provide highly precise control of intravenous fluid volume, drop volumes do not vary enough to create significant errors.

The left side of Fig. 15.8 shows the third technique for infusion of fluids: the motor-driven syringe. A mechanism that slowly and uniformly advances the piston expels the fluid from the syringe. A geared-down constant speed motor rotates a lead screw, which advances the piston. Varying the gear ratio varies the rate of infusion. In another technique, a fixed drive device uses a stepping motor. A major limitation with a syringe pump is that the syringe has limited capacity and, once it has been emptied, it must either be manually refilled or replaced. This requires

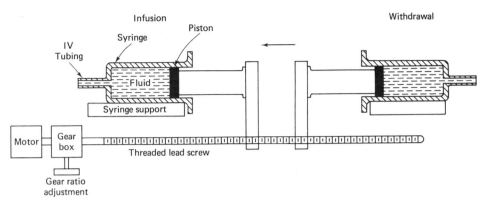

**FIGURE 15.8.** A driven syringe neonatal exchange transfusion pump.

more human intervention than do the other types of pumps, but it controls the rate of infusion more accurately than the other two types of pumps.

### Feeding the Premature Infant

In addition to maintaining fluid and electrolyte balance, the infant must take in appropriate fuels for maintaining energy production and growth. Gastric feeding of mother's milk or formula is the only way to fully achieve this, although intravenous hyperalimentation can, in some cases, approach this goal. The small preterm infant has special problems that must be considered when feeding. Often their suck is not adequate or of sufficiently long duration to provide sufficient intake. They frequently also have uncoordinated swallowing reflexes, which again limit their ability to transport material to the stomach. These infants run the risk of aspiration of stomach contents into the lungs, which is a serious problem.

Feeding these infants through oral gastric tubes placed in the esophagus, so that formula can be administered directly into the stomach, helps to minimize these problems, but the risk of aspiration is still present. We must ascertain the maximum volume for stomach contents for which the risk of regurgitation is still small and then feed accordingly. This can be a difficult problem in some neonates because their nutritional requirements are greater than the amount of material that we can safely administer when we consider stomach volume and emptying rate. In such infants, we have no recourse other than to augment the feeding with intravenous therapy. At the present time, feeding regimens are based upon the previously mentioned criteria and what the clinician feels the capacity of the neonate might be. A need exists to be able to monitor the neonatal gastric contents to allow maximum nutritional intake while minimizing the risk of aspiration.

## 15.8 NEONATAL JAUNDICE

Jaundice or icterus is the yellow coloration of tissue due to the presence of excessive amounts of the substance bilirubin. This discoloration is observed in the sclera (whites of the eyes) and the skin. In the neonate, concentrations of greater than 5 mg/100 ml are necessary to produce observable jaundice. Nevertheless, serum bilirubin concentrations of greater than 2 mg/100 ml are considered excessive and patients with bilirubin concentrations greater than this should be carefully watched.

## Bilirubin Metabolism

Bilirubin is produced in the biochemical degradation of the heme portion of the hemoglobin molecule (heme moity). In adults, the primary source of bilirubin is the degradation of hemoglobin from aging red blood cells. There are other proteins that contain the heme moity that also produce bilirubin in their degradation. These include the precursors of the heme moity itself, myoglobulin, and the cytochromes. This form of bilirubin is known as unconjugated bilirubin and enters the circulation. It is of extreme importance in the neonate because it can be transported to and enter cells in the central nervous system and cause their demise. Thus, uncontrolled, high unconjugated bilirubin concentrations in the blood can produce brain damage. The normal elimination of bilirubin from the body involves three organs. The liver converts unconjugated bilirubin to conjugated bilirubin, which is excreted in the bile into the intestine. Here, it is converted into a form that can be reabsorbed and eliminated in the urine by the kidneys or converted into another form that passes from the body in the stool.

## Hyperbilirubinemia

Elevated blood level of unconjugated bilirubin is known as hyperbilirubinemia, Considering the pathway of bilirubin synthesis and elimination described previously, it is easy to see the basic conditions that produce elevated levels. Either there is such a great source of bilirubin resulting from the degradation of heme that the liver cannot handle the load, or there is a problem in the liver, intestine, or kidneys that limits the rate at which unconjugated bilirubin can be eliminated. Either situation can lead to brain damage and must be carefully watched. The first situation occurs in normal infants and is referred to as physiologic jaundice of the newborn. It is more severe in premature neonates than in those delivered at term. Although we do not fully understand the mechanisms producing the elevated bilirubin, it is thought that it comes from a source of heme being rapidly degraded. The serum unconjugated bilirubin generally peaks at three days of age and then the level decreases. Levels greater than 10–20 mg/100 ml should be avoided because neuronal damage can occur. We can eliminate this condition, known as kernicterus, by modern therapeutic technology.

## Photography

Exposure to blue light in the wavelength band from 420–500 nm oxidizes bilirubin to compounds that are more easily eliminated. Thus, we can use this photo-oxidation to assist the neonate in eliminating bilirubin from the blood and tissues.

This is done by means of a phototherapy unit consisting of a group of eight or ten 20-W fluorescent lamps spaced 30–40 cm above the unclothed infant. This light penetrates the skin and helps to oxidize and hence eliminate bilirubin. Practical units fit above the clear plastic hood of an incubator and illuminate the infant through it. A clear plastic cover on the phototherapy lamp unit serves as a mechanical shield and absorbs ultraviolet light emanating from the fluorescent tubes. Because the light output in the blue range decreases with the age of the fluorescent tube, phototherapy units frequently have elapsed time meters on them so that the lamps can be changed when their effective energy output begins to drop.

Phototherapy units must be used cautiously because they have complications. The effect of the radiation on the neonatal eyes is not well understood, and so it is essential to have eye protection for the infants receiving this form of treatment. There is also a 40–190% increase in insensible water loss for small premature infants receiving phototherapy (Bell and Oh, 1979), and so it is necessary to compensate for this by providing fluids to the patient. In some neonates, the phototherapy produces a dark brown pigment in the serum, skin, and urine. This gives the child a bronzelike appearance and the condition is sometimes referred to as the bronze baby syndrome. When it occurs, phototherapy should be stopped and the hyperbilirubinemia treated by other means. Phototherapy units also supply radiant heat to the neonate, and this must be taken into account in determining thermal balance. $Q_r$ in equation 15.1 is much smaller when the lights are on; thus, the incubator does not have to supply as much heat.

Because all effects of phototherapy are not well understood and we do not know what additional complications could arise from prolonged exposure to radiation from fluorescent lamps, it is important that the neonate receive only the minimum effective amount of radiation. Therefore, we must determine the amount of radiated energy in the 420–500-nm band so that we can calculate the minimal exposure time. Instruments to do this consist of a small probe containing a photosensor, which can be held just above the neonate so that the energy incident on it will be similar to the energy incident on the neonatal skin. It is important that this probe have a field of view similar to that of the neonatal skin so that we can make an accurate energy measurement. The electrical signal from the probe drives a readout circuit consisting of an appropriately scaled amplifier and either an analog or digital readout. Most instruments are small and battery-operated for maximum convenience.

### Exchange Transfusion

Another method to eliminate bilirubin from the neonatal blood is to perform an exchange transfusion. This procedure, which is used to treat other neonatal blood and metabolic disorders as well, involves the removal of blood from the infant and replacement with donor blood. Because the neonatal blood volume is small, the best method of exchange is the simultaneous infusion and withdrawal of blood. Of course, some of the fresh blood is withdrawn along with the contaminated blood, but we cannot exchange a patient's blood as we would change the oil in an automobile by draining it all out before replacement. Figure 15.8 shows a special exchange pump generally used in exchange transfusions. Two equal-sized syringes are used in the pump, and the pistons of each are driven at the same velocity by the motor, but in opposite directions. Thus, at the beginning of the procedure, one syringe is filled with the donor blood and the other is empty and, at the end of the procedure, the empty syringe is filled with blood from the patient. By exchanging in this way, the neonatal blood volume remains constant.

## 15.9 THERAPEUTIC DEVICES IN OBSTETRICS AND GYNECOLOGY

Not only have therapeutic devices made significant contributions in the field of neonatology, but they also have been important in obstetrics and gynecology as well. Many of these devices have been covered in other chapters of this book and need not be repeated here. There are, however, some devices or applications of devices that are unique to obstetrics and gynecology. We briefly consider some of these in this section.

### *Fertility Enhancement*

An important area in obstetrics and gynecology is fertility control in the human. Although a large amount of publicity is received by devices, drugs, and techniques to diminish fertility or terminate pregnancy, an equal effort towards enhancing fertility goes relatively unnoticed. Important strides are being made in this area. Two problems that cause infertility in the female are failure to ovulate and failure to transport the fresh ovum to the site of fertilization in the fallopian tube and the fertilized zygote onto the uterus, where it can implant in the endometrium at the appropriate time. The laparoscope is an important device that allows the physician to study patients and determine if problems in ovulation or problems in transport are present and to make some changes to effect improvement. It permits direct observation of the ovary and fallopian tube by transabdominal endoscopy, and allows the physician to observe the ovary to determine if ovulation has taken place. The physician can also determine if there are mechanical defects that prevent the fallopian tube from picking up the freshly ovulated ovum and transporting it. The device can also be used to collect freshly ovulated ova for in vitro fertilization, a highly controversial and poorly understood procedure at the present time.

Laparoscopic examination may show mechanical defects that prevent approximation of the end of the fallopian tube against the ovary for collection of ova, or fibrotic constrictions obstructing or partially obstructing the lumen of the tube. Then, through the laparoscope, surgical correction, such as cutting the fibrous bands or repositioning the tube in an attempt to correct the problems can be done. If blockage of the fallopian tube is diagnosed, it is sometimes possible to excise the blocked portion of the tube and surgically connect the remaining sections to reestablish an open lumen. Sometimes, prosthetic devices, known as tubal stents, are placed in the lumen to help line up the sides being connected. These hollow plastic tubes are placed in the lumen and the two sides of the fallopian tube are sutured together over the stent. Although they generally maintain an open lumen to the tube, they often interfere with the normal physiology of tubal transport and produce a functional, if not physical, blockage. Improved microsurgical techniques are now being developed that will hopefully eliminate the need for the stent.

## Contraception

The other aspect of fertility control is to diminish fertility to the extent that unwanted pregnancies do not occur. Although there is some controversy as to whether this constitutes therapy or not, we wish to avoid that question and briefly look at some of the devices for achieving contraception without commenting on their moral, ethical, religious, or sociologic aspects. One principle of contraception is to prevent fertilization by blocking the production or transport of either the sperm or ovum. Another principle involves incapacitating one or the other gamete so that fertilization cannot take place. A third principle is accelerating transport of the fertilized zygote so that it is washed from the uterus before implantation is possible.

Only pharmacologic techniques can be used to block production, but various devices as well as drugs and surgical procedures can be used to interfere with transport. Rubber-membraned devices such as the condom and diaphragm can prevent mingling of sperm and ova, and in some experimental animal work, silicone rubber plugs have been used to occlude the fallopian tube, thereby inhibiting sperm transport to the site of fertilization. A more permanent form of interruption of transport is obtained by surgical ligation (cutting) of the vas deferens in the male or the fallopian tube in the female. Surgical procedures have recently been developed for ligation of the fallopian tube through the laparoscope. In one technique, a segment of tube is destroyed by fulguration (Chapter 11) using a special electrosurgical probe that is passed and observed through the laparoscope. A second procedure involves crimping the fallopian tube as we would crimp a garden hose to stop the flow of water. The tube is then maintained in this position by passing a silicone rubber ring over the crimped section. Both procedures can be carried out using the laparoscope; thus, only a small incision around the umbilicus is needed to enter the abdominal cavity. This can be done under local anesthesia, and the risk of visceral involvement is minimized by first inflating the abdomen with carbon dioxide to raise the anterior wall above the viscera. The entire procedure can be done on an outpatient basis.

Implantation of the fertilized zygote can be blocked by the presence of a foreign body in the uterus. Intrauterine contraceptive devices have been developed and are widely used to prevent pregnancy in this way. Figure 15.9 shows that these devices come in various shapes. They are generally made of polymeric materials such as silicone rubber or polypropylene, but some devices also include copper or copper salts. Recently, devices have been developed that contain hormones that slowly leak out to further aid in the prevention of pregnancy.

The design of an intrauterine contraceptive device must include several features. The device must be easily sterilized and maintained in the sterile state. It must be possible to easily insert it into the uterus with minimal trauma or discomfort to the patient. It must be of such a design that it will remain in the uterus. This often conflicts with the requirement of easy insertion. Thus, most devices come

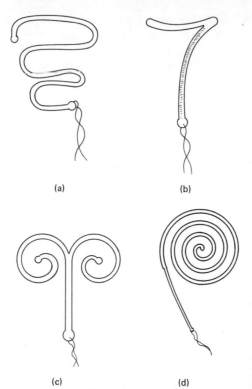

(a)                                (b)

(c)                                (d)

**FIGURE 15.9.** Examples of the shapes of various types of intrauterine contraceptive devices. (a) Lippes loop, (b) copper 7, (c) Saf-T-Coil, and (d) Bernberg bow.

prepackaged in an insertion tube in which they are collapsed. The insertion tube is passed through the uterine cervix, and then the intrauterine contraceptive device is extruded from the tube, at which time it assumes its normal shape. For example, the Lippes loop with its multiple S-shaped curves is stretched out into a straight line in its insertion tube to allow easy passing of the tube through the cervix. Pushing the device out of the insertion tube allows it to assume its characteristic shape so that it will remain in the uterus.

Another requirement in the design of intrauterine contraceptive devices is that they can be removed when the patient or the physician desires to have this done. Thus, the devices must have a small tail that is usually a flexible plastic fiber that extends out of the cervix into the vagina. Not only does this tail serve the purpose of a means of removal of the device, but it also is a simple, although crude, diagnostic check to make sure that the device remains in the uterus after insertion. If, upon routine pelvic examination, the obstetrician does not see the tail extending through the cervix, he must suspect that the device has either come out of the uterus or perforated the uterus and is in the abdominal cavity. Because uterine perforation is a possible complication with intrauterine contraceptive devices, it is important to design them in such a way that their extrauterine location can be determined. They should be x-ray opaque and visible to ultrasonic tomographic scans.

Finally, these devices should be designed in such a way that they do not promote infection or inflammation of the female reproductive tract. Although it is necessary for the tail to protrude into the vagina, a nonsterile environment, the tail should be designed so that pathogens cannot ascend it into the uterine cavity. One intrauterine contraceptive device that was frequently used several years ago was found to have a tail design that promoted wicking of vaginal fluid into the uterus. In several women, this was thought to be the cause of pelvic inflammatory disease, which went on to provide serious complications and permanent sterilization.

## Assisted Abortion

Another method of birth control that has had widespread application in the United States and some other countries is assisted abortion. Outpatient clinics that specialize in this procedure exist in major centers of population in this country. Early abortion can be achieved by a procedure known as dilation and curettage. In this case, the cervix is first dilated and the contents of the uterus are removed by either suction or scraping. Tapered blunt instruments are generally used to dilate the cervix, starting with one of the smallest diameter and passing it through the cervical canal. This is followed by passing larger and larger sized dilators until the cervix is open enough to allow the abortion to be performed. It is thought that this dilation technique can produce damage to the cervix and result in a situation known as an incompetent cervix, which will prevent the cervix from containing a later, desired pregnancy in the uterus. Alternate methods of cervical dilation have thus been considered. A laminaria tent made from natural Japanese reeds can be placed in the cervical canal the night before the procedure is to be done. This material slowly takes up water from the cervical mucus and swells, causing the cervix to slowly dilate, minimizing the possible damage. Balloons have been employed to effect similar results.

In suction curettage, a tube connected to a vacuum pump is introduced into the uterus through the dilated cervix. This device then withdraws the contents of the uterus, thereby terminating the pregnancy. Curettage can also be accomplished by mechanically scraping the lining of the uterus using special instruments.

## Control of Labor

The majority of this chapter has been concerned with the intensive care of the premature neonate. It would be better to eliminate the need for this care than to develop improved techniques and devices. Thus, a major problem in obstetrics is the prevention of premature labor. Our understanding of what causes premature labor, or even term labor for that matter, is still very limited, and this is one of the major areas in which additional studies are needed. At present, there is no effective way to prevent most premature labor.

The other aspect of control of labor involves inducing labor when this is deemed to be necessary. Labor can be induced by the continuous infusion of drugs that stimulate the uterus. Generally, this is done by the intravenous infusion of the appropriate materials using pumps, such as described in Section 15.6. These drugs, however, can overstimulate the uterus, producing a tetanic contraction that is extremely risky to the fetus as well as sometimes producing side effects. Thus, it is important when inducing labor to minimize the amount of drug given while getting optimal response. Steer (1979) has developed a feedback control system for the administration of oxytocin, a uterine stimulant. He determines the uterine activity from recording intrauterine pressure and uses this to set the rate of oxytocin infusion. He was able to demonstrate a significant reduction in the amount of oxytocin required to achieve effective labor in his patients.

# REFERENCES

AMERICAN ACADEMY OF PEDIATRICS (1971). *Hospital care of newborn infants,* 5th ed. Evanston, IL.

BEHRMAN, R. E. (1977). *Neonatal-perinatal medicine: Diseases of the fetus and infant,* 2nd ed. St. Louis: Mosby.

BELL, E. F., and W. OH (1979). Fluid and electrolyte balance in very low birth weight infants. *Clin. Perinatol.,* 6: 139–50.

BOYLE, R. J. and W. OH (1978). Respiratory distress syndrome. *Clin. Perinatol.,* 5: 283–98.

BRÜCK, K. (1961). Temperature regulation in the newborn infant. *Biol. Neonate,* 3: 65.

DAVIS, R. H., H. A. PLATT, D. K. MOONKA, and J. B. KESSEL (1979). Chronic occlusion of the monkey fallopian tube with silicone polymer. *Obstet. Gynecol.,* 53: 527.

GLUCK, L. (1970). Design of a perinatal center. *Pediatr. Clin. North Am.,* 17: 777.

KLAUS, M. H., R. JERAULD, N. C. KREGER, W. MCALPINE, M. STEFFA, and J. H. KENNELL (1972). Maternal attachment: Importance of the first post-partum days. *N. Eng. J. Med.,* 286: 460.

NEUMAN, M. R. (1973). Two simple safety devices for use with I-A and I-V lines on neonates. *Proc. Annu. Conf. Eng. Med. Biol.,* 15: 243.

NEUMAN, M. R. (1979). The biophysical and bioengineering bases of perinatal monitoring — Part V: Neonatal cardiac and respiratory monitoring. *Perinatology/Neonatology,* 3(2): 17–23.

PERLSTEIN, P. H., N. K. EDWARDS, and J. M. SUTHERLAND (1970). Apnea in premature infants and incubator-air-temperature changes. *N. Eng. J. Med.,* 282: 461.

STEER, P. J. (1979). *The quantitation of uterine activity and the control of induced labour.* Personal communication (submitted for publication).

STERN, L. (1973). The use and misuse of oxygen in the newborn infant. *Pediatr. Clin. North Am.,* 20: 447.

# STUDY QUESTIONS

15.1 How might the color of the walls of a neonatal intensive care unit affect the diagnosis of neonatal jaundice?

15.2 In one hospital design, there are glass windows between the neonatal intensive care unit and a waiting room for parents that has no outside windows. Discuss whether you think this will affect radiant heat balance from infants in the intensive care unit.

**15.3** When it is absolutely essential to have a window to the outside in a neonatal intensive care unit either because the unit is placed in an existing room that already has outside windows or the clinical staff insists on it, how can this be done to minimize radiative heat gain or heat loss from the patients? Describe several techniques that could be used.

**15.4** Explain why it is not practical for every hospital to have its own neonatal intensive care unit. What alternate approaches can be taken?

**15.5** The infant chamber in an incubator measures 78 × 45 × 32 cm. It is made of Plexiglas that is 6 mm thick. If the infant chamber temperature is maintained at 34°C and the nursery room temperature is 25°C, how much heat loss is there through the hood over the infant chamber? *Note:* The thermal conductivity of Plexiglas may be taken as 4 BTU$\cdot$h$^{-1}\cdot$ft$^{-2}$ at a temperature gradient of 1°F/in. (For those of you concerned about this not being in S. I. units, this is the way that engineering data of this type are usually found in catalogs and tables,)

**15.6** An early form of neonatal incubator consisted of a double-walled chamber made of glass, metal, and wood with the walls separated by approximately 2 in. Heated water was circulated in the space between the two walls. Consider this design from the standpoint of caring for a premature infant and keeping him in a neutral thermal environment and discuss the relative merits and demerits of such a design.

**15.7** The text mentions several factors that affect the neonatal neutral thermal environment. Consider each of these and describe how these either raise or lower the energy requirements of the infant.

**15.8** Radiant warmers are used only with infants who are receiving some acute form of treatment and require considerable handling. Explain why it is undesirable to use a radiant warmer for the long-term care of premature infants. What problems exist, and why do these make it difficult to use the radiant warmer for chronic care?

**15.9** The air temperature directly over the head of a neonate in an incubator was measured to be 33.7°C, while the temperature just beyond the feet of the infant was 36.4°C. Why is there a temperature difference between the head and feet of the infant? What can be done to minimize this temperature difference? If the incubator has proportional electronic temperature control, where would be the best place to put the temperature sensor? Consider the placement of the thermometer in the incubator in Fig. 15.1. Is this location the best for determining the temperature for the neutral thermal environment of the infant?

**15.10** Explain what changes have to be made in an adult ventilator to make it appropriate for use with a neonate.

**15.11** A nasal cannula for administering continuous positive air pressure (CPAP) as shown in Fig. 15.3 can be modeled as several circular cylinders. The nasal cannulae themselves have a 3.5-mm diameter lumen and are each 12 mm long. They are connected to an 8-mm diameter tube that is 18 mm long. This, in turn, is connected to a larger fitting that has an internal diameter of 12 mm and is 15 mm long. How much dead space does this add to the neonatal breathing circuit? Assuming the neonate has a lung volume of 50 ml, what percentage of this volume is the additional dead space?

**15.12** In problem 15.11, you calculated the additional dead space added to the neonatal pulmonary system by the use of the CPAP nasal cannula. Considering the design of this cannula, can you suggest ways that this dead space can be minimized?

**15.13** Why is it necessary to nebulize or humidify the air–oxygen mixture administered to the neonate through an oxygen hood? *Hint:* Be sure to review Chapter 13 before answering this question.

**15.14** Design an instrument that can be used to measure the radiant power from a phototherapy unit. Carry your design out to the block-diagram stage and explain the function of each block in your system. What blocks are critical to the function of the instrument and what are these critical factors? What practical considerations must you make in your design to achieve an instrument that can be conveniently used in the neonatal intensive care unit?

**15.15** What safety features should be incorporated into a neonatal phototherapy unit before it is certified for use in the neonatal intensive care unit?

**15.16** Derive an expression for the volume, $V$, of fresh blood received by a neonate who is undergoing exchange transfusion. The neonatal blood volume is $V_B$ and the rate of infusion (and withdrawal) is $\alpha$. You may assume rapid mixing in the neonate. How much blood must be administered to completely change 50% of the neonate's original blood? How much fresh blood is required to effect a 90% exchange?

**15.17** How may you carefully weigh an infant to determine whether he is in water balance? What errors can occur when this is the only method used to monitor water balance?

**15.18** In Fig. 15.7, the block labeled *electronic control circuit* is not well defined. Design in block diagram form the electronic control circuit for a device for maintaining a constant rate of intravenous fluid infusion and explain the operation of the system.

**15.19** How can each of the therapeutic devices described in this chapter affect water loss from the neonate?

**15.20** What advantages does laparoscopic tubal sterilization have over the conventional method of surgical ligation?

# 16 Radiation Therapy

*Philip H. Heintz*
*David R. Asche*

## 16.1 LEARNING OBJECTIVES

Upon completing this chapter you will be able to:

- Define cancer and describe its mechanism of growth and spread.
- Describe the principles of cancer treatment by radiation therapy.
- Describe the basic principles of radiation biology and physics.
- Define and discuss the design of equipment for radiation therapy.

## 16.2 WHAT IS CANCER?

Cancer is a large variety of malignant tumors with lethal potential. Cancer cells can arise in any body tissue at any age. Characteristically, they can invade local tissues by direct extension, or they can spread throughout the body through vessels.

Patterns and incidence of disease vary with sex, age, race, and geographic location. In females, the most common cancers are those of breast, colon, uterus, and skin. In males, the common lesions are those of lungs, gastrointestinal tract, skin, prostate, oral cavity, larynx, pharynx, and bladder (Rubin, 1978).

The exact cause of cancer remains undetermined; however, there is increasing evidence to indicate that cancer may arise from genetic mutations. Cancer seems to arise from normal tissue. Unless cancer cells are always present in normal tissue, normal tissue must be transformed into cancer.

The primary goal of cancer therapy is to cure the patient of the disease, but if the disease is judged to be incurable, then to implement palliative therapy. Palliative therapy relieves life-threatening symptoms and improves the overall quality of life.

## 16.3 FUNDAMENTALS OF CANCER TREATMENT

### Modes of Treatment

There are four modes of treatment open to the cancer patient: surgery, chemotherapy, radiation therapy, and a combination of two or all three of these. Surgery is the oldest and most widely used method for the treatment of malignant diseases. In surgery, we excise the local lesion, plus a generous margin of normal tissue, along with the regional lymph nodes. Chemotherapy seeks to control systemic spread of cancer by the use of drugs. The anticancer drugs interfere with the growth and spread of malignant cells. Radiation therapy employs the use of ionizing radiation, such as x radiation, to completely eradicate cancerous tissue. The cancer patient today usually receives a multimodal course of treatment. That is, he receives at least two of these modalities during his course of treatment.

### The Interaction of Radiation with Matter

Many forms of radiation produce biological effects, but radiation therapy is concerned only with the application of ionizing radiation. Figure 16.1 shows how biological damage may occur. The incident radiation, usually x rays or gamma rays, produces fast electrons, which in turn produce secondary ionization, which produces free radicals. The free radicals then produce chemical changes by breaking molecular bonds, thereby producing the end biological effect.

   **Physics.** Ionizing radiations are subdivided into two groups: electromagnetic radiations and particulate radiations. There are two types of electromagnetic radiations: x rays and gamma rays. Particulate radiations include beta particles (electrons), alpha particles, neutrons, and heavy nuclei. Electromagnetic radiation is the most widely used mode of treatment for radiation therapy. Electron beams are also used to a limited extent.

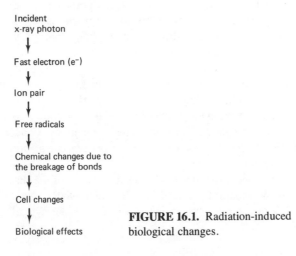

Incident
x-ray photon

Fast electron (e⁻)

Ion pair

Free radicals

Chemical changes due to
the breakage of bonds

Cell changes

Biological effects

**FIGURE 16.1.** Radiation-induced biological changes.

The terms *x rays* and *gamma rays* are used to describe ionizing electromagnetic radiation. Although these radiations are identical, the name characterizes their respective origins. X rays originate from electron interactions outside the nucleus, whereas gamma rays are radiation emitted spontaneously by radioactive nuclei undergoing nuclear transitions. The term *photon* is often used to describe both x rays and gamma rays. The energy of the photon is given by

$$E = h\nu \qquad (16.1)$$

where $\nu$ is the frequency of the electromagnetic radiation. Energy is measured in electron volts (eV). An electron volt is the energy acquired by an electron when it falls through a potential difference of 1 V. $h$ represents Planck's constant, $6.62 \times 10^{-34}$ J·s.

*Example 16.1:* Calculate the energy of a gamma ray with a wave length ($\omega$) of 10 pm.

$$E = h\nu = \frac{hc}{\omega}$$

$$E \text{ (keV)} = \frac{(6.62 \times 10^{-34} \text{ J·s}) (3 \times 10^8 \text{ m/s})}{(10\text{pm}) (10^{-12} \text{ m/pm}) (1.6 \times 10^{-16} \text{ J/keV})}$$

$$E = \frac{1241}{10 \text{ pm}} = 124 \text{ keV}$$

X rays are generated by accelerating electrons through some potential, allowing them to strike a target and, in turn, to interact with target nuclei. The predominate mode of interaction is by the bremsstrahlung reaction in which the electron slows down from coulombic interaction with the target nuclei. Electrons are slowed and deflected, which produces an energy loss. The loss of energy is released in the form of x rays. A monoenergetic electron beam produces a spectrum of x-ray energies through this reaction. The energy of the x-ray beam is given the unit kVp or kV, corresponding to the energy of the electron beam (in keV).

Photon sources are usually small and may be considered point sources. If the source is emitted freely in air unperturbed by matter, its intensity decreases inversely as the square of the distance from the source. This principle is called the inverse square law.

*Example 16.2:* An x-ray beam emits 2,000 photons/s at 1 m. What is its intensity at 2 m?

$$\text{intensity} = I = \left(\frac{d_2}{d_1}\right)^2 \times I_0$$

$$I \text{ at 2 m} = \left(\frac{1 \text{ m}}{2 \text{ m}}\right)^2 \times 2,000 \text{ photon/s}$$

$$I = 500 \text{ photons/s}$$

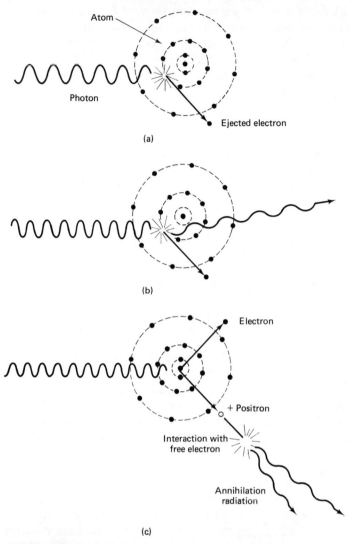

**FIGURE 16.2.** The interaction of electromagnetic radiation with matter (a) photoelectric effect (b) Compton effect (c) pair production.

Electromagnetic radiation interacts with a medium by one of three processes: photoelectric effect, Compton effect, and pair production. Their relative importance varies with the energy of the incident photon and the nature of the absorber. The fast-moving electrons released by these reactions produce further ionization and the biological effect. Figure 16.2 shows these reactions.

The photoelectric effect occurs when a photon of energy less than 100 keV strikes one of the innermost electrons. The entire energy of the photon is transferred to the electron, which is ejected from the atom. The Compton effect, or Compton scattering, is the dominant reaction of photons between 30 kVp and 30 MeV. In this reaction, the photon scatters off one of the loosely bound orbiting electrons, transferring only part of its energy to the ejected electron. The process of pair production occurs with photons above 1.02 MeV, where the photon interacts near the nucleus of the atom, producing two particles: a positive electron (positron) and a negative electron. The incident photon completely disappears, but its energy reappears in the form of two particles. Excess energy above 1.02 MeV is transferred to the particles in the form of kinetic energy.

Microscopically, photons can undergo one, two, or all three of these reactions when interacting with a tissue medium. From a macroscopic point of view, we are only concerned with the total number of interactions, or the absorption of the beam, not the type of reactions. If a parallel beam of photons is incident upon an absorber, the intensity $N_0$ (photon $\cdot$ cm$^{-2}$ $\cdot$ s$^{-1}$) of the radiation is reduced to a value $N$ at some depth $r$ cm in the slab. The reduction of photons is due to interactions of photons with the individual atoms of the absorber. The absorption is described by

$$N = N_0 e^{-\mu r} \qquad (16.2)$$

where $\mu$ is the linear attenuation coefficient for a particular absorber and photon energy. The linear attenuation coefficient is the fraction of energy lost per centimeter of absorber by the photons.

*Example 16.3:*    A beam of x rays of intensity 100 photons $\cdot$ cm$^{-2}$ $\cdot$ s$^{-1}$ is reduced to 50 photons $\cdot$ cm$^{-2}$ $\cdot$ s$^{-1}$ by a slab of tissue 10 cm thick. What is the linear attenuation coefficient of the tissue?

$$N = N_0 e^{-\mu r}$$

$$\ln \frac{N}{N_0} = -\mu r$$

$$\mu = \frac{-1}{r} \cdot \ln \frac{N}{N_0} = \frac{-1}{10 \text{ cm}} \cdot \ln \left( \frac{50}{100} \right) = 0.0693 \text{ cm}^{-1}$$

The thickness of a slab of matter required to reduce the intensity of a photon beam to one half is the half value layer (HVL) or the half value thickness (HVT). HVL is found by letting $N$ equal $N_0/2$ and $r$ equal HVL in equation 16.2.

$$\text{HVL} = \frac{0.693}{\mu} \qquad (16.3)$$

The half value layer describes the (quality) or the penetrability of the beam.

As a beam of radiation passes through tissue, energy from the beam is absorbed. Two quantities have been defined to express the amount of radiation present: *exposure* and *absorbed dose*. Equation 16.4 defines radiation exposure, $X$. $Q$ represents charge liberated as x or gamma rays interact with a small volume of air of mass $m$.

$$X = \frac{Q}{m} \qquad\qquad\qquad (16.4)$$

The unit of radiation exposure is the *roentgen* (R).

$$1 \text{ R} = 2.58 \times 10^{-4} \text{ C/kg of air}$$

The absorbed dose $D$ is defined by equation 16.5.

$$D = \frac{E}{m} \qquad\qquad\qquad (16.5)$$

where $E$ is the absorbed energy and $m$ is the mass. The unit of absorbed dose is the *rad*.

$$1 \text{ rad} = \frac{0.01 \text{ J}}{\text{kg}}$$

The energy absorbed in air from 1 R is equal to 0.869 rads. However, in radiation therapy, we are interested in the absorbed dose in tissue, not in air. If 1 R of radiation is incident upon a small volume of tissue, the absorbed dose is close to 1 rad; that is, for cobalt 60 irradiation, 1 R equals 0.957 rads.

*Example 16.4:*   A dose of 6,000 rads is delivered uniformly throughout a tumor volume. If the tumor has a mass of 10 g, what is the total absorbed energy in joules?

$$D = \frac{E}{m}$$

or

$$E = mD$$

$$E = 6{,}000 \text{ rads} \times \frac{10^{-2} \text{ J}}{\text{kg} \cdot \text{rad}} \times 10 \text{ g} \times \frac{\text{kg}}{1000 \text{ g}}$$

$$E = 0.6 \text{ J}$$

Another quantity used to express the amount of energy absorbed is the *rem*. This unit accounts for the different biological effects of particulate radiation. For x and gamma radiation, a rem is equal to a rad. For neutrons and alpha particles, the rem may be 2–10 × greater than the absorbed dose in rads (Johns and Cunningham, 1969).

**Radioactive Decay.**   The atoms of radioactive material are unstable and spontaneously undergo radioactive decay. They emit either electromagnetic radiation or particles, or both. The rate of decay is referred to as the *activity* of the sample. The unit of activity is the curie (Ci) defined as: 1 Ci = $3.7 \times 10^{10}$ disintegrations per second.

The disintegration rate or activity is proportional to the number of radioactive atoms of the sample present.

$$A = -\lambda N \qquad (16.6)$$

$\lambda$ is the decay constant and is characteristic for a particular radioisotope. The activity $A$ is expressed mathematically as a function of time as follows:

$$A = A_0 e^{-\lambda t} \qquad (16.7)$$

where $t$ is the time and $A_0$ is the initial activity. $\lambda$ can be expressed in terms of half-life $t_{\frac{1}{2}}$ of a radioisotope as shown in equation 16.8.

$$\lambda = \frac{0.693}{t_{\frac{1}{2}}} \qquad (16.8)$$

*Half-life* is the time it takes for $^1/_2$ the radioactive atoms present at any time to decay ($A = ^1/_2 A_0$).

**Biology.** It is the high-speed electrons that start the chain of events that ultimately result in the biological changes. Next in the chain is the interaction of the high-speed electrons with the molecules in the tissue irradiated. About 85% of living tissue is made of water. Therefore, the most probable interaction of radiation is on water, producing highly reactive H and O ions. The irradiated water ions in turn produce the chemical changes in the sensitive macromolecules of the cell system (RNA and DNA molecules).

Chemical changes ultimately result in damage to cells. Cell damage depends upon the amount of energy absorbed and on the spatial distribution. Figure 16.3 shows a typical survival curve for mammalian cells. Cell survival shown here is for mitotic death. The frequency of cell division is the most important factor influencing cell survival: more divisions—more sensitivity to radiation.

The effects of radiation on organs and organ systems depend upon (1) the volume of tissue irradiated, (2) the anatomical site irradiated, (3) radiation absorbed dose, (4) rate at which radiation is delivered, and (5) dose fractionation. (Fractionation is the division of the prescribed dose into daily fractions.) We must consider these factors when designing a course of radiation therapy for the cancer patient (Pizzarello and Witcofski, 1972).

## Radiation Safety and Protection

Persons working around equipment that produces radiation have the potential of being exposed. Because all ionizing radiation kills cells and has a potential to cause cancer, governmental agencies have established the *maximum permissible dose* (MPD) levels for persons working around sources of radiation. The MPD is 5 rem per year, or 1.25 rem per quarter. For the general public, the limit is 0.5 rem per

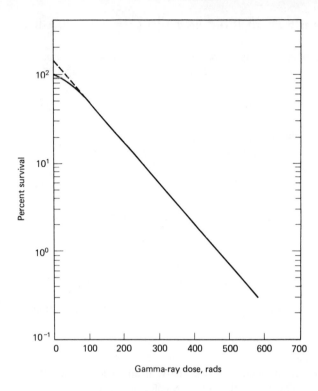

**FIGURE 16.3.** Typical mammalian cell survival curve for single acute gamma ray exposure.

The y-axis is labeled "Percent survival" with values $10^2$, $10^1$, $10^0$, $10^{-1}$. The x-axis is labeled "Gamma-ray dose, rads" with values 0, 100, 200, 300, 400, 500, 600, 700.

year. It is important to point out that the maximum permissible dose does not mean a completely safe dose. It means that, in light of the present knowledge, this dose is not expected to cause appreciable bodily injury to a person at any time during his lifetime. Effort must be maintained at all times to keep all occupational exposures to a minimum. There are three significant concepts to be utilized in the reduction of exposure. The first is *time*—the shorter the duration of exposure to ionizing radiation, the lower the dose. The second is *distance*. Because we are dealing primarily with point sources, the greater the distance between the individual and the radiation source, the lower the exposure (inverse square law). The third is *shielding*. The total exposure can be reduced by providing adequate shielding between the individual and the radiation source.

## 16.4 OVERVIEW OF RADIATION THERAPY

The aim of radiation therapy is to eradicate all of the malignant cells in a tumor or to render them permanently incapable of further cell division, without producing excessive damage to the normal tissue surrounding the tumor. Ionizing radiations have the same effect on both normal and malignant cells, but, fortunately, the malignant cells are generally more sensitive to radiation than normal cells. It is this difference and the fact that normal cells, under homeostatic control, can repopulate faster than cancer cells, that make it possible to use ionizing radiation to destroy malignant cells without producing excessive damage to normal cells surrounding the tumor.

We start radiation therapy by localizing the tumor. Tumor localization is particularly important in radiation therapy because we must know the extent of the tumor in order to treat the entire volume and to know the anatomical relationship of the tumor to neighboring radiosensitive organs such as spine, lung, and eyes. Following tumor localization, we decide upon the modality of radiotherapy. Therapeutic modalities are usually divided into two categories: external beam therapy and implant therapy.

## External Beam Therapy

In external beam therapy, we treat the tumor by a beam of radiation from an external source of radiation. Radiation beams of varying energy and penetrating power are available and the choice of radiation beam varies with the anatomical site of the tumor. We treat skin and superficial lesions with x-ray beams of energy in the 40–300 kV range. We treat deeper lesions by beams of higher energy, such as those produced by linear accelerators of 4–25 MV or a cobalt 60 unit.

We adjust the dimensions and shape of the radiation beam by the use of collimators placed around the exit of the beam from the treatment unit and by the insertion of suitably shaped lead blocks placed in the path of the beam. We may combine two or more converging beams to achieve uniform irradiation of a deep or asymmetrically shaped tumor volume. Figure 16.4 shows several possible combinations of beams appropriate for varying locations of tumors.

We give external beam treatments with the patient lying on a motorized table or couch. We move the couch to position the patient under the beam of radiation. The unit projects a light field demarcating the extent of the treatment field onto the patient for localization. We perform final positioning of the patient by aligning the marks on the patient's skin with the localizing field and setting up the proper treatment distance. The technologist remains outside the shielded room during treatment and monitors the patient with a closed-circuit television system and intercom.

We rarely give single treatments in external beam therapy and generally give daily fractions over a period of 4–6 weeks. Total tumor dose for such a course of treatment could vary from 3,000–7,000 rads.

## Implant Therapy

We divide implant therapy into two categories: interstitial therapy and intracavitary therapy. In both types of implant therapy, the tumor is treated by implantation of radioactive sources. In interstitial therapy, we geometrically arrange the radioactive sources so that a uniform dose of radiation is delivered to the entire tumor volume. This technique is generally used only for superficial lesions such as carcinoma of the tongue, skin, breast, and so on. In intracavitary therapy, the tumor is irradiated by the radioactive sources maintained in suitable applicators or molds. Most intra-

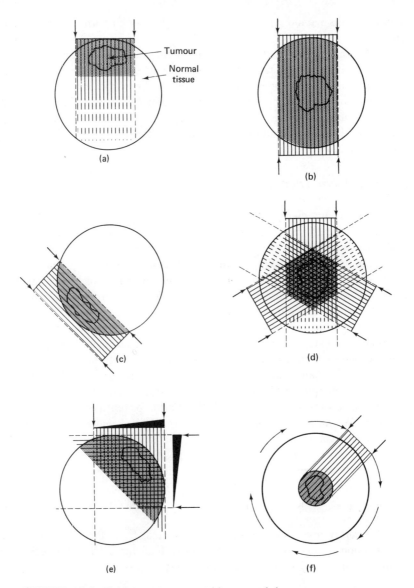

**FIGURE 16.4.** Field arrangements with external beam radiation therapy (a) Stationary single field (b) Parallel opposed fields (c) Tangential fields (d) Multiple isocenter fields (e) Converging wedged fields (f) Rotating single field.

cavitary therapy involves gynecological treatments, where the radioactive sources can be placed in the middle of the tumor (Barnes and Rees, 1972).

A typical implant for either type of therapy produces a uniform dose rate of about 1,000 rads per day to the entire tumor volume. Because the implant is usually left in for several days, the tumor dose can vary from 2,000 to 7,000 rads.

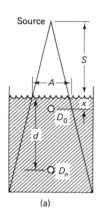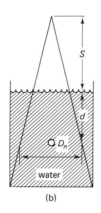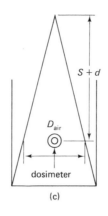

**FIGURE 16.5.** (a) Definition of %DD. (b&c) Definition of TAR (see text).

## 16.5 EXTERNAL BEAM TREATMENT PLANNING AND DOSIMETRY

### Simulation

Before a patient starts external radiation therapy, we must localize the radiation field on a simulator. A simulator is identical to a treatment unit mechanically, except that a diagnostic x-ray tube replaces the radiation source. Thus, we may take radiographs with the unit in the treatment position to confirm the accurate localization of the treatment fields and the tumor volume. If the prescribed radiation plan is complex, that is, something other than simple anterior–posterior opposed fields, then we must gather more information during simulation. This usually includes taking orthogonal (anterior–posterior and lateral) x-ray films of the tumor volume and obtaining the patient's cross-sectional contour through the middle of the tumor to be treated. The additional simulator information is used to plan the treatment.

### Treatment Planning and Dose Calculation

Planning complex radiation therapy techniques requires the definition of new physics terms. Figure 16.5 shows the depth dose $D_n$ as the radiation dose delivered at some point within a patient. The fractional depth dose is the ratio of $D_n$ to the absorbed dose $D_0$ at the surface or at maximum depth dose along the central axis of the beam. The *percentage depth dose* %DD is the fractional depth dose multiplied by 100.

$$\%DD = \frac{D_n}{D_0} \times 100$$

$$(16.9)$$

Figure 16.6 plots percentage depth dose for beams of various energies as a function of depth below the surface of a patient. The percentage depth dose increases rapidly from the surface until an equilibrium depth is reached. Beyond the equilibrium depth, it decreases slowly. The slope of this curve beyond the equilibrium depth is

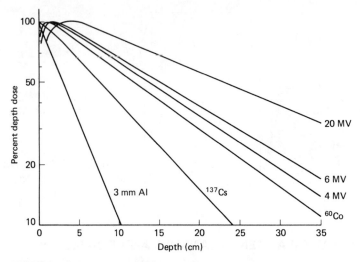

FIGURE 16.6. Percent depth dose for x and gamma ray
beams of different energies, plotted as a function of depth
in tissue. 100% point is depth of dose maximum.

a measure of the penetrability. The higher the energy of the machine, the shallower
the slope of the curve and the more penetrating the beam.

*Example 16.5:* We desire an absorbed dose of 180 rads per day for a tumor
located 8 cm below the surface. An 8 × 8 cm cobalt 60 beam is used at 80-
cm source skin distance (SSD). What is the dose per treatment at the depth of
dose maximum (0.5 cm deep)? If the exposure rate is 55 R/min at dose
maximum, what treatment time should we use? (%DD @ 8 cm = 62.7).

$$\%DD = \frac{D_n}{D_0} \times 100$$

or

$$D_0 = \frac{D_n}{\%DD} \times 100 = \frac{180}{62.7} \times 100 = 287 \text{ rads}$$

Dose rate at 0.5 cm deep = 55 R/min × 0.957 rad/R

= 52.6 rad/min

$$\text{Time} = \frac{287 \text{ rad}}{52.6 \text{ rad/min}} = 5.45 \text{ min}$$

If we treat the tumor by rotating the source around the patient, for example, 360°,
then we position the center of the tumor at the axis of rotation. We compute

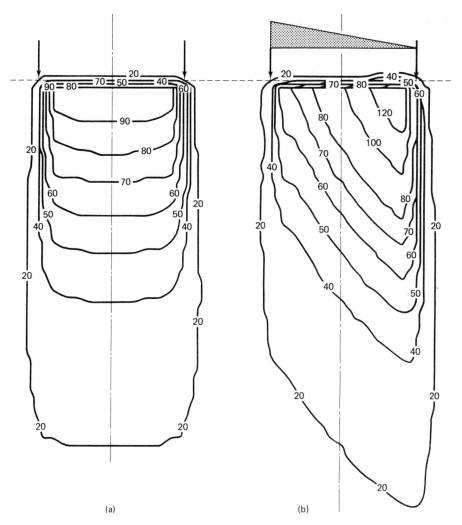

**FIGURE 16.7.** (a) Isodose distribution for a $10 \times 10$ field at 80 cm SSD (a) for cobalt 60 teletherapy unit and (b) with a 45 degree wedge on a cobalt teletherapy unit.

radiation dose delivered to the tumor with *tissue–air ratio*. The tissue–air ratio, or TAR, is

$$\text{TAR} = \frac{D_\text{n}}{D_\text{air}} \qquad (16.10)$$

where $D_\text{n}$ is the absorbed dose at the axis of rotation in a tissue and $D_\text{air}$ is the absorbed dose to soft tissue at the same location with the tissue removed. The tissue–air ratio is similar to the fractional depth dose, except that we determine the reference absorbed dose in air at the center of rotation (the isocenter) instead of the surface of the medium. To compute the absorbed dose to an off-axis location, an isodose distribution for the photon beam is necessary. Figure 16.7a shows an isodose distribution for a $10 \times 10$ cm cobalt 60 beam at 80-cm SSD (source skin distance). The shapes of the isodose curves are determined by the uniformity of the primary beam leaving the treatment machine and by the contribution of scattered radiation to the absorbed dose along the edge of the beam (Hendee, 1970).

Photon beams are mixed in various ways to furnish isodose patterns that are useful for certain procedures in radiation therapy. If a proposed radiation therapy treatment plan calls for the angle of intersection of two beams to be other than parallel, it may be necessary to alter the uniformity of the radiation field to achieve a homogeneous dose within the tumor volume. In this case, we may introduce a wedge filter in the beam between the source and the patient to slope the isodose curves. Figure 16.7b shows the effect of such a wedged filter on the $10 \times 10$ cm isodose curve.

Using the information just described and the patient's contour obtained during simulation, we can determine the pattern of radiation dose within the patient. By putting the patient's contour, tumor location, and inhomogeneities such as air cavities, bone, and so on, into the computer, along with the measured isodose data, the computer very accurately determines the dose distribution for virtually any plan desired. Many commercial treatment-planning computers are now on the market. Such computer systems are so sophisticated that graphics are totally interactive, some being capable of optimizing treatment plans without operator intervention.

## 16.6 EXTERNAL BEAM THERAPY EQUIPMENT

The basic features of a machine used in external beam therapy include a radiation source, collimation to shape the beam, and a patient-support assembly or couch. Each type of machine to be discussed employs different design parameters, but the basic parts are the same. All external beam machines, and especially the mega-voltage units, are capable of delivering potentially lethal doses of radiation to patients or personnel. As a result, the design uses a "fail-safe" philosophy. Interlocks turn off the therapy beam (or prohibit its coming on) if a problem or forbidden condition exists in one of the monitored systems. To aid in servicing the equipment, most machines provide a visual indication of the problem area at the operator's console. A good example of a safety interlock system is found at the treatment-room door. Switches are placed at each door. These switches require that the door be closed before the unit can be turned on, thus preventing medical personnel and the patient from receiving accidental exposure. The size of the treatment field is defined by a collimator. The collimator allows the definition of all rectangular beams from $0 \times 0$ cm to fields greater than $30 \times 30$ cm. If fields other than rectangles are prescribed, then we must provide additional external blocking of the beam.

We must also provide a means of localizing the beam during the setup on the patient when a beam is not present. We normally accomplish this by the use of a light field that is coincident with the emitted radiation field. Crosshairs locate the center of the field.

The geometry and the intensity of the beam change with distance from the apparent source of radiation (inverse square law). Therefore, an optical distance indicator permits aligning the patient at the proper distance.

Stationary and rotational units are available commercially. Rotational units are designed to rotate about a point in space, termed isocenter, such that the source remains at a fixed distance from this point as it rotates. This variation is generally specified to be within ±1 mm of true isocenter throughout the full 360° rotation. Rotational units have the advantage of rotating with the radiation beam on or lessening the setup time when used to set up patients with multiple stationary fields. These advantages are highlighted when the facility also employs the use of ceiling and lateral wall lights, aligned to intersect at the axis of rotation.

All therapy machines have radiation shielding. Because photons are produced in all directions, only the useful radiation must be allowed to escape. This is achieved by surrounding the radiation source with lead or tungsten shielding. The only radiation to leave the shielded volume is through the collimator. In order to protect the treatment personnel from radiation exposure, the machine is surrounded by concrete or lead walls that reduce the radiation levels as low as possible. Typical wall thickness may be 1–2 m thick concrete.

## Cobalt Teletherapy Unit

Cobalt 60 units are the simplest of all megavoltage therapy devices. The radioactive cobalt is contained within a doubly encapsulated stainless steel cylinder. The source size is approximately 1–2 cm in diameter and 3 cm high. The beam is turned on by moving the source to a position where part of the shielding is removed, thus permitting the radiation to escape the shielded container. To terminate the beam the source is moved back to the fully shielded position. This is usually accomplished by a source drawer or tray to which the source is physically attached. The drawer slides in and out in a horizontal direction driven by a pneumatic system.

Pneumatic systems are often chosen for use in cobalt units due to their relative simplicity and high reliability. The pressure in the pneumatic system is monitored at all times, and should it fall below a preset level, the source is automatically retracted regardless of the timer setting.

The system for controlling patient exposure is a timing device that is designed such that the starting of the timer initiates the movement of the source. Likewise, the termination of the timer terminates the exposure by returning the source to the off position.

Special controls are necessary if we use rotational therapy. We must control the direction and the rate of source rotation, as well as the time during which the source is on or off. Through the use of electrical commutators, most cobalt units are capable of continuous rotation. Figure 16.8 shows a typical cobalt unit.

## Linear Accelerator

Figure 16.9 shows that the medical linear accelerator looks like a cobalt unit. It has the same basic features, including shielding, collimation, and a patient-support

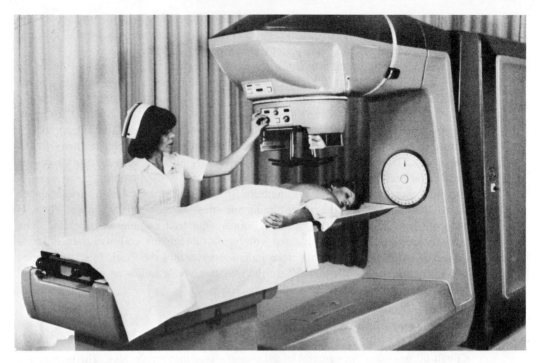

**FIGURE 16.8.** Rotational cobalt teletherapy unit. (Courtesy AECL Medical, Division of Atomic Energy of Canada Limited.)

device. What makes the linear accelerator different is its source of radiation. It uses an assembly of electromechanical systems to produce high energy x-ray and electron beams. Figure 16.10 shows a block diagram of the device (Karzmark and Pering, 1973).

An accelerator guide operating at microwave frequencies (2–3 GHz) accelerates electrons to the desired energy and then bombards a target with the electron beam. The electrons interact by the bremsstrahlung reaction and produce electromagnetic radiation or x rays. A klystron or a magnetron produces the microwave power used in the accelerator guide. The modulator pulses this microwave tube with a high dc pulse. A high-voltage power supply is necessary to charge the modulator circuitry. A control unit adjusts power levels and timing necessary for efficient acceleration and x-ray production.

**Microwave Cavities.** When operating at microwave frequencies above 1 GHz, we can design very high-efficiency circuits. To understand the derivation of the microwave cavity, we review a low-frequency LC circuit. This circuit consists of a discrete lumped constant capacitor and inductor connected in parallel. When properly energized, this circuit oscillates at a single frequency. To increase resonant frequency, we reduce the value of both the capacitor and the inductor. As we tune this circuit to the microwave frequencies, the parallel plates of the capacitor begin to merge on their periphery with a large number of parallel, partially turned inductors. When totally enclosed, the circuit becomes a resonant cavity. Although

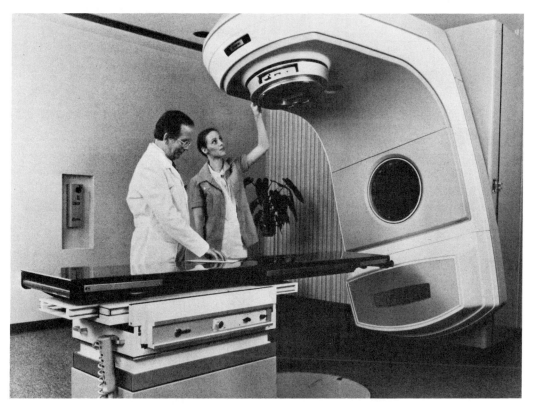

**FIGURE 16.9.** A 6-MV medical linear accelerator. (Courtesy of Varian Associates, Palo Alto, CA.)

true microwave cavities are capable of oscillating at an infinite number of resonant frequencies, we usually employ the lowest frequency in accelerator technology. Because this microwave cavity is totally enclosed, it cannot radiate energy in free space and, consequently, if resistive losses are low, the cavity has a high $Q$. If the cavity consists of copper and is operated at 3 GHz, a typical unloaded value of $Q$ would be 15,000. The power of the cavity is defined by the electric and magnetic intensities.

**Accelerator Guide.** The accelerator guide consists of a series of colinear microwave cavities (see Fig. 16.11). In traveling wave accelerator guides, the high-energy microwaves sequentially excite the cavities. As the wave travels down the guide, it develops high-intensity electric fields in the direction of the acceleration across each cavity. Electrons are injected into the accelerator guide and essentially ride this wave, much as a surfboard rider would catch a wave and ride it. In standing wave accelerator guides, the incident wave reflects off the end of the guide such that it returns in phase with the incident wave. Because the coupled cavities are spaced with a $\Pi/2$ phase shift, alternating cavities are located at electric field nodes. Because these cavities have essentially zero field at all times, they have no effect on the acceleration. These cavities may then be moved off axis to provide a

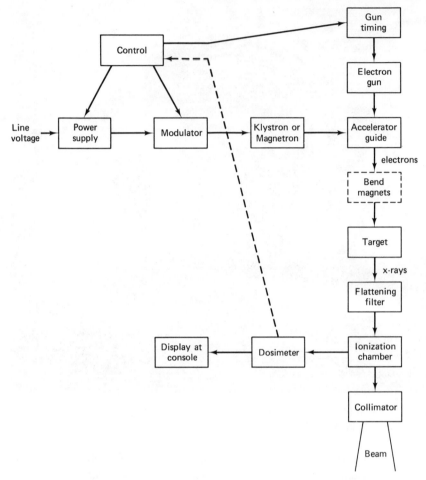

**FIGURE 16.10.** Functional block diagram of a simplified linear accelerator.

bimodal structure, which consists of the central accelerating cavities and the side-coupled cavities. The standing waveguide technology provides a much shorter accelerating guide with equivalent energy output.

**Microwave Power Generation.** The klystron and magnetron have the opposite operation to that described in the function of the accelerator guide. These tubes generate microwave power by extracting energy from electrons accelerated by a dc potential and injected into a resonant cavity whose decelerating electric field slows the electron bunch. Because energy must be conserved, the kinetic energy lost by the electron is transferred to the resonant electromagnetic field of the cavity, thereby producing RF power.

**Support Systems.** The accelerator guide, klystron, and magnetron deal with very high-energy electron beam currents. As a result, they must operate in a high

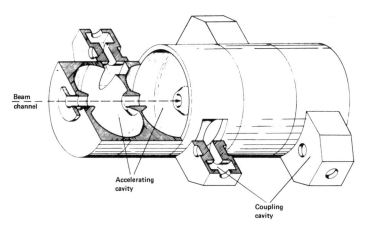

**FIGURE 16.11.** Cross section of standing wave guide for a medical linear accelerator. (Courtesy of Varian Associates; reprinted from Karmark and Pering, *Phys. Med. Biol.,* 18:330, 1973, © The Institute of Physics, 1973 with permission.)

Beam channel

Accelerating cavity

Coupling cavity

vacuum, typically $10^{-10}$ mmHg. The large electron currents require water cooling to all critical RF components to maintain thermal stability.

The modulator provides power to the microwave power tubes. The 100-kV dc pulse is provided by charging a series resonant circuit and pulsing it by switching a thyratron into a high-voltage transformer. The modulator operates at a voltage of 12 kV and a frequency of 30–360 Hz.

The gun injects electrons into the accelerator guide. The gun is a grid-controlled cathode pulsed in phase with the RF pulse of the accelerator guide. In high-energy machines, the accelerator guide may be too long to permit vertical mounting. In this case it is mounted horizontally and a bend magnet directs the accelerated electron beam into the target.

**Beam Monitoring** Following production, the "raw" x-ray beam enters the treatment head assembly, where it is flattened and scattered to produce a nearly uniform x-ray beam across the collimator opening. The ionization chamber then monitors the flattened or scattered beam. The chamber has minimal effects on the final therapeutic beam. Its primary function is to measure the radiation emitted by the accelerator. A dosimetry circuit converts the signal from the ionization chamber to a display at the operator's console. The console displays both the dose rate and the integrated dose. Termination of a treatment is by coincidence of the integrated dose with a preset dose set at the operator's console.

The ionization chamber is divided into four quadrants that are capable of independently recording radiation dose. Opposite quadrants of the chamber provide redundant dosimetry and evaluate the symmetry of the beam. Should the beam become asymmetric, the signal from one of these four quadrants would exceed the others and the interlock system would terminate exposure. This is an example of the fail-safe design in the linear accelerator.

In summary, linear accelerators are extremely complex devices, which makes in-house service difficult. As a result of this complexity, their reliability is not as good as cobalt and they have higher maintenance costs. The linear accelerator has a high dose rate, which allows very rapid treatment of patients. Linear accelerators are able to provide higher energies than cobalt for better depth penetration. They may provide electron beams as an alternate mode of therapy. Because there is no natural source of radiation, the fail-safe design philosophy has been heavily emphasized in its technology, and the medical linear accelerator has been designed to be a safe device.

### Betatron

**X-Ray Production.** Betatrons are similar to the linear accelerator, except that they accelerate electrons in a circular orbit using a time-varying magnetic flux. A hollow circular evacuated tube provides a frictionless path. This tube is made of glass or porcelain and is referred to as the "donut." The donut is mounted between the poles of an electromagnet that is energized by an alternating voltage, which oscillates between 50 and 180 Hz. The magnetic field generated by this electromagnet performs two functions. First, as the magnetic field changes, it induces the accelerating voltage and, second, because charged particles moving through a magnetic field are bent, it serves to create the circular path of the electrons within the betatron. The magnet creates an electron path of constant radius known as the "equilibrium orbit." An electron gun injects electrons into the donut with an energy of about 50 keV. Electrons accelerated to the proper energy are released from the equilibrium orbit by a brief reduction in the magnetic field intensity. This allows the electron orbit to expand and strike the target.

**Control Systems.** Control systems utilized in therapeutic betatrons parallel those used in linear accelerators with modifications for the different technologies. For example, the energy of the beam in a linear accelerator requires the control of the RF power injected into the accelerator guide. In the betatron, the instantaneous amplitude of the magnetic field determines the energy of the electrons in the equilibrium orbit. In multienergy machines, the beam-extraction circuits may be activated earlier in the cycle if a lower energy is desired. To maintain a beam of uniform energy, the extraction circuitry must be very carefully controlled so as to extract the electrons at the same point in the cycle.

For photon energies greater than 25 MV, the betatron is the primary device currently available.

### Kilovoltage Therapy Units

Kilovoltage therapy units are x-ray generating devices that normally operate between 100 and 500 kV. These are the simplest of the x-ray generating devices and were the first used in radiation therapy.

**X-Ray Generation.** The source of electrons is a filament in which a current flows. The current heats the filament and the electrons are boiled off through a process of thermionic emission. The filament is located within the cathode, which is negatively charged and is constructed to help focus the electrons emitted by the filament. Electrons are accelerated from the cathode to the anode by a positive accelerating voltage on the anode (target). At these energies, the accelerating voltage can be supported between the cathode and the anode without electrical breakdown. The electrons impinge upon the target, where x rays are produced. The electrons undergo the bremsstrahlung reaction, producing an x-ray beam. The peak photon energy obtained is equivalent to the peak voltage between the cathode and the anode. This reaction must take place in a vacuum to reduce the interaction of the electron beam with gas molecules. A typical vacuum is $10^{-5}$ mm Hg ($6.6 \times 10^{-3}$ Pa).

**Target.** The x-ray production efficiency of the tungsten target bombarded by 100-kV electrons is only 0.6%. This means that less than 1% of the energy deposited at the target is realized in the energy of the x-ray beam. Most of the energy is deposited as heat and, therefore, the target material must have a high melting point (tungsten melts at 3,330°C). The tube must be designed to remove the heat that accumulates from electron beam bombardment. Oil baths and water cooling coils help dissipate the excess anode heat.

**Control Systems.** We must consider three basic parameters when controlling the beam from a kilovoltage unit: energy, intensity, and the treatment time. The voltage between the cathode and the anode determines the energy of the beam. This is displayed at the operator's console as kV and is monitored from the primary side of the high-voltage transformer. On most units kV is adjustable from the operator's console. The current in the filament controls intensity. An adjustment for this current is also available at the console and displayed in terms of beam current. A timer similar to that used on cobalt units controls beam current. The timer activates the on–off switch, which applies voltage to the primaries of the high-voltage transformer. When timed out, it opens the switch and terminates the beam. Control circuits have been employed to regulate both kV and mA but, because there is no direct monitoring of the radiation produced by the machine, the output of kilovoltage units generally varies by a larger percentage than that of linear accelerators.

## 16.7 IMPLANT THERAPY—BRACHYTHERAPY

### Radioactive Sources

Implant therapy is performed with sealed sources of radioactive material placed near the cancer. The radioactive material employed most frequently has been radium ($^{226}$Ra). Artificially produced radioactive isotopes such as $^{137}$cesium, $^{192}$iridium, and $^{125}$iodine are being used with increasing frequency. The physical configuration of the radioactive sources falls into three categories: needles and tubes, wires, and seeds; $^{137}$Cs and $^{226}$Ra are primarily configured as needles and tubes. The radioactive materials combine with an inert filler to form a cylindrical cell. Figure 16.12 shows that the cells are doubly encapsulated in platinum or stainless steel tubing. Radioactive wires, usually $^{192}$Ir and $^{182}$Ta are produced as radioactive wire surrounded by a thin-wall tubing of stainless steel. Seeds are made from wire cut into small pieces 2–3 mm long.

Because radioactive sources constantly emit radiation, they must be stored in a shielded container between treatments. The most commonly used storage device is a lead safe with drawers to hold each of the different radioactive sources. This lead

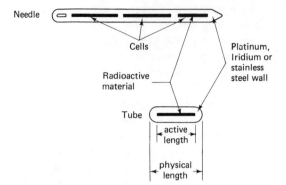

Needle

Cells

Platinum,
Iridium or
stainless
steel wall

Radioactive
material

Tube

active
length

physical
length

**FIGURE 16.12.** A needle and tube containing radioactive radium or cesium.

safe provides permanent protection to personnel while the sources are not in use. However, the use of radioactive sources inevitably involves some radiation danger to staff personnel and we must take care in the proper handling and the use of such sources.

## Interstitial Therapy

Interstitial therapy is a treatment modality in which the radioactive material in the form of needles or wires is directly implanted into the tumor. The type of implant used depends on the thickness and the size of the tumor mass.

Almost all implants are performed in surgery. In order to minimize radiation exposure to personnel, hollow tubes or guides are placed in the patient during surgery. The radioactive material is inserted after the patient has regained consciousness and has returned to his room.

In actual practice, it is extremely difficult to achieve the planned source distribution. Therefore, postoperative radiographs of all implants are taken. Orthogonal radiographs and/or stereoradiographs are taken of the implant to determine the true location of the needles and wires. Inspection of the radiographs enables the needle distribution to be visualized and to see if any serious malplacement has occurred, which results in hot or cold spots. Using either pair of radiographs, we can make calculations from the films to determine the actual radiation dose distribution through the tumor volume. These calculations are done either manually or, more precisely and faster, using computer programs.

Not all interstitial implants are temporary implants for which radioactive material is removed before the patient leaves the hospital. Some interstitial implants are permanent implants. Two such radioactive isotopes used for permanent interstitial implants are $^{125}I$ and $^{198}Au$. Permanent implants are generally used for deep-seated tumors that require long surgical procedures to localize the lesion. Once the patient is surgically open, the radioactive material, in the form of seeds, is injected into the tumor volume. The patient is closed and kept in the hospital until the activity of the radioactive material has decayed to less than 30 mCi. The patient is then allowed to convalesce at home and then goes on with a normal life, maintaining this radioactive material in him for the rest of his life.

## Intracavitary Therapy

Intracavitary therapy involves a system that maintains a radioactive material in a relatively rigid relationship with the anatomy. The physical relationship of the applicator is two ovoids positioned in the vagina and an intrauterine tube. Insertions of this type are performed in surgery under general anesthesia. We insert the hollow applicator and pack it to push the normal anatomy away from the applicator inside the patient, place dummy sources inside the hollow tubes of the applicator, and take orthogonal x rays of the implant. We place radiopaque dyes in the bladder and rectum to localize them with respect to the implant. From these x rays, we can calculate the dose distribution of the application.

## 16.8 CALIBRATION DOSIMETRY

Because the dose required to "cure" a cancer is specified and critical, it is the goal of calibration dosimetry to accurately define the characteristics of the radiation source. In the case of the external beam-therapy machine, we must maintain these characteristics within ±5%. The two primary characteristics that need definition are energy and radiation output. If a radioactive isotope is the source of radiation, the energy is defined by the decay process. For machines that generate radiation electrically, we generally specify the energy by measuring the half-value layer of the beam. In all cases, we must measure the radiation output of the machine.

### Equipment

Figure 16.13 shows the primary tools utilized in calibration dosimetry. These tools consist of an ionization chamber, an electrometer, and an appropriate scattering medium or phantom. The phantom usually consists of a large tank filled with water, which represents tissue.

**Ionization Chamber.** The ionization chamber is schematically represented as two parallel plates bounding an air cavity. When placed in a beam of radiation, the radiation interacts with the air molecules and creates ions. The number of ions produced is directly proportional to the amount of radiation passing through the chamber. If a voltage is placed across the two plates or electrodes in the chamber, the ions are attracted to one or the other of the plates, depending upon the sign of the charge. The charge collected is measured by an electrometer. The charge is proportional to the absorbed dose at the point where the ionization chamber is placed. If the ionization chamber is placed within the water phantom, the absorbed dose at any given point or at any position in the beam can be determined. By careful experimental setup, we determine such factors as machine output, TAR, %DD, beam flatness, and symmetry. To ease the physicist in collection of these data, many devices are now available to increase the speed and accuracy of positioning the ionization chamber. Beam scanners have been developed that simultaneously move the ionization chamber and allow collection of the appropriate data. An extension of this concept is to tie the controls into a computer. It then becomes

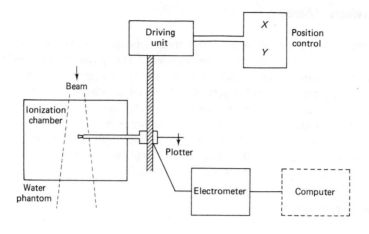

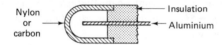

**FIGURE 16.13.** Ionization chamber, electrometer and water phantom.

feasible for the computer to control a whole series of measurements and simultaneously run the calculations, store the data, and print out a calibration report.

### Standardization

Because physical characteristics between ionization chambers vary, the sensitivity of ionization chambers varies. For this reason, the National Bureau of Standards recognizes regional calibration laboratories where ionization chambers and electrometers may be sent and calibrated against the national standard. In this way, all ionization chambers can be corrected to read equivalently.

### Routine Checks

Radiation therapy units are thoroughly calibrated at least once a year. In addition, routine daily and weekly checks are performed to assure that the machine is still functioning according to that calibration. The output of megavoltage machines should be checked each morning before they are utilized to further ensure this quality control.

## 16.9 FUTURE TRENDS

The major new thrusts in the treatment of cancer are in the field of chemotherapy. Multiagent chemotherapy regimes have been developed to test the hundreds of new cancer drugs developed. Clinical trials worldwide are underway to test these agents, either by themselves or in combination with radiation and surgery.

We can divide future trends in radiation therapy into four categories: fractionation, radiation sensitizers, particle therapy, and hyperthermia.

Studies are presently under way to establish the best fractionation scheme for treatment of cancer. The initial results of studies indicate that present fractionation schemes for many cancer treatments can be altered, thereby increasing the effectiveness of the treatment.

One difficulty in conventional photon therapy is that many tumors have a core of hypoxic cells. These oxygen-starved cells are more resistant to radiation than fully oxygenated cells. Two methods are being developed to overcome this problem: chemotherapy and particulate radiation therapy. Drugs such as Misonidazole have been developed to sensitize hypoxic cells in tumors. Misonidazole and others are being tested today in clinical trials with the hope of improving the sensitivity of the hypoxic tumor cells. Particle therapy using neutrons, protons, or heavy nuclei in place of conventional x rays is being developed to achieve the same goal. By replacing the photon with one of these heavy particles, the oxygen effect can be reduced and hopefully eliminated. Charged particles such as protons and pions have the additional potential to provide a better dose distribution and allow a higher tumor dose with a minimum dose to the surrounding normal tissues.

In a separate area of research, heat is being used to treat tumors. There is some clinical evidence today that malignancies respond to heat treatment as either a stand-alone therapy or in conjunction with radiation or chemotherapy. This response appears to be predicated on the higher thermal sensitivity of neoplastic cells compared with normal cells. To achieve this selective destruction, the treatment temperature must be closely controlled to range of 42–43°C. Methods for inducing local hyperthermia include microwaves, radiofrequency radiation, and ultrasound.


# REFERENCES

BARNES, P., and D. REES (1972). *A concise textbook of radiotherapy.* Philadelphia: Lippincott.

BOUCHARD, R., and N. F. OWENS (1972). *Nursing care of the cancer patient.* St. Louis: C. V. Mosby.

CHRISTENSEN, E. E., T. S. CURRY, and J. E. DOWDY (1978). *An introduction to the physics of diagnostic radiology.* Philadelphia: Lea and Febiger.

FOWLER, J. F. (1977). Developments in radiotherapy other than heavy particle beams. *Int. J. Rad. Onc.,* 3: 351–58.

GLASSER, O. (ed) (1950). *Medical physics,* 2. Chicago: Year Book Medical Publishers.

HENDEE, W. R. (1970) *Medical radiation physics.* Chicago: Year Book Medical Publishers.

JOHNS, H. E., and J. R. CUNNINGHAM (1969). *The physics of radiology.* Springfield: IL: Charles C Thomas.

KARZMARK, C. J., and N. C. PERING (1973). Electron linear accelerator for radiation therapy: History, principles, and contemporary developments. *Phys. Med. Biol.,* 18: 321–54.

PIZZARELLO, D. J., and R. L. WITCOFSKI (1972). *Medical radiation biology*. Philadelphia: Lea and Febiger.

RUBIN, P. (ed) (1978). *Clinical oncology for medical students and physicians*. New York: American Cancer Society.

## STUDY QUESTIONS

**16.1** What are the three modes of cancer treatment and how do they differ?

**16.2** Name and describe three types of reactions that a photon can undergo when interacting with a tissue media. Describe how they depend on the energy of incident radiation.

**16.3** A beam of 1-MV photons interacts with a lead wall resulting in a transmission of 1.6%. How thick is the wall if the HVL equals 8 mm?

**16.4** A tumor at a depth of 10 cm is irradiated with a cobalt 60 beam having dimensions 15 × 15 cm at the tumor. The dose rate at this position in free space is 150 rads/min. Find the tumor dose rate. A dose of 180 rads is to be delivered each day. What is the treatment time?

**16.5** Name three radioisotopes used in implant therapy.

**16.6** For most radioactive sources, the rate of emission of gamma rays decreases continuously. What quantity is used to describe this rate of change? What are the units?

**16.7** Name three types of megavoltage therapy machines. Outline the basic principles of operation.

**16.8** Name and describe the main components of a linear accelerator.

**16.9** $^{131}$Iodine has a half life of 8 days. If the activity was 100 mCi on the day it arrived, what is the activity 4 and 16 days later?

**16.10** Draw a schematic diagram of a medical linear accelerator.

**16.11** How do x rays and gamma rays differ from each other and from particulate radiations?

**16.12** Define the terms *rad, rem, half-value layer* and *roentgen*. How are the rem and rad related for electromagnetic and particulate radiations?

**16.13** What factors influence the effects of radiation on specific organs or organ systems?

**16.14** What are the three concepts utilized to provide radiation safety?

**16.15** What are the two types of implant therapy and when are they used?

**16.16** Find the frequency of a 10-MeV x ray.

**16.17** A cobalt 60 source emits 100 photon/s at 1 m; at what distance will the intensity drop to 10 photon/s?

**16.18** In problem 16.17, how much concrete would be needed to reduce the intensity to 10 photon/s at 1 m if the linear attenuation coefficient is 11.2 m$^{-1}$?

# Index

*Page numbers in boldface type indicate the location of an illustration.*

# A

**Kidney function (cont.)**
   functional unit, **494**
   glomerular filtration rate, 493
   regulatory function, 495
Kilovoltage therapy units, 570-571
Knee replacement, 320-323
   anatomy, **322**
   design, 321
   problems, 323
   summary, **324**
Kurzweil reading machine, 169


**L**


Language
   aphasias, 154
   structure, 154
Laser blade scalpel, 396-**397**
Laser cane, **172-173**
Laser scalpel
   argon, 396
   articulating arm, **398**
   carbon dioxide, 394-395
   coagulation, **395**
   Nd:YAG, 396
Lasers for surgery
   carbon dioxide, 400-**401**
   coagulation, **387**
   coherent light, 384
   delivery systems, **401**
   mirrors, 386
   photocoagulator, **392**, 399-**400**
   types, **385**
Left heart bypass
   clinical experience, 120
   energy converters, 118-119
   pumps, 118-**119**
Linear accelerator, **567-568**
   accelerator guide, 567, **569**
   beam monitoring, 569
   microwave cavities, 566
   power generation, 568
Lower limb orthoses
   ankle-foot, 271
   cast braces, 272

drop lock, **273**
enhancing function, 274
gait cycle, 270
knee, 273
line of gravity, **271**


**M**


Mammoplasty, 329-330
Materials compatibility
   arterial grafts, 115
   bone implants, 313-314
   metals, 99
   polymers, 99, 111
   pyrolytic carbon, 99
   silicone rubber, 99
Materials for implants
   ceramics, 312-313
   cobalt alloys, 308
   compositions, **309**
   polymers, 310, **311**-312
   stainless steel, 305, 308
   tissue response, 313-314
   titanium, 308
Micturation reflex, 146
Mobility aids
   blind, 170-177
   *see also* Electronic travel aids
Models
   lung, 24
   problems, 24
Modified vehicles
   powered lifts, 288-**289**
   wheelchair tie-downs, 288, **291**
Monitoring, 3
   examples, 4
Mowat Sensor, 177


**N**


Neonatal intensive care unit
   features, 524
   high-risk patient, 523-524

Prostheses, external, 8
  construction, 245
  energy consumption, 246-**247**
  fit, 244
  locomotion, 245
  *see also* Above-knee, Below-
    knee, Upper limb
Prostheses, internal
  biocompatibility, 303
  corrosion, 304
  encapsulation, 304-305, **306-307**
  mechanical requirements,
    302-303
  problems, 330-331
  standards, 302
  toxicity, 304
  *see also* Fracture fixation, Hip
    Prostheses, Knee replace-
    ment, Materials for implants
Pump, drug, implantable, **9**
Pump-oxygenator
  oxygenators, 103-109
  roller pump, 102-103

# R

Radiation therapy
  depth dose, **561-562**
  external beam, 559-**560**
  implant, 559-560
  isodose distribution, **563**-564
  tissue-air ratio, 563
  *see also* Ionizing radiation
Reading aids
  Kurzweil reading machine, 169
  magnification, 161
  Optacon, **165-168**
  optical character recognition,
    168-**169**
Renal failure
  access routes, 501
  acute, 496
  end-stage, 497
  freedom of movement, 499-500

therapy, 497-499
Respiratory therapy
  humidifier, 447, **454**
  nebulizer, 447, 454-**455**
  neonatal, 449
  oxygenators, 448
  oxygen tent, 449
  positive pressure, 448
  resuscitator, 446-**447**
  suction, 446-447
Rheobase, 130

# S

Sensory substitution
  auditory, 160-161
  tactile, 158-160
  visual, 161
Speech
  compression, 163
  dysarthia, 153
  production, 153
Spinal cord
  injury, 148
  stimulation, 140-141
Spinal orthoses
  cervical, 276
  Halo, 276-**277**
  Milwaukee brace, 277-**278**
  stabilization, 275
  thoracic, 276-277
Strength-duration curve
  cardiac muscle, 73, **74-76**
  nerve and muscle, 129, **130**
Surgery, 7

# T

Technical aids, **285**
  dressing, 285-286
  eating, 284-**286**
  grooming, 286